REAL-WORLD NURSING SURVIVAL GUIDE:
PHARMACOLOGY

D1416192

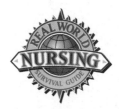

REAL-WORLD NURSING SURVIVAL GUIDE SERIES

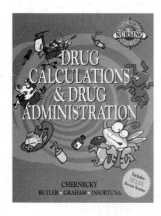

CHERNECKY
BUTLER · GRAHAM · INFORTUNA

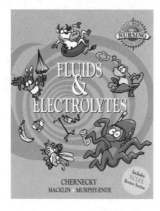

CHERNECKY
MACKLIN · MURPHY-ENDE

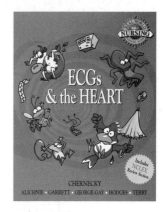

CHERNECKY
ALICHNIE · GARRETT · GEORGE-GAY · HODGES · TERRY

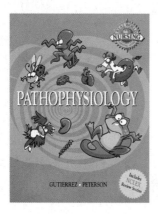

GUTIERREZ · PETERSON

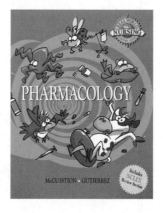

McCUISTION · GUTIERREZ

REAL-WORLD NURSING SURVIVAL GUIDE:
PHARMACOLOGY

LINDA E. McCUISTION, PhD, RN, ANP, CNS
Professor, Division of Nursing
Our Lady of Holy Cross College
New Orleans, Louisiana

KATHLEEN JO GUTIERREZ, PhD, RN, ANP, CNS
Independent Practice, Internal Medicine
Littleton, Colorado
Affiliate Faculty
Regis University
Denver, Colorado

W. B. SAUNDERS COMPANY
Philadelphia London Montreal Sydney Tokyo Toronto

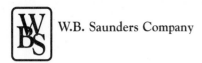
W.B. Saunders Company

The Curtis Center
Independence Square West
Philadelphia, Pennsylvania 19106-3399

Vice President and Publishing Director, Nursing: Sally Schrefer
Acquisitions Editor: Robin Carter
Developmental Editor: Gina Hopf
Project Manager: Catherine Jackson
Designer: Amy Buxton
Cover Designer and Illustrator: Chris Sharp, GraphCom Corporation

NOTICE

Nursing is an ever-changing field. Standard safety precautions must be followed, but as new research and clinical experience broaden our knowledge, changes in treatment and drug therapy may become necessary or appropriate. Readers are advised to check the most current product information provided by the manufacturer of each drug to be administered to verify the recommended dose, the method and duration of administration, and the contraindications. It is the responsibility of the licensed prescriber, relying on the experience and knowledge of the patient, to determine dosages and the best treatment for each individual patient. Neither the publisher nor the editor assumes any liability for any injury or damage to persons or property arising from this publication.

The Publisher

REAL-WORLD NURSING SURVIVAL GUIDE:

PHARMACOLOGY ISBN 0-7216-9047-5

Copyright © 2002 by W.B. Saunders Company

All rights reserved. No part of this publication may be reproduced or transmitted in any form or by any means, electronic or mechanical, including photocopy, recording, or any information storage and retrieval system, without permission in writing from the publisher.

Printed in the United States of America

Last digit is the print number: 9 8 7 6 5 4 3 2

About the Authors

Dr. Linda E. McCuistion is a professor in the Division of Nursing at Our Lady of Holy Cross College. Dr. McCuistion is licensed as an advanced practice nurse and has 35 years of nursing experience, including acute care and home health nursing. She is a past advisory board member, consultant, and reviewer of a software preparation company for the state licensure examination. Dr. McCuistion has served as coordinator for the "Graduate Plus Internship" program for new nursing graduates to ease their transition into the workforce. Dr. McCuistion has served as a legal nurse consultant and as a member of a medical review panel and is past advisory board member of a school for surgical technicians. She has served as a consultant to improve the quality of nursing care and to assist in the preparation for accreditation of acute care facilities. Dr. McCuistion is a past president, vice-president, and faculty advisor of the Sigma Theta Tau International Honor Society in Nursing, Xi Psi chapter-at-large, as well as past associate editor of the *NODNA Times*, which is the New Orleans District Nurses' Association newsletter. Dr. McCuistion was chosen as a "Great One Hundred Nurse" by the New Orleans District Nurses' Association in 1993. She has lectured regionally and nationally on a variety of nursing topics and has published articles in nursing journals and written chapters in several textbooks.

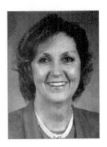

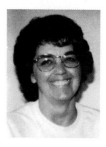

Dr. Kathleen Jo Gutierrez completed an associate degree in nursing from the Community College of Denver, a bachelor of science degree in nursing from Metropolitan State College of Denver, and a master of science degree from the University of Colorado Health Sciences Center. She also completed a post-master's program as an adult nurse practitioner through Beth El College in Colorado Springs. Her interest in education and professional development compelled her to obtain a doctorate degree in education from the University of Denver.

Dr. Gutierrez is currently a primary health care provider in an internal medicine office in the Denver area. During the 15 years before entering private practice, she was an associate professor with the Department of Nursing at Regis University in Denver. She remains active with the National League for Nursing Accreditation Commission as a program evaluator and member of the program review panel.

In addition to her work on *Real-World Nursing Survival Guide: Pharmacology*, Dr. Gutierrez is the author and editor of *Pharmacotherapeutics: Clinical Decision-Making in Nursing* and a co-author for the *Real-World Nursing Survival Guide: Pathophysiology*. She has published numerous journal articles, the latest of which is a research article describing the prescribing behaviors of Colorado's advanced practice nurses.

Dr. Gutierrez has been named in "Who's Who in American Nursing," "Who's Who in American Education," and "Who's Who in Medicine and Health Care." She is board certified as both an adult nurse practitioner and medical-surgical clinical nurse specialist. She is a member of the American Nurses Association, the National Organization of Nurse Practitioner Faculties, American Academy of Nurse Practitioners, and Sigma Theta Tau, the International Honor Society of Nursing.

Contributors

Marie M. Adorno, APRN, MN, CNS
Assistant Professor of Nursing
Our Lady of Holy Cross College
New Orleans, Louisiana

Deborah S. Anderson, RPh, PharmD, BS(Pharm.)
Clinical Pharmacist, Internal Medicine
Ochsner Foundation Hospital
Clinical Assistant Professor, Pharmacy Practice
Xavier University of Louisiana College of Pharmacy
Adjunct Faculty, Nursing Practitioner Program
Loyola University of New Orleans
City College, School of Nursing
New Orleans, Louisiana

Joanne M. Bullard, BSN, MN, APRN
Assistant Professor of Nursing
Our Lady of Holy Cross College
New Orleans, Louisiana

Jennifer S. Couvillon, MSN, RN, BSN
Instructor of Nursing
Adult Health, Critical Care
Louisiana State University Health Sciences Center School
    of Nursing
New Orleans, Louisiana

Lynn J. Drummond, MSN, BS, RN
Nurse Educator and Clinical Manager
Community Health Agency
Southfield, Michigan

Pamela B. Egan, MN, RN,C-FNP,C-ANP, CS
Family Nurse Practitioner
Covington Family Health Clinic
Covington, Louisiana
Owner and President
Egan Healthcare Services
Home Health, Medical Equipment, Pharmacy
Metairie, LaPlace, Covington, and Plaquemine Parish,
    Louisiana

Kathleen Jo Gutierrez, PhD, RN, ANP, CNS
Independent Practice, Internal Medicine
Littleton, Colorado
Affiliate Faculty
Regis University
Denver, Colorado

Annette M. Knobloch, RN, BSN, MPH, LCCE
Associate Professor of Nursing
William Carey College
New Orleans, Louisiana

Linda Eilee Schmidt McCuistion, PhD, RN
Professor, Division of Nursing
Our Lady of Holy Cross College
New Orleans, Louisiana

Karen K. Mullins, BSN
Charge Nurse Med-Surg
Med-Surg Nursing
Dukes Memorial Hospital
Peru, Indiana

Mary Ann Nemcek, DNS, RN
Assistant Professor of Nursing
Loyola University
New Orleans, Louisiana
Continuing Education Coordinator
Home Care Services
Egan Health Care Services
Metairie, Louisiana

Phyllis G. Peterson, RN, MN, AOCN
Assistant Professor
Division of Nursing
Our Lady of Holy Cross College
New Orleans, Louisiana

Susan S. Rick, DNS, RN, CNS
Assistant Professor of Nursing
Louisiana State University Health Sciences Center
New Orleans, Louisiana

Jennifer C. Robinson, MSN, RN
Instructor of Nursing
Southeastern Louisiana University
Hammond, Louisiana

Linda J. Rubino, MSN
Assistant Administrator
Egan Health Care
Metairie, Louisiana

Eileen H. Stoll, MSN, RN, CCRN
Assistant Professor
Division of Nursing
Our Lady of Holy Cross College
New Orleans, Louisiana

Annette Walton, RN, BSN
Renaissance Home Health Care
Southfield, Michigan

Faculty & Student Reviewers

FACULTY

Nancy Henne Batchelor, MSN, RNC, CNS
Northern Kentucky University
Highland Heights, Kentucky

Stephanie Lynn Boots, RN, BSN

David Derrico, MSN, RN, OCN
Assistant Clinical Professor
College of Nursing
University of Florida
Gainesville, Florida

Margaret H. Doherty, MSN, RN, CCRN
Instructor, Department of Nursing
Sonoma State University
Rohnert Park, California

Diane Marie Ford, RN, MS, FNP, CS, CCRN
Andrews University
Berrien Springs, Michigan

Margaret M. Gingrich, MSN, RN
Harrisburg Area Community College
Harrisburg, Pennsylvania

Margie J. Hansen, PhD, RN
Clinical Associate Professor of Nursing
University of North Dakota
Grand Forks, North Dakota

Joan Klemballa, PhD, RN, FNP-C
The College of West Virginia
Beckley, West Virginia

Sharon Mitchell, LPN, BS
Canadian Valley Technology Center
El Reno, Oklahoma

Mary Ellen Mitchell-Rosen, RN, BSN
RTM Star Center
Dania Beach, Florida

Harry Peery, RN, MS, BS
Lecturer, Departments of Pharmacology, Toxicology, and Medical Chemistry
Division of Nursing Practice, College of Nursing
College of Pharmacy
University of Arizona
Tucson, Arizona

Kimberly R. Pugh, MSEd, RN, BSN
Nurse Consultant
Baltimore, Maryland

Dottie Roberts, MSN, RN, C, MACI, ONC CNS
Penrose—St. Francis Health Services
Colorado Springs, Colorado

Susan B. Stillwell, MSN, RN
Clinical Associate Professor
Arizona State University
Tempe, Arizona

Christine L. Vandenhouten, MSN, RN, CNOR
Bellin College of Nursing
Green Bay, Wisconsin

Janis Waite, EdD, MSN, RN
Associate Professor
St. Francis Medical Center College of Nursing
Peoria, Illinois

James Joseph Wojcik, BA, BSN, MBA
Instructor
Virginia College of Huntsville
Huntsville, Alabama

STUDENTS

Evelyn DeMoss, ADN
Austin Community College
Austin, Texas

Mary Jo Lampart, RN, BSN
Geisinger Medical Center
Danville, Pennsylvania
Former Student
Bloomsburg University
Bloomsburg, Pennsylvania

Clifford (Troy) Shaffer Jr., EMT
Medical College of Georgia
   School of Nursing
Augusta, Georgia

The following students from Our Lady of Holy Cross College and Charity Delgado School of Nursing, New Orleans, Louisiana, helped the editors shape the vision of this reference through focus group reviews and breakout sessions:

Kenya Michelle Alexander
Brian Badeaux
Deana Bell
Cynthia G. Bienvenu
Anastasia Erb
Bernard Fernandes
Faith A. Fray
Bridgette Rowena Gasaway
Elizabeth Gonzalez
Heather G. Herbert

Thomas J. Higgins, Jr.
Joy Jones
Mae Crovetto Juan
L. Michelle Keller
Jana Kellogg
Ronni McCaskill
Amy E. McDonald
Kimberly A. Palmisano
Shawn R. Passons
Shanny M'Lee Pierce

Robin Richoux
Francine S. Ricks
Catherine Roark
Gretchen Rothenberger
Erica Saia
Melissa Tefft
Rachel Till
Sharon Nance Vincent

FACULTY

Edwina A. McConnell, PhD, RN, FRCNA
Professor
School of Nursing
Texas Technical University Health Sciences Center
Lubbock, Texas
Consultant
Gorham, Maine

Judith L. Myers, MSN, RN
Health Sciences Center
St. Louis University
School of Nursing
St. Louis, Missouri

FEATURED STUDENTS

Shayne Michael Gray, RN, was born in Little Rock, Arkansas, and graduated with a BSN degree from the University of Arkansas for Medical Sciences (UAMS) in 1999. He has spent a year working at the University as an Intensive Care Nurse and has also applied for a medical commission in the Naval Reserve. Future plans include becoming a CRNA. Before nursing school, Shayne played drums in a band that eventually signed with a record label and was distributed by Polygram and Phillips Multimedia; this afforded him the opportunity to tour the United States and Canada for 3 years. Following that, he left the band and earned a leading role in an independent film that was shown at the prestigious Sundance Film Festival. It is the earnings from this movie role that Shayne credits with helping him finish his nursing school prerequisites at the University of Arkansas at Little Rock, and he married his wife Michelle in 1996, just as he was being accepted into the nursing program. He spent 2 years serving as a volunteer for the Arkansas Lung Association, speaking about the dangers of smoking to local school children, and has also been a volunteer for many of UAMS's fundraisers and community clean-up projects. A former Helicopter Flight Medic in the Army National Guard, Shayne is a certified scuba diver and loves the outdoors, playing guitar, and writing. He is also ACLS qualified and hopes to participate in nursing/medical research in the future.

For **Jill Hall,** attending nursing school has been the fulfillment of a childhood dream. Before that opportunity, she served an apprenticeship as a Mechanical and Production Engineer with British Aerospace. She then spent 2 years as a stay-at-home mother for her two children. When her husband accepted a job in California, the family moved from northern England to Huntington Beach, where Jill began taking prerequisite nursing classes at Golden West College. Once into the nursing program, she knew she had found what she was meant to do. She became involved in the Student Nurses' Association, and a trip to the mid-year NSNA convention in Dallas sparked her enthusiasm to run for national office. At the annual convention in Pittsburgh, she was elected to the Nominations and Elections Committee, and her year in office involved conventions in both Charlotte and Salt Lake City. In her own community, she is a member of the United Methodist Church and the high school PTO. She has been a Girl Scout leader, Sunday school teacher, soccer coach, and soccer camp coordinator, as well as a volunteer in the emergency room of a local hospital. She is currently employed in the Pediatric ICU at Miller Children's Hospital in Long Beach, California. She also plans to pursue both BSN and MSN degrees. She offers special thanks to two instructors who have served as mentors during her time in the nursing program at Golden West College, Nadine Davis and Marcia Swanson: "Their standards of excellence have inspired me to achieve more than I ever thought I could. Gracious thanks for all they have done for me."

Elizabeth J. Hoogmoed, RN, BSN, recently graduated from William Paterson University and is currently a neurological nurse at Valley Hospital in Ridgewood, New Jersey. She serves on the Executive Board of Sigma Theta Tau as Corresponding Secretary for the Iota Alpha chapter. She also served as Membership and Nominations Chair for New Jersey Nursing Students from 1998 to 1999 and continues to be a sustaining member of the organization. She has also been a volunteer for her local ambulance corps for 7 years. She has been accepted into the program at New York University, where she will complete her Masters degree to become a Nurse Practitioner. Her hope is to promote the profession of nursing and show its importance to the future of health care. In this era of computers and technology, she believes it is reassuring to know that a select number of individuals continue to follow the inner call to care for people and promote wellness in society: "These are the nurses."

Katie Scarlett McRae, BA, BSN, says that if you talk to her for more than a few minutes, you'll be sure to hear her say, "I love my job." She serves as a staff RN on the cardiovascular/telemetry floor at Oregon Health Sciences University (OHSU) in Portland, caring for patients who have had heart transplants or other cardiac/vascular surgeries or who suffer from congestive heart failure, diabetes, or arrhythmias. Working with many experienced nurses "great at sharing their insights and knowledge," Katie loves the teaching hospital environment and jokes that nursing is her "second career"; when she graduated from the OHSU nursing program in 1999, it was actually her second Bachelor's degree, but "the two degrees were 24 years apart!" Katie credits the rigorous OHSU program with giving her the confidence to know she could practice nursing safely. During nursing school, she was active in student government, and she is also a current member of the Oregon Nurses' Association, the ANA, and the AACN. She plans to return to OHSU soon to begin work on a Master's degree in Adult Health and Illness, with a focus on diabetes, and her ideal career would be to create and manage a comprehensive diabetes management for the state of Oregon.

STUDENTS

Joy Kutlenios Amos, RN, BSN
Piedmont Medical Center
Rock Hill, South Carolina
Former student
Wheeling Jesuit University
Wheeling, West Virginia

Angela M. Boyd, AS
University of Tennessee at Martin
Martin, Tennessee

Jennifer Hamilton
University of Virginia
Charlottesville, Virginia

Preface

An understanding of pharmacologic concepts provides a solid foundation for the nurse to administer drugs, provide patient teaching, monitor desired body responses and drug effects, and intervene to make drug therapy more tolerable by managing adverse effects. It is important for the nurse to be aware of pharmacologic and biologic entities, such as mechanisms of action, appropriate use, toxicities, drug interactions, and nursing responsibilities.

Patient teaching is of prime importance for the nurse in the management of drug therapy. It may involve informal teaching such as the monitoring of vital signs, deciding whether to take a drug with food, and determining the duration of drug treatment; or patient teaching may involve formal classes that teach drug self-administration. Detailed and enthusiastic patient teaching on the part of the nurse enhances patient compliance and adherence to a prescribed regimen.

This book is one in a series created in response to input from nursing students. Focus groups held at the National Student Nurses' Association convention identified helpful methods to achieve mastery of new information. Their responses were used to design the basic structure and approach behind the *Real World Nursing Survival Guide Series*. In addition, throughout the development of this book, student nurses met to evaluate and critique its content and progress.

The drug information in this book is presented in a manner that promotes a clear understanding of drug actions and body responses. Because there are literally thousands of drugs, it is impossible to memorize all specific information for each drug. This book organizes drugs with similar characteristics into classifications or families to help the learner assimilate the information. Great care has been taken to organize the drug information into an easily understandable format.

We include many features in the margins to help the reader focus on the most important information needed to succeed in the classroom and in the clinical setting. TAKE HOME POINTS are composed of both study tips for classroom tests and "pearls of wisdom" to assist you in caring for patients. Both are drawn from our many years of combined academic and clinical experience. Content marked with a caution icon is vital and usually involves nursing actions that may have life-threatening consequences or significantly affect patient outcomes. The lifespan icon and the culture icon highlight variations in treatment that may be necessary for specific age or ethnic groups. A calculator icon will draw your eye to important equations and examples that will help you calculate proper medication dosages. A web links icon will direct you to sites on the Internet that give more detailed information on a given topic. Each of these icons will specifically help you focus on real-world patient care, the nursing process, and positive patient outcomes.

We created a special icon just for use in this book of the series. A cross-reference icon will refer you to further information in the *Real-World Nursing Survival Guide: Pathophysiology* regarding the physical disorders that are treated with the discussed drug class. This information is not absolutely necessary to your understanding of a specific drug or its associated nursing responsibilities, but it will give you a more rounded view of drug classes, actions, and uses.

We also use consistent headings that emphasize specific nursing actions. "What It IS" describes the action and use of the drugs in a given classification. Most drug class discussions include a box that focuses on the most common drugs in the category, highlighting prototype drugs in color. "What You NEED TO KNOW" summarizes contraindications and precautions, drug interactions, and adverse effects of the drug classification. "What You DO" includes bulleted lists of nursing interventions and responsibilities because, as professionals, we are responsible for providing expert, comprehensive care for our patients. Under this heading you will find special apple bullets that highlight the patient teaching necessary as part of the plan of care. Finally, "Do You UNDERSTAND?" provides questions and exercises that are both entertaining and useful to reinforce the topic's concepts. This four-step approach both provides you with information and helps you learn how to apply it in the clinical setting.

We hope this book will make a difficult topic easier and will provide you with new insights and understanding about drug classes and their uses. Share the knowledge you gain with others, and most of all, use this information to make a positive difference in the lives of your patients.

This book is dedicated to my friends and family, especially Bob, Gerald, Joanne, Donna, Barbara, Jean, Cynthia, Patti, and Cherie.

Linda E. McCuistion

To my husband and soul-mate, Pat, who stands beside me through thick and thin, maintains our home, nourishes me, and helps me to keep my sanity—I don't know what I would do without you.

To my daughter, Pam, and son-in-law, Brad, whose ability to be forthright and honest helps keep my life in perspective, especially through life's challenges.

And to my son, Michael, who remains the most honest, compassionate, devoted, nonjudgmental individual I have ever known.

Kathleen J. Gutierrez

Acknowledgments

I would like to express my deep appreciation to Dr. Gerald DeLuca and Sister Bernardine Hill, who have helped me develop my writing style with their expert guidance.

A very special thanks is extended to my family and several friends for their support, encouragement, and advice: Dr. Robert Ekas, Jr., Joanne Bullard, Phyllis Peterson, Donna Deffner, Jean Hyver, Barbara Power, Sister Cynthia Knowles, Patricia Smart, Cherie Caznavette, Brielle Bullard, Cynthia Chernecky, Dana Peick, Robin Carter, and Gina Hopf. To these people I offer my sincere appreciation.

I would also like to acknowledge the nursing students who graciously volunteered to read and evaluate this book and to provide honest feedback. Their invaluable assistance in this endeavor is immensely appreciated.

Linda E. McCuistion

No author writes a book alone. My thanks to the many students, nurse educators, and health care providers for their collaboration over a number of years. Thanks to Phyllis Peterson and Linda McCuistion for the opportunity to participate in this dual project. My continued thanks and appreciation to Robin Carter, Executive Editor, and Gina Hopf, Developmental Editor, for their patience and understanding, continually sound advice, marketing savvy, and most importantly, friendship. The wonderful people at W.B. Saunders once again made an important contribution to nursing resources come to fruition.

Kathleen J. Gutierrez

Contents

1 Drugs Affecting the Immune System, *1*
Section A—Antibiotics, *LINDA E. MCCUISTION*, *1*
Section B—Antivirals and Antifungals, *PAMELA B. EGAN & LINDA E. MCCUISTION*, *24*
Section C—Biologic Response Modifiers, *LINDA E. MCCUISTION*, *38*
Section D—Antineoplastic Agents, *PHYLLIS G. PETERSON*, *49*

2 Drugs Affecting the Nervous System, *62*
Section A—Sympathetic Nervous System Agents, *EILEEN H. STOLL*, *62*
Section B—Parasympathetic Nervous System Agents and Antiparkinsonism Agents, *EILEEN H. STOLL*, *69*
Section C—CNS Stimulants and Skeletal Muscle Relaxants, *LINDA E. MCCUISTION*, *81*
Section D—Anticonvulsants, *LINDA J. RUBINO & LINDA E. MCCUISTION*, *91*
Section E—Anesthetics, *LINDA E. MCCUISTION*, *103*
Section F—Psychotherapeutic Agents, *LYNN J. DRUMMOND & ANNETTE WALTON*, *107*

3 Drugs Affecting the Hematologic System, *131*
MARY ANN NEMCEK

4 Drugs Affecting Blood Pressure and Blood Flow, *140*
Section A—Antihypertensives, *LINDA E. MCCUISTION*, *140*
Section B—Antihyperlipidemics, *LINDA E. MCCUISTION*, *160*

5 Drugs Affecting the Cardiac System, *169*
Section A—Agents Affecting Cardiac Output, *LINDA E. MCCUISTION*, *169*
Section B—Antiarrhythmics, *EILEEN H. STOLL*, *178*

6 Drugs Affecting the Respiratory System, *193*
Section A—Agents Affecting Upper Respiratory Disorders, *JOANNE M. BULLARD*, *193*
Section B—Antihistamines, *JOANNE M. BULLARD*, *201*
Section C—Antiasthmatics and Bronchodilators, *JOANNE M. BULLARD*, *208*

7 Drugs Affecting the Endocrine System, *221*
Section A—Pituitary and Adrenal Hormones, *KATHLEEN JO GUTIERREZ*, *221*
Section B—Thyroid and Parathyroid Agents, *SUSAN S. RICK*, *235*
Section C—Antidiabetics, *JOANNE M. BULLARD*, *242*

8 Drugs Affecting the Gastrointestinal System, *257*
Section A—Agents Affecting Hyperacidity, Gastric Mucosa, Motility, and Flatulence,
JENNIFER C. ROBINSON & LINDA E. MCCUISTION, *257*
Section B—Antiemetics, Emetics, and Agents Used for Digestive Problems, *MARY ANN NEMCEK*, *271*
Section C—Laxative and Antidiarrheal Agents, *JENNIFER C. ROBINSON & LINDA E. MCCUISTION*, *283*

9 Drugs Affecting the Genitourinary Tract and Renal Disorders, 300
Section A—Agents Used in Urinary Tract Disorders and to Improve Renal Output, MARY ANN NEMCEK, 300
Section B—Agents Used in Renal Failure, DEBORAH S. ANDERSON & LINDA E. McCUISTION, 313

10 Drugs Affecting the Reproductive System, 323
Section A—Male and Female Hormones, JENNIFER S. COUVILLON, 323
Section B—Agents Affecting Uterine Motility, MARIE M. ADORNO & LINDA E. McCUISTION, 335

11 Drugs Affecting the Musculoskeletal System, 343
Section A—Antiinflammatory Agents, KAREN K. MULLINS & LINDA E. McCUISTION, 343
Section B—Antigout Agents, KAREN K. MULLINS & LINDA E. McCUISTION, 352

12 Drugs for Nutritional Imbalances, 359
JOANNE M. BULLARD

13 Drugs Affecting the Sensory System, 369
Section A—Ophthalmics and Otics, KATHLEEN JO GUTIERREZ, 369
Section B—Dermatologics, JENNIFER S. COUVILLON, 384

14 Agents Used for Pain Relief, 395
Section A—Opioid Agents, ANNETTE M. KNOBLOCH, 395
Section B—Antimigraine Agents, LINDA E. McCUISTION, 401

References, 407
NCLEX Section, 411

Drugs Affecting the Immune System

SECTION A
ANTIBIOTICS

This chapter reviews drugs that are used to treat infectious diseases. An antibiotic is a chemical substance that is derived from mold or bacteria with the ability to inhibit the growth or destroy one or more causative pathogens in the treatment of infectious conditions. Generally, antibiotic monotherapy (single-drug therapy) is sufficient; however, in some instances, multidrug therapy is necessary to eradicate the infectious process.

β-Lactam Antibiotics

β-Lactam antibiotics have a β-lactam ring in their molecules and exhibit some cross-sensitivity. Penicillins and cephalosporins are β-lactam antibiotics that inhibit enzymes that are required for the synthesis of bacterial cell walls. In a weakened cell wall, bacteria are destroyed as a result of swelling from osmotic pressure (osmotic lysis).

What IS a Penicillin Antibiotic?

Penicillin Types	Trade Names	Uses
Natural penicillin penicillin G potassium [pen-ih-SILL-in]	Megacillin	Treatment of moderate-to-severe systemic infections
Penicillinase-resistant penicillin oxacillin [ox-uh-SILL-in]	Prostaphlin	Treatment of staphylococcal infections
Aminopenicillin amoxicillin [uh-MOX-ih-sill-in]	Amoxil	Treatment of mild-to-moderate infections
Extended-spectrum penicillin ticarcillin [TIE-car-sill-in]	Timentin	Treatment of septicemia, intraabdominal, skin, soft tissue, and respiratory and GU tract infections

Action

The penicillin classification is separated into four groups: natural, penicillinase-resistant, aminopenicillins, and extended-spectrum penicillins. Natural penicillins inhibit enzymes that are required for bacterial cell wall synthesis, thus they kill bacteria.

Bacteria that are initially sensitive to natural penicillins may develop a protective enzyme (**penicillinase**) and become resistant to therapy. Penicillinase splits open the β-lactam ring of the antibiotic molecule and renders the bacteria resistant to natural penicillins, thereby inactivating natural penicillin antibiotics. Penicillinase-resistant penicillins overcome bacterial resistance because they are stable against penicillinase or β-lactamase enzymes that break down natural penicillins. Other newly developed penicillins include aminopenicillins, which have an amino group attached to their penicillin nucleus that enhances their activity against gram-negative bacteria. Extended-spectrum penicillins have a wider spectrum of activity than do the other types of penicillin.

Penicillins are bactericidal (i.e., inhibit the action of enzymes that are necessary for bacterial cell wall formation, thereby killing bacteria). Normally, a microorganism's cell wall lies outside the cytoplasmic membrane and is stiff, penetrable, and meshlike. The high osmotic pressure within the organism's cytoplasmic membrane creates a strong gradient that attracts water thus the cell swells. Without the stiff cell wall, water would be absorbed to such a degree that the organism would burst. Penicillins suppress substances that are necessary for bacterial cell wall rigidity, making the bacterial cells osmotically unstable, which results in excessive water intake, swelling, and rupture of the bacterial cell, causing bacterial death. Because human cells lack a similar cell wall, the penicillins have virtually no direct effect on host cells.

Uses

Penicillins affect gram-positive and gram-negative aerobes, anaerobes, streptococci, staphylococcus, bacilli, and enterococci. Penicillins are used for the treatment of pharyngitis, tonsillitis, otitis media, pneumonia, endocarditis, soft-tissue infections, meningitis, scarlet fever, rat-bite fever, diphtheria, anthrax, urinary tract infections, syphilis, and gonorrhea. Prophylactically, penicillins may be given before surgery or dental procedures in patients with a history of rheumatic fever.

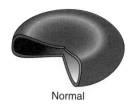

Normal

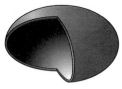

Swollen

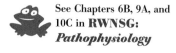 See Chapters 6B, 9A, and 10C in **RWNSG:** *Pathophysiology*

  Caution is to be observed when penicillins are given to patients who are pregnant and lactating or those with anemia, thrombocytopenia, granulocytopenia, bone marrow depression, or renal insufficiency.

 # What You NEED TO KNOW

Contraindications/Precautions

Penicillins are contraindicated for patients with a history of allergic reaction to any penicillin or cephalosporins.

Drug Interactions

The effectiveness of penicillin and penicillinase-resistant groups is decreased when given with tetracyclines. Aminoglycosides are inactivated when given with penicillins. Probenecid slows the excretion of penicillins. Penicillins are thought to decrease the effectiveness of oral contraceptives. The serum level of beta blockers is decreased when given with ampicillin.

Adverse Effects

Penicillins are the most common cause of drug allergy. Allergic reactions vary from minor rashes to life-threatening anaphylaxis. The severe reactions are most likely to occur with parenteral use. Immediate penicillin reactions occur within the first 30 minutes after drug administration. Delayed reactions may take days or weeks to develop. Hypersensitivities may appear in the form of rash, pruritus, fever, wheezing, severe dyspnea, stridor, nausea, vomiting, tachycardia, sweating (**diaphoresis**), vertigo, hypotension, loss of consciousness, or death. Because of cross-sensitivity, patients who are allergic to one type of penicillin are generally considered allergic to all penicillins.

The adverse effects of penicillins generally involve the gastrointestinal (GI) system with glossitis, mouth sores (**stomatitis**), anorexia, heartburn, gastritis, abdominal pain, nausea, vomiting, and mild-to-severe diarrhea. Taste alterations, sore mouth, and discolored tongue (i.e., black, furry tongue) are primarily a result of the loss of normal flora and the subsequent opportunistic infections called superinfections. More serious effects are neurologic, nephrologic, or hematologic toxicities. Neurologic reactions include lethargy, twitching, confusion, difficulty swallowing (**dysphasia**), agitation, hyperreflexia, depression, hallucinations, psychosis, convulsions, and coma. Hematologic toxicity includes neutropenia, thrombocytopenia, hemolytic anemia, and prolonged bleeding time. Other adverse effects include fever, macular rash, eosinophilia, proteinuria, hematuria, and leukocyturia, which can progress to renal failure.

What You DO

Nursing Responsibilities

When administering penicillins, the nurse's prime concern is to be aware of the potential for allergic reactions.

Some penicillins are well absorbed following oral administration. However, penicillin G is unstable in acid, and the majority of an oral dose is destroyed in the stomach. Food slows gastric emptying thus prolonging exposure of the penicillin to gastric acid. Consequently, to produce blood levels comparable in effec-

TAKE HOME POINTS

Women who are taking oral contraceptives should be advised to practice an alternate form of birth control throughout penicillan antibiotic therapy.

  Penicillins, when given with anti-coagulants, increase bleeding time.

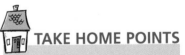

TAKE HOME POINTS

Observe for anaphylactic reactions, which are common in penicillin therapy, and immediately treat with epinephrine, antihistamines, and corticosteroid administration.

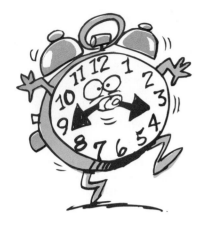

tiveness to parenteral administration, the oral dose must be four to five times greater, and the drug must be taken on an empty stomach. When administering oral penicillins, the nurse should encourage the patient to take penicillins at the prescribed dose and at evenly spaced intervals. Because of rapid clearance, around-the-clock administration is required for drug efficacy.

All forms of penicillin may be given intramuscularly (IM), but various penicillins (e.g., sodium, potassium, procaine, benzathine) are absorbed at different rates. For example, the sodium and potassium forms of penicillin G are rapidly absorbed, with peak blood levels reached in 15 to 30 minutes after injection. In contrast, procaine and benzathine forms are absorbed at a decreased rate. The average peak penicillin drug effect is reached in 4 hours after administration. When administering penicillin, the nurse should:

- Monitor the intravenous (IV) sites for phlebitis, and apply warm compresses when they become painful and swollen.
- Discontinue the IV access, and restart another line on discovery of phlebitis.
- Monitor the patient who is receiving sodium or potassium penicillin drugs for electrolyte imbalance because hyperkalemia can lead to cardiac arrest.
- Examine laboratory results for renal dysfunction, bone marrow depression, and prolonged bleeding time to detect toxicities early.
- Teach patients about the need for additional contraception throughout the duration of penicillin therapy.
- Instruct the patient to report the following to the health care provider: any unusual bleeding or bruising, severe headaches, dizziness, weakness, sudden fever elevation, chills, sore throat, mouth sores, vaginal itching, hives, rash, severe diarrhea, or difficulty breathing.
- Instruct the patient to take oral doses of penicillin on an empty stomach (1 hour before or 2 hours after meals) with a full glass of water. Fruit juices and soft drinks should be avoided with oral penicillin.
- Inform the patient that antibiotics should be continued for the full course of therapy, usually 10 days, at equally spaced times around the clock for efficacy, even when the infection has subsided.
- The patient should take adequate hydration to replace fluids that are lost from diarrhea.

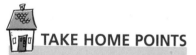

TAKE HOME POINTS

Offer frequent mouth care, ice chips, or sugarless candy to suck, which helps relieve discomfort from stomatitis.

Do You UNDERSTAND?

DIRECTIONS: **Provide appropriate responses to the following questions
and statement.**

1. What is the most unique adverse effect of penicillin therapy?

   _____

   _____

2. Hypersensitivity responses to penicillin include what?

   _____

   _____

3. List four types of penicillins and one example of each.

   _____   _____

   _____   _____

   _____   _____

   _____   _____

What IS a Cephalosporin?

Cephalosporin	Trade Names	Uses
First generation cefazolin [seff-UH-zoe-lin]	Ancef Kefzol	Treatment of respiratory, GU, and biliary tract, skin, bone, and joint infections
Second generation cefamandole [SEFF-uh-MAN-dahl]	Mandol	Treatment of lower respiratory, GU tract, skin, bone, and joint infections, septicemia, and peritonitis
Third generation Cefotaxime [seff-oh-TAX-eem]	Claforan	Treatment of lower respiratory, skin, bone, joint, pelvic, and intraabdominal infections, and perioperative prophylaxis
Fourth generation cefepime [SEFF-eh-pim]	Maxipime	Treatment of pneumonia, and skin and GU infections

Action

Cephalosporins are semisynthetic antibiotics that are organized into four generations based on their order of development. Each generation has increasing activity against gram-negative bacteria and anaerobes. Cephalosporins are bactericidal and act on bacteria by interfering with bacterial cell wall synthesis. The bacterial cell walls weaken, swell, and burst from increased osmotic pressure within the cell, causing bacterial cell death.

Answers: 1. Black, furry tongue; 2. rash, pruritus, fever, wheezing, severe dyspnea, stridor, nausea, vomiting, tachycardia, diaphoresis, vertigo, hypotension, loss of consciousness, and death; 3. natural penicillin (penicillin G), penicillinase-resistant penicillins (oxacillin), aminopenicillins (amoxicillin), extended spectrum penicillins (ticarcillin).

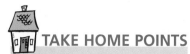

TAKE HOME POINTS

Cephalosporins are similar to penicillins in structure and activity.

First-generation cephalosporins are used for gram-positive cocci infections. Second-generation cephalosporins are active against bacteria that are susceptible to the first-generation cephalosporins and gram-negative bacteria. Third-generation cephalosporins are active against bacteria that are susceptible to first- and second-generation cephalosporins and unusual strains of enteric bacteria. Fourth-generation cephalosporins have a greater spectrum of antibiotic activity and greater stability against β-lactamase enzymes than third-generations. Fourth generations are also active against both gram-positive and gram-negative bacteria and unusual strains of enteric bacteria.

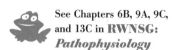

See Chapters 6B, 9A, 9C, and 13C in **RWNSG:** *Pathophysiology*

Uses

Cephalosporins are effective treatment for sinusitis, pharyngitis, laryngitis, tonsillitis, bronchitis, otitis media, skin infections, urinary tract infections, abdominal infections, pelvic inflammatory disease, septicemia, meningitis, and osteomyelitis. They are used prophylactically in patients involving the GI and genitourinary (GU) tracts, bone, and skin surgeries.

Cautious use is taken for patients with renal failure. Preexisting renal failure may interfere with drug excretion and lead to toxic levels.

Caution should also be taken in pregnant and lactating women because of the potential risk to the fetus or infant.

What You NEED TO KNOW

Contraindications/Precautions

Because of the cross-sensitivity, cephalosporins are contraindicated for patients with known allergies to cephalosporins or penicillins.

Drug Interactions

Consuming alcohol while taking cefamandole, cefoperazone, or cefotetan will induce a disulfiram-like reaction. A disulfiram reaction involves tremors, nausea, severe vomiting, diarrhea, and either hypotension or hypertension. This reaction may occur up to 72 hours after the drug is discontinued. Drugs that promote anticoagulation may increase bleeding time when used concurrently with cephalosporins. Probenecid delays renal excretion of some cephalosporins and prolongs their effect. Cephalosporins given concurrently with aminoglycosides may lead to an increased risk of nephrotoxicity.

Adverse Effects

Cephalosporins are usually tolerated well and are one of the safest types of antibiotics. Five to ten percent of penicillin-sensitive patients are also sensitive to cephalosporins because the structural similarity between the two classes of drugs. Common systemic hypersensitivity reactions involve rash, pruritus, fever, chills, urticaria, joint pain or inflammation, edema, erythema, and eosinophilia.

The most common adverse effects of cephalosporins involve the GI effects of anorexia, nausea, flatulence, vomiting, abdominal pain, and diarrhea. Other GI adverse effects that may occur are taste alteration, decreased salivation, dyspepsia, glossitis, flatulence, abdominal pain, and hepatic dysfunction. Additional adverse effects include dizziness, hallucinations, malaise, fatigue, nightmares, headache, bleeding tendencies, paresthesia, menstrual irregularities, vaginitis, genital pruritus, vaginal moniliasis, and nephrotoxicity. An overgrowth of non-susceptible microorganisms (superinfection) is associated more frequently with third-generation cephalosporins compared with the other generations.

What You DO

Nursing Responsibilities

Many cephalosporins can be administered orally, but others must be administered parenterally. Cephalosporin drug therapy is usually continued for 48 to 72 hours after the patient reaches an asymptomatic state. Perioperative prophylaxis is usually discontinued within 24 to 48 hours after surgery. When administering cephalosporins, the nurse should:

- Monitor the IM site for evidence of local abscess and the IV site for phlebitis. Discontinue the IV site and restart at another location when phlebitis occurs. Warm compresses relieve the pain and edema of a local abscess.
- Schedule cephalosporins at equally spaced times throughout a 24-hour period.
- Monitor renal and hepatic function studies throughout cephalosporin therapy because they have been shown to cause transient alterations in various test results, including blood urea nitrogen (BUN), alanine aminotransferase (ALT), serum glutamic pyruvic transaminase (SGPT), aspartate aminotransferase (AST), alkaline phosphatase, lactate dehydrogenase (LDH), and bilirubin levels.
- Teach the patient who is taking cephalosporin to continue the full course of treatment.
- Instruct the patient to take the medication with a small meal or snack to decrease GI effects.
- Inform the patient to perform adequate hydration to replace fluids that are lost with diarrhea. Frequent oral care and sucking ice chips or sugarless candy may relieve stomatitis discomfort.
- Counsel the patient to avoid consuming alcohol until 72 hours after drug discontinuation to avoid the "disulfiram reaction."
- Monitor prothrombin times for appropriate dose adjustment when oral anticoagulants are administered concurrently with cephalosporins.
- Instruct the patient to report bleeding gums or bruising, which requires a reduction of the oral anticoagulant dose.
- Advise the patient to report difficulty breathing, severe headache, severe diarrhea, dizziness, weakness, and superinfections to the health care provider.

TAKE HOME POINTS

- Cephalosporin antibiotic therapy requires equidistant spacing to maintain an effective blood level.
- Cephalosporins may cause false-positive results for the Coombs' test, and cefotetan can cause falsely elevated serum and urine creatinine concentrations. When cephalosporins are taken concurrently with aminoglycosides, the patient should be monitored frequently for nephrotoxicity (elevated BUN and creatinine levels) to determine any needed dose adjustment.
- Cephalosporin therapy should be continued 48 to 72 hours after the patient reaches an asymptomatic state (usually 10 days) or 24 to 48 hours after surgery when used for perioperative prophylaxis.
- Cefamandole, cefoperazone, and cefotetan will induce a disulfiram-like reaction when taken with alcohol.
- Monitor prothrombin times when administering cephalosporins because concurrent administration of anticoagulants may increase bleeding time.

Do You UNDERSTAND?

DIRECTIONS: Fill in the blanks with appropriate responses to the following question and statements.

1. Which generation cephalosporin is most associated with superinfections?

   _____

2. List five signs of a disulfiram-like reaction.

   _____

   _____

   _____

   _____

   _____

3. Ceftriaxone (Rocephin) is a _____-generation drug and is used against _____ microorganisms.

4. Cefazolin (Ancef) is a _____-generation drug and is used against _____ microorganisms.

What IS a Sulfonamide?

Sulfonamide	Trade Names	Uses
sulfisoxazole [sull-fih-SOX-uh-zole]	Gantrisin	Treatment of conjunctivitis, otitis media, UTI, and meningococci
trimethoprim-sulfamethoxazole [try-METH-oh-prim– suhl-fuh-meth-OX-uh-zole]	Bactrim Septra	Treatment of UTI, otitis media, and bronchitis
sulfasalazine [SULL-fuh-SAL-uh-zeen]	Azulfidine	Treatment of ulcerative colitis

Action

Sulfonamides (sulfa drugs) are synthetic derivatives that are bacteriostatic, which means they have the ability to inhibit the formation of new bacteria but have no effect on bacteria that are already formed. Sulfonamides compete with para-aminobenzoic acid (PABA) and prevent PABA from uniting with folic acid to form new bacteria, thereby preventing the growth of bacteria. The sulfonamides, rather than PABA, enter the reaction, competing for the enzyme involved and causing the formation of nonfunctional derivatives of folic acid. Because bacteria require PABA to unite with folic acid—an agent that is required for the synthesis of deoxyribonucleic acid (DNA), ribonucleic acid (RNA), and proteins—bacterial cell replication is halted. Therefore sulfonamides stop growth, development, and multiplication of new bacteria but do not kill mature, fully formed bacteria. Bacteria that can use preformed folic acid are unaffected by sulfonamides. Therefore the growth of human or host cells are unaffected by sulfonamides because they can use preformed folic acid.

TAKE HOME POINTS

Some bacteria are able to alter their metabolic pathways to use precursors or other forms of folic acid, thereby developing resistance to the antibacterial action of sulfonamides. After resistance to one sulfonamide develops, cross-resistance to other sulfonamides is common.

Answers: 1. third; 2. tremors, nausea, severe vomiting, diarrhea, hypotension or hypertension; 3. third, gram-positive and negative cocci and unusual strains of enteric microorganisms; 4. first, gram-positive cocci.

Uses

Sulfonamides are bacteriostatic against a wide range of gram-positive and gram-negative bacteria. Sulfonamides are indicated for the treatment of otitis media, bronchitis, urinary tract infections (UTIs), ulcerative colitis, chlamydia, gonorrhea, and other sexually transmitted diseases (STDs), as well as typhoid fever, dermatitis herpetiformis, pneumocystis carinii pneumonia, toxoplasmosis, brucellosis, and shigellosis. Sulfonamides are also used prophylactically in patients with a history of rheumatic fever, penicillin allergies, granulocytopenia, in children who are infected with human immunodeficiency virus (HIV), and in patients with traveler's diarrhea. Because of the emergence of resistant bacteria and the development of newer antibiotics, sulfonamides are no longer used to a great extent. Sulfonamides remain inexpensive, thus when cost is an issue, they are used for UTIs and chronic contagious conjunctivitis (**trachoma**).

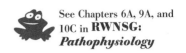

See Chapters 6A, 9A, and 10C in **RWNSG:** *Pathophysiology*

What You NEED TO KNOW

Contraindications/Precautions

Sulfonamides are contraindicated for patients with any known allergy to sulfonamides, sulfonylureas, or thiazide diuretics because of the possibility of cross-sensitivity. Sulfonamides are also contraindicated for patients with blood dyscrasias, porphyria, or those who are within 2 to 3 weeks of an acute gout attack.

Drug Interactions

When administered concurrently with sulfonamides, several drug interactions occur. Alcohol combined with a sulfonamide leads to increased blood urate levels. When taken with a sulfonamide, salicylates decrease uricosuric activity. Concurrent drugs that increase the risk of hypoglycemia include sulfonylurea agents or those that stimulate insulin release. Warfarin increases the effects of anticoagulants and may cause bleeding when taken with sulfonamides. Other interactions include decreased renal excretion of methotrexate and decreased hepatic clearance of phenytoin, barbiturates, tolbutamide, and uricosurics; increased thrombocytopenia when taken with thiazide diuretics; and increased nephrotoxicity when taken with cyclosporine.

Adverse Effects

Sulfonamide adverse effects have varying degrees of severity and may include hypersensitivity reactions. The most common adverse effects of sulfonamides include rash, headache, fever, anorexia, nausea, vomiting, abdominal pain, and diarrhea. Other adverse effects include urticaria, weakness, flushing, drowsiness, dizziness, stomatitis, glossitis, photosensitivity, ataxia, convulsions, depression, peripheral neuritis, hematuria, oliguria, anuria, uric acid kidney stones, and exacerbations of gout. Older sulfonamides have low solubility and present a high risk for crystalluria, resulting in renal damage. Newer sulfonamides have increased solubility but the potential for crystalluria remains.

 Sulfonamides are contra-indicated during pregnancy and lactation.

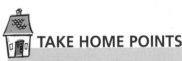 **Sulfonamide antibiotics should be used cautiously in patients with a history of peptic ulcers or renal disorders because these drugs tend to irritate the gastric mucosa and have a potential for nephrotoxicity.**

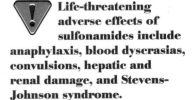 **TAKE HOME POINTS**

Cross-sensitivity may exist among sulfonamides, sulfonylureas, or thiazide diuretics.

Life-threatening adverse effects of sulfonamides include anaphylaxis, blood dyscrasias, convulsions, hepatic and renal damage, and Stevens-Johnson syndrome.

What You DO

Nursing Responsibilities

Sulfonamides are usually administered orally, on an empty stomach, 1 hour before or 2 hours after meals, and with a full glass of water. If GI distress occurs, sulfonamides may be taken with small, frequent meals or snacks. Frequent oral care and sucking on ice chips or sugarless candy may relieve discomfort of stomatitis. After oral administration, peak plasma levels are generally reached within 4 hours. In severe infections, sulfonamides are given IV for a faster response. The peak action after IV administration occurs in 1 hour. When administering sulfonamides, the nurse should:

- Monitor complete blood count (CBC) for early detection of bone marrow depression and the development of blood dyscrasias.
- Monitor renal and liver function tests before and throughout administration of sulfonamides to assure adequate functioning of these organs.
- Monitor glucose levels of patients who are taking sulfonylurea agents or other drugs that stimulate insulin release because dose adjustments of the antidiabetic agents may be required.
- Teach the patient to increase fluid intake to prevent crystalluria and replace fluids that are lost from diarrhea.
- Teach the patient to store sulfonamides in a tight, light-resistant container at room temperature.
- Advise the patient to avoid sunlight, use a sunscreen, and wear protective clothing to prevent sunburns.
- Instruct the patient to adhere to the full treatment length for therapeutic effects and to prevent a superinfection.
- Instruct patients to notify their health care provider in the event of hypersensitivity reaction, difficulty breathing, rash, ringing in the ears, fever, sore throat, and blood in the urine.

Do You UNDERSTAND?

DIRECTIONS: Indicate in the space provided whether the statement is *true* or *false*.

_____ 1. Sulfamethoxazole (Gantanol) may have cross-sensitivity with thiazide diuretics.

_____ 2. Sulfasalazine (Azulfidine) should be taken for 5 days to prevent superinfections.

_____ 3. A unique adverse effect of sulfonamides that is linked to their low solubility is crystalluria.

TAKE HOME POINTS

- Antibiotics require appropriate spacing between doses to maintain a certain blood level for effectiveness.
- Teach the patient to increase fluid intake to 2 liters per day to prevent crystalluria and replace fluids.

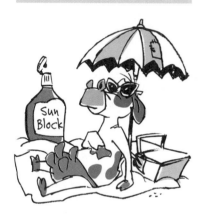

Counsel patients to avoid driving or operating dangerous machinery because of the adverse effects of dizziness, lethargy, and ataxia.

Answers: 1. true; 2. false; they should be taken for 10 days; 3. true.

What IS an Aminoglycoside?

Aminoglycosides	Trade Names	Uses
gentamicin sulfate [JEN-tuh-MY-sin]	Garamycin	Treatment of serious infections, especially gram-negative
amikacin sulfate [am-ih-KAY-sin]	Amikin	Treatment of infections, especially gram-negative
kanamycin sulfate [kan-uh-MY-sin]	Kantrex	Treatment of serious infections, especially gram-negative
tobramycin sulfate [TOE-bruh-MY-sin]	Nebcin	Treatment of serious infections, especially gram-negative

Action

Aminoglycosides are bactericidal; they bind irreversibly to both the 30S and 50S ribosomes to prevent bacterial protein synthesis. When ribosomes stop functioning, protein synthesis is disrupted and the bacterial cell eventually dies.

Uses

Because aminoglycosides are potent, they are usually reserved for more serious, life-threatening infections. These medications kill aerobic gram-positive and gram-negative bacteria, mycobacteria, aerobic gram-negative bacilli, and some protozoa. Aminoglycosides are used to treat serious nosocomial infections (e.g., gram-negative bacteremia, peritonitis, pneumonia).

A synergistic effect may be achieved by administering aminoglycosides in combination therapy with cephalosporins, penicillins, or vancomycin for greater effectiveness. Gentamicin is usually combined with penicillin to treat amebic dysentery. Extended-spectrum penicillins are usually combined with an aminoglycoside to treat serious pseudomonas infections.

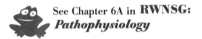

See Chapter 6A in **RWNSG:** *Pathophysiology*

What You NEED TO KNOW

Contraindications/Precautions

Aminoglycosides are contraindicated for patients with known allergies, renal or hepatic disease, preexisting hearing loss, active herpes, mycobacterial infections, myasthenia gravis, and parkinsonism.

Drug Interactions

The concurrent administration of dimenhydrinate can mask aminoglycoside toxicity. Co-administrating aminoglycosides and a neuromuscular blocking agent can lead to peripheral nerve toxicity and paralysis. Co-administration

Aminoglycosides should be administered with caution in neonates because of their immature renal systems. Fetal damage may occur when these drugs are given to pregnant or lactating women.

Aminoglycosides are contraindicated during lactation.

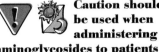

Caution should be used when administering aminoglycosides to patients who are pregnant.

with potent diuretics increases the incidence of ototoxicity, nephrotoxicity, and neurotoxicity. Because aminoglycosides decrease intestinal vitamin K synthesis, concurrent use of oral anticoagulants can increase bleeding time.

Adverse Effects

Adverse effects from aminoglycosides include nausea, vomiting, stomatitis, diarrhea, weight loss, headache, paresthesia, neuromuscular blockade, dizziness, vertigo, skin rash, fever, and superinfections.

Aminoglycosides are potent antibiotics and are capable of producing potentially serious toxicities. Common toxicities that may result from aminoglycosides are nephrotoxicity and ototoxicity. Symptoms of ototoxicity or eighth cranial nerve damage include dizziness, tinnitus, vertigo, nystagmus, ataxia, and hearing loss. Gentamicin and streptomycin are the primary culprits that cause toxicity to the vestibular portion of the eighth cranial nerve. Kanamycin, amikacin, and netilmicin primarily are associated with cochlear toxicity, although tobramycin may cause both types of ototoxicity. Nephrotoxicity involves symptoms of urinary casts, proteinuria, and increased BUN and serum creatinine levels. Patients at higher risk for nephrotoxicity are those with preexisting renal impairment and those who are taking other concurrent nephrotoxic drugs. Depressed bone marrow toxicity may result from aminoglycosides, leading to eosinophilia and immune suppression. Toxicity damage is usually associated with high doses, high trough levels, or prolonged therapy.

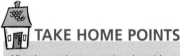

TAKE HOME POINTS

Allergic reactions to aminoglycosides are rare. Evidence of an allergic reaction involves a rash, urticaria, pruritus, generalized burning, and fever.

What You DO

Nursing Responsibilities

Aminoglycosides have negligible GI absorption. When an aminoglycoside is ordered for IV administration, refrigerate the prepared solution until use, and infuse over at least 30 minutes. When administering aminoglycosides, the nurse should:

- Administer aminoglycosides and penicillins at least 2 hours apart.
- Draw peak and trough levels periodically throughout aminoglycoside therapy to evaluate effectiveness and early detection of toxicity. A serum trough level is typically drawn 15 minutes before drug administration and the peak level is drawn 30 minutes after.
- Monitor renal function tests (creatinine, BUN, and urinalysis) at least every other day in patients with impaired renal function and at least once a week in patients with normal renal function to detect toxicity early.
- Monitor CBCs for evidence of bone marrow suppression.

An IV aminoglycoside should not be mixed in solution with extended-spectrum penicillins because the aminoglycoside will be inactivated.

- Instruct the patient to consume adequate fluids to overcome fluid loss from diarrhea and to decrease nephrotoxicity.
- Teach the patient safety precautions (e.g., avoidance of driving or operating hazardous machinery).
- Instruct the patient to report any difficulty breathing, severe headache, loss of hearing or tinnitus, or a decreased urine output to the health care provider.
- Instruct the patient to report bleeding to the health care provider immediately because aminoglycosides decrease intestinal vitamin K, and concurrent use of oral anticoagulants can increase bleeding time.

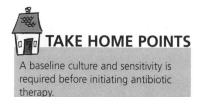

TAKE HOME POINTS

A baseline culture and sensitivity is required before initiating antibiotic therapy.

Do You UNDERSTAND?

DIRECTIONS: Provide an accurate response to each of the following statements.

1. List five possible signs of ototoxicity.

   _____

   _____

   _____

   _____

   _____

2. List three possible signs of nephrotoxicity.

   _____

   _____

   _____

3. Identify one nursing measure that can be used to prevent nephrotoxicity with aminoglycoside therapy.

   _____

4. Identify one antibiotic that should not be mixed with an aminoglycoside and should be spaced at least 2 hours apart.

   _____

Answers: 1. dizziness, tinnitus, nystagmus, ataxia, and hearing loss; 2. proteinuria, increased BUN and creatinine levels, and urinary casts; 3. encourage fluids for adequate hydration; 4. extended-spectrum penicillin.

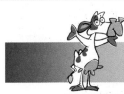

What IS a Tetracycline?

Tetracyclines	Trade Names	Uses
tetracycline [the-truh-SIGH-kleen]	Achromycin	Treatment of gram-positive and gram-negative infections
doxycycline [DOX-ee-SIGH-kleen]	Vibramycin	Treatment of gram-positive and gram-negative infections
demeclocycline [dem-e-klo-SIGH-kleen]	Declomycin	Treatment of gram-positive and gram-negative infections

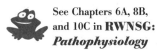

Because the targeted bacterial protein is similar to a protein found in human cells, tetracyclines in high concentrations can be toxic to humans.

Action

Tetracyclines are bacteriostatic, semisynthetic antibiotics that enter bacterial cells by passive diffusion and an active transport system. Tetracyclines compete for the binding of the 30S subunit site of the RNA ribosome to decrease bacterial growth, repair, and multiplication, thereby obstructing protein cell wall synthesis in susceptible bacteria. Tetracyclines may be bactericidal in high concentrations or against highly susceptible bacteria.

Uses

Because broad-spectrum antibiotics are effective against both gram-positive and gram-negative bacteria, tetracyclines are useful in treating several uncommon infections. Tetracyclines are considered the first-line drug defense for Rocky Mountain spotted fever and other rickettsial infections, as well as typhus, trachoma, lymphogranuloma venereum, urethritis, cervicitis, pneumonia, peptic ulcer disease, brucellosis, and cholera. Doxycycline has proven to be effective against malaria.

See Chapters 6A, 8B, and 10C in **RWNSG:** *Pathophysiology*

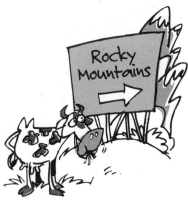

Additional uses for tetracyclines include acne, sinusitis, cystitis, tetanus, rat-bite fever, tropical sprue (bacterial infection of the intestine found in tropical regions, characterized by weakness, weight loss, and malabsorption of essential nutrients), tularemia (an acute plague-type infection from an infected tick, other infected insect or animal, or infected food or water), anthrax, yaws (infectious disease that is caused by a spirochete), and plague. When patients are allergic to penicillin, tetracyclines are frequently used to treat certain STDs, urinary and respiratory tract infections, and meningitis.

What You NEED TO KNOW

Tetracyclines are contra-indicated for women during pregnancy and lactation and for children under 8 years of age.

Contraindications/Precautions

Tetracyclines are contraindicated for patients with renal and hepatic dysfunction and bile duct obstruction.

Drug Interactions

With the exception of doxycycline and minocycline, absorption of tetracyclines is compromised when taken with dairy products and concurrent administration of antacids that contain calcium, magnesium, aluminum, or iron. Because these products prevent tetracycline absorption, antibacterial efficacy is decreased.

When tetracyclines are taken with penicillin, the bactericidal action of penicillin is decreased. Concurrent use of doxycycline with barbiturates, carbamazepine, and phenytoin increases the metabolism of tetracyclines. Cimetidine, taken concurrently, decreases the absorption of tetracyclines. Nephrotoxicity may occur when tetracyclines are taken with the general anesthetic methoxyflurane. When tetracyclines are given concurrently with digitalis, the risk of digitalis toxicity is increased.

Adverse Effects

The most common adverse effects of tetracyclines are nausea, abdominal cramping and distention, vomiting, diarrhea, and superinfections. A red rash upon exposure to sunlight is more common with demeclocycline and doxycycline compared with other tetracyclines; however, photosensitivity reactions may occur with any tetracycline.

Minocycline may evoke dizziness and vestibular reactions. A rash, glossitis, dermatitis, sore throat, dysphagia, hemolytic anemia, eosinophilia, neutropenia, thrombocytopenia, leukopenia, leukocytosis, and hepatotoxicity are other adverse effects of tetracyclines. Rare effects are hemolytic anemia and bone marrow depression. Hypersensitivity reactions include fever, headache, impaired vision, papilledema, intracranial hypertension, and anaphylaxis.

 # What You DO

Nursing Responsibilities

Absorption can be enhanced when taken on an empty stomach because alterations in gastric pH may decrease the absorption. Ideally, tetracyclines are given 1 hour before meals or 2 hours after meals with a full glass of water. However, when GI upset occurs, a small meal may be consumed with the drug to minimize distress. When administering tetracyclines, the nurse should:

- Space antacid doses at least 3 hours after tetracycline administration when the patient is taking both drugs.
- Provide the patient who is taking tetracyclines with adequate hydration to compensate for fluid loss from diarrhea.
- Check the dose and rate carefully when tetracycline is administered IV.
- Monitor CBCs, urinalysis, and liver and kidney function tests. Several laboratory values may be altered from tetracycline therapy. Elevated BUN, creatinine, bilirubin, alkaline phosphatase, ALT and AST, and urinary levels of catecholamines and protein may be present. Additionally, hemoglobin and

Tetracyclines should be used cautiously in patients with asthma, myasthenia gravis, or those who are malnourished.

Concurrent use of tetracycline with oral contraceptives leads to breakthrough bleeding, altered GI bacterial flora, decreased contraceptive effectiveness, and increased risk of pregnancy.

Because tetracyclines have a high affinity for calcium, prolonged use during the fourth fetal month through the eighth year of life when tooth development occurs may cause inadequate calcium deposit and discoloration of both deciduous and permanent teeth.

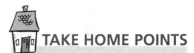 TAKE HOME POINTS

- Instruct patients to avoid tetracyclines during the fourth fetal month through the eighth year of life and during lactation periods to prevent discoloration of teeth.
- Instruct patients that adequate absorption is prevented when tetracyclines are taken with dairy products, antacids, or iron.

High-dose IV tetracycline that exceeds 2 g/day has been associated with liver failure and death.

TAKE HOME POINTS

Advise patients that a drug interaction between tetracyclines and contraceptives increases the risk of pregnancy and breakthrough bleeding when taken concurrently. When tetracyclines are necessary for the woman who is taking oral contraceptives, additional barrier contraceptives must be used.

platelet values may be decreased, and urine glucose results may be falsely positive or falsely negative.

🍎 Instruct the patient that tetracyclines should be avoided during pregnancy and lactation.

🍎 Instruct patients to use protective clothing and sunscreen to protect themselves from sunlight and ultraviolet light exposure because of a possible photosensitivity reaction. The sunscreen should not contain PABA.

🍎 Inform patients that outdated tetracyclines should not be ingested because degraded drugs are highly nephrotoxic.

🍎 Teach the patient to report any difficulty breathing, rash, itching, cramps, severe diarrhea, or a decrease in urine to the health care provider.

Do You UNDERSTAND?

DIRECTIONS: **Indicate in the space provided whether the statement is** *true* **or** *false.*

_____ 1. Iron interacts with tetracyclines and decreases absorption.

_____ 2. A drug interaction of tetracyclines with oral contraceptives may lead to an increased risk of pregnancy.

_____ 3. The maximal IV tetracycline dose is 4 grams per day.

_____ 4. The patient who is taking tetracyclines should use a sunscreen with PABA.

What IS a Macrolide?

Macrolides	Trade Names	Uses
erythromycin [eh-RITH-row-MY-sin]	E-Mycin	Treatment of ocular infections
azithromycin [UHZ-ith-row-MY-sin]	Zithromax	Treatment of respiratory tract, pelvic, skin infections, and STDs
clarithromycin [kluh-RITH-row-MY-sin]	Biaxin	Treatment of respiratory tract and skin infections
dirithromycin [die-RITH-row-MY-sin]	Dynabac	Treatment of respiratory tract and skin infections

Action

Macrolides are bacteriostatic or bactericidal, depending on their concentration and the offending bacteria. Macrolides bind to the 50S ribosomal subunits and inhibit polypeptide synthesis, thereby inhibiting protein synthesis. By binding to bacterial cell membranes, macrolides change protein function and cause cell death or prevent cell division.

Answers: 1. true; also milk, dairy products, antacids, and cimetidine; 2. true; 3. false; high doses over 2 grams per day have been associated with liver failure and death; 4. false; use sunscreen without PABA.

Uses

Macrolides are used in treating mild-to-moderate infections and are effective against gram-positive and gram-negative cocci. Macrolides are also used to treat mild-to-moderate infections of the respiratory tract, sinuses, skin, GI tract, and soft tissue, as well as diphtheria, STDs, and impetigo contagiosa. Macrolides are also the drug of choice in pertussis, diphtheria, Legionnaires' disease, atypical viral pneumonia, syphilis, and *Chlamydia*. Macrolides are also given prophylactally before dental procedures in patients with valvular heart disease to prevent endocarditis. Erythromycin is also used to treat anthrax infection.

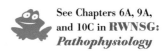

See Chapters 6A, 9A, and 10C in **RWNSG:** *Pathophysiology*

What You NEED TO KNOW

Contraindications/Precautions

Macrolides are contraindicated for patients with preexisting liver disease and a known allergy to any macrolide because cross-sensitivity occurs. Ocular macrolides are contraindicated for patients with eye infections that may be exacerbated by the loss of normal bacterial flora.

Drug Interactions

The absorption of macrolides is decreased when they are taken with antacids. Increased effects of anticoagulants, digoxin, carbamazepine, triazolam, astemizole, corticosteroids, theophylline, valproate, alfentanil, bromocriptine, cyclosporine, terfenadine, tacrolimus, and ergot alkaloids are present when macrolides are given concurrently. Macrolides may decrease the effects of zidovudine.

Adverse Effects

Macrolides are considered to have low toxicity among antibiotics and have relatively few adverse effects. The most common adverse effects of macrolides include dose-related anorexia, abnormal taste, heartburn, nausea, vomiting, abdominal cramping, stomatitis, flatulence, diarrhea, pruritus ani, reversible hearing loss, allergic reactions, and mild acute pancreatitis. These adverse effects usually resolve with continued therapy. Other adverse effects of erythromycin include headache, vertigo, dizziness, confusion, abnormal thinking, uncontrollable emotions, somnolence, tinnitus, palpitations, chest pain, bilateral hearing loss, and superinfections.

Hepatotoxicity with jaundice occurs with estolate and ethylsuccinate forms of erythromycin. Additionally, cholestatic hepatitis (from obstruction of bile flow) has been associated with erythromycin when drug therapy lasts longer than 10 days or when the drug is given repeatedly.

 Macrolides should be administered with caution in patients with impaired liver function and in women during pregnancy and lactation.

 Safety and efficacy of macrolides has not been established for patients under 12 years of age.

When macrolides are given concurrently with astemizole, terfenadine, or cisapride, potentially fatal cardiac dysrhythmias may occur.

What You DO

Nursing Responsibilities

Macrolides may be inactivated by gastric acid, thus they are enteric coated or buffered. Ideally, macrolides should be taken 1 hour before or 2 hours after meals for better absorption. However, because of the high incidence of GI distress, macrolides may be taken with a small snack. When administering macrolides, the nurse should:

- Not give erythromycin IM because of the pain upon injection and the potential formation of sterile abscess.
- Teach the patient about safety precautions and using caution when driving vehicles or operating machinery.
- Monitor liver function tests to ensure adequate functioning.
- Be certain that culture and sensitivity tests are performed before macrolide therapy to ensure that the most effective drug is given.
- Monitor the patient for phlebitis during IV infusion.
- Be aware that aminoglycosides and tetracyclines should not be given together because they have similar actions and compete with each other.
- Monitor digoxin levels because increased levels occur when the drug is taken concurrently with macrolides. The digoxin dose may need to be adjusted throughout macrolide therapy.
- Inform patients that frequent mouth care and sucking on ice chips or sugarless candy may relieve discomfort.
- Instruct the patient to drink an adequate amount of fluids and maintain nutrition to compensate for any nausea, vomiting, and diarrhea.
- Instruct patients to report changes in hearing, signs of cholestatic hepatitis (e.g., nausea, vomiting, abdominal pain, jaundice, rash), and allergic reactions to the health care provider.

 Erythromycin stearate should not be administered with food. Macrolides should not be mixed for IV use with incompatible drugs (e.g., vitamin B complex, vitamin C, cephalothin, tetracycline, heparin, colistimethate sodium, flurosemide, metaraminol bitartrate, metoclopramide hydrochloride).

 TAKE HOME POINTS

A baseline culture and sensitivity is required before initiating antibiotic therapy. IV solutions should be administered within 4 hours after reconstitution.

Do You UNDERSTAND?

DIRECTIONS: Provide accurate responses to the following statements and question.

1. List three of the most common adverse effects of macrolides.

   _____

   _____

   _____

2. Macrolides are contraindicated for patients with what condition?

   _____

3. List two preferred routes of macrolide administration.

   _____

   _____

Answers: 1. GI distress, anorexia, abnormal taste; 2. preexisting liver disease; 3. orally, IV.

What IS a Fluoroquinolone?

Fluoroquinolones	Trade Names	Uses
ciprofloxacin [sip-ROW-FLOX-ah-sin]	Cipro	Treatment of lower respiratory and GU infections, bone, skin, joint, and STDs
levofloxacin [lee-voe-FLOX-ah-sin]	Levaquin	Treatment of respiratory, GU, and skin infections

Action

Fluoroquinolones are a relatively new classification of antibiotics and are bactericidal against a broad spectrum of bacteria. Fluoroquinolones interfere with DNA gyrase, which is an enzyme that is required to synthesize bacterial DNA and for growth and reproduction.

Uses

Fluoroquinolones are active against a wide range of gram-positive and gram-negative bacteria and are used to treat infections involving the respiratory, urinary, and GI tracts, infections of the sinus, skin, soft tissue, bones, joints, and prostate, as well as anthrax infection, infectious diarrhea, and STDs. Newer fluoroquinolones—gatifloxacin and moxifloxacin—are available for once-a-day treatment of community-acquired pneumonia, acute bacterial exacerbations of chronic bronchitis, and acute sinusitis.

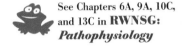
See Chapters 6A, 9A, 10C, and 13C in **RWNSG:** *Pathophysiology*

What You NEED TO KNOW

Contraindications/Precautions

Fluoroquinolones are contraindicated for women during pregnancy and lactation and for children under 18 years of age.

Drug Interactions

Fluoroquinolones increase xanthine effects of theophylline and caffeine, both of which predispose a patient to seizures. When given concurrently with fluoroquinolones, the effects of anticoagulants are increased. Probenecid interferes with renal tubular secretion. Sucralfate and antacids that contain magnesium or aluminum hydroxide decrease the effect of fluoroquinolones. The risk of nephrotoxicity may be increased when fluoroquinolones are taken concurrently with cyclosporine. Nitrofurantoin may interfere with the antibacterial effects of norfloxacin. The elimination of fluoroquinolones may be decreased by cimetidine. When fluoroquinolone administration is combined with nonsteroidal antiin-

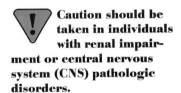
Caution should be taken in individuals with renal impairment or central nervous system (CNS) pathologic disorders.

flammatory drugs (NSAIDs), an increased risk of CNS stimulation occurs. Additionally, dairy products and food reduce the absorption of ciprofloxacin. Food also delays the absorption of lomefloxacin.

Adverse Effects

Fluoroquinolones may cause mild-to-moderate adverse effects, which usually disappear after the drug is discontinued. Common adverse effects include nausea, vomiting, abdominal discomfort, headache, dizziness, insomnia, confusion, restlessness, and depression. Other adverse effects include fever, skin rash, photosensitivity, photophobia, flushing, dry mouth, unpleasant taste, anorexia, pruritus, urticaria, visual difficulty, superinfections, and renal impairment. Crystalluria may occur with large doses of fluoroquinolone. The most serious adverse effects are seizures and tendon injury. Rare adverse effects include tendonitis, vasculitis, palpitations, syncope, atrial flutter, myocardial infarction (MI), respiratory difficulty, leukopenia, eosinophilia, anaphylaxis, and heart attack. Cross-sensitivity among fluoroquinolones may occur. Serious adverse effects may occur after a single dose.

What You DO

Nursing Responsibilities

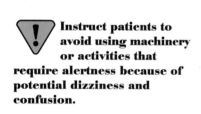

Instruct patients to avoid using machinery or activities that require alertness because of potential dizziness and confusion.

Ciprofloxacin is the most widely used fluoroquinolone and can be administered in oral, injectable, and topical forms. When administering ciprofloxacin IV, the drug should be infused over 60 minutes. When administration is too rapid, seizures may occur. When giving fluoroquinolones, the nurse should:

- Instruct the patient to complete the full course of treatment to prevent the development of resistant strains of bacteria.
- Monitor theophylline and warfarin levels because these drugs may require dose adjustment.
- Monitor renal function tests for impairment and possible dose reduction.
- Instruct patients to maintain an adequate fluid intake to compensate for diarrhea and to prevent crystalluria.
- Instruct the patient to avoid milk products, antacids, iron, or sucralfate because these agents decrease the fluoroquinolone effect.
- Instruct patients to use protective clothing and sunscreen to protect themselves from exposure to sunlight and ultraviolet light.
- Instruct patients to report difficulty breathing, severe headache, severe diarrhea, fainting, and heart palpitations to the health care provider.
- Be aware that taking fluoroquinolones concurrently with drugs that prolong the Q-T interval or cause torsades de pointes (e.g., quinidine, procainamide, amiodarone, sotalol, bepridil, erythromycin, terfenadine, astemizole, cisapride, pentamidine, tricyclics, phenothiazines) may lead to fatal cardiac dysrhythmias.
- Monitor patients who are taking fluoroquinolones and NSAIDs for seizures.

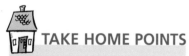

TAKE HOME POINTS

Frequent mouth care and sucking on ice chips or sugarless candy may relieve discomfort.

Do You UNDERSTAND?

DIRECTIONS: **Match the statements from Column A to the corresponding responses in Column B.**

Column A

_____ 1. Peak fluoroquinolone serum level
_____ 2. Concurrent fluoroquinolones and NSAIDs can lead to these
_____ 3. IV Cipro should be infused over
_____ 4. Adverse effect of large doses of fluoroquinolones

Column B

a. 60 minutes
b. Crystalluria
c. 1 to 3 hours
d. Seizures

What IS a Miscellaneous Antibiotic?

Miscellaneous Antibiotics	Trade Names	Uses
aztreonam [azz-TREE-oh-nam]	Azactam	Treatment of urinary and lower respiratory tract, skin, intra-abdominal infections
clindamycin [KLIN-duh-MY-sin]	Cleocin	Treatment of serious abdominal and pelvic infections
imipenem-cilastatin [ih-mih-PEN-em–SIGH-luh-STAT-in]	Primaxin	Treatment of serious urinary and lower respiratory tract, skin, bone, joint, and intraabdominal infections
vancomycin [van-koe-MY-sin]	Vancocin	Treatment of serious infections

Action

Several other antibiotics that do not fit into the previous classifications are discussed in this section. Aztreonam disrupts cell wall synthesis of bacteria that cause a leakage of intracellular contents and cell death. This drug is bactericidal against gram-negative aerobic bacteria, thus it has a narrow spectrum of activity. Clindamycin is an example of the lincosamide antibiotic classification, which binds to the 50S subunit of the bacterial ribosomes and inhibits protein synthesis.

Imipenem/cilastatin is composed of imipenem (a β-lactam antibiotic) and cilastatin (an inhibitor of dipeptidase inactivation of imipenem). Imipenem is bacteriocidal because mucopeptide synthesis in bacterial cell walls is inhibited, which leads to cell death. This drug has the greatest spectrum of any β-lactam antibiotic. Vancomycin inhibits bacterial cell wall synthesis and promotes bacterial lysis and death. Vancomycin also binds to the molecules that serve as precursors for cell wall biosynthesis, thereby disrupting the bacterial cell wall.

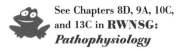

See Chapters 8D, 9A, 10C, and 13C in **RWNSG:** *Pathophysiology*

Uses

Aztreonam is indicated in the treatment of skin, intraabdominal, urinary tract, and gynecologic infections, and septicemia. Clindamycin is used in severe anaerobic infections outside the CNS. Clindamycin is a preferred drug for abdominal and pelvic infections and is also used for acne vulgaris and bacterial vaginosis. Imipenem/cilastatin is used to treat serious infections in the respiratory tract, urinary tract, bones, joints, skin, intraabdominal area, gynecologic system, endocarditis, and bacterial septicemia. Vancomycin is used to treat life-threatening infections and is the choice treatment of antibiotic-associated pseudomembranous colitis (AAPC).

What You NEED TO KNOW

Contraindications/Precautions

Clindamycin is contraindicated for patients with lincosamide hypersensitivity, regional enteritis, and ulcerative colitis. Imipenem/cilastatin is contraindicated for patients with hypersensitivity. Vancomycin is contraindicated for patients with hypersensitivity, previous hearing loss, and concurrent ototoxic or nephrotoxic drugs.

The most severe toxicity of clindamycin is AAPC, which is a superinfection with profuse, watery diarrhea of up to 10 to 20 stools per day. The condition may be fatal without treatment. Rapid IV administration may cause hypotension, dysrhythmias, and cardiac arrest.

Drug Interactions

Probenecid slows renal elimination of aztreonam when given concurrently. When clindamycin is given with neuromuscular blocking agents, the neuromuscular blocking action is enhanced. Clindamycin, erythromycin, and chloramphenicol may antagonize the effects of each other when given together because the ribosomal sites (at which the lincosamides bind) overlap. The antibiotic effect of imipenem/cilastatin may be antagonized by aztreonam, penicillin, or cephalosporins. Vancomycin leads to the risk of otic and renal toxicities when given concurrently with aminoglycosides, amphotericin B, colistin, polymyxin B, and other ototoxic or nephrotoxic drugs.

Aztreonam should be used with caution in patients with a hypersensitivity to penicillin or cephalosporins and renal or hepatic dysfunction.

Aztreonam is contraindicated for women during pregnancy and lactation and for children. Clindamycin is contraindicated for women during pregnancy and lactation and for infants under 1 month of age. Imipenem/ cilastatin is contraindicated for women during pregnancy and for children under 12 years of age. Vancomycin is contraindicated during pregnancy.

Adverse Effects

Because aztreonam is well tolerated, adverse effects are few. The most common adverse effects are pain and thrombophlebitis at the injection site. Other adverse effects include headache, dizziness, confusion, tinnitus, nasal congestion, sneezing, diplopia, nausea, vomiting, diarrhea, paresthesia, insomnia, seizures, urticaria, rash, superinfections, elevation of liver function tests, and eosinophilia. Because aztreonam differs greatly in structure from β-lactam antibiotics, little cross-allergenicity exists between aztreonam with penicillins and cephalosporins. Therefore aztreonam appears to be a safe alternative for patients with β-lactam allergies.

Adverse effects of clindamycin include hypersensitivity, rash, skin dryness, loss of taste, nausea, vomiting, abdominal pain, flatulence, diarrhea, abnormal liver function tests, and blood dyscrasias.

Imipenem/cilastatin is well tolerated. Adverse effects include hypersensitivity, rash, pruritus, fever, nausea, vomiting, and diarrhea. Rare adverse effects from imipenem/cilastatin include superinfections and seizures. Vancomycin can cause highly toxic adverse effects. Adverse effects that are associated with vancomycin include superinfections, ototoxicity, and renal failure. "Red man syndrome" or "red neck syndrome" can also occur, which is a result of an increase in histamine release following an infusion that is too rapid. Fever, rash, chills, paresthesia, tachycardia, sudden and severe hypotension, and flushing or redness on the neck and back are characteristics of "red man syndrome."

Clindamycin should be given cautiously to patients with asthma, eczema, hay fever, GI disorders, renal or hepatic dysfunction, and older adults. Imipenem/cilastatin should be used with caution in patients with seizures, head injuries or other CNS disorders, renal impairment, penicillin hypersensitivity, and in lactating women. Vancomycin should be given cautiously to neonates and patients with renal dysfunction.

What You DO

Nursing Responsibilities

When administered IM, aztreonam should be injected deeply into large muscle mass. (Refer to *Real World Nursing Survival Guide: Drug Calculations and Drug Administration* for injection sites.) Clindamycin is unaffected by food and may be given orally, IM, or IV. When given orally, clindamycin should be followed by a full glass of water. AAPC usually begins in the first week of treatment but may develop 4 to 6 weeks after treatment. AAPC is treated with oral vancomycin or metronidazole, with the diarrhea subsiding in 3 to 5 days. Vancomycin can be administered orally or IV. Infusions should be administered slowly for 60 minutes or more. The vancomycin IV site should be monitored for thrombophlebitis. When administering antibiotics, the nurse should:

- Be certain that culture and sensitivity tests are performed before administering an antibiotic to ensure that the most effective drug is given.
- Draw peak and trough levels periodically throughout vancomycin therapy to evaluate effectiveness and to detect toxicity. A serum trough level is typically drawn 15 minutes before administering the drug, and the peak level is drawn 30 minutes after administration.
- Monitor hepatic and renal function tests throughout the course of treatment for early detection of dysfunction and necessary dose alteration.
- Prevent thrombophlebitis from IV antibiotic infusions by diluting the drug appropriately and frequently changing the infusion site.
- Instruct the patient to report more than five watery stools per day for the early detection of AAPC.

TAKE HOME POINTS

Baseline culture and sensitivity is required before initiating antibiotic therapy.

Do You UNDERSTAND?

DIRECTIONS: Answer the following questions with the appropriate responses.

1. Which miscellaneous antibiotic is likely to cause AAPC?

   _____

2. Which miscellaneous antibiotic causes "red neck syndrome?"

   _____

3. Which miscellaneous antibiotic causes severe ototoxicity?

   _____

SECTION B

ANTIVIRALS AND ANTIFUNGALS

This section reviews selected antivirals, including protease inhibitors, nucleoside reverse transcriptase inhibitors, nonnucleoside reverse transcriptase inhibitors, and nucleoside analogs. The antifungals that are discussed include polyenes and azoles.

Antivirals

Viruses are intracellular parasites with no metabolic machinery of their own; they lack both a cell wall and a cell membrane and do not carry out metabolic processes. To replicate, viruses must attach to and enter a living host cell—animal, plant, or bacteria—and use its metabolic processes. Viral replication requires DNA or RNA synthesis and synthesis of viral proteins and glycosylation.

All viruses require cells to replicate. Most antiviral drugs must penetrate cells that are already infected to produce a therapeutic antiviral response. Few drugs are sufficiently selective to prevent viral replication without injury to the host. Some drugs discriminate sufficiently between cellular and viral reactions to be effective and yet relatively nontoxic. Unfortunately, only a few viral groups respond to these drugs. Many antiviral agents inhibit single steps in the viral replication cycle. These agents are considered virustatic and do not destroy a given virus but temporarily halt replication. Optimal antiviral effectiveness requires a competent host immune system that can eliminate or effectively halt virus replication.

TAKE HOME POINTS

Retrovirus is a common name for the family of RNA-containing tumor viruses. These viruses induce tumors such as sarcomas, leukemias, and lymphomas. These viruses contain reverse transcriptase, which is essential for the production of a DNA molecule from RNA.

What IS a Protease Inhibitor Antiretroviral?

Protease Inhibitors	Trade Names	Uses
saquinavir [sack-KWIN-uh-vihr]	Invirase	Treatment of advanced HIV infection
nelfinavir [nell-FIN-ah-veer]	Viracept	Treatment of HIV infection

Action

Aspartate proteinase is essential for the final step of viral proliferation and is encoded with the HIV genome, thus it is absent in uninfected CD4 cells. These agents interfere with HIV protease, thereby impeding the viral replication of retroviruses, including HIV type I (HIV-1) and type II (HIV-2). The active enzyme generates proteins, which are necessary to the virus. The HIV protease inhibitors interfere in this process and lead to the assembly of nonfunctional virions. Protease inhibitors interfere with the multiplication of the virus and slow the progression of the disease, which possibly prolongs survival.

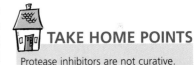

TAKE HOME POINTS

Protease inhibitors are not curative.

Uses

Protease inhibitors are used to treat HIV infection in adults.

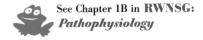

See Chapter 1B in **RWNSG:** *Pathophysiology*

What You NEED TO KNOW

Contraindications/Precautions

Protease inhibitors are contraindicated for patients with hypersensitivity or hemophilia.

Drug Interactions

Because the hepatic cytochrome P-450 family of enzymes metabolizes protease inhibitors, they interact with other drugs, leading to further interactions. When more than one protease inhibitor is given together, liver metabolism may be inhibited, or a synergistic or antagonistic action may occur. Prolonged sedation, cardiac dysrhythmias, neurotoxicity, or elevated indinavir levels may occur when indinavir is taken concurrently with ergot alkaloids, triazolam, or midazolam. Rifampin markedly reduces the plasma concentration and action of protease inhibitors. Ketoconazole, clarithromycin, and quinidine sulfate increase indinavir levels when given concurrently. Indinavir increases isoniazid levels when given together. Anticonvulsants decrease nelfinavir levels.

  When administering these agents, caution should be taken in patients with diabetes mellitus, renal or hepatic dysfunction, and in older adults.

Adverse Effects

Although protease inhibitors are usually well tolerated, headache, alopecia, dizziness, rash, dry skin, fatigue, cough, taste alteration, nausea, vomiting, diarrhea, back pain, hyperglycemia, and paresthesias around the mouth may occur. More serious adverse effects include nephrolithiasis, anaphylaxis, hepatic failure, and Stevens-Johnson syndrome. Elevated hepatic aminotransferase, serum glutamicoxaloacetic transaminase, SGPT, and triglyceride levels have been reported.

What You DO

Nursing Responsibilities

When administering protease inhibitors, the nurse should:

- Instruct the patient to take protease inhibitors with water or milk 1 hour before meals or 2 hours after meals. If the patient develops GI distress, then the medication may be taken with a light snack, such as dry toast with jelly.
- Instruct the patient to avoid mixing nelfinavir with an acidic juice or food because of the bitter taste.
- Advise the patient to drink at least 1.5 liters of fluids within a 24-hour period when taking protease inhibitors to prevent nephrolithiasis.
- Instruct the patient to take protease inhibitors at least 1 hour apart from didanosine.
- Instruct the patient to take the full dose of medication as ordered. These drugs must be given in doses sufficiently high to completely suppress viral replication; otherwise, resistant viruses can emerge. Cessation of treatment results in reemergence of the virus.
- Instruct the patient that when a dose of protease inhibitors is missed, disregard that dose and take the next dose at the usual time.

Do You UNDERSTAND?

DIRECTIONS: Indicate in the space provided whether the statement is true or false.

_____ 1. Protease inhibitors interfere with the first step of viral proliferation.

_____ 2. Protease inhibitors eliminate aspartate proteinase.

_____ 3. Protease inhibitors are curative.

_____ 4. Protease inhibitors should be given at the lowest possible dose to prevent adverse effects.

_____ 5. Protease inhibitors are safe to use, with rare drug interactions.

TAKE HOME POINTS

Advise the patients that when they are unable to swallow tablets, the tablets may be dissolved in water and mixed with milk or chocolate milk.

Answers: 1. false; 2. true; 3. false; 4. false; 5. false.

What IS a Nucleoside Reverse Transcriptase Inhibitor Antiretroviral?

Nucleoside Reverse Transcriptase Inhibitors	Trade Names	Uses
zidovudine (AZT) [sid-OH-vue-deen]	Retrovir	Treatment of HIV infection
didanosine [die-DAN-oh-SEEN]	Videx	Treatment of HIV infection

Action

Nucleoside reverse transcriptase inhibitors (NRTIs) interfere with viral RNA-directed DNA polymerase (reverse transcriptase), thereby impeding the replication of retroviruses, including HIV. NRTIs exert a virustatic effect against retroviruses.

Zidovudine is also known as azidothymidine (AZT) and is an analogue of thymidine, which is a nucleoside present in DNA. In retroviruses (e.g., HIV), zidovudine is an active inhibitor of reverse transcriptase. This drug is combined with triphosphate by cellular enzymes. The triphosphate form competes with equivalent cellular triphosphates, which are the essential basis for the formation of proviral DNA by viral reverse transcriptase (viral RNA-dependent DNA polymerase). The incorporation of this substance into growing viral DNA strands results in chain termination. Mammalian alpha DNA polymerase is relatively resistant to the effect. However, gamma DNA polymerase in the host cell mitochondria is fairly sensitive to the compound, which may be the basis of unwanted effects.

Because of rapid mutation, the virus is a constantly moving target, thus the therapeutic response decreases with long-term usage, particularly in the later stage of the disease. Resistant strains can be transferred between individuals. Another factor that contributes to the loss of drug efficacy includes increased viral load resulting from a reduction in immune mechanisms.

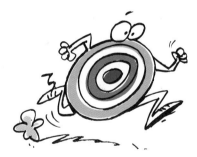

Uses

NRTIs are used in the treatment of HIV infection in adults or children over 3 months of age. Retroviral therapy should be started before immunodeficiency becomes evident. The aim is to reduce plasma viral concentration as much as possible and for as long as possible. NRTIs have greater effectiveness in the treatment of HIV-acquired immunodeficiency syndrome (AIDS) when used in combination of at least three drugs (e.g., two reverse transcriptase inhibitors and one protease inhibitor). When plasma viral concentration increases, the health care provider can change to a new regimen.

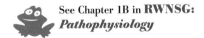

See Chapter 1B in **RWNSG:** *Pathophysiology*

What You NEED TO KNOW

NRTIs are contraindicated for women during pregnancy and lactation.

Contraindications/Precautions

NRTIs are contraindicated for patients with hypersensitivity. NRTIs should be used with caution in patients with peripheral vascular disease, neuropathy, chronic pancreatitis, and renal or liver dysfunction.

Drug Interactions

When didanosine is taken with aluminum and magnesium antacids, the adverse effects are increased. When they are taken with zalcitabine, an additive neuropathy may develop. NRTIs decrease the effectiveness of dapsone. When zidovudine is taken with acetaminophen, bone marrow suppression may occur. The risk of AZT toxicity is increased when taken with amphotericin B, aspirin, dapsone, indomethacin, interferon, and vincristine.

Adverse Effects

Common adverse effects associated with NRTIs include anemia and neutropenia, particularly with long-term administration. Other adverse effects include dizziness, headache, fever, insomnia, confusion, nervousness, anxiety, depression, dry mouth, cough, dyspnea, weakness, poor coordination, seizures, abdominal pain, nausea, vomiting, diarrhea, constipation, paresthesias, myopathy, and liver dysfunction. Influenza-like syndrome, hypocalcemia, hypokalemia, hypomagnesemia, elevated hemoglobin and white blood count, visual disturbance, palpitations, and dysrhythmias have also been reported. The short-term prophylactic use in relatively healthy adults who have specific exposure to the virus is associated with only minor reversible adverse effects.

What You DO

Nursing Responsibilities

When administering NRTIs, the nurse should:
- Be aware that NRTIs are administered orally or IV.
- Administer oral NRTIs on an empty stomach, either well before or well after meals.
- Instruct the patient to take oral NRTIs with water, not a fruit juice or an acidic liquid. Tablets should be chewed thoroughly or crushed to disperse in 30 ml of water and swallowed immediately.

- Monitor the patient's plasma viral load, CD4 count, CBC, renal and liver function studies throughout NRTIs therapy. When the plasma viral count increases in a patient who is taking NRTIs, a new treatment regime is indicated.
- Instruct the patient that when a dose is missed, avoid doubling the next dose. Rather, take the missed dose only when it is greater than 4 hours before the next dose.

Do You UNDERSTAND?

DIRECTIONS: **Select the word(s) from the italicized list below to complete the following statements.**

1. When a patient is taking an NRTI, the nurse should monitor

_____.

2. The most common adverse effect of NRTIs is

_____.

polycythemia	*liver function tests*	*cough*
anemia	*K level*	

What IS a Nonnucleoside Reverse Transcriptase Inhibitor Antiretroviral?

Nonnucleoside reverse transcriptase inhibitors	Trade Names	Uses
nevirapine [nuh-VEER-uh-peen]	Viramune	Treatment of HIV infection
delavirdine [dell-ah-VIR-deen]	Rescriptor	Treatment of HIV-1 infection

Action

A nonnucleoside reverse transcriptase inhibitor (NNRTI) antiviral is different from an NRTI in structure and action. NNRTIs bind to the active center of reverse transcriptase to block RNA and DNA polymerase activities. This action causes a disruption of the enzyme's catalytic site and prevents replication of HIV-1 virus.

Uses

NNRTIs are used in the treatment of HIV infection. Usually, treatment with NNRTIs is in combination with other antiviral agents.

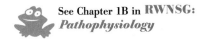

See Chapter 1B in RWNSG: *Pathophysiology*

What You NEED TO KNOW

  NNRTIs are contra-indicated for women during lactation.

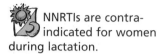 **NNRTIs should be used with caution in children, in patients with hepatic dysfunction and CNS disorders, and in women during pregnancy.**

Contraindications/Precautions

NNRTIs are contraindicated for patients with hypersensitivity.

Drug Interactions

Antacids and didanosine decrease absorption of delavirdine. When given concurrently, delavirdine increases serum levels of indinavir, saquinavir, alprazolam, midazolam, dapsone, quinidine, clarithromycin, warfarin, ergot alkaloids, calcium channel blockers, and antiarrhythmics. Nevirapine decreases concentrations of protease inhibitors and oral contraceptives when given together. Rifampin and rifabutin decrease the action of nevirapine.

Adverse Effects

The most common adverse effect of NNRTIs is a rash, which can be benign or life threatening. The rash may be associated with fever, conjunctivitis, blistering, oral lesions, muscle or joint pain, erythema multiforme, and Stevens-Johnson syndrome. Other common adverse effects include headache, fatigue, nausea, vomiting, and diarrhea. Anemia and neutropenia may also develop.

What You DO

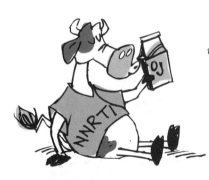

Nursing Responsibilities

NNRTIs may be given with or without food. Delavirdine should be mixed with at least 3 ounces of water before administration. Antacids and didanosine should not be administered within 1 hour of delavirdine. Because acidity enhances absorption, these agents may be given with an acid beverage, such as orange or cranberry juice. When administering NNRTIs, the nurse should:

- Monitor the liver enzymes, which may elevate in the patient who is taking NNRTIs.
- Monitor renal function studies for early detection of renal dysfunction.
- Monitor CBC for early detection of blood dyscrasias.
- Warn the patient that drowsiness and fatigue may occur when taking NNRTIs and that safety must be considered when operating hazardous equipment.
- Instruct patients who are taking NNRTIs to withhold the drug and notify the prescribing health care provider immediately when a severe rash occurs. A severe rash may indicate erythema multiforme or Stevens-Johnson syndrome.

Do You UNDERSTAND?

DIRECTIONS: Indicate in the space provided whether the statement is
true or *false*.

_____ 1. NNRTIs are used primarily in the treatment of herpes simplex.

_____ 2. Delavirdine decreases serum levels of warfarin.

What IS a Nucleoside Analog Antiviral?

Nucleoside Analogs	Trade Names	Uses
acyclovir [A-SIKE-low-vihr]	Acycloguanosine	Treatment of herpes simplex viruses, varicella zoster, and genital herpes
famciclovir [fam-Cl-clo-vihr]	Famvir	Treatment of herpes simplex, herpes zoster, and genital herpes

Action

Acyclovir acts by being converted by the viral cell into its active form of triphosphate and inhibits viral DNA polymerase. Acyclovir preferentially interferes with DNA synthesis of herpes simplex types 1 and 2 and varicella-zoster virus.

Uses

Nucleoside analog antivirals are used to inhibit viral replication of herpes, types 1 and 2 herpes simplex, and varicella (chickenpox) viruses. These agents also exert antiviral activity against Epstein-Barr virus (infectious mononucleosis) and cytomegalovirus.

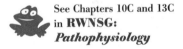 See Chapters 10C and 13C in RWNSG: *Pathophysiology*

What You NEED TO KNOW

Contraindications/Precautions

Nucleoside analog antivirals are contraindicated for patients with hypersensitivity and blood dyscrasias.

Drug Interactions

Nucleoside analog antivirals have some drug interactions with other drugs. When probenecid is given with acyclovir, the action of acyclovir is prolonged. Zidovudine causes increased acyclovir levels increasing the risk of toxicity.

  Nucleoside analog antivirals should be used with caution in patients with neurologic and renal dysfunction, dehydration, in older adults, and in patients who are taking nephrotoxic drugs.

Answers: 1. false; NNRTIs prevent replication of the HIV-1 virus; 2. false; delavirdine increases serum levels.

Adverse Effects

The adverse effects of acyclovir include headache, confusion, tremors, rash, malaise, nausea, vomiting, and diarrhea. Other more serious adverse effects include hallucinations, hematuria, seizures, and coma.

What You DO

Nursing Responsibilities

Nucleoside analog antivirals are given orally or via IV infusion but not subcutaneously (SC), IM, IV bolus, or opthalmically. The absorption of nucleoside analog antivirals is unaffected by food. When administering the nucleoside analog antivirals, the nurse should:

- Monitor the IV site carefully during administration and for several days after drug completion. An infusion pump and a microdrip infusion set are preferred to avoid inflammation, phlebitis, extravasation, or sloughing of tissues at the injection site.
- Be certain that the patient is well hydrated for 2 hours after drug infusion to prevent renal damage.
- Monitor the patient's creatinine and BUN levels because these values may elevate after drug infusion.
- Inform the patient that these drugs can only manage the disease; they can neither cure it nor keep it from spreading to others.
- Instruct the patient to avoid sexual intercourse when either partner has evidence of a herpes infection.
- Instruct the patient to report any unexplained redness or pain in the eye. An untreated eye infection can lead to corneal keratitis and blindness.

Do You UNDERSTAND?

DIRECTIONS: **Indicate in the space provided whether the statement is**
true or _false._

_____ 1. Nucleoside analog antivirals are used in the treatment of chickenpox.
_____ 2. Probenecid decreases the action of acyclovir.

TAKE HOME POINTS

Administer an IV dose of nucleoside analog antivirals over 1 hour to prevent renal damage. Be certain that the patient who is taking nucleoside analog antivirals is well hydrated.

TAKE HOME POINTS

Other precautions must be taken to prevent spreading viruses. Teach the patient that after herpes simplex virus is controlled, latent viruses can be activated by exposure to sunlight, fever, stress, menstruation, sexual intercourse, and trauma.

Answers: 1. true; 2. false; probenecid prolongs its action.

Antifungals

Fungal infections may be superficial or systemic. Systemic infections occur mostly in the immunocompromised, such as patients with AIDS or those who are taking corticosteroids or anticancer drugs.

Three main groups of fungi can cause disease in humans:

1. Molds (filamentous fungi) grow as long filaments that intertwine to form a mycelium. Examples of molds are the dermatophytes and *Aspergillus fumigatus*. Dermatophytes (given their name because of their ability to digest keratin) cause infections of the skin, nails, and hair. *Aspergillus fumigatus* may cause pulmonary or disseminated aspergillosis.

2. True yeast is either unicellular round or oval fungus. An example of a type of yeast is *Cryptococcus neoformans*, which may cause cryptococcal meningitis or pulmonary infections, usually in immunocompromised patients.

3. Yeast and fungi are similar to yeasts but may also form nonbranching filaments, which cause a wide range of diseases, including oral thrush, vaginitis, endocarditis, and fatal septicemia.

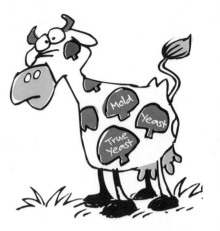

Currently, few effective antifungal drugs exist, and the first-line drug that is used in severe and potentially fatal systemic mycoses is highly toxic. Flucytosine is much less toxic than is amphotericin, but its use is limited because of its narrow spectrum, and resistance can develop rapidly during therapy. Flucytosine is converted in fungal cells into fluorouracil, which inhibits DNA synthesis. Flucytosine fails to undergo this conversion in human cells. The imidazoles, which are widely used topically, are broad-spectrum antifungal drugs that inhibit ergosterol synthesis. The triazoles are newer drugs, structurally similar to the imidazoles, but with a wider range of antifungal activity. These agents have a lower incidence of adverse effects because they are much more specific inhibitors of lanosterol x-demethylase action that results in inhibition of ergosterol synthesis.

What IS a Polyene Antifungal?

Polyene Antifungals	Trade Names	Uses
amphotericin B [am-foe-TER-ih-sin B]	Amphotec	Treatment of systemic fungal infections
nystatin [nye-STAT-in]	Mycostatin	Treatment of Candida infections

Action

Amphotericin B is an amphoteric polyene macrolide antibiotic that exerts its antifungal action primarily by binding to sterols, such as ergosterol, in the fungal cell membrane. The fungal cell membrane is then no longer able to function as a selective barrier. As a result, cell membrane permeability is changed, allowing leakage of intracellular components and causing cell death. The drug is selectively toxic because in human cells, the major sterol is cholesterol rather than ergosterol. The binding to sterols in cells (e.g., kidney cells, erythrocytes) may account for some of the toxicities. Nystatin (another polyene) is too toxic for parenteral use.

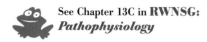

See Chapter 13C in **RWNSG:** *Pathophysiology*

Uses

The first-line antifungal drug is amphotericin B. This agent is used for most pathogenic fungi, including yeasts and protozoa. Amphotericin B is a wide-spectrum antifungal drug that is used to treat potentially fatal systemic infections from *Aspergillus, Candida,* or *Cryptococcus.* Nystatin is used primarily for *Candida albicans* infections of the skin and mucous membranes and has little systemic effect.

What You NEED TO KNOW

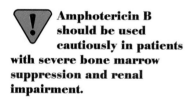

Polyene antifungals are contraindicated for women during pregnancy and lactation.

Contraindications/Precautions

Polyene antifungals are contraindicated for patients with hypersensitivity.

Drug Interactions

Amphotericin B interacts with corticosteroids and digitalis to increase the risk of hypokalemia. Concurrent use of amphotericin B with furosemide, vancomycin, aminoglycosides, capreomycin, carboplatin, and cisplatin increase the risk of nephrotoxicity.

Amphotericin B should be used cautiously in patients with severe bone marrow suppression and renal impairment.

Adverse Effects

The adverse effects of amphotericin B are common; most patients develop fever, chills, anorexia, nausea, vomiting, dyspepsia, and abdominal cramping. Long-term therapy inevitably causes renal damage, which is reversible only when detected early. Additionally, amphotericin B may cause headache, hypotension, weight loss, hypokalemia, malaise, arthralgia, ototoxicity, anemia, and thrombocytopenia. Local irritation, burning, and thrombophlebitis at the IV site may also occur.

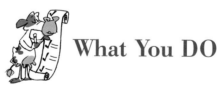

What You DO

Nursing Responsibilities

Amphotericin B is poorly absorbed orally and is given by IV infusion or intrathecally when the CNS is involved. When administering the polyene antifungals, the nurse should:

- Protect amphotericin B IV solutions from light exposure, particularly when given over 8 hours. This drug is usually infused slowly over a minimum of 6 hours.
- Be aware that heparin and saline should not be used to flush the amphotericin B IV line. Long-term therapy with amphotericin B usually requires placement of a central line.

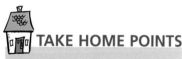

TAKE HOME POINTS

When a test dose of amphotericin B is given (usually 1 mg over 20 to 30 minutes), the vital signs should be monitored every 30 minutes for at least 4 hours.

- Administer nystatin oral suspension by rinsing the mouth or by using a "swish and swallow" technique. The solution should then be kept in the mouth as long as possible (at least 2 minutes).
- Instruct the patient to avoid food or drink for 30 minutes after oral administration of nystatin.
- Instruct the patient to remove dentures before oral administration and at night because infections are more likely to occur in patients who wear dentures 24 hours per day.
- Insert vaginal suppositories and creams high into the vagina.
- Instruct the patient to lie recumbent for 10 to 15 minutes after vaginal insertion.
- Instruct patients to continue suppository-cream therapy during menses.
- Inform the patient that topical or vaginal administration should be discontinued when sensitivity or rash occurs; otherwise, the treatment should be continued for the full course to eradicate the fungus and to prevent reoccurrence.
- Monitor intake and output and the daily weight (checking for weight loss or gain).
- Monitor electrolytes, hepatic and renal function, and hematological studies frequently, and compare with baseline studies for early detection of dysfunction.
- Withhold amphotericin B and report to the health care provider when the BUN exceeds 40 mg/dl or when the serum creatinine is elevated above 3 mg/dl.
- Monitor vital signs frequently during the beginning phase of therapy.
- Instruct the patient to report tinnitus, vertigo, unsteady gait, or hearing loss because ototoxicity is common with amphotericin B administration.

Some prescribing health care providers take prophylactic measures by ordering aspirin or acetaminophen, antiemetics, antihistamines, and corticosteroids 1 hour before amphotericin B infusion to reduce intensity of adverse reactions.

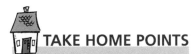

TAKE HOME POINTS

Potassium supplements are usually given concurrently with amphotericin B to prevent hypokalemia.

Febrile reactions of fever, chills, headache, and nausea usually occur in up to 90% of patients who receive amphotericin B and generally begin 1 to 2 hours after initiation of infusion subsiding within 4 hours after the drug is discontinued.

Do You UNDERSTAND?

DIRECTIONS: Provide appropriate responses to the following statement and question.

1. Identify two other drug or drug groups that increase the risk of hypokalemia when given concurrently with amphotericin B.

   _____

   _____

2. Amphotericin B should be administered IV in over a minimum of how many hours?

   _____

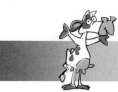

What IS an Azole Antifungal?

Azole Antifungals	Trade Names	Uses
fluconazole [flew-KOE-nuh-zole]	Diflucan	Treatment of candidal infections and cryptococcal meningitis
ketoconazole [KEY-toe-KOE-nuh-zole]	Nizoral	Treatment of systemic and cutaneous fungal infections
clotrimazole [kloe-TRIM-a-zole]	Lotrimin	Treatment of skin, oropharyngeal, and vulvovaginal candidiasis
oxiconazole [ox-I-CON-a-zole]	Oxistat	Treatment of tinea pedis, tinea cruris, and tinea corporis

Action

Azoles are wide-spectrum antifungal drugs to which resistance rarely develops. These agents bind to sterols in the fungal cell membrane, which changes cell membrane permeability. Azoles can be fungistatic or fungicidal, depending on the drug concentration and the organism. Ketoconazole is classified as an imidazole antifungal, while fluconazole is classified as triazole antifungal.

Uses

See Chapter 13C in RWNSG:
Pathophysiology

Fluconazole is used for cryptococcal meningitis, systemic fungal infections, and prophylactically to decrease the incidence of candidiasis in patients with bone marrow transplants. Triazoles have been used successfully in a wide range of superficial and systemic mycoses (not *Aspergillus*). Ketoconazole has been used in the treatment of local and systemic mycoses. Clotrimazole is widely used topically in the treatment of dermatophyte and *Candida albicans* infections. Oxiconazole is used to treat cutaneous candidiasis, tinea pedis, tinea cruris, and tinea corporis. Tinea is a fungal skin infection occurring on various body parts (e.g., pedis affects the foot and is commonly called athlete's foot; cruris affects scrotal, anal, or genital areas and is commonly called jock itch; corporis affects the body and is commonly called ringworm).

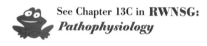 Azole antifungals are contraindicated for women during pregnancy or lactation.

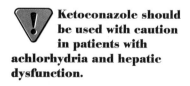 **Ketoconazole should be used with caution in patients with achlorhydria and hepatic dysfunction.**

What You NEED TO KNOW

Contraindications/Precautions

Azole antifungals are contraindicated for patients with hypersensitivity. Ketoconazole is contraindicated for patients with chronic alcoholism and fungal meningitis.

Drug Interactions

When fluconazole is given concurrently with cimetidine and rifampin, fluconazole levels are reduced. An increase in fluconazole level occurs when given concurrently with hydrochlorothiazide. Fluconazole increases the level of cyclosporine, phenytoin, and theophylline when given together. Itraconazole decreases the efficacy of oral contraceptives and increases the effects of alfentanil, zolpidem, vinca alkaloids, tacrolimus, benzodiazepines, corticosteroids, ritonavir, losartan, protease inhibitors, and felodipine.

Antacids, anticholinergics, H$_2$ blockers, didanosine, and sucralfate decrease the absorption and action of ketoconazole. Ketoconazole may increase the effects of protease inhibitors, tricyclic antidepressants, carbamazepine, quinidine, sulfonylureas, benzodiazepines, buspirone, donepezil, nisoldipine, vinca alkaloids, zolpidem, warfarin, corticosteroids, cyclosporine, and tacrolimus. When given together with ketoconazole, oral contraceptive efficacy may be reduced, as well as the effects of theophylline.

Co-administration of itraconazole with pimozide, triazolam, oral midazolam, and quinidine may cause life-threatening dysrhythmias.

Adverse Effects

Most adverse effects of azole antifungals are mild-to-moderate. Common adverse effects include hypersensitivity, headache, dizziness, depression, nausea, vomiting, abdominal pain, and diarrhea. Other adverse effects include photophobia, taste perversion, tinnitus, hypertension, fainting, orthostatic hypotension, insomnia, myalgia, menstrual disorders, impotence, gynecomastia, suicidal tendencies, thrombocytopenia, leukopenia, hemolytic anemia, angioedema, decreased secretion of adrenal corticosteroids, and hepatic dysfunction. Anaphylactic reactions rarely occur.

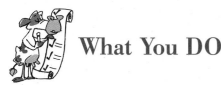

What You DO

Nursing Responsibilities

When fluconazole is given as an IV infusion, the maximal rate is 200 mg/hr. IV admixtures of other drugs are not recommended. When administering azole antifungals, the nurse should:

- Administer itraconazole capsules after a full meal (oral solutions should be taken without food).
- Instruct the patient to report evidence of liver dysfunction (e.g., unusual fatigue, anorexia, nausea, vomiting, dark urine, pale stools, jaundice).
- Apply topical administration sparingly and protect hands with latex gloves when applying the drug. Occlusive dressings should be avoided, unless otherwise directed. Before topical use, cleanse the skin according to the prescribing health care provider's orders. Dry skin thoroughly before applying the drug. Avoid contact with eyes.
- Monitor hepatic function studies, BUN, and serum creatinine periodically for 1 month or when suggestive symptoms occur for early detection of dysfunction.

- Obtain fungal culture specimens before initiating drug therapy.
- Avoid administering ketoconazole concurrently with antacids, anticholinergics, or H$_2$ blockers.
- Allow clotrimazole oral lozenge to dissolve slowly in the mouth over 15 to 30 minutes for maximal effectiveness.
- Be aware that itraconazole capsules and oral solution cannot be used interchangeably.
- Instruct the patient that when a dose is missed, the next dose should not be doubled. Rather, take the missed dose only when the next scheduled dose is more than 4 hours away.

Do You UNDERSTAND?

DIRECTIONS: **Indicate in the space provided whether the statement is** *true* **or** *false.*

_____ 1. Azoles that are absorbed systemically require monitoring of hepatic function studies.

_____ 2. Topical skin application of clotrimazole and miconazole should be applied sparingly.

SECTION C
BIOLOGIC RESPONSE MODIFIERS

Biologic response modifiers augment and use the body's immune system to counteract the side effects of various treatments, particularly cancer chemotherapy. The selected pharmacologic agents that are discussed in this section include immunosuppressants and immunomodulators, such as interferons, interleukins, colony-stimulating factors, and monoclonal antibodies.

What IS an Immunosuppressant?

Immunosuppressants	Trade Names	Uses
azathioprine [AZE-uh-THIGH-oh-preen]	Imuran	Prevents rejection of kidney transplantation
cyclosporine [SIGH-kloe-spore-EEN]	Sandimmune	Prolongs survival of transplants involving skin, heart, kidneys, pancreas, bone marrow, small intestine, liver, and lungs
muromonab-CD3 [MYOO-row-MOE-nab-CD3]	Orthoclone OKT3	Treats rejection of heart, renal, and liver transplantation

Answers: 1. true; 2. true.

Action

An immunosuppressant acts to suppress the body's natural immune response to an antigen. Azathioprine, cyclosporine, and tacrolimus inhibit T-helper cells and T-suppressor cells, thereby suppressing humoral immunity and cell-mediated immune reactions (e.g., delayed hypersensitivity, T-cell effects, allograft rejection, collagen-induced arthritis). Azathioprine also alters antibody production.

Uses

Immunosuppressants are given primarily to prevent rejection of transplanted organs. Muromonab-CD3 treats rejection of heart, renal, and liver transplantation that is resistant to standard steroid therapy.

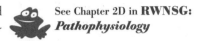 See Chapter 2D in **RWNSG:** *Pathophysiology*

 # What You NEED TO KNOW

Contraindications/Precautions

Immunosuppressants are contraindicated for patients with hypersensitivity.

Cyclosporine is contraindicated for patients with renal dysfunction, uncontrolled hypertension or malignancies, and psoriasis. Muromonab-CD3 is contraindicated for patients with infection, chickenpox, herpes zoster, and a 3% weight gain before treatment.

Drug Interactions

Azathioprine decreases the action of anticoagulants, decreases cyclosporine levels, reverses neuromuscular blockers, induces severe leukopenia when given with angiotensin converting enzyme (ACE) inhibitors, increases action and toxic effects of allopurinol, and increases 6-MP metabolite levels when given together.

When cyclosporine is given with other nephrotoxic drugs (e.g., antiinflammatories, antibiotics, antifungals, GI agents), the risk of renal dysfunction is increased. When given with lovastatin, increased digoxin levels, severe myopathy, or rhabdomyolysis may occur. Androgens, amiodarone, azole antifungals, calcium channel blockers, macrolide antibiotics, metoclopramide, and oral contraceptives increase cyclosporine levels. Anticonvulsants may decrease cyclosporine levels. Colchicine and corticosteroids increase the adverse effects and toxicities of cyclosporine.

Adverse Effects

Immunosuppressants commonly cause nausea, vomiting, diarrhea, rash, fever, and malaise. Azathioprine may also cause joint and muscle pain, hypotension, temporary infertility, and fetal damage. This drug may lead to dose-related severe leukopenia, thrombocytopenia, macrocytic anemia, and severe bone marrow depression. Additional adverse effects of cyclosporines include photosensitivity, anxiety, confusion, depression, increased LDLs, diabetes mellitus, nephrotoxicity, hepatotoxicity, CNS toxicity, convulsions, tremors, hirsutism, hypertension, gum hyperplasia, chest pain, MI, and malignancies.

 TAKE HOME POINTS

T and B cells are the two major types of lymphocytes, forming approximately 20% of white blood cells. Several different types of T cells exist, including T-helper cells and T-suppressor cells. T-helper cells carry out different immune functions, such as assisting in the reproduction of memory cells that provide long-lasting immunity against specific antigens. T-suppressor cells have immunosuppressive and regulatory functions. B cells produce antibodies against an antigen and have antibody-type receptors on their cell surface, which assists in immunity.

Most immunosuppressants are contraindicated for children and for women during pregnancy and lactation.

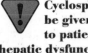 **Cyclosporine should be given with caution to patients with hepatic dysfunction, diabetes mellitus, elevated low-density lipoproteins (LDLs), and cancer.**

Adverse effects of muromonab-CD3 include tachycardia, wheezing, dyspnea, chest pain, pulmonary edema, and increased susceptibility to *Pneumocystosis carinii*, cytomegalovirus, and *Serratia*.

What You DO

Nursing Responsibilities

Azathioprine is usually administered with food or in divided doses to decrease gastric distress. This medication is usually initiated 1 to 3 days before and repeated within 24 hours after transplantation. When giving immunosuppressants, the nurse should:

- Monitor the patient's CBC weekly during the first month of therapy, every 2 weeks during the second and third months, and monthly thereafter.
- Monitor periodic renal and hepatic function tests and electrolytes.
- Teach the patient who is taking azathioprine to report any abnormal bleeding or signs of infection immediately.
- Instruct patients to avoid contact with people who have known infections, thereby protecting themselves and preventing infections.
- Be aware that cyclosporine is given as a single dose, initially 4 to 12 hours before transplantation. Cyclosporine may be given IV when the patient is unable to tolerate the drug orally.
- Mix oral solutions of cyclosporine with milk, chocolate milk, or orange or apple juice in a glass container (never plastic) at room temperature. Grapefruit juice should be avoided because it affects the metabolism of cyclosporine.
- Instruct patient to thoroughly stir oral cyclosporine solutions, take immediately, and follow with more diluent in the same glass to ensure that the entire dose is consumed.
- Instruct patient to take cyclosporine on a consistent schedule every day.
- Carefully monitor the patient who is receiving IV cyclosporine for at least 30 minutes after initiating drug administration and frequently thereafter for hypersensitivity and other adverse effects.
- Monitor the patient who is receiving IV cyclosporine for infection, nephrotoxicity, and neurotoxicity.
- Monitor renal and liver function tests and potassium before therapy as a baseline and periodically thereafter for comparison and early detection of toxicity.
- Instruct the patient who is taking cyclosporine to wear sunscreen and protective clothing thus limiting exposure to sunlight.
- Instruct patients who are taking cyclosporine to practice thorough oral hygiene and to inspect the mouth daily for swollen gums, sores, and white patches.
- Inform patients who are taking cyclosporine that hirsutism is reversible after drug therapy is discontinued.
- Warn women to use effective contraception before immunosuppressant therapy, during therapy, and up to 6 weeks after this drug has been discontinued.

TAKE HOME POINTS

Azathioprine should be discontinued or the dose reduced at the first indication of abnormally large or continued decrease in leukocytes or platelets to avoid irreversible bone marrow depression.

TAKE HOME POINTS

Instruct patient who is taking azathioprine to report fever, sore throat, unusual bruising, bleeding, pale stools, or darkened urine immediately.

 Instruct patients who are taking immunosuppressants to report evidence of infection, hematuria, and peripheral edema.

- Be aware that cyclosporine must be discontinued at least 24 hours before initiating tacrolimus.
- Be aware that muromonab-CD3 is given by IV bolus. IV methylprednisolone sodium succinate should be given before muromonab-CD3 administration and IV hydrocortisone sodium succinate should be given 30 minutes after drug administration to reduce the occurrence of a first-dose reaction.
- Assess the patient for fever. If the patient has a fever of 37.8° C (100° F) or pulmonary edema or both, then the health care provider should be consulted before muromonab-CD3 treatment to prevent acute pulmonary edema and possible death.

First-dose reaction usually occurs 45 to 60 minutes after the first and second doses. Monitor the patient who is taking muromonab-CD3 for early signs of acute pulmonary edema and have resuscitation equipment available (e.g., intubation, oxygen, corticosteroids).

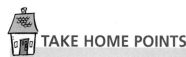

TAKE HOME POINTS

Monitor the patient who is taking muromonab-CD3 for 48 hours after first dose for early signs of first-dose reaction (e.g., high fever, chills, malaise, dyspnea).

Do You UNDERSTAND?

DIRECTIONS: Indicate in the space provided whether the statement is
true or false.

_____ 1. Immunosuppressants are given primarily to prevent rejection of transplanted organs.

_____ 2. Immunosuppressants are contraindicated for women during pregnancy.

_____ 3. Immunosuppressants predispose patients to infection.

Immunomodulators

Immunomodulators have the ability to change immune responses. The selected immunomodulators that are discussed in this section include interferons, interleukins, and colony-stimulating factors.

What IS an Interferon?

Interferons	Trade Names	Uses
interferon α-2a [IN-ter-FEAR-ahn]	Roferon-A	Treatment of hairy cell and chronic myelogenous leukemia, and Kaposi's sarcoma
interferon α-2b [IN-ter-FEAR-ahn]	Intron A	Treatment of hairy cell leukemia, malignant melanoma, condylomata acuminata, Kaposi's sarcoma, and chronic hepatitis B and C

Action

An interferon acts on the body by exerting antitumor activity. The mechanism is not clearly understood. The belief is that interferons modulate the host's immune response and prevent tumor cells from reproducing.

Uses

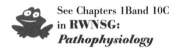

See Chapters 1Band 10C in **RWNSG:** *Pathophysiology*

Interferon α-2a is indicated in the treatment of hairy cell leukemia, AIDS-related Kaposi's sarcoma, and chronic myelogenous leukemia. Interferon α-2b is used in the treatment of hairy cell leukemia, malignant melanoma, condylomata acuminata (genital and perianal warts), AIDS-related Kaposi's sarcoma, and chronic hepatitis B and C.

What You NEED TO KNOW

Contraindications/Precautions

Interferon α-2a is contraindicated for patients with a known hypersensitivity.

Interferon α-2a should be given with caution to patients with cardiac disease, severe renal or hepatic impairment, seizure disorders, myelosuppression, and compromised CNS function.

Interferon α-2b is contraindicated for any patient with a hypersensitivity, thyroid abnormality, or preexisting psychiatric condition or history of a severe psychiatric disorder. Caution should be used when giving interferon α-2b to patients with thrombocytopenia, influenza symptoms, pneumonia, cardiovascular disease, retinal damage, hepatic impairment, autoimmune diseases, hyperglycemia, and infertility.

Drug Interactions

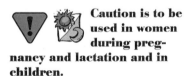

Caution is to be used in women during pregnancy and lactation and in children.

The effects of theophylline and aminophylline are exacerbated when interferon α-2a and interferon α-2b are given concurrently. When interferon α-2a is given concurrently with interleukin-2, a potential risk for renal failure exists. When interferon α-2b is given with zidovudine, the patient may have an increased risk of neutropenia.

Adverse Effects

Serious adverse effects include suicidal ideation, GI hemorrhage, life-threatening anemia, renal or hepatic impairment, and cardiac dysrhythmias.

Adverse effects of interferon α-2a and interferon α-2b include fever, fatigue, headache, chills, weight loss, photosensitivity, dizziness, rash, diaphoresis, anxiety, lethargy, alopecia, and itching. Other adverse effects include depression, paresthesia, sleep disturbance, decreased mental status, anorexia, nausea, vomiting, diarrhea, bone and joint pain, coughing, and dyspnea. Adverse effects may be severe to the extent that these drugs must be discontinued.

What You DO

Nursing Responsibilities

Interferon α-2a is given SC or IM. After the initial dose, maintenance doses are usually given three times weekly. Interferon α-2b is given IV, SC or IM but should not be given IM to patients with thrombocytopenia and platelet counts less than 60,000/mm. This population may receive interferon α-2b SC as a substitute. When administering interferons, the nurse should:

- Monitor frequent CBCs, platelet counts, blood chemistries, electrolytes, thyroid-stimulating hormone (TSH) levels, liver function tests, chest x-ray studies, and electrocardiogram (ECG) data in patients who are receiving interferon.
- Instruct the patient who is taking interferon to report any hives, itching, cough, difficulty breathing, wheezing, tightness in the chest, dizziness, or suspected pregnancy to the health care provider.
- Recommend contraceptive measures during interferon therapy.
- Warn patients who are taking interferon α-2a to avoid changing brands of interferon because changes in the dose may result.
- Advise patients who are taking interferon α-2a to maintain adequate hydration.
- Instruct the patient that photosensitivity may occur and to take precautions in sunlight.
- Instruct the patient to use caution when driving or operating hazardous machines that require alertness and coordination because interferon may cause drowsiness or dizziness.

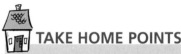

TAKE HOME POINTS

Instruct the patient who is taking interferon to use sunscreens and protective clothing and to decrease ultraviolet exposure until tolerance is determined.

Do You UNDERSTAND?

DIRECTIONS: Indicate in the space provided whether the statement is *true* or *false*.

_____ 1. Patients who are taking interferon should take precautions regarding ultraviolet light exposure.

_____ 2. Patients should not receive interferon when the platelet count is less than 100,000/mm.

What IS an Interleukin?

Interleukins	Trade Names	Uses
Interleukin-11 [IN-ter-LU-kin]	Oprelvekin	Prevent severe thrombocytopenia in myelosuppression
Interleukin-2 or proleukin [IN-ter-LU-kin]	Aldesleukin	Treatment of metastatic melanoma or renal cell carcinoma

Action

Oprelvekin is a thrombopoietic growth factor that stimulates platelet production. Aldesleukin is a recombinant protein that enhances lymphocyte mitogenesis, stimulates long-term growth of human interleukin-2–dependent cell lines, enhances lymphocyte cytotoxicity, and induces interferon-gamma production. Interleukins activate cellular immunity with profound lymphocytosis, eosinophilia and thrombocytopenia, the production of cytokines (including tumor necrosis factor, interleukin-1, and gamma interferon), and inhibit tumor growth.

Uses

See Chapter 3A in **RWNSG:** *Pathophysiology*

Oprelvekin is indicated in the prevention of severe thrombocytopenia; it can also be used to reduce the need for platelet transfusions following myelosuppressive chemotherapy. Interleukin-11 and interleukin-2 are used in the treatment of metastatic renal-cell carcinoma.

What You NEED TO KNOW

 Interleukin-1 should be given with caution to patients with autoimmune diseases because the conditions may be exacerbated.

Contraindications/Precautions

Interleukins are contraindicated for patients with hypersensitivity, abnormal thallium stress test, pulmonary function tests, uncontrolled dysrhythmias, pericardial tamponade, angina, or MI.

Drug Interactions

Interleukin-1 may cause leakage of plasma proteins and fluid into the extravascular space and loss of vascular tone leading to hypovolemia, significant hypotension, tachycardia, and hypoprofusion. This agent may also cause mental changes, renal and hepatic toxicity, infertility, allograft rejection in transplant patients, and thyroid impairment. When interleukin-2 is given with other nephrotoxic or hepatoxic drugs, the risk of toxicity in increased. Antihypertensives increase the hypotension caused by interleukin-2.

 Interleukin-11 should be used with caution in patients with congestive heart failure, and papilledema, as well as women during pregnancy and lactation and in children. Interleukin-2 should not be given to children under 18 years of age.

Adverse Effects

Most adverse effects following interleukin-11 administration are mild or moderate in severity and reversible after the drug is discontinued. These adverse effects include blurred vision, chills, nervousness, alopecia, asthenia, anorexia, dyspepsia, constipation, abdominal pain, ecchymosis, muscle and bone pain, and infection. Other adverse effects include nausea, vomiting, dyspnea, cough rhinitis, edema, headache, rash, eye hemorrhage, amblyopia, paresthesia, skin discoloration, and exfoliative dermatitis.

Interleukin-2 may cause many cardiovascular adverse effects, including dysrhythmias, MI, congestive heart failure (CHF), cardiac arrest, stroke, pericardial effusion, and thrombosis. Interleukin-2 may also cause pulmonary congestion, wheezing, apnea, pneumothorax, respiratory failure, GI bleeding, intestinal perforation, coma, seizures, coagulation disorders, thrombocytopenia, and electrolyte disturbances.

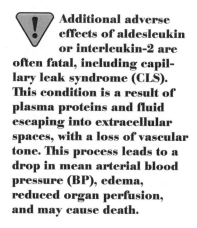 **Additional adverse effects of aldesleukin or interleukin-2 are often fatal, including capillary leak syndrome (CLS). This condition is a result of plasma proteins and fluid escaping into extracellular spaces, with a loss of vascular tone. This process leads to a drop in mean arterial blood pressure (BP), edema, reduced organ perfusion, and may cause death.**

 # What You DO

Nursing Responsibilities

Interleukin-11 is administered by an IV infusion over 15 minutes every 8 hours and is administered SC as a single dose in the abdomen, thigh, hip, or upper arm. Drug administration may begin at least 6 hours after the completion of chemotherapy. When giving interleukins, the nurse should:

- Monitor platelet counts periodically to assure effectiveness of therapy. Interleukin therapy should continue until the platelet count postnadir is greater than 50,000 cells/µl. A treatment course of more than 21 days is not recommended.
- 🍎 Teach the patient who is self-administering interleukin at home about proper reconstitution and administration techniques, proper caution, and disposal of materials.

Reconstituted solution may be stored at 36° to 46° F until used, but do not freeze. The reconstituted interleukin solution should be used with 3 hours. Do not use when the solution is discolored or contains particles.

 TAKE HOME POINTS

When reconstituting solution, gently swirl vial, but do not shake the solution.

 # Do You UNDERSTAND?

DIRECTIONS: Fill in the blanks to complete the following statements.

1. Interleukin-11 is given to stimulate _____ cell production.
2. Interleukin-11 therapy is usually initiated at least _____ hours after chemotherapy is completed.

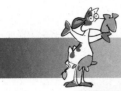

What IS a Colony-Stimulating Factor?

Colony-Stimulating Factor	Trade Names	Uses
erythropoietin [e-RITH-roe-po-E-tin]	Epogen	Treatment of low hematocrit levels in anemia
filgrastim [fil-GRASS-tim]	Neupogen	Treatment of neutropenia
sargramostim [sar-GRA-mos-tim]	Leukine	Restore red bone marrow after transplantation

Action

Erythropoietin is a serum protein that promotes monocyte differentiation. A colony-stimulating factor called erythropoietin is a glycoprotein (a compound of carbohydrate and protein) that stimulates red blood cell production. Normally, erythropoietin is produced primarily in the kidneys in response to hypoxia;

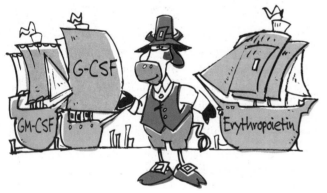

however, in chronic renal failure (CRF), erythropoietin production is impaired. The impaired erythropoietin production is the main cause of anemia in CRF. Erythropoietin stimulates erythropoiesis and is indicated in patients with anemia. After administration, the reticulocyte count is usually increased within 10 days. The red cell count, hemoglobin, and hematocrit are usually increased within 2 to 6 weeks. Filgrastim (G-CSF) is a glycoprotein that regulates the production of neutrophils. Sargramostim (GM-CSF) is a hematopoietic growth factor that stimulates neutrophils, monocytes, and macrophages.

Uses

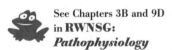

See Chapters 3B and 9D in RWNSG: *Pathophysiology*

Erythropoietin is indicated in patients with anemia and zidovudine-treated HIV-infected patients with cancer who are taking chemotherapy, as well as those on postsurgical status. Erythropoietin is also used in patients with CRF, whether they require dialysis or not. This agent decreases the number of transfusions that are usually required in patients with CRF, as well as improves cardiovascular status, cognitive function, exercise tolerance, and quality of life. G-CSF is used to promote a regeneration of neutrophils, thereby decreasing the incidence of infection in patients who are receiving myelosuppressive anticancer drugs. GM-CSF is effective in the treatment of bone marrow deficiency from cancer chemotherapy or bone marrow transplantation. Sargramostim is used to restore red bone marrow following bone marrow transplantation.

What You NEED TO KNOW

Contraindications/Precautions

Erythropoietin is contraindicated for patients with uncontrolled hypertension and known hypersensitivity. GM-CSF is contraindicated for patients with excessive leukemic myeloid blasts in the bone marrow.

Drug Interactions

When corticosteroids and lithium are given with GM-CSF, myeloproliferative effects may be increased. Myeloproliferative effects are a rapid reproduction of bone marrow elements. When erythropoietin is given concurrently with heparin, anticoagulation effects may decrease.

Adverse Effects

Elevated BP is an adverse effect of erythropoietin, which may require antihypertensive medication. Seizures and hypertensive encephalopathy have occurred in patients who are taking erythropoietin and those with CRF. Other adverse effects of erythropoietin include headache, dizziness, anxiety, fatigue, sweating, hypertension, insomnia, fever, nausea, vomiting, diarrhea, constipation, joint pain, clotting of arteriovenous (AV) fistula, and seizures.

Adverse effects from G-CSF include bone pain, transient decrease in BP, nausea, vomiting, diarrhea, and fatigue. First-dose syndrome from G-CSF is an adverse effect that includes respiratory distress, hypoxia, flushing, syncope, tachycardia, hypotension, neutrophils above 20,000/mm or a platelet count greater than 500,000/mm. Other adverse effects include peripheral edema, stomatitis, nausea, vomiting, diarrhea, abdominal pain, GI hemorrhage, blood dyscrasia, hyperglycemia, fever, chills, malaise, weight loss, asthenia, muscle and bone pain, and hypertension.

Cardiovascular adverse effects from GM-CSF include hypertension, hypotension, edema, tachycardia, and MI. Other adverse effects include dyspnea, paresthesia, insomnia, anxiety, fever, rash, itching, alopecia, anorexia, nausea, vomiting, diarrhea, abdominal pain, stomatitis, GI bleeding, bilirubinemia, blood dyscrasias, and hyperglycemia.

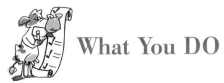

What You DO

Nursing Responsibilities

Erythropoietin can be given SC or IV three times a week. Dose adjustment should not be made more than once a month. When administering colony-stimulating factors, the nurse should:

- Monitor the BP before erythropoietin therapy. Hypertension may occur as an adverse effect, particularly when the hematocrit is rising quickly.

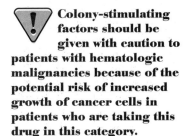

Colony-stimulating factors should be given with caution to patients with hematologic malignancies because of the potential risk of increased growth of cancer cells in patients who are taking this drug in this category.

Caution should be taken when administering erythropoietin to children and women who are pregnant or lactating. G-CSF should be given with caution to patients with hypothyroidism, pregnant or lactating women, and children. This agent should be given with caution to patients with cardiovascular or respiratory disease, renal or hepatic impairment, and those with fluid retention.

Because lithium may cause the release of neutrophils, G-CSF should be given with caution to patients who require both drugs. Because lithium and corticosteroids may cause myeloproliferative effects, caution should be used with GM-CSF.

 TAKE HOME POINTS

Do not shake the solution because this may denature the glycoprotein, making it biologically inactive. Erythropoietin doses should be decreased if the hematocrit elevates more than four points in a 2-week period. The BP should be closely monitored and controlled in patients who are receiving erythropoietin.

TAKE HOME POINTS

When necessary, G-CSF may be diluted in 5% dextrose solution but never in saline because the medication may precipitate.

TAKE HOME POINTS

- Monitor the hematocrit twice weekly after beginning erythropoietin therapy (until the dose is stabilized) and throughout therapy; the risk for seizures is greater when the hematocrit increases rapidly.
- Premature discontinuation of G-CSF is not recommended before recovery from the expected neutrophil nadir.

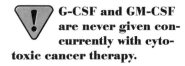

G-CSF and GM-CSF are never given concurrently with cytotoxic cancer therapy.

- Discard any unused portion of the vial, because erythropoietin contains no preservatives.
- Monitor the hematocrit, fluid and electrolyte balance, and renal function. After reaching target hematocrit or when the hematocrit rises more than four points in a 2-week period, notify the health care provider for dose reduction. When the hematocrit fails to rise five to six points or is still below target range after 8 weeks of therapy, notify the health care provider for dose increase.
- Be aware that patients who are taking erythropoietin and those undergoing hemodialysis treatment may require heparin anticoagulation to prevent arteriovenous shunt clotting.
- Instruct patients to avoid driving or engaging in hazardous activity when the possibility of seizures is present.
- Be aware that G-CSF should not be given within 24 hours of cytotoxic chemotherapy. G-CSF is usually given daily for 2 weeks until the neutrophil count reaches 10,000/mm.
- Monitor a baseline CBC and platelet count drawn before G-CSF therapy. Following initiation of therapy, these tests should be monitored two times a week during therapy. G-CSF should be discontinued after neutrophil counts remain at normal levels for at least 3 days.
- Administer GM-CSF over a 2-hour IV infusion for a 21-day treatment at least 24 hours after the last chemotherapy dose and 12 hours after the last radiation dose.
- Monitor the CBC with differential two times a week during therapy. When the neutrophils increase 20,000/mm or the platelet count is greater than 500,000/mm, GM-CSF therapy should be interrupted or the dose reduced by one half.

Do You UNDERSTAND?

DIRECTIONS: Fill in the blanks with the appropriate responses.

1. The first-dose syndrome of GM-CSF involves symptoms that include

   _____
   _____
   _____
   _____
   _____

2. GM-CSF should be discontinued or the dose reduced by one half when the neutrophil reaches _____
   or the platelet count is _____.

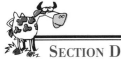

SECTION D
ANTINEOPLASTIC AGENTS

Antineoplastic agents are used to treat a wide variety of diseases and disorders, including many different types of cancers and autoimmune disorders. Cytotoxic agents tend to interfere with growth and replication of rapidly dividing cells. Normal tissue that is characterized by rapid growth and replication includes the hair follicles, the bone marrow, and the lining of the GI tract that extends from the mouth to the anus. Cancer therapy affects these parts of the body in varying degrees. Nearly all chemotherapeutic agents have potential organ-specific toxicities that the nurse should identify before administration thus appropriate evaluation and monitoring may be implemented before, during, and after the drugs are given. Because of the high toxicity profile, the dosing schedule of these drugs is calculated according to the patient's body surface area, which is calculated based on height and weight.

Currently, chemotherapy drugs are not tumor specific; therefore, they can exert damaging effects on normal healthy cells in addition to cancer cells. Antineoplastic drugs are prescribed with one of three goals in mind: to cure, control, or obtain palliation of malignant disease.

Chemotherapy agents are classified according to their mechanism of action, the point at which they act within the cell's life cycle, and their chemical structure. To maximize therapeutic outcomes, combination regimens consist of two or more drugs. Most cancer treatment protocols use drugs that act at different points within the cell cycle, maximizing tumor cell kill and decreasing the severity of adverse effects. The term cell cycle refers to the reproductive process that occurs in both normal and malignant cells. The cell cycle or replication of body cells is a predetermined sequence of events that occurs in the interval between the origination of the cell and its division into two new cells.

The cell cycle involves several phases:

1. G_0 is the resting phase during which the cell performs all functions except replication.
2. G_1 is the first active phase during which RNA and enzymes that are required for the creation of DNA are developed.
3. S is the phase during which DNA is synthesized for chromosomes.
4. G_2 is the phase during which RNA is synthesized and the mitotic spindle is formed.
5. M is the last phase during which mitosis occurs, allowing the cell to split into two cells.

A broad range of potentially dangerous complications and safety issues exists that are associated with antineoplastic therapy treatment. Only a registered nurse with special educational preparation may assume responsibility for preparing and administering antineoplastic drugs.

Because antineoplastic agents are also classified as biohazardous substances, special precautions must be taken when preparing, handling, and administering

> **The nurse must use extreme caution when administering chemotherapy drugs, many of which have potentially serious, even lethal, adverse effects and toxicities.**

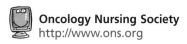

Oncology Nursing Society
http://www.ons.org

these drugs. In the event of an accidental spill, special cleaning procedures must be observed. These safety procedures are beyond the scope of this book but are available on-line.

Because these drugs are potentially lethal, the nurse must always ensure that the patient has given informed consent before therapy can begin.

What IS an Antimetabolite Agent?

Antimetabolite Agents	Trade Names	Uses
cytarabine [sye-TARE-a-been]	ARA-C	Treatment of leukemias
5-fluorouracil [flure-oh-YOUR-a-sil]	5FU	Treatment of carcinoma
floxuridine [flox-YOUR-i-deen]	FUDR	Treatment of carcinoma
methotrexate [meth-oh-TREX-ate]	MTX	Treatment of leukemia, lymphoma, and neoplasms .
capecitabine [cap-e-SI-ta-been]	Xeloda	Treatment of breast cancer

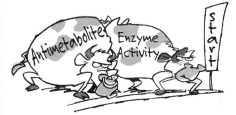

Action

Antimetabolites are similar in structure to normal metabolites. These agents compete for enzyme activity within the cell and prevent the synthesis of DNA. Cellular division is stopped, which results in cell death. These drugs act within the S phase of the cell's life cycle.

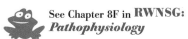

See Chapter 8F in RWNSG:
Pathophysiology

Uses

Because of the limited time in the cell's life cycle during which these drugs are effective, antimetabolites are typically prescribed for rapidly growing tumors, such as leukemias and lymphomas. Antimetabolites are useful in the treatment of many different types of tumors, including acute and chronic leukemias and some solid tumors.

What You NEED TO KNOW

Contraindications/Precautions

5-Fluorouracil is contraindicated for women during pregnancy and lactation. Floxuridine is contraindicated during pregnancy.

Antimetabolite agents are contraindicated for patients with hypersensitivity. Floxuridine is contraindicated for patients with a current or recent viral infection. 5-Fluorouracil is contraindicated for patients with malnutrition and myelosuppression.

Drug Interactions

Patients who use over-the-counter medications, herbal and vitamin preparations, and other alternative therapies may encounter drug interactions when taking antimetabolite therapy (e.g., folic acid decreases the effect of methotrexate). When cytarabine is given together with digoxin, decreased serum levels of digoxin may occur. Serum levels of fluorouracil are increased, which then leads to fluorouracil toxicity when fluorouracil is given with cimetidine or α-interferon. Increased methotrexate toxicity may occur when methotrexate is given with aspirin, NSAIDS, or sulfonamides. When thioguanine is given concurrently with myelosuppressants, an increased risk of toxicity, bleeding, and liver damage may occur.

Adverse Effects

Antimetabolite drugs tend to exert their main toxicities in the bone marrow, the lining of the GI tract, and hair follicles. High doses of these drugs may also cause renal and neurologic damage.

Similar to most chemotherapy agents, these drugs tend to reach their lowest point (**nadir**) 10 to 14 days after administration. When renal and hepatic functions are normal, the body gradually resumes normal function approximately 21 days after these drugs are last administered.

Cellular debris is thought to cause increased inflammation and hypermotility of the GI tract, which causes abdominal pain, cramping, and diarrhea. Mucosal surfaces of the GI tract tend to develop ulcers because the body is unable to replace cells that are worn away by the normal processes of eating and digestion. When the patient has visible mouth ulcers, the intestines are likely to be similarly affected.

Temporary suppression of bone marrow function may occur. The degree and duration of suppression is a function of the dose and the patient's overall health status. White blood cells are most likely to show a decrease in number, placing the patient at risk for a variety of infections. A decrease in white blood cells leaves the patient unable to mount a normal immunologic or inflammatory response to tissue injury or infection.

Patients may experience delayed wound healing, tissue repair, and life-threatening infections. Early signs and symptoms of infection in these patients include mild-to-moderate fever, chills, malaise, weakness, fatigue, and inadequate oxygenation. In patients with neutropenia, these symptoms may be subtle and easily overlooked.

> ⚠ **5-Fluorouracil should be used cautiously in patients who have had major surgery within 1 month. Floxuridine should be used with caution in patients who are malnourished or have bone marrow depression. Capecitabine should be used with caution in patients with infections. Caution should also be used for antimetabolite drugs in patients with renal or hepatic dysfunction.**

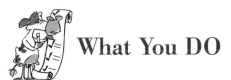

What You DO

Nursing Responsibilities

When administering antimetabolites, the nurse should:
- Provide the patient with written and verbal explanation about possible toxic effects, precautions, and measures to manage and minimize adverse effects.

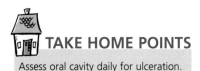

TAKE HOME POINTS

Assess oral cavity daily for ulceration.

- Confirm that the patient has given informed consent before therapy begins.
- Evaluate CBC, BUN, creatinine clearance, and liver function studies before initiating therapy. The patient with preexisting organ damage or bone marrow suppression may not be a candidate for this category of drugs or may require a dose reduction.
- Establish reliable IV access before therapy begins.
- Monitor all chemotherapy infusions carefully for patency of the IV site because these drugs may cause pain and tissue damage during infiltration.
- Assess patients who have already received treatment for evidence of chemotherapy-related mouth ulcers (**stomatitis**), GI distress (particularly vomiting and diarrhea), and symptoms of infection.
- Evaluate patients carefully for evidence of infection.
- Before discharge, teach the patient the proper way to avoid potential sources of infection. Reinforce the need for ongoing medical follow-up visits.
- Assess the patient for GI distress and changes in bowel habits.
- Monitor intake and output of patients with diarrhea because they may require fluid replacement and treatment with antidiarrheal agents.
- 🍎 Teach patients about the importance of maintaining good oral care and of avoiding potential sources of infection.
- Adjust the patient's diet as necessary to maximize oral intake. Small portions of soft, bland, room-temperature food are generally tolerated.

Do You UNDERSTAND?

DIRECTIONS: **Indicate in the space provided whether the statement is** *true* **or** *false***.**

_____ 1. Antimetabolites compete for enzymatic activity within the cell and prevent DNA synthesis.

_____ 2. Antimetabolites particularly cause toxicity of the cardiovascular system.

What IS a Mitotic Inhibitor?

Mitotic Inhibitors	Trade Names	Uses
vincristine [vin-KRIS-teen]	Oncovin	Treatment of carcinoma, Hodgkin's disease, acute lymphoblastic leukemia, and Wilms' tumor
paclitaxel [pac-li-TAX-el]	Taxol	Treatment of breast cancer or ovarian cancer
topotecan [toe-po-TEE-can]	Hycamtin	Treatment of metastatic ovarian, lung, and colorectal cancers
etoposide [e-toe-PO-side]	Toposar	Treatment of testicular and small cell lung carcinoma

Answers: 1. true; 2. false; antimetabolites cause renal, neurologic, GI, and bone marrow damage.

Action

Mitotic inhibitors are all plant derivatives that are grouped into four classes: vinca alkaloids, taxines, camptothecins, and podophyllotoxins. Most of the drugs in this category are cell-cycle specific and act either within the G or S phase of cellular reproduction.

The vinca alkaloids (e.g., vincristine, vinblastine, vinorelbine, vindesine) are cell-cycle specific that inhibit the formation of the mitotic spindle and the replication of DNA and RNA, thereby stopping cell mitosis. Taxines (e.g., docetaxel, paclitaxel) inhibit the division of tumor cells in the M and G phases of the cell cycle. Camptothecins (**Topoisomerase I inhibitors**), such as irinotecan and topotecan, produce irreparable breaks in the cell's DNA, thereby causing cell death. These agents inhibit the enzyme that is needed for DNA replication. Podophyllotoxins (**Topoisomerase II inhibitors**), such as etoposide and teniposide, act in the G_2 phase of the cell cycle to prevent mitosis, thereby stopping cellular replication.

Uses

Mitotic inhibitors are used to treat tumors of various body parts, such as the lung, breast, testes, and ovaries. Vincristine is used to treat Hodgkin's disease, acute lymphoblastic leukemia, oat cell carcinoma of the lung, and Wilms' tumor. Paclitaxel is used for the treatment of advanced breast and ovarian cancers. Topotecan is used for lung, ovarian, and colorectal cancer. Etoposide is used for small cell lung and testicular cancer.

See Chapter 6D in **RWNSG:** *Pathophysiology*

 # What You **NEED TO KNOW**

Mitotic inhibitors are contraindicated for women during pregnancy and lactation and for children.

Contraindications/Precautions

Mitotic inhibitors are contraindicated for patients with hypersensitivity. Paclitaxel is also contraindicated for patients with a neutropenia count of less than 1500 cells/mm^3. Topotecan is further contraindicated for patients with acute infection. Etoposide is contraindicated for patients with severe bone marrow depression, current or recent infection, and severe renal and hepatic dysfunction.

Drug Interactions

Vinca alkaloids may cause severe bone marrow suppression. Vinblastine reaches a nadir 4 to 10 days after administration. When vinblastine is given concurrently with mitomycin, bronchospasms may occur. When paclitaxel and ketoconazole are given together, serious toxicities may occur.

Topoisomerase I inhibitors and vincristine are all capable of causing severe peripheral neuropathy and autonomic neuropathy, which may be permanent if dose reductions are not implemented when the symptoms first appear. When irinotecan is taken with laxatives, severe, prolonged diarrhea may occur, leading to volume depletion and electrolyte imbalances. When irinotecan is taken with

Vincristine should be used cautiously in patients with infection, leukopenia, bone marrow suppression, chickenpox, current neurologic or neuromuscular disorders, and hepatic dysfunction. Paclitaxel should be used with caution in patients with cardiac dysrhythmias. Topotecan should be used cautiously in patients with a history of bleeding disorders, previous radiation therapy, and myelosuppression. Etoposide should be used with caution in patients with gout.

Decadron, an increased risk of hyperglycemia and decreased lymphocyte count occur. When prochlorperazine is taken within 24 hours of irinotecan, an increased risk of akathisia may occur. Topoisomerase II inhibitors may cause dose-limiting bone marrow suppression and stomatitis. Topotecan may cause stomatitis, nausea, vomiting, and headache. Myelosuppression is the major dose-limiting toxicity for the taxines.

Adverse Effects

Mitotic inhibitors are all plant derivatives, thus they have a relatively high incidence of allergic reactions. All of the vinca alkaloids are vesicants, which means that these drugs are capable of causing permanent tissue damage and necrosis when allowed to extravasate into tissues.

What You DO

Nursing Responsibilities

When giving vesicant drugs via a peripheral IV route, extreme caution must be taken to establish reliable IV access that has not been subjected to recent venipuncture. Vinca alkaloids (**vesicant drugs**) can cause leakage of drug into soft tissues around the venipuncture site (**extravasation**). When administering mitotic inhibitors, the nurse should:

- Establish protocol for administration of antidotes and application of heat or cold before administrating a vesicant drug thus treatment may be provided immediately in the event of an extravasation. Research indicates that heat or cold applications or both, depending on the drug, may minimize tissue damage.
- Administer antidotes to minimize the damage caused by extravasation. Some, but not all, vesicant drugs have antidotes.
- Verify that informed consent has been given before beginning treatment.
- Check the patient's laboratory and diagnostic studies before beginning therapy, with special attention being given to the CBC, platelet count, and liver function studies. Counts that are unacceptably low or reflective of organ dysfunction may indicate the need to delay treatment or decrease the dose, particularly when the patient has recently received previous treatment with cytotoxic agents.
- Monitor the patient for evidence of treatment-related toxicities, particularly bone marrow depression and peripheral neuropathy.
- Teach the patient about signs and symptoms of peripheral neuropathy, including paresthesias in the hands or feet, difficulty with fine-motor skills, and numbness. Other signs and symptoms include constipation, paralytic ileus, urinary retention, and jaw pain.
- Instruct the patient to report any of these complaints immediately to the health care provider, who will generally choose either to delay treatment or to decrease the dose.

TAKE HOME POINTS

Obtain reliable IV access with an intact vein to decrease the risk of tissue damage from extravasation of vesicant agents. Remember "V" for vesicant and take precautions!!

- Vincristine
- Vinblastine
- Velban
- Vindesine

TAKE HOME POINTS

Always check laboratory studies and diagnostic test results before starting therapy, even when the patient has never received previous treatment.

Failure to report peripheral neuropathy immediately may result in irreversible neurologic damage.

● Teach the patient about measures to prevent constipation and decrease the risk of infection.

● Teach the patient the proper way to manage adverse effects and the point at which to seek medical assistance.

Do You UNDERSTAND?

DIRECTIONS: Fill in the blanks to complete the following statements.

1. Mitotic inhibitors are used to treat tumors in the _____,
_____, _____, _____.

2. The nurse should carefully monitor the patient for evidence of adverse effects that include _____
and _____.

What IS an Alkylating Agent?

Alkylating Agents	Trade Names	Uses
cyclophosphamide [sye-kloe-FLOSS-fa-mide]	Cytoxan	Treatment of neoplasms
busulfan [byoo-SUL-fan]	Myleran	Treatment of chronic myelogenous leukemia

Action

Alkylating agents cause single- and double-strand breaks in DNA, thereby preventing cellular replication. Although these drugs are cell-cycle nonspecific, they tend to be most effective against rapidly dividing cells.

Uses

This group of agents has demonstrated activity against lymphoma, Hodgkin's disease, breast cancer, and multiple myeloma.

What You NEED TO KNOW

Contraindications/Precautions

Alkylating drugs are contraindicated for patients with serious infections and myelosuppression.

Answers: 1. lung, breast, testes, ovaries; 2. bone marrow suppression, neuropathy.

Alkylating drugs should be used with caution in patients with gout, urate renal stones, or patients who have undergone recent radiation or cytotoxic drug therapy. Cyclophosphamide should be used with caution in patients with renal or hepatic dysfunction, leukopenia, and thrombocytopenia, or patients who are undergoing steroid drug therapy.

Alkylating drugs are contraindicated for patients of childbearing age and women during pregnancy and lactation.

Birth defects in the children of patients who have been treated with alkylating drugs are not uncommon.

TAKE HOME POINTS

- Lomustine and carmustine are noted for prolonged nadirs of 5 to 6 weeks, which makes receiving comprehensive education regarding self-care measures and adequate medical care and follow-up after discharge important.
- Adverse effects of alkylating agents include severe nausea, vomiting, hair loss, and sterile hemorrhagic cystitis.

Drug Interactions

When cyclophosphamide is given with succinylcholine, prolonged neuromuscular blocking activity may occur. Doxorubicin may increase cardiac toxicity when given together with cyclophosphamide. When busulfan is given concurrently with probenecid and sulfinpyrazone, uric acid levels may increase.

Adverse Effects

Alkylating agents are highly effective against a wide variety of cancers. However, when given in high doses, these agents appear to increase the patient's risk of developing a second primary cancer. After repeated doses, these drugs may produce cumulative myelosuppression, with a prolonged recovery period.

Cisplatin is considered as one of the most emetogenic (i.e., capable of causing nausea and vomiting) drugs. Gonadal atrophy may occur in varying degrees, according to the age of the patient at the time that the agents are administered. Decreased sperm production is frequently observed in men and may be permanent, depending on the age of the individual at the time of treatment and the size of the dose that is administered. Chemotherapy-related alopecia is frequently severe with this class of drugs, although the hair growth typically returns to normal soon after the drugs are discontinued. The by-product of cyclophosphamide may cause sterile hemorrhagic cystitis that can be severe to the extent that surgical removal of the bladder is required.

What You DO

Nursing Responsibilities

Melphalan is a vesicant and should be administered with extreme care when a peripheral IV is used. Carmustine and lomustine deserve special mention because they are associated with an extremely long nadir of 3 to 5 weeks after the drugs are administered; it may continue for several weeks afterward. When administering an alkylating agent, the nurse should:

- Validate that laboratory and diagnostic studies are within acceptable limits before initiating chemotherapy.
- Monitor the therapy tolerance of patients who are receiving highly emetogenic therapy (e.g., cisplatin) and report adverse effects to the health care provider immediately.
- Provide treatment with antiemetic drugs before nausea and vomiting become severe.

Nursing care is directed toward preventing damage that is associated with antineoplastic therapy and maximizing the patient's comfort.

- Prepare patients for their eventual hair loss, and encourage them to shop for attractive head coverings and wigs before the hair loss is noticeable. Hair loss from antineoplastic therapy may be particularly devastating for some patients because hair loss is a visible reminder of a life-threatening illness.

- Provide vigorous hydration before, during, and after cyclophosphamide administration.
- Instruct the patient who is taking the oral form to do so early in the day and to empty the bladder at least every 2 hours to avoid damaging the bladder mucosal lining.

Do You UNDERSTAND?

DIRECTIONS: Fill in the blanks to complete the following statements.
1. One of the most emetogenic drugs is _____.
2. Melphalan is a vesicant that should be administered by the _____ route.

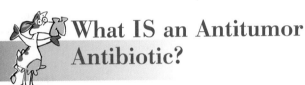

What IS an Antitumor Antibiotic?

Antitumor Antibiotic	Trade Names	Uses
doxorubicin [dox-oh-ROO-bi-sin]	Adriamycin	Treatment of neoplasms
dactinomycin [dak-ti-know-MY-sin]	Actinomycin-D	Treatment of neoplasms

Action

Antitumor antibiotics were derived originally from fungi in soil and are cell-cycle, nonspecific drugs. These agents exert their mechanism of action by combining with cell DNA to form complexes, which inhibit DNA activity.

Uses

Antitumor antibiotics are highly effective in the treatment of a wide variety of tumors, including malignancies of the breast, lymphatics, and ovaries.

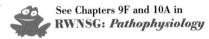

See Chapters 9F and 10A in
RWNSG: *Pathophysiology*

What You NEED TO KNOW

Contraindications/Precautions

Doxorubicin is contraindicated for patients with myelosuppression, jaundice, and cardiac or pulmonary dysfunction. Additionally, dactinomycin is contraindicated for patients with viral infections.

Answers: 1. cisplatin; 2. peripheral IV.

Antitumor antibiotics should be used with caution in patients with renal or hepatic dysfunction and those with antineoplastic or radiation therapy within 3 to 6 weeks. Dactinomycin should be used with caution in patients who are obese or those with gout.

 Antitumor antibiotics are contraindicated for pregnant or lactating women and for infants under 6 months of age.

Risk factors for cardiac toxicity include certain dosing schedules, children, adults over the age of 50, and patients with previous cardiac damage or previous radiation therapy to the chest wall.

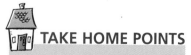 **TAKE HOME POINTS**

Most antitumor antibiotics are toxic to the heart and lungs.

Drug Interactions

When doxorubicin is given with barbiturates, body metabolism may be increased, which may necessitate an increased dose of doxorubicin. Conversely, streptozocin may prolong doxorubicin, necessitating a dose reduction. Because dactinomycin may elevate uric acid level, dose adjustments may be required when given together with antigout drugs. Effects of dactinomycin may be increased when given concurrently with other myelosuppressants or radiation. Dactinomycin decreases the effects of vitamin K, leading to an increased risk of hemorrhage.

Adverse Effects

Because antitumor antibiotics are derived from a naturally occurring substance, they have the potential to cause anaphylaxis. Alopecia, stomatitis, nausea, and vomiting are the most commonly occurring nonorgan-specific adverse effects. Daunorubicin and doxorubicin may cause dose-limiting myelosuppression. The anthracyclines may cause severe irreversible cardiac and pulmonary toxicity. Bleomycin and mitomycin-C may cause severe pulmonary toxicity. When reconstituted, daunorubicin and doxorubicin have a bright, reddish-orange color, which causes the patient's urine to turn a similar color. Dactinomycin is a radiation sensitizer and may cause a phenomenon called radiation recall. This condition means that tissue that was damaged by radiation may become reddened and inflamed in response to antineoplastic therapy.

What You DO

Nursing Responsibilities

Because cardiac toxicity is well documented for doxorubicin, recommendations are that patients should not exceed a cumulative lifetime dose of 550 mg/m² or 450 mg/m² when previous radiation therapy to the chest has been administered.

The cardiac health of all patients should be carefully evaluated before initiating treatment. Currently, a radiologic examination of the heart (known as a gated blood pool scan) is used to measure the left ventricular ejection fraction. This test provides information on the pumping ability of the heart and correlates well with cardiac damage. In most cases, by the time the patient manifests cardiac symptoms, irreversible damage has occurred. Patients in high-risk groups may require a decrease in the dose. When administering antitumor antibiotics, the nurse should:

- Evaluate the patient's cardiopulmonary status thoroughly before initiating antitumor antibiotic therapy and before each treatment. Patients who need a prolonged treatment regimen or those who require large doses of doxorubicin may benefit from the concurrent administration of a cardioprotective agent called dexrazoxane.
- Obtain a baseline evaluation of cardiac and pulmonary function before beginning therapy.

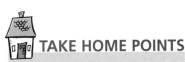

- Monitor the patient for early signs and symptoms of CHF and progressive cardiomyopathy (e.g., dry cough, tachycardia, dyspnea at rest) and report all abnormal findings to the health care provider immediately.
- Evaluate the patient's CBC, platelet count, and serum chemistry studies before starting treatment.
- Administer antitumor antibiotics with the appropriate precautions to avoid tissue damage because these drugs are vesicants.
- Administer antiemetics before starting therapy because of the potential for nausea and vomiting.
- Provide the patient with antiemetics that are suitable for home use before discharge.
- Provide the patient a detailed verbal and written explanation of the proper way to manage adverse symptoms (e.g., fatigue, food aversion, appetite changes, nausea, vomiting) before discharge.
- Provide the patient with a written list of symptoms that require immediate medical intervention.

TAKE HOME POINTS

- Monitor the patient's CBC and chemistry laboratories because a low white blood cell count or inadequate renal function may indicate the need to delay or stop therapy.
- Provide comprehensive patient education on management of symptoms and the point at which to seek medical care. Many antitumor antibiotics are vesicants and must be administered with the appropriate precautions.

Do You UNDERSTAND?

DIRECTIONS: **Indicate in the space provided whether the statement is true or false. If false, rewrite the statement in the margin to the right to make it true.**

_____ 1. Antitumor antibiotics are toxic to the GI tract and kidneys.

_____ 2. A low red blood cell count or inadequate renal function may indicate the need to delay or stop therapy.

What IS a Miscellaneous Antineoplastic Drug?

Miscellaneous Antineoplastics	Trade Names	Uses
hydroxyurea [hye-DROX-ee-yoo-ree-ah]	Hydrea	Palliative treatment of CML or metastasis
asparaginase [a-SPAR-a-gi-nase]	L-Asparaginase	Treatment of acute lymphocytic leukemia
procarbazine [pro-CAR-ba-zeen]	Matulane	Palliative treatment of Hodgkin's disease

Action

Not all antineoplastic agents can be neatly classified. The exact mechanism of action in some drugs is unknown or the chemical structure is not well understood. Hydroxyurea is a cell-cycle–specific drug that inhibits DNA synthesis. In some patients, hydroxyurea appears to act as a radiation sensitizer, although this effect does not consistently occur and is poorly understood. Asparaginase exerts

Answers: 1. false; toxic to the heart and lungs; **2.** false; low white blood cell count.

its mechanism of action by depriving cells of an essential nutrient (asparagines). Procarbazine disrupts chromatin arrangement in the cell and interfering with mitosis.

Uses

Hydroxyurea is used in palliative treatment of chronic myelocytic leukemias (CML). Asparaginase is helpful in the treatment of myeloproliferative disorders. This drug is commonly used in conjunction with vincristine and prednisone as induction therapy for acute lymphocytic leukemia. Procarbazine is used for palliation of Hodgkin's disease and advanced carcinoma of the adrenal cortex.

What You NEED TO KNOW

Contraindications/Precautions

Miscellaneous antineoplastics are contraindicated for patients with myelosuppression. Asparaginase is also contraindicated for patients with herpes infections and pancreatitis.

Drug Interactions

Asparaginase decreases the hypoglycemic effects of sulfonylureas and insulin. When asparaginase is given concurrently with corticosteroids or vincristine, the risk for toxicity is increased. When asparaginase is given concurrently with methotrexate, the antitumor effect is counteracted. Procarbazine is a monoamine oxidase inhibitor (MAOI) and may precipitate a hypertensive crisis when the patient consumes foods that contain tyramine. CNS depression is increased when given with alcohol, phenothiazines, or other CNS depressants.

Adverse Effects

Adverse effects of hydroxyurea include headache, malaise, fever, chills, dizziness, anorexia, nausea, vomiting, diarrhea, constipation, seizures, hallucinations, and bone marrow suppression. Asparaginase is a naturally occurring compound that has the potential to cause hypersensitivity reactions ranging in severity from itching to anaphylaxis. Asparaginase is different from most antineoplastic agents in that it does not usually cause myelosuppression or hair loss (alopecia). Asparaginase may cause prolonged bleeding times, pancreatitis, hepatic dysfunction, and acute renal insufficiency. Adverse affects of procarbazine include bone marrow suppression, nausea, vomiting, and neuropathy.

Miscellaneous antineoplastics are contraindicated for women during pregnancy and lactation.

Miscellaneous antineoplastics should be given with caution to patients with renal or hepatic dysfunction, diabetes mellitus, and those who have undergone radiation or antineoplastic therapy within 1 month. Hydroxyurea should be given with caution to patients with asthma, epilepsy, migraines, cardiac dysfunction, or mental depression. Asparaginase should be given with caution to patients with gout. Procarbazine should be given with caution to patients who are undergoing concurrent CNS depressant therapy.

What You DO

Nursing Responsibilities

When administering antineoplastics, the nurse should:

- Obtain baseline clotting, renal, and hepatic function tests before asparaginase therapy begins.
- Have resuscitation equipment and emergency drugs readily available.
- Monitor the patient carefully, particularly when the drug is infused IV.
- Instruct the patient to report any unusual symptoms immediately, particularly those suggestive of hypersensitivity (e.g., itching, respiratory distress, rash).
- Check glucose levels daily and anticipate orders for subcutaneous doses of vitamin K to restore normal clotting function.
- Monitor the CBC and platelet count routinely for the patient who is undergoing procarbazine therapy.
- Assess the patient carefully for evidence of neuropathy or poor oral intake.
- Report any abnormal findings or laboratory values to the health care provider before beginning treatment.
- Be aware that MAOIs should be discontinued 14 days before initiating procarbazine therapy. Some foods that must be avoided when given concurrently with procarbazine include cheese, chocolates, and red wine.

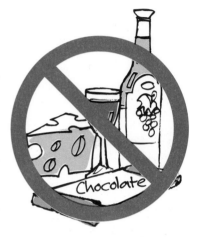

Do You UNDERSTAND?

DIRECTIONS: **Fill in the blanks to complete the following statements.**

1. _____ does not usually cause myelosuppression or alopecia.

2. _____ is a drug that disrupts chromatin arrangement in the cell and interferes with mitosis. This agent is used for palliation of Hodgkin's disease and advanced carcinoma of the adrenal cortex.

Drugs Affecting the Nervous System

SECTION A
SYMPATHETIC NERVOUS SYSTEM AGENTS

Hormones (norepinephrine and epinephrine) activate the sympathetic nervous system. Sympathetic nerves release both of these hormones, while the adrenal gland also releases epinephrine. Norepinephrine and epinephrine stimulate three types of receptor sites found in autonomic nerve pathways: α-adrenergic, β_1-adrenergic, and β_2-adrenergic receptors. Several physiologic responses result when each type of receptor is activated. The nurse must be aware of the different receptor sites and the associated responses, thus the effects of the agents can be predicted. These responses include:

α-Receptors effect:
- Pupil dilation
- Gastrointestinal (GI) tract motility
- Vasoconstriction of arterioles (increases blood pressure)

β_1-Receptors effect:
- Heart rate, contractility, automaticity, and conduction

β_2-Receptors effect:
- Bronchodilation
- Vasoconstriction of arterioles (increases blood pressure)
- Conversion of glycogen to glucose

Sympathetic nervous system agents either stimulate or inhibit α- or β-receptors or both. Most agents either stimulate or inhibit more than one receptor but usually activate one more strongly than it does the other. Sympathetic nervous system agents are classified as adrenergic agonists (stimulators) and adrenergic antagonists (inhibitors).

For further explanation of adrenergics, refer to Chapters 5E and 5F in RWNSG: *Pathophysiology*

For further information on antiadrenergics, see Chapters 4C and 10A in RWNSG: *Pathophysiology*

Adrenergic Agonists

What IS an Adrenergic Agonist?

Adrenergic Agonists	Trade Names	Receptor Site	Primary Use
albuterol [al-BYOO-ter-ahl]	Proventil Ventolin	beta primarily β2	Bronchospasm associated with asthma or bronchitis
dobutamine [doe-BYOOT-uh-meen]	Dobutrex	β1	Inotropic support in congestive heart failure and cardiogenic shock
dopamine [DOE-puh-meen]	Intropin	α and β1 dopaminergic	Hypotension associated with any shock state and renal insufficiency
ephedrine [eh-FED-rin]	Ephedsol Ectasule Vatronol	α and β	Temporary relief of nasal and sinus congestion
isoproterenol [eye-so-pro-TER-uh-nahl]	Isuprel	beta	Unresponsive bradycardia
pseudoephedrine hydrochloride [soo-doe-e-FED-rin]	Sudafed	α and β	Nasal, sinus, and eustachian tube congestion

Action

Adrenergic agonists (**adrenergics** or **sympathomimetic agents**) can stimulate any one or any combination of α- or β-receptors.

Adrenergic agonists that stimulate only one type of receptor can be further classified as either an α-agonist or β-agonist. α-Agonists constrict arterioles, thereby elevating blood pressure (BP).

Adrenergic agonists that stimulate β-receptors are called β-adrenergic agonists. The type of β-receptor they primarily stimulate further classifies them as selective or nonselective agents. β_1-agonists speed conduction and automaticity and increase myocardial contractility, which restores cardiac rhythm. β_2-agonists cause bronchodilation in the presence of asthma, bronchospasm, emphysema, and anaphylactic reactions.

Uses

Adrenergic agonists are used primarily for three reasons: hemodynamic compromise (e.g., hypotension resulting from any type of shock, acute congestive heart failure, or depressed cardiac rhythm), bronchospasm, and nasal or sinus congestion.

The adrenergic agonists agents that are commonly used for hypotension include dopamine, norepinephrine, ephedrine, and phenylephrine. α-Agonists

TAKE HOME POINTS

Most adrenergic agonists frequently stimulate more than one adrenergic receptor site, producing a variety of effects.

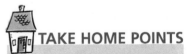

TAKE HOME POINTS

Many of the adrenergic agents are emergency agents that are used to treat cardiovascular collapse or arrest.

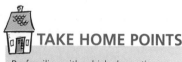

TAKE HOME POINTS

Be familiar with which drug stimulates which receptor site to predict the effects of different adrenergic agonists.

are used to treat shock. β_1-Agonists are used to restore cardiac rhythm in profound bradycardia, second-degree type II heart block, or complete heart block until the insertion of a pacemaker, as well as acute congestive heart failure and cardiogenic shock. β_2-Agonists are used primarily for pulmonary disorders and to treat or prevent bronchospasm by causing bronchodilation.

Dopamine is a unique drug and different from the other adrenergic agonists because its actions depends on the dose. Doses of 5 to 10 µg/kg/min stimulate β_1-receptors, and doses greater than 10 µg/kg/min stimulate α-receptors. Doses of 2 to 3 µg/kg/min stimulate dopaminergic receptors, causing dilation of the mesenteric and renal arteries. Dopamine is frequently used to increase blood flow to the kidneys when renal insufficiency is present or to prevent renal failure from shock.

What You NEED TO KNOW

Contraindications/Precautions

Because α-agonists cause pupil dilation (**mydriasis**), they are contraindicated for patients with narrow-angle glaucoma.

Drug Interactions

The adrenergic agonists should be avoided in patients with coronary artery disease because these agents may precipitate angina or myocardial infarction (MI).

Agents that increase the effects of adrenergic agonists on the cardiovascular and central nervous system (CNS) include monoamine oxidase inhibitors (MAOIs), theophylline, and tricyclic antidepressants. Antihistamines and atropine increase the risk of tachycardia. Digoxin, when taken with adrenergic agonists, increases the risk of ventricular dysrhythmias.

Adverse Effects

The most common adverse effects of all adrenergic agonists involve the cardiovascular and CNS. Cardiovascular effects include tachycardia, ectopic beats, tachydysrhythmias, hypertension, and myocardial ischemia. CNS effects include nervousness, tremors, and anxiety. Adrenergic agonists also elevate blood glucose levels. α-Agonists cause pupil dilation. Additive adverse effects may occur when more than one adrenergic agent is administered together.

What You DO

Nursing Responsibilities

Gastric acid inactivates many adrenergic agonists thus most are given intravenously (IV) or through inhalation or both. When given IV, the effects are usually immediate or within minutes. After the agents enter the bloodstream, they are rapidly metabolized. The rapid metabolism results in a short duration of action for these agents.

All the adrenergic agonists that are used for hemodynamic compromise are given IV, but some may be given intramuscularly (IM) or subcutaneously (SC). The IV route may be given by direct IV or diluted and given only as a continuous infusion.

When an adrenergic drug is given as a continuous infusion, it should be titrated until the desired effect is achieved. The prescribing health care provider will order the desired effect or dose range. Titration of these agents should be done slowly (e.g., 2 to 3 ml every 3 to 5 minutes). Continuous infusions should not be discontinued abruptly, but rather, titrated down slowly.

Do not abruptly halt continuous infusions of adrenergic agonists. Rather, slowly titrate down. Sudden discontinuation may cause extreme fluctuations in BP and heart rate. All continuous infusions should be infused through microdrip tubing via an infusion pump. Macro-drip tubing and manual rate control does not ensure accurate titration.

Most adrenergic agonists that are used to treat bronchospasm are given by inhalation therapy. Inhalation therapy includes use of a nebulizer, intermittent positive-pressure breathing (IPPB), and metered-dose inhaler (MDI). Albuterol may be given orally. These agents are commonly found as over-the-counter (OTC) oral preparations or nasal sprays. Many of these agents are absorbed into the systemic circulation from the respiratory tract, thus cardiovascular and CNS effects may be observed during or after an inhalation treatment.

When administering adrenergic agonists to treat hemodynamic compromise or bronchospasm, the nurse should:

- Monitor for cardiovascular and CNS effects during and after inhalation treatments because these are the most common adverse effects of adrenergic agonists.
- Monitor blood glucose levels closely, particularly in patients with diabetes.
- Avoid giving α-agonists to patients with narrow-angle glaucoma because they increase intraocular pressure.
- Teach patients with ischemic heart disease that they should check with the health care provider before taking any OTC adrenergic agonists.

Most adrenergic agents that are used to treat nasal and sinus congestion are given intranasally or orally. These agents consist of common OTC "cold medicines." Similar to other adrenergic agonists, these agents may also cause cardiovascular and CNS effects, thus they should be avoided in the presence of ischemic heart disease.

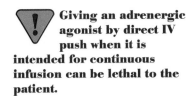

Giving an adrenergic agonist by direct IV push when it is intended for continuous infusion can be lethal to the patient.

TAKE HOME POINTS

- Be aware of which adrenergic agents may be given by direct IV push and which should be diluted and given only by continuous infusion.
- Slowly titrate continuous infusions until the desired effect (e.g., increased BP or myocardial contractility) or dose is achieved to promote hemodynamic stability.

Agents such as norepinephrine and dopamine can cause a serious local reaction when they infiltrate into the surrounding tissues. Infiltration of these agents can cause extravasation and sloughing of local tissues. When an IV infiltrates with any of these agents, a local antidote must be given to prevent tissue necrosis. The antidote is 5 to 10 mg of phentolamine in 10 ml of normal saline that is injected into the infiltrated tissue through multiple injections with a tuberculin needle. This procedure should be performed within 12 hours after an infiltration is suggested, preferably immediately.

Do You UNDERSTAND?

DIRECTIONS: **Fill in the blanks with the name of the receptor that produces the effect listed.**

1. Stimulating _____-receptors results in bronchodilation.
2. Stimulating _____-receptors increases myocardial contractility.
3. Stimulating _____-receptors increases BP.
4. Stimulating _____-receptors decreases GI motility.

Adrenergic Antagonists

Adrenergic antagonists inhibit or block the effects of the sympathetic nervous system neurotransmitters and are antagonists to the adrenergic agonists. Adrenergic antagonists are also called adrenergic blockers or sympatholytic agents because they block sympathetic effects throughout the body (lyse). Agents that block sympathetic receptors produce responses similar to those occurring when parasympathetic receptors are activated. Adrenergic antagonists do not occur naturally in the body. Dissimilar to adrenergic agonists, which can stimulate more than one receptor type, most adrenergic antagonists block only one type of receptor, either the α- or β-receptors. These adrenergic antagonist agents can be further classified as either α-antagonists or β-antagonists.

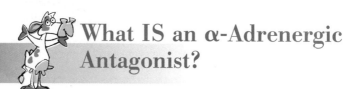

What IS an α-Adrenergic Antagonist?

α-Adrenergic Antagonists	Trade Names	Uses
doxazosin mesylate [dox-A-zo-sin]	Cardura	Treatment of hypertension
tolazoline hydrochloride [toe-LAZ-a-leen]	Priscoline	Treatment of vasospastic disorders
tamsulosin hydrochloride [TAM-su-lo-sin]	Flomax	Treatment of benign prostatic hypertrophy

Action

α-Adrenergic antagonists block receptors throughout the body. The following responses result when these sites are blocked:

- Pupil constriction (miosis)
- Increased GI tract motility
- Vasodilation of arterioles (decreases BP)

The primary effects of α-adrenergic antagonists involve the cardiovascular system. Because the α-receptors are blocked, the arterioles dilate, which decreases BP and peripheral vascular resistance.

Answers: 1. β₂; 2. β₁; 3. α, β₂; 4. α.

Uses

α-Adrenergic antagonists are used primarily to treat five conditions: hypertension, migraine headaches, Alzheimer's disease, benign prostatic hypertrophy, and vasoactive disorders. Most agents are used for only one condition.

α-Adrenergic antagonists can be used to treat benign prostatic hypertrophy because they dilate blood vessels along the urinary tract and enhance urine outflow. Ergoloid mesylate is used to treat Alzheimer's disease by increasing cerebral blood flow via vasodilation of the cerebral arteries. Tolazoline is one type of agent that is used to treat vasoactive disorders, such as Raynaud's disease and Berger's disease because it helps increase peripheral blood flow.

 # What You NEED TO KNOW

Contraindications/Precautions

α-Adrenergic antagonists, except doxazosin, prazosin, and terazosin, should be avoided in patients with ischemic heart disease.

Drug Interactions

The only specific drug interactions with α-antagonists involve the use of agents that are classified as α-agonists because they counteract the desired effects.

Adverse Effects

The major adverse effect of α-adrenergic antagonists is orthostatic hypotension. The sympathetic nervous system is stimulated when a person stands up quickly, causing vasoconstriction to prevent blood from pooling in the legs. When a person is taking an α-adrenergic antagonist, the vessels are unable to constrict because α-receptors are blocked. As a result, BP rapidly falls, and blood flow to the brain decreases, causing the person to become dizzy and develop syncope. The decrease in BP from most α-adrenergic antagonists also tends to cause reflexogenic cardiac stimulation. This reflex causes tachycardia and an increase in the force of myocardial contractions. Therefore the cardiac stimulation may increase the workload of the heart and result in myocardial ischemia or MI.

Doxazosin, prazosin, and terazosin are the only types of α-adrenergic antagonists that cause minimal cardiac stimulation. These agents usually do not cause the reflex tachycardia because they block only one type of α-receptor ($α_1$) and not the type ($α_2$) that causes cardiac stimulation. α-Adrenergic antagonists used for migraine headaches (ergot alkaloids) may also cause bradycardia and hypotension.

Other adverse effects are also related to blocking of α-receptor sites, including an increase in GI motility, miosis, increase in lacrimation, mucus secretion in the upper respiratory tract, and impaired ejaculation.

> ⚠ **When other antihypertensive agents are used, α-antagonists should be used cautiously to prevent hypotension. Avoid α-adrenergic antagonists, except doxazosin, prazosin, and terazosin, in patients with ischemic heart disease.**

TAKE HOME POINTS

- Monitor for orthostatic hypotension, particularly after the initial doses of α-adrenergic antagonists.
- Administer α-adrenergic antagonists, when used as antihypertensive agents, in equally divided doses during an entire 24-hour period to regulate BP. Administer agents for migraine headaches immediately after the onset of the headache to optimize effectiveness.
- Administer phentolamine immediately or at least within 12 hours to treat a dopamine or norepinephrine IV infiltration.

What You DO

Nursing Responsibilities

When administering α-adrenergic antagonists, the nurse should:

- Monitor for orthostatic hypotension, particularly after the initial dose. Instruct patients to rise to a standing position slowly and to sit immediately when dizziness or light-headedness occurs to prevent falling.
- Monitor patients who are taking α-adrenergic antagonists for tachycardia.
- Advise patient to avoid participating in any activity that may be dangerous (e.g., driving) until the drug response is determined.
- Instruct patient to report any weakness or dizziness immediately to the health care provider.
- Administer an α-adrenergic antagonist, given for hypertension, at the same time every day and spaced equally throughout a 24-hour period to optimize its effect on BP. For example, administering the drug every 8 hours is preferable to three times during the day (tid).
- Instruct the patient that agents used to relieve migraine headaches are more effective when administered immediately after the onset of the headache.

Place the patient with a migraine headache in a quiet, dark environment. Phentolamine is the drug of choice to prevent tissue extravasation in the event of either a dopamine or a norepinephrine IV infiltration. Usually, 5 to 10 mg is diluted in 10 ml of normal saline. A tuberculin-size needle is used to make multiple injections into the infiltrated tissue. This procedure must be performed within 12 hours of the infiltration, otherwise tissue extravasation and sloughing may occur. Phentolamine is most effective when given immediately after the infiltration.

Do You UNDERSTAND?

DIRECTIONS: Fill in the blanks with appropriate responses.

1. _____ should be closely monitored after the initial dose of an α-adrenergic antagonist.
2. _____ is the drug of choice for a norepinephrine IV infiltration.
3. _____ is an α-adrenergic antagonist that is used to treat Alzheimer's disease.

What IS a β-Adrenergic Antagonist?

Refer to page 147 for a discussion of β-adrenergic antagonist.

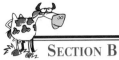

SECTION B
PARASYMPATHETIC NERVOUS SYSTEM AGENTS AND ANTIPARKINSONISM AGENTS

The parasympathetic nervous system is concerned primarily with conserving energy and promoting digestion. Several responses occur when the parasympathetic nervous system is stimulated:

- Pupil constriction (**miosis**)
- Lacrimation
- Salivation
- Bronchoconstriction
- Decrease in heart rate, conduction, and automaticity
- Stimulation of gastric secretions and increase in GI motility
- Contraction of bladder and relaxation of the sphincter

Several groups of agents that affect parasympathetic activity are discussed in this section. Most of these agents either enhance or inhibit the parasympathetic nervous system receptors. Direct-acting cholinergic agonists and cholinesterase inhibitors enhance parasympathetic activity. Agents that reduce or inhibit parasympathetic activity are classified as anticholinergics.

Agents that are used to treat Parkinson's disease will also be reviewed in this section. These agents are generally classified as antiparkinsonism agents. Selective anticholinergic agents and dopaminergics are used to relieve some of the major symptoms that are associated with Parkinson's disease.

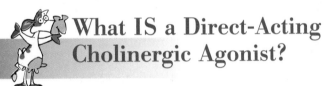

What IS a Direct-Acting Cholinergic Agonist?

Direct-Acting Cholinergic Agonists	Trade Names	Uses
bethanechol chloride [beth-AN-ih-kole KLOR-ide]	Urecholine	Treatment of urinary retention
dexpanthenol [dex-PAN-the-nole]	Ilopan	Prevention or treatment of post operative abdominal distention, intestinal atony, and paralytic ileus
metoclopramide [MET-oh-KLOE-pra-mide]	Reglan	Treatment of gastroparesis, nausea and vomiting associated with antineoplastics and gastroesophageal reflux

Action

Acetylcholine (ACh) is the primary neurotransmitter that is involved in the parasympathetic nervous system. ACh stimulates cholinergic receptors that are classified as either muscarinic or nicotinic. Muscarinic receptors are located in the CNS, heart, glands, and smooth muscle of organs. The response of muscarinic receptors is generally inhibitory, except for stimulation of glandular secretions (e.g., stimulation of gastric secretions, salivation). Nicotinic receptors are located in skeletal muscle cells and autonomic ganglia. The nicotinic response is an excitatory effect (e.g., increase in GI motility). Direct-acting cholinergic agonists affect primarily the muscarinic receptors. These agents act similarly to ACh in stimulating muscarinic receptors and producing parasympathetic responses or cholinergic effects. Direct-acting cholinergic agonists are also called parasympathomimetic agents and cholinergic agonists.

Uses

Bethanechol is used for urinary retention because it contracts the bladder, allowing the bladder to empty. Several of the direct-acting cholinergic agonists are used to treat GI disturbances because they increase GI motility. Dexpanthenol is used to prevent or treat postoperative abdominal distention, intestinal atony, and paralytic ileus. Metoclopramide is effective in relieving gastroparesis, nausea, and vomiting that are associated with antineoplastic agents and gastroesophageal reflux.

What You NEED TO KNOW

Contraindications/Precautions

Direct-acting cholinergics are contraindicated for patients with asthma because they can precipitate bronchospasm. These agents are also contraindicated for patients with mechanical obstruction in either the GI or the urinary tract because stimulation may cause tearing of body tissues.

Drug Interactions

Several agents can alter the effects of direct-acting cholinergic agonists. Cholinesterase inhibitors can augment the cholinergic effects. Procainamide, quinidine, atropine, and epinephrine antagonize the effects of cholinergic agents. Alcohol and CNS depressants enhance sedation. Metoclopramide can cause extrapyramidal symptoms (e.g., acute dystonia), and phenothiazines may increase the potential of these symptoms.

Adverse Effects

Most of the adverse effects that are associated with direct-acting cholinergic agonists are related to the parasympathetic responses that they produce. These effects include dry mouth, sedation or drowsiness, excessive lacrimation, miosis, decreased BP with reflex tachycardia, excessive salivation, diarrhea, cramping, and abdominal pain.

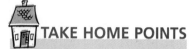

TAKE HOME POINTS

Be familiar with the parasympathetic responses that are produced by direct-acting cholinergic agonists to ensure safe administration.

See Chapter 9B in **RWNSG:** *Pathophysiology*

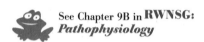

TAKE HOME POINTS

Be aware that alcohol and CNS depressants can enhance sedation.

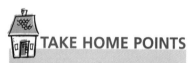

What You DO

Nursing Responsibilities

When direct-acting cholinergics are used for GI tract symptoms, they should be given before meals and at bedtime for optimal effect. Metoclopramide should be given 30 minutes before meals.

When administering direct-acting cholinergics, the nurse should:

- Monitor the patient for signs and symptoms of cholinergic overdose, including salivation, sweating, flushing, abdominal cramps, and nausea.
- Administer the antidote or antagonist for cholinergic overdose (atropine sulfate), which is administered IM, slow IV, or SC and repeated every 2 hours as needed.
- Monitor respiratory status of patients who are taking direct-acting cholinergic agonist therapy and immediately report dyspnea to the health care provider.
- Direct-acting cholinergics that are used for GI disorders should be given before each meal and at bedtime.

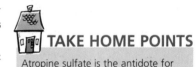

TAKE HOME POINTS

Atropine sulfate is the antidote for cholinergic overdose.

Do You UNDERSTAND?

DIRECTIONS: Place a check next to the responses that occur with direct-acting cholinergic agonists.

_____ 1. Decreased salivation
_____ 2. Decreased heart rate
_____ 3. Increased gastric motility
_____ 4. Increased cardiac conduction

What IS a Cholinesterase Inhibitor?

Cholinesterase Inhibitors	Trade Names	Uses
ambenonium chloride [am-be-NOE-nee-um KLOR-ide]	Mytelase	Maintenance treatment of myasthenia gravis
edrophonium chloride [eh-droe-FOE-nee-uhm]	Tensilon	Diagnoses myasthenia gravis; differentiates between myasthenic and cholinergic crisis
neostigmine bromide [nee-oh-STIG-meen]	Prostigmin	Diagnoses myasthenia gravis; differentiates between myasthenic and cholinergic crisis

Continued

Answers: decreased heart rate; increased gastric motility.

Cholinesterase Inhibitors—cont'd	Trade Names	Uses
donepezil hydrochloride [dawn-EPP-uh-zill]	Aricept	Treatment of Alzheimer's disease
rivastigmine tartrate [riv-ah-STIG-meen]	Exelon	Treatment of Alzheimer's disease

Action

Cholinesterase inhibitors are also referred to as acetylcholinesterase inhibitors. ACh is released in the peripheral nerves, as well as the central nerves. When released in the peripheral nerves, ACh reacts with target cells to stimulate the skeletal muscles. Immediately after ACh interacts with target cells, the enzyme acetylcholinesterase (AChE) stops its action on the target cells. Cholinesterase inhibitors are agents that inhibit AChE. Inhibiting this enzyme allows the actions of ACh to be prolonged and more intense (e.g., excess vasodilation can lead to shock).

Uses

Because cholinesterase inhibitors prolong the effect of ACh, most of these agents are used to restore skeletal muscle function from either myasthenia gravis or from nonpolarizing skeletal muscle relaxants. Some of these agents are used to improve memory in patients with Alzheimer's disease. Ambenonium chloride is used for maintenance therapy in treating myasthenia gravis. Edrophonium chloride and neostigmine have a short duration of action, thus they are not used for maintenance therapy in treating myasthenia gravis, but rather, to diagnose myasthenia gravis and to differentiate between a myasthenic and cholinergic crisis.

A myasthenic crisis occurs when the dose of a cholinesterase inhibitor is subtherapeutic, therefore skeletal muscle function declines. When doses of a cholinesterase inhibitor become toxic, a cholinergic crisis results, leading to cholinergic effects. Donepezil hydrochloride and rivastigmine are used to improve memory in patients with Alzheimer's disease.

The nurse should know the difference between a cholinergic and myasthenic crisis. Cholinesterase inhibitor underdosing may lead to a myasthenic crisis. Overdosing may lead to a cholinergic crisis.

Edrophonium and neostigmine are used to reverse the neuromuscular blockade effects produced by nonpolarizing skeletal muscle relaxants that are commonly used to produce paralysis during surgery.

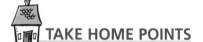

TAKE HOME POINTS

Cholinesterase inhibitors inhibit AChE, thereby improving skeletal muscle function.

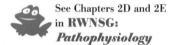

See Chapters 2D and 2E in RWNSG: *Pathophysiology*

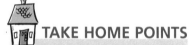

TAKE HOME POINTS

Cholinesterase inhibitors are used primarily to restore skeletal muscle function, particularly in patients with myasthenia gravis.

Edrophonium and neostigmine should be used cautiously in patients with bronchial asthma. Donepezil should be used cautiously in patients with a history of ulcers and GI bleeding.

What You NEED TO KNOW

Contraindications/Precautions

Donepezil and neostigmine are contraindicated for patients with bradycardia or hypotension. Donepezil, edrophonium, and neostigmine are contraindicated for patients with urinary tract and intestinal obstruction.

Drug Interactions

Several drug interactions may occur with cholinesterase inhibitors. Depolarizing muscle relaxants, such as succinylcholine and decamethonium, have prolonged action when administered with cholinesterase inhibitors. Tubocurarine, atracurium, vecuronium, pancuronium, procainamide, quinidine, and atropine, as well as any drug with anticholinergic properties (e.g., antihistamines, antidepressants, phenothiazines, disopyramide), inhibit the effects of cholinesterase inhibitors. Procainamide, quinidine, mecamylamine, and succinylcholine can intensify the toxicity of ambenonium. The metabolism of donepezil is inhibited by ketoconazole and quinidine, and its elimination is increased by carbamazepine, dexamethasone, phenobarbital, phenytoin, and rifampin.

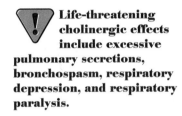

TAKE HOME POINTS

The nurse should know which agents enhance or antagonize the effects of cholinesterase inhibitors.

Adverse Effects

Common adverse effects that are associated with cholinesterase inhibitors are related to excessive cholinergic stimulation. These effects include salivation, sweating, flushing, abdominal cramps, and nausea. Rivastigmine has few adverse effects, which include anorexia, nausea, vomiting, diarrhea, and dizziness. Food may affect the absorption of cholinesterase inhibitors. Food decreases the rate and extent of tacrine absorption.

Life-threatening cholinergic effects include excessive pulmonary secretions, bronchospasm, respiratory depression, and respiratory paralysis.

What You DO

Nursing Responsibilities

Two problems can develop in patients with myasthenia gravis who are receiving cholinesterase inhibitor therapy. Either a myasthenic crisis from underdosing or a cholinergic crisis from overdosing of a cholinesterase inhibitor can develop. Both conditions are difficult to differentiate because they have similar symptoms of skeletal muscle weakness and respiratory depression. An edrophonium test (Tensilon test) is performed (usually by the health care provider) to differentiate between a myasthenic crisis and a cholinergic crisis. Edrophonium is administered IV, and improvement is observed within 1 minute when the patient is experiencing a myasthenic crisis. When the condition worsens, the problem is a cholinergic crisis. No response indicates an optimal treatment regimen.

Ambenonium should be given with food to minimize cholinergic effects. Laboratory testing of liver enzymes must be monitored for patients who are taking tacrine because of its hepatotoxicity.

When administering cholinesterase inhibitors, the nurse should:
- Place atropine sulfate at the bedside for immediate administration to reverse the cholinergic effects when a cholinergic crisis is present before the Tensilon test is performed.

- Be certain that intubation equipment is available in the event of a respiratory depression or arrest. Atropine is an anticholinergic drug that antagonizes the cholinergic stimulation that is produced by cholinesterase inhibitors.
- Immediately report any respiratory distress or depression.
- Teach the patient to recognize adverse effects of ambenonium and adjust the dose accordingly.
- Warn patients that they may become resistant to ambenonium when on long-term treatment. However, when the drug is withdrawn for several days or the dose is reduced, individuals usually become responsive again.
- Protect the patient who is taking donepezil or rivastigmine because dizziness and fainting episodes may occur.
- Teach patients who are taking donepezil to report any signs of GI ulceration or bleeding immediately.

Do You UNDERSTAND?

DIRECTIONS: Indicate in the space provided whether each statement is true or false.

_____ 1. AChE inhibits the actions of ACh.

_____ 2. Inhibiting AChE causes less stimulation of skeletal muscles.

_____ 3. ACh stimulates skeletal muscles.

_____ 4. Cholinesterase inhibitors intensifies and prolongs the action of ACh.

What IS an Anticholinergic?

Anticholinergics	Trade Names	Uses
atropine sulfate [A-troe-peen]	Isopto Atropine	Treatment of GI hyperacidity, hypermotility, and spasms; preoperative drug to dry secretions
glycopyrrolate [glye-koe-PYE-roe-late]	Robinul	Treatment of GI hyperacidity, hypermotility, and spasms; preoperative drug to dry secretions
oxybutynin chloride [ox-I-BYOO-ti-nin]	Ditropan	Treatment of neurogenic bladder; relieves bladder spasms
propantheline bromide [proe-PAN-the-leen]	Pro-Banthine	Treatment of GI hyperacidity, hypermotility, and spasms; preoperative drug to dry secretions
scopolamine [skoe-POL-a-meen]	Hyoscine	Controls spasticity; preoperative drug to dry secretions; relieves motion sickness

Action

Anticholinergics block muscarinic receptors, thereby antagonizing the effects of ACh and inhibiting parasympathetic actions. Anticholinergics are also called parasympatholytic and antimuscarinic agents. Because these agents block the actions of the parasympathetic nervous system, the effects produced mimic many of the sympathetic effects. Anticholinergic agents produce the following responses:

- Pupil dilation (mydriasis)
- Decreased lacrimation
- Increased heart rate, automaticity, conduction, and contractility
- Decreased GI motility and gastric acid secretion
- Decreased salivary gland secretion
- Decreased sweat gland activity
- Bladder muscle contraction and relaxation of sphincter

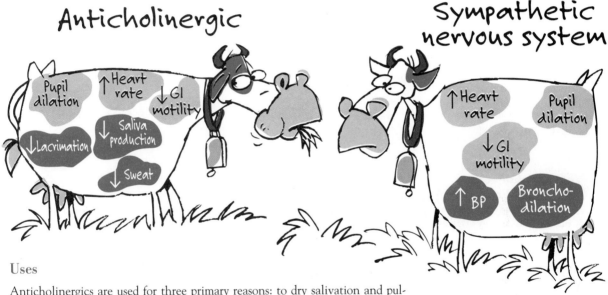

Uses

Anticholinergics are used for three primary reasons: to dry salivation and pulmonary secretions; to relieve symptoms that are associated with Parkinson's disease; and to relieve spasms of the GI tract, genitourinary (GU) tract, and those associated with menstrual cramps. Some agents may be used for one or more of the three primary uses.

Agents that dry secretions are used as preoperative medications to dry salivation, perspiration, and respiratory secretions during surgery. In addition to use as a "drying" agent, scopolamine is also used for a sedative effect in obstetric patients and to relieve motion sickness.

Atropine is used as an agent to dry secretions, as well as an antidote to treat cholinergic overdose that is produced by other medications (e.g., cholinesterase inhibitors, direct-acting cholinergic agonists) and to treat a cholinergic crisis in patients with myasthenia gravis. Another important use for atropine is its use in

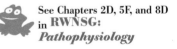

See Chapters 2D, 5F, and 8D in **RWNSG:** *Pathophysiology*

emergency cardiovascular situations. Atropine increases the heart rate in patients who have sinus bradycardia, second-degree type II atrioventricular block, complete heart block, or asystole. Atropine is also an antidote for organophosphate poisoning from insecticides, and it dries excessive pulmonary secretions that organophosphates produce.

Anticholinergic agents, used as antispasmodics, help relieve symptoms that are associated with GI disorders that produce hyperacidity, hypermotility, and spasms (e.g., peptic ulcer, irritable bowel syndrome, neurogenic bowel disorder, pylorospasms, spasms of the biliary tract). Some anticholinergics, used as antispasmodics, are also used to relieve symptoms that are associated with dysmenorrhea or various GU disorders (e.g., bladder spasms, nocturnal enuresis, neurogenic bladder). Orphenadrine is used to relieve spasms of the musculoskeletal system.

Another group of anticholinergics are used as antiparkinsonism agents. These anticholinergics are used as an adjunct to the dopaminergic agent levodopa, particularly in the advanced stages of Parkinson's disease. These agents relieve some of the extrapyramidal symptoms that are associated with Parkinson's disease, such as drooling, tremors, and rigidity.

What You NEED TO KNOW

Contraindications/Precautions

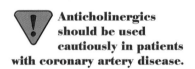

Anticholinergics should be used cautiously in patients with coronary artery disease.

Anticholinergics are contraindicated for patients with narrow-angle glaucoma because they cause pupil dilation. Anticholinergics are also contraindicated for male patients who have an enlarged prostate and for patients with myasthenia gravis because they inhibit the effects of ACh.

Drug Interactions

Several agents affect or can be affected by anticholinergics. Antihistamines, tricyclic antidepressants, quinidine, procainamide, disopyramide, and amantadine may increase the anticholinergic effects. Anticholinergics decrease the antipsychotic effects of phenothiazines. Methotrimeprazine may precipitate extrapyramidal symptoms when taken with an anticholinergic. Alcohol enhances the sedative effects of anticholinergics, particularly in anticholinergics that are used to treat Parkinson's disease (e.g., benztropine, biperiden, procyclidine, scopolamine, trihexyphenidyl). Antacids decrease the absorption of anticholinergics.

Adverse Effects

Several adverse effects are associated with anticholinergics, most of which are related to antimuscarinic properties. Common adverse effects include dry mouth, tachydysrhythmias, hypertension, decreased sweating, constipation, drowsiness, nervousness, confusion, blurred vision, and mydriasis. Because anticholinergics increase the heart rate, conduction, contractility, and automaticity, an increase in myocardial oxygen demand may occur, resulting in myocardial ischemia. Anticholinergics may cause acute urinary retention in patients with an enlarged prostate or benign prostatic hypertrophy.

 # What You DO

Nursing Responsibilities

When administering anticholinergics, the nurse should:

- Space 1 hour between administering an antacid and an anticholinergic.
- Decrease doses in patients with hepatic or renal dysfunction because most anticholinergics are metabolized by the liver and eliminated through the kidneys.
- Advise patients who are taking an anticholinergic to avoid high temperatures because their ability to perspire is inhibited, making them susceptible to heat stroke.
- Warn patients to avoid driving or engaging in any activity that requires alertness until the sedative effects of the anticholinergic is determined.
- Instruct patients to avoid concurrent use of alcohol and other depressants.
- Instruct patients to check with the health care provider before taking any OTC agents, particularly any antihistamines because they increase anticholinergic effects.
- Instruct patients to perform frequent mouth care to relieve dry mouth.
- Instruct patients to report any anticholinergic adverse effects (e.g., urinary retention, constipation, drowsiness, confusion) to the health care provider.

When administering atropine, the nurse should:

- Use atropine only when the patient with ischemic heart disease is symptomatic. Atropine increases the myocardial oxygen demand and should be used to treat symptomatic bradycardia (not asymptomatic bradycardia), particularly in patients with coronary artery disease. When atropine is used for treatment of bradycardia, a minimum IV dose of 0.5 mg should be given to the adult patient because a dose less than 0.5 mg may cause paradoxical bradycardia.
- Immediately inform the health care provider about any patient who complains of chest pain and who is receiving atropine or an anticholinergic.
- Be aware that atropine is the drug of choice for treatment of bradydysrhythmias and heart blocks.
- Be aware that atropine is used to treat an overdose of cholinesterase inhibitors (**cholinergic crisis**) and direct-acting cholinergic agonists. Atropine is also used to treat organophosphate poisoning. The nurse should be aware of the doses for atropine when used as an antidote for these conditions.

 TAKE HOME POINTS

- Antacids decrease the absorption of anticholinergics, thus 1 hour should be spaced between administering an antacid and an anticholinergic. Alcohol enhances the sedative effects in anticholinergics.
- Atropine should be used to treat symptomatic and not asymptomatic bradycardia.

Do You UNDERSTAND?

DIRECTIONS: Match the following appropriate responses in Column A
with the items listed in Column B.

Column A

_____ 1. May precipitate extrapyramidal effects
when taken with an anticholinergic.

_____ 2. May increase the anticholinergic effects
of anticholinergics.

_____ 3. Decrease(s) the absorption of
anticholinergics.

_____ 4. Increase(s) the sedative effects in
anticholinergics.

Column B

a. antacids

b. methotrimeprazine

c. alcohol

d. antihistamines

What IS a Dopaminergic?

Dopaminergics	Trade Names	Uses
amantadine hydrochloride [a-MAN-ta-deen]	Symmetrel	Treatment of Parkinson's disease and drug-induced extra-pyramidal symptoms
bromocriptine mesylate [BROE-moe-KRIP-teen MEH-sih-LATE]	Parlodel	Treatment of Parkinson's disease
carbidopa-levodopa [CAR-bih-doe-puh]	Sinemet Sinemet-CR Lodosyn	Treatment of Parkinson's disease
levodopa [LEE-voe-DOE-puh]	Dopar, Larodopa	Treatment of Parkinson's disease

Action

A variety of pharmacologic actions exist among the dopaminergic agents, but all
optimize the availability of dopamine in the brain. Levodopa is a metabolic precursor of dopamine. Amantidine releases dopamine from dopaminergic neurons.
Amantidine also has antiviral properties and is used to treat symptoms that are
associated with influenza A. Bromocriptine, pramipexole, ropinirole, and pergolide are dopamine agonists. Selegiline inhibits the enzyme that degrades
dopamine.

Uses

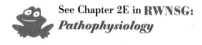

See Chapter 2E in **RWNSG:**
Pathophysiology

Dopaminergics are used to treat Parkinson's disease. This disease is progressive
and chronic, involving the areas of the brain that control balance, posture, and
coordination. Three primary symptoms that are observed in Parkinson's disease
include rigidity, tremors, and slow movements (**bradykinesia**). These symptoms

result because of a deficiency of dopamine in the brain's extrapyramidal system and basal ganglia. Dopaminergic nerves are either degenerated or a depletion of the neurotransmitter stores occurs.

Levodopa is a common, primary dopaminergic that is used to treat Parkinson's disease because it is identical to the chemical in the body, called dihydroxyphenylalanine (DOPA). The enzyme DOPA decarboxylase converts to dopamine. One way to enhance the effects of levodopa without increasing the dose is to administer the drug in a preparation combined with carbidopa, which inhibits DOPA decarboxylase in the GI tract. This inhibition prevents the conversion of levodopa to dopamine before the latter reaches the brain, thus more dopamine becomes available in the brain. Some of the dopaminergics are ineffective alone, thus they are used only as adjuncts to levodopa. These adjunctive agents include bromocriptine, pergolide, and selegiline.

What You NEED TO KNOW

Contraindications/Precautions

Administration of dopaminergics is also contraindicated within 2 weeks of administering MAOIs. Amantidine should be avoided in patients with a history of seizures because it may precipitate seizure activity.

Drug Interactions

Several agents interact with dopaminergics. Anticholinergics may increase the anticholinergic effects of amantidine. Alcohol may increase CNS depression caused by dopaminergics.

MAOIs may precipitate a hypertensive crisis, particularly with levodopa and levodopa-carbidopa. Pyridoxine, MAOIs, benzodiazepines, phenytoin, and phenothiazines antagonize the effects of levodopa. Butyrophenones, metoclopramide, and phenothiazines antagonize the effects of the dopaminergic agents, bromocriptine, pramipexole, ropinirole, and pergolide. Selegiline with opioids may result in possible life-threatening reactions, including excitation, sweating, rigidity, hypertension, hypotension, and coma.

Adverse Effects

A variety of adverse effects may occur with dopaminergics. All of the dopaminergics may become toxic and produce CNS effects, such as involuntary movements, ataxia, twitching, confusion, delusions, depression, hallucinations, and agitation. Dopaminergics may also produce cardiovascular effects, including orthostatic hypotension, rhythm disturbances, and palpitations. Additionally, dopaminergics frequently cause a dry mouth. Levodopa or carbidopa-levodopa may cause blurred vision, mydriasis, leukopenia, and hemolytic anemia. Amantidine may precipitate seizure activity in patients with a history of seizures.

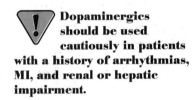

Dopaminergics should be used cautiously in patients with a history of arrhythmias, MI, and renal or hepatic impairment.

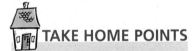

TAKE HOME POINTS

- Consumption of alcohol or other depressants with a dopaminergic drug increases CNS depression, thus these drug combinations should be avoided.
- When selegiline is taken with opioids, life-threatening reactions may result.

What You DO

Nursing Responsibilities

The doses of dopaminergics that are metabolized by the liver and eliminated by the kidneys should be decreased in patients with either hepatic or renal failure. When administering dopaminergics, the nurse should:

- Assess possible extrapyramidal and parkinsonian symptoms before initiating dopaminergics and throughout therapy. Symptoms include akinesia, tremors, rigidity, shuffling gait, twisting motions, and drooling. Worsening of symptoms may indicate drug toxicity.
- Monitor the patient's BP for hypotension, particularly when the patient rises to a standing position.
- Warn patients to make postural changes slowly.
- Monitor complete blood counts, including white blood cell counts, hemoglobin and hematocrit, in patients who are taking either levodopa or carbidopa-levodopa because these agents may cause leukopenia and hemolytic anemia.
- Instruct patients to avoid driving or any activity that requires alertness until the sedative response is determined.
- Advise patients who are taking dopaminergics to avoid alcohol and other depressants.
- Inform patients to avoid abrupt discontinuation of dopaminergics because sudden parkinsonian symptoms may occur.
- Instruct patients to report any symptoms of mental changes or dizziness, thus doses may be decreased.

TAKE HOME POINTS

- When administering dopaminergics, monitor for postural hypotension.
- Levodopa or carbidopa-levodopa may cause leukopenia or hemolytic anemia, thus complete blood counts should be monitored.

Do You UNDERSTAND?

DIRECTIONS: **Indicate in the space provided whether each statement is**
true or _false_.

_____ 1. Dopaminergics optimize the availability of dopamine in the brain.

_____ 2. Selegiline inhibits the enzyme that degrades dopamine.

_____ 3. Bromocriptine is used as a single agent to treat Parkinson's disease.

_____ 4. Amantidine is a metabolic precursor of dopamine.

Answers: 1. true; 2. true; 3. false; 4. false.

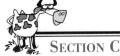

SECTION C

CNS STIMULANTS AND SKELETAL MUSCLE RELAXANTS

This section reviews pharmacologic agents that stimulate the CNS and relax skeletal muscles. Some CNS stimulants can produce severe psychologic dependence. The Controlled Substances Act of 1970 classifies these drugs as schedule II drugs. Continuous use of CNS stimulants may lead to drug tolerance and dependence.

CNS stimulants are used in the treatment of narcolepsy and obesity, as well as attention-deficit/hyperactivity disorder (ADHD) (attention-deficit disorder [ADD] or hyperkinetic syndrome). The medications that are discussed in this section include psychomotor stimulants, anorexiants, analeptics, centrally acting muscle relaxants, and peripherally acting muscle relaxants. Xanthines (e.g., theophylline) are also CNS stimulants. However, prescription use of xanthines as CNS stimulants is rare, thus xanthines will be discussed in Chapter 6, Section C as a treatment of respiratory disorders.

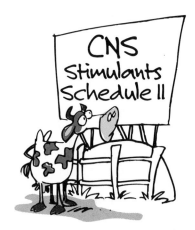

What IS a Psychomotor Stimulant?

Psychomotor Stimulants	Trade Names	Uses
amphetamine sulfate [am-FET-uh-meen]	Adderall	Treatment of narcolepsy and ADHD
dextroamphetamine sulfate [DEX-troe-am-FET-uh-meen]	Dexedrine	Treatment of narcolepsy and ADHD
Methylphenidate [meth-ill-FEN-ih-date]	Ritalin	Treatment of narcolepsy and ADHD

Action

Psychomotor stimulants affect the CNS. These drugs cause a release of brain neurotransmitters involving serotonin, dopamine, and norepinephrine. Small doses of amphetamines tend to act selectively to increase alertness, concentration, metabolism, improve motor performance, elevate mood, decrease perception of fatigue, reduce appetite, and stimulate the respiratory and cardiovascular systems. Large doses of amphetamines tend to stimulate the entire CNS and produce restlessness, insomnia, tremors, and motor performance deterioration. By exerting a direct blocking action on central receptors for serotonin, psychomotor stimulants affect the individual psychologically by increasing initiative and self-confidence. Physiologic effects include systolic and diastolic BP elevation, bronchial relaxation, increased sphincter tone in urinary bladder, increased peristalsis, and suppressed rapid eye movement (REM) sleep.

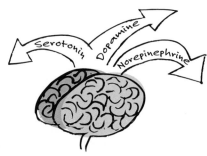

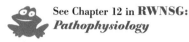

See Chapter 12 in **RWNSG**: *Pathophysiology*

Methylphenidate is used in treating ADHD in children and narcolepsy in adults. Pemoline is a schedule IV controlled drug and is used only in treating ADHD in children.

Psychomotor stimulants are contraindicated for women during pregnancy and lactation. Psychomotor stimulants are not recommended for children under 6 years of age for ADHD or in children under 12 years of age for appetite suppression.

Caution must be taken when administering amphetamines to older patients with malnutrition, restlessness, insomnia, or diabetes mellitus.

When initiating drug administration or in subsequent titrations, extended-release or resin preparations should not be used.

TAKE HOME POINTS

Instruct the patient that meticulous oral hygiene with gentle brushing of the tongue is required because decreased saliva may lead to demineralization of tooth surfaces and oral mucosal erosion.

Uses

The therapeutic uses of amphetamines include treatment of narcolepsy, exogenous obesity, and ADHD.

What You NEED TO KNOW

Contraindications/Precautions

Psychomotor stimulants are contraindicated for patients with hypertension, cardiovascular disease, anxiety, agitation, glaucoma, psychopathologic disorders, hyperthyroidism, and Gilles de la Tourette's syndrome. These agents are contraindicated for patients with suicidal tendencies or those who are homicidal. These agents are also contraindicated during or within 14 days of MAOI therapy.

Drug Interactions

When amphetamines are taken concurrently with adrenergic or tricyclic antidepressants, the adrenergic effects are intensified. Taking MAOIs and phenothiazines together with amphetamines can lead to a hypertensive crisis. The effects of antihypertensives may be antagonized when given with amphetamines. Phenothiazines decrease the effect of amphetamines. When amphetamines are taken with anticonvulsants, the anticonvulsant effects are delayed. Psychomotor stimulants cause an alteration in insulin requirements. Acid urine promotes drug elimination, and when the urine is alkaline (promoted by cranberry juice consumption), reabsorption is promoted and the drug action is prolonged.

Adverse Effects

Adverse effects of amphetamines include irritability, restlessness, nervousness, anxiety, headache, perceptual disturbances, hallucinations, euphoria, insomnia, tremors, and hyperactive reflexes. GI adverse effects include dry mouth, metallic taste, anorexia, nausea, vomiting, abdominal cramps, diarrhea, and constipation. More serious adverse effects include cardiac stimulation, angina, palpitations, tachycardia, hypertension, dysrhythmias, seizures, psychosis, and hepatic failure.

What You DO

Nursing Responsibilities

After the dose of psychomotor stimulant is stabilized, the extended-release preparations are safe and convenient. The first dose of the day should be administered early in the day and the last dose given no later than 6 hours before bedtime to avoid insomnia. When administering psychomotor stimulants, the nurse should:

• Instruct patients to rinse the mouth frequently with clear water and increase fluid intake to prevent dryness.

Instruct patients to avoid using psychomotor stimulants to overcome fatigue and sleep deficit (e.g., students studying for tests, athletes, or long-distance drivers). The stimulating drug effect masks fatigue. After the exhilaration has disappeared, fatigue and depression are usually greater than previously experienced, requiring a longer rest period.

Inform patients that use of these drugs may impair the ability to engage in hazardous activities, such as operating an automobile or machinery.

Warn patients to anticipate that height and weight suppression occurs as a result of appetite suppression.

• Monitor liver function for early detection of hepatic failure.

• Monitor glucose in patients with diabetes who are taking psychomotor stimulants for potential dose adjustments of insulin.

Instruct patients to avoid concurrent intake of caffeine and psychomotor stimulants to prevent intensified effects.

• Interrupt therapy periodically to evaluate the patient's need for continued drug use and to allow for normal growth and development. Prolonged therapy is inappropriate because of a potential risk of drug tolerance with long-term usage.

Do You UNDERSTAND?

DIRECTIONS: Place checks next to the descriptions that demonstrate adverse effects of psychomotor stimulants.

_____ a. Shaking (tremors)

_____ b. Coughing

_____ c. Opening door to bathroom

_____ d. Drinking large glass of water

_____ e. Sleeping soundly

 Children should be given psychomotor stimulants after meals to minimize appetite suppression and interference with nutrition and growth.

 TAKE HOME POINTS

Psychomotor stimulants should be gradually withdrawn after prolonged use to avoid profound depression or other psychopathologic conditions that may last several weeks

Closely monitor children who are taking psychomotor stimulants because long-term effects are unknown. Older patients are likely to experience mental confusion, anxiety, nervousness, and insomnia from psychomotor stimulants.

What IS an Anorexiant?

Anorexiants	Trade Names	Uses
diethylpropion [die-ETH-uhl-PRO-pee-ahn]	Tepanil	Treatment of exogenous obesity
benzphetamine [benz-FET-uh-meen]	Didrex	Treatment of exogenous obesity
mazindol [MAY-zin-dole]	Sanorex	Treatment of exogenous obesity
phenmetrazine [fen-MET-ra-zeen]	Preludin	Treatment of exogenous obesity

Action

The action of anorexiants is unknown, but they are thought to stimulate the satiety center in the hypothalamus. Appetite receptors in the satiety center respond specifically to hunger messages and trigger a feeling of fullness, reducing the need to consume food.

Uses

 See Chapter 12 in **RWNSG:** *Pathophysiology*

Anorexiants are used for short-term treatment in the adjunctive management of exogenous obesity. Adjunctive treatment modalities include exercise, diet, and behavior modification.

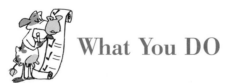

What You NEED TO KNOW

Contraindications/Precautions

 Anorexiants are contraindicated for patients with hypersensitivity, glaucoma, severe cardiovascular disease, hyperthyroidism, and agitation.

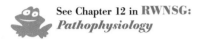 Anorexiants are contra-indicated for children under 12 years of age.

Drug Interactions

Drug interaction between anorexiants and insulin leads to a reduction of insulin requirements. When anorexiants are given concurrently with guanethidine, the hypotensive effect of guanethidine is decreased. When given concurrently or within 14 days of MAOIs, a hypertensive crisis may be triggered. Other CNS depressants (e.g., alcohol, general anesthetics) create an intensified effect to anorexiants.

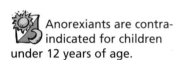 **Caution should be taken in older adults who require anorexiant therapy.**

Adverse Effects

Adverse effects of anorexiants include dyspnea, restlessness, vomiting, diarrhea, menstrual irregularities, and rash. Cardiovascular related adverse effects include dizziness, fatigue, palpitations, tachycardia, hypertension, and dysrhythmias. Psychologically related adverse effects include euphoria, insomnia, confusion, depression, and psychosis.

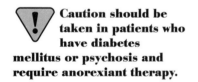 **Caution should be taken in patients who have diabetes mellitus or psychosis and require anorexiant therapy.**

What You DO

Nursing Responsibilities

A single anorexiant dose is usually taken mid-morning or mid-afternoon, depending on the patient's eating habits. Anorexiants should be given on an empty stomach, approximately 30 to 60 minutes before meals. To avoid insomnia, the daily dose should be administered no later than 6 hours before bedtime.

When administering anorexiants, the nurse should:

- Teach the patient who is taking anorexiants about safety from potential dizziness.
- Carefully monitor patients with diabetes who are taking both insulin and an anorexiant because dose adjustments may be necessary.
- Inform the patient that the anorexiant effect is temporary and seldom lasts more than a few weeks. Because this tolerance may occur, short-term use is appropriate.
- Inform the patient that a potential exists for dependence on these drugs.
- Inform the patient that abrupt withdrawal of the drug following prolonged high doses may result in GI distress, abdominal cramping, tremors, extreme fatigue, and mental depression.

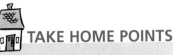

TAKE HOME POINTS

Warn patients to avoid driving any vehicle or operating hazardous machinery until the reaction to the drug is determined. Anorexiant therapy should not exceed 12 weeks.

 Advise patient to avoid abrupt discontinuation of anorexiants.

Do You UNDERSTAND?

DIRECTIONS: **Match the appropriate phrase in Column A with the word(s) in Column B.**

Column A

____ 1. When given concurrently or within 14 days, this drug can trigger hypertensive crisis.

____ 2. Anorexiants typically cause this alteration in the heart rate.

____ 3. The best time of day to take an anorexiant.

Column B

a. Alcohol
b. MAOIs
c. Bradycardia
d. Tachycardia
e. Bedtime
f. Mid-morning

What IS an Analeptic?

Analeptics	Trade Names	Uses
caffeine [kaf-EEN]	Caffedrine Vivarin	Promotes mental alertness and wakefulness
doxapram [DOX-a-pram]	Dopram	Treatment of postanesthesia and drug-induced respiratory depression

Action

Analeptics release epinephrine and norepinephrine from the adrenal medulla, producing CNS stimulation. These agents (e.g., caffeine, doxapram) inhibit the phosphodiesterase enzyme, which results in higher concentrations of cyclic adenosine monophosphate (cAMP). In small doses, caffeine stimulates the cerebral cortex, reducing drowsiness and fatigue while increasing awareness. Higher doses stimulate respiratory, medullary, vasomotor, and vagal centers. The peak time of caffeine effects is 15 to 45 minutes.

Answers: 1. b; 2. d; 3. f.

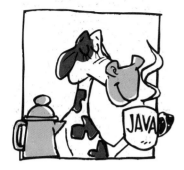

Uses

Analeptics are used as mild CNS stimulants to restore mental alertness and aid in remaining awake. Doxapram stimulates the CNS at all levels, but clinical use is generally for stimulating respirations. Doxapram promotes arousal and the return of pharyngeal and laryngeal reflexes and is generally used for short-term adjunctive therapy of respiratory depression from drugs or anesthesia. Caffeine is found in many beverages, such as coffee, tea, cola, and chocolate. Caffeine is also an ingredient in many OTC headache medications (e.g., Anacin, Excedrin).

What You NEED TO KNOW

Contraindications/Precautions

Caffeine is contraindicated for patients with depression, duodenal ulcers, and diabetes mellitus. Doxapram is contraindicated for patients with seizures, flail chest, pneumothorax, acute chronic obstructive pulmonary disease (COPD), severe hypertension, coronary artery disease, head injury, and cerebral vascular accident (CVA).

Drug Interactions

Caffeine increases CNS effects when taken concurrently with cimetidine, ciprofloxacin, enoxacin, phenylpropanolamine, disulfiram, and oral contraceptives. Doxapram produces increased effects when given with anesthetics (e.g., halothane, cyclopropane, enflurane). When doxapram is given concurrently with MAOIs or sympathomimetics, hypertensive effects are increased. The effects of caffeine are reduced when taken while the patient is smoking. When caffeine is taken together with iron, it decreases the absorption of iron.

Adverse Effects

The adverse effects of analeptics include headache, dizziness, tachycardia, nausea, vomiting, and diarrhea. Additional adverse effects following caffeine use include restlessness, nervousness, insomnia, abdominal pain, and diuresis. Adverse effects of doxapram include flushing, disorientation, sweating, hyperactivity, increased reflexes, elevated BP, seizures, laryngospasm, and bronchospasm.

 Caffeine is contra-indicated for women during lactation.

Doxapram should be used with caution during pregnancy and lactation.

Doxapram should also be given cautiously to patients who have dysrhythmias, hyperthyroidism, pheochromocytoma, cerebral edema, increased intracranial pressure, peptic ulcers, and acute agitation.

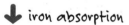 ↑ caffeine consumption = ↓ iron absorption

What You DO

Nursing Responsibilities

When administering analeptics, the nurse should:
* Delay doxapram treatment at least 10 minutes following discontinuation of anesthetics.

 Instruct patients to take iron at least 2 hours before or after caffeine in the form of coffee, tea, cola, and chocolate.

 Instruct patients that caffeine withdrawal effects include headache, anxiety, and increased muscle tension.

Do You UNDERSTAND?

DIRECTIONS: Provide appropriate responses to the following statements.

1. List three beverages that contain caffeine.

_____

_____

_____

2. List an OTC medication that contains caffeine.

_____

3. State the peak time for caffeine effects.

_____

4. List at least three adverse effects of analeptics or caffeine.

_____

_____

_____

What IS a Centrally Acting Muscle Relaxant?

Central Muscle Relaxants	Trade Names	Uses
cyclobenzaprine [SIGH-kloe-BEN-zuh-preen]	Flexeril	Treatment of muscle spasms
baclofen [BACK-low-fen]	Lioresal	Treatment of muscle spasms
carisoprodol [car-eye-so-PRO-dole]	Soma	Treatment of muscle spasms and rigidity
chlorzoxazone [klor-ZOX-uh-zone]	Parafon Forte	Treatment of muscle spasms and pain
methocarbamol [meth-oh-CAR-buh-mahl]	Robaxin	Treatment of muscle spasms

Action

The exact action of centrally acting muscle relaxants is unknown. However, these drugs are thought to produce CNS depression of the thalamus, brainstem, basal ganglia, and spinal cord. These agents may also block nerve impulses that lead to increased skeletal muscle tone and contraction.

Answers: 1. coffee, tea, cola; 2. Anacin or Excedrin; 3. 15 to 45 minutes; 4. headache, dizziness, tachycardia, nausea, vomiting, diarrhea, restlessness, nervousness, insomnia, abdominal pain, diuresis, flushing, disorientation, sweating, hyperactivity, increased reflexes and BP, seizures, laryngospasm, and bronchospasm.

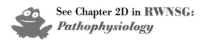
See Chapter 2D in RWNSG: *Pathophysiology*

Uses

Centrally acting muscle relaxants are used primarily to reduce muscle spasms. Baclofen inhibits neurotransmission at the spinal level and is used in the management of detrusor sphincter incoordination that is associated with spinal cord disease and reduction of severe spasticity of multiple sclerosis or cerebral palsy.

What You NEED TO KNOW

Contraindications/Precautions

Centrally acting muscle relaxants are contra-indicated for children under 12 years of age and for women during pregnancy or lactation.

Centrally acting muscle relaxants are contraindicated for patients with porphyria (a rare inherited disorder of porphyrin metabolism).

Drug Interactions

Centrally acting muscle relaxants are used with caution in patients with impaired liver or kidney function.

When alcohol, antihistamines, CNS depressants, or MAOIs are taken concurrently with central muscle relaxants, the interaction intensifies CNS depression. Intensified CNS depression increases the risk of hepatotoxicity. Drug interaction with MAOIs and centrally acting muscle relaxants may also lead to a hypertensive crisis. When orphenadrine and propoxyphene are taken together, the patient may experience increased confusion, anxiety, and tremors. An increased hypotensive effect occurs when centrally acting muscle relaxants are taken together with antihypertensives.

Adverse Effects

Adverse effects from centrally acting muscle relaxants include visual disturbances, headache, dizziness, hypotension, weakness, fatigue, drowsiness, ataxia, nervousness, irritability, dry mouth, taste alterations, nausea, vomiting, diarrhea or constipation, and urinary retention. The adverse effects of tizanidine include hallucinations, bradycardia, and prolonged Q-T intervals. Baclofen may cause nasal congestion, slurred speech, confusion, tinnitus, nystagmus, anorexia, abdominal pain, dysuria, muscle stiffness, urgency, and male sexual dysfunction.

What You DO

Nursing Responsibilities

TAKE HOME POINTS

Assist with or supervise ambulation because the initial loss of spasticity may affect the patient's ability to stand or walk.

Centrally acting muscle relaxants should be discontinued over a 2-week or greater period. Abrupt withdrawal after prolonged administration leads to anxiety, agitation, tachycardia, seizures, hallucinations, and exacerbation of spasticity. When administering centrally acting muscle relaxants, the nurse should:

- Administer the drug with food or milk when the patient experiences GI distress.

- Institute safety measures to compensate for the potential of causing drowsiness in the patient.
- Warn the patient to avoid driving or operating hazardous equipment until the response to the drug is known.
- Warn the patient that CNS depression is intensified by alcohol.
- Monitor liver function for early detection of hepatotoxicity.
- Instruct the patient to report drowsiness, dizziness, or ataxia because most of these adverse effects can be decreased by dose reduction.
- Inform the patient that centrally acting muscle relaxant drugs may elevate blood glucose levels, necessitating dose adjustments in oral hypoglycemics and insulin.

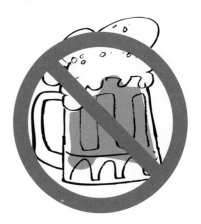

Older patients are especially sensitive to centrally acting muscle relaxants and may develop confusion, depression, and hallucinations.

Do You UNDERSTAND?

DIRECTIONS: **Indicate in the space provided whether each statement is** *true* **or** *false.*

_____ 1. Centrally acting muscle relaxants are used in the treatment of spasticity in patients with multiple sclerosis or cerebral palsy.

_____ 2. Alcohol exacerbates this drug class and relaxes muscles but stimulates the CNS.

_____ 3. When discontinuing centrally acting muscle relaxants, they should be tapered over a 4-day period.

What IS a Peripherally Acting Muscle Relaxant?

Peripheral Muscle Relaxants	Trade Names	Uses
dantrolene [dan-troe-LEEN]	Dantrium	Treatment of spasticity associated with spinal cord injury, CVA, cerebral palsy, and multiple sclerosis
quinine [KWIE-nine]	Quinamm Quiphile	Prevention and treatment of nocturnal leg cramps

Action

Peripherally acting muscle relaxants exert their actions in different methods. Dantrolene inhibits calcium release from sarcoplasmic reticulum, thereby reducing muscle contractility. Quinine acts similarly to salicylates and exerts a curarelike skeletal muscle relaxation.

Uses

Dantrolene is used in the management of spasticity from upper motor neuron (UMN) disorders, spinal cord, or cerebral disease, as well as perioperative management of malignant hyperthermia. Quinine is used primarily in the treatment of nocturnal leg cramps.

See Chapter 2D in RWNSG: *Pathophysiology*

Answers: 1. true; 2. false; alcohol exacerbates CNS depression; 3. false; taper over 2 weeks or more.

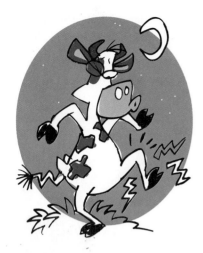

 Peripherally acting muscle relaxants are contra-indicated for women during pregnancy and lactation and for children under 5 years of age.

 What You NEED TO KNOW

Contraindications/Precautions

Peripherally acting muscle relaxants are contraindicated for patients with hepatic dysfunction.

Drug Interactions

CNS depression is intensified when alcohol and CNS depressants are taken concurrently with dantrolene. The interaction of estrogens and dantrolene leads to an increased risk of hepatotoxicity. When calcium channel blockers are taken with dantrolene, an increased risk of ventricular fibrillation occurs. Quinine increases the effects of oral anticoagulants, digoxin, anticholinergics, and neuromuscular blockers. Anticonvulsants, barbiturates, and rifampin increase the metabolism of quinine, reducing its effectiveness. Conversely, sodium bicarbonate, carbonic anhydrase inhibitors, and antacids decrease quinine excretion, increasing the risk of toxicity.

Peripherally acting muscle relaxants are used with caution in patients with impaired cardiac or pulmonary function and those over the age of 35, particularly women.

Adverse Effects

Adverse effects of peripherally acting muscle relaxants include headache, dizziness, euphoria, blurred vision, confusion, tachycardia, severe itching, hives, nausea, vomiting, and diarrhea. The specific adverse effects of dantrolene include nervousness, insomnia, weakness, speech disturbances, photophobia, urinary frequency or retention, nocturnal diuresis, erectile dysfunction, depression, and seizures. Prolonged high doses of dantrolene can lead to hepatotoxicity. Specific adverse effects of quinine use include anxiety, fever, rash, tinnitus, ototoxicity, angina, acute asthmatic episodes, blood dyscrasias, hypothermia, cardiovascular collapse, coma, and death.

 What You DO

Nursing Responsibilities

When administering peripherally acting muscle relaxants, the nurse should:
- Monitor IV administration carefully to avoid extravasation because the IV solution is extremely irritating to the tissues.
- Monitor liver function studies for early detection of hepatotoxicity.
- Monitor coagulation studies resulting from the interaction with warfarin.
- Instruct the patient who is concurrently taking oral anticoagulants to report increased bruising or bleeding.
- Monitor digoxin levels resulting from a drug interaction with quinine.

 TAKE HOME POINTS

Carefully monitor digoxin levels in the patient who is concurrently taking quinine.

Do You UNDERSTAND?

DIRECTIONS: Fill in the blanks with appropriate responses.

1. Identify two spasticity disorders in which peripherally acting muscle relaxants might be used as a treatment.

_____

2. List the disorder for which quinine therapy is used.

_____

Section D
ANTICONVULSANTS

This section reviews drugs that manage seizure disorders. The primary aim of treatment is seizure control. The two types of seizure disorders include isolated events as observed in a febrile illness and recurrent events, such as in epilepsy. Anticonvulsant drugs decrease the excess firing, inhibit the spread of nerve impulses, and elevate the seizure threshold, thereby promoting the stabilization of abnormal brain cells. No single drug is available that controls all types of seizures; drug choice is individualized for each patient. This section explains the various anticonvulsant medications, which include hydantoins, barbiturates, benzodiazepines, succinimides, valproic acid, carbamazepine, and gabapentins.

What IS a Hydantoin?

Hydantoins	Trade Names	Uses
phenytoin [FEN-ih-toyn]	Dilantin	Controls grand mal and psychomotor seizures
mephenytoin [me-FEN-ih-toyn]	Mesantoin	Controls grand mal, psychomotor, focal, and jacksonian seizures

Action

The mechanism of action in anticonvulsants is not completely known. Theories suggest that anticonvulsants stabilize neuronal membranes and limit the spread of neuronal or seizure activity. Hydantoins appear to act on the motor cortex. Anticonvulsants inhibit seizure activity by promoting sodium outward flow (efflux) from neurons and inhibiting the production of repetitive action potentials at synapses. Because hyperexcitability is a result of excessive stimulation or environmental changes, which reduces the membrane sodium gradient, hydantoins tend to stabilize the hyperexcitability threshold. Hydantoins lower the activity of brain stem centers, which controls the tonic phase of grand mal seizures.

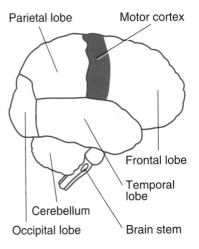

Parietal lobe
Motor cortex
Frontal lobe
Temporal lobe
Cerebellum
Occipital lobe
Brain stem

Answers: UMN disorders, spinal cord or cerebral disease; 2. nocturnal leg cramps.

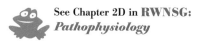

See Chapter 2D in **RWNSG:**
Pathophysiology

Uses

Hydantoins are used primarily to control grand mal (tonic-clonic) and psychomotor seizures. Phenytoin is the oldest and most well known of the hydantoins. Phenytoin remains one of the most effective and commonly used anticonvulsants. Phenytoin is also used in the prevention and treatment of seizures in patients who are undergoing neurosurgery and has been effective in controlling status epilepticus. Because of their efficacy, hydantoins are used in all age groups. In addition to controlling grand mal and psychomotor seizures, mephenytoin is used to control focal or jacksonian seizures.

What You NEED TO KNOW

Hydantoins are contra-
indicated for pregnant
and nursing women.

Contraindications/Precautions

Hydantoins are contraindicated for patients with hypersensitivity. Ethotoin is contraindicated for patients with hepatic and hematologic disorders. Phenytoin is contraindicated for patients with sinus bradycardia, sinoatrial block, second- and third-degree atrioventricular block, and Adams-Stokes syndrome.

Drug Interactions

Several drugs interact adversely with hydantoins, particularly phenytoin. Prolonged use of acetaminophen together with hydantoins may increase the risk of hepatotoxicity. Because hydantoin anticonvulsants may increase serum glucose concentrations, the possibility of hyperglycemia exists for patients who are receiving antiglycemic agents. Therefore these individuals may require medication adjustments. Concurrent use of antacids may affect the efficacy of phenytoin.

TAKE HOME POINTS

Carefully monitor patients with cardiac function impairment, such as Stokes-Adams, second- and third-degree atrioventricular block, sinoatrial node block, and sinus bradycardia because of the antiarrhythmic effect of phenytoin.

Adverse Effects

Hydantoins have varying degrees of adverse effects. The most frequent adverse effects include constipation, headache, dizziness, drowsiness, nausea, vomiting, diarrhea, and enlargement of facial features. Other adverse effects occurring at high plasma levels include CNS toxicity including ataxia, confusion, nystagmus, slurred speech, stuttering, trembling of hands, excitement, nervousness, irritability, and gingival hyperplasia. Peripheral neuropathies and blood dyscrasias (e.g., agranulocytosis) are rare adverse effects.

Adverse effects are more likely to occur in the geriatric population compared with the younger populations.

TAKE HOME POINTS

Although rare, the occurrence of blood dyscrasias may be a significant adverse effect of treatment.

What You DO

Nursing Responsibilities

Anticonvulsants are usually administered orally; however, some of the hydantoins may be given IM or IV in emergency situations. When administering hydantoins, the nurse should:

- Monitor periodic blood studies to ensure therapeutic plasma levels, particularly in the initial stages of therapy.
- Observe the patient closely for possible adverse reactions to anticonvulsants, particularly at the initiation of therapy.
- Monitor periodic hepatic and hematologic laboratory studies to identify potential adverse reactions.
- Provide clear and accurate information for the proper use of hydantoins, thus patients can self-administer their medication successfully and achieve seizure control. The proper dose, compliance with therapy, and taking medications as prescribed are three important aspects of therapy.
- Teach the patient the proper way to address missed doses of medication. The patient should be advised to contact the health care provider when doses are missed for 2 or more days in a row.
- Advise the patient on precautions (e.g., older patients tend to metabolize hydantoins slowly). Other medication should not be taken concurrently, nor should the brand or dose forms of phenytoin be changed without contacting the health care provider.
- Instruct patients to avoid alcoholic beverages and other CNS depressants when taking hydantoins.
- Advise the patient to avoid abrupt discontinuation of the medication. A gradual dose reduction is required to maintain seizure control and should be designed by the health care provider.
- Instruct patients to take oral hydantoin immediately after meals to lessen gastric irritation.
- Provide the patient with information on obtaining MedicAlert information.

TAKE HOME POINTS

Monitor laboratory tests for therapeutic hydantoin levels, hepatic function, and hematologic status. Instruct patients that if a dose is omitted, the next dose should not be doubled. Impress on the patient the importance of avoiding abrupt discontinuation of the medication.

Older patients tend to metabolize hydantoins slowly, increasing the potential for toxic serum levels. Older patients frequently require decreased doses and subsequent dose adjustment.

Do You UNDERSTAND?

DIRECTIONS: Indicate in the space provided whether the statement is *true* or *false.*

_____ 1. Hydantoins are used to control petit mal and psychomotor seizures.

_____ 2. Adverse effects are more likely to occur in the geriatric population.

_____ 3. Older patients frequently require higher doses of hydantoins because of this population's metabolism.

_____ 4. Hydantoins should not be discontinued abruptly.

What IS a Barbiturate?

Barbiturates	Trade Names	Uses
phenobarbital [fee-noe-BAR-bi-tal]	Luminal	Long-term treatment of grand mal and partial seizures; controls status epilepticus, eclampsia, and febrile convulsions in children

Continued

Answers: 1. false; 2. true; 3. false; 4. true.

Barbiturates—cont'd	Trade Names	Uses
mephobarbital [me-foe-BAR-bi-tal]	Mebaral	Controls grand mal and petit mal seizures
metharbital [Meth-ARE-bi-tal]	Gemonil	Controls grand mal and petit mal seizures

Action

Phenobarbital was the first widely effective, long-acting antiepileptic drug. The primary anticonvulsant mechanism is the decrease of nerve transmission and excitability of the nerve cell. Barbiturates also increase the threshold for electrical stimulation of the motor cortex.

Uses

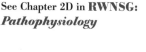

See Chapter 2D in **RWNSG:** *Pathophysiology*

Barbiturates are indicated in long-term anticonvulsant therapy for the treatment of generalized tonic-clonic seizures and simple-partial seizures. Mephobarbital and metharbital are indicated as alternatives to phenobarbital. Although other more effective, selective, and less sedating anticonvulsants are available, barbiturates may still be used because of their efficacy in seizure reduction.

What You NEED TO KNOW

Contraindications/Precautions

Barbiturates are contraindicated for patients with hypersensitivity, severe respiratory dysfunction, renal impairment, or those with a history of porphyria.

Drug Interactions

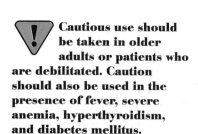

Cautious use should be taken in older adults or patients who are debilitated. Caution should also be used in the presence of fever, severe anemia, hyperthyroidism, and diabetes mellitus.

Several drugs interact with barbiturates. The effects of anticoagulants may be decreased when used concurrently with barbiturates. Bleeding may result when the barbiturate is discontinued, thus periodic monitoring of prothrombin time may be indicated. The concurrent use of another hydantoin anticonvulsant may result in its unpredictable metabolism. Barbiturates may also reduce the contraceptive reliability of estrogen-containing oral contraceptives. Alcohol or other CNS depressants may increase the depressant effect of either of the previously mentioned substances.

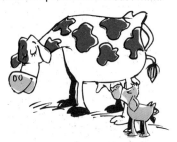

Barbiturates are contraindicated for women who are pregnant and lactating.

Barbiturates cross the placenta and are present in breast milk.

Adverse Effects

Barbiturates are depressants of both respiratory and GI motility, although the degree of depression is dose dependent. Common adverse effects include drowsiness, lethargy, vertigo, headache, and CNS depression. Withdrawal symptoms may occur after as little as 2 weeks of uninterrupted barbiturate therapy. Allergic reactions, exfoliative dermatitis, hallucinations, hypotension, and blood dyscrasias (e.g., agranulocytosis, thrombocytopenia) may occur in rare instances.

What You DO

Nursing Responsibilities

Barbiturates are administered orally, rectally, or parenterally. Emergency treatment of status epilepticus may require IV administration. When administering barbiturates, the nurse should:

- Monitor seizure activity for changes with regard to character, frequency, and duration.
- Warn the patient about concurrent use of other CNS depressants (e.g., analgesics, antihistamines, alcohol).
- Advise the patient to seek medical approval before taking OTC cold or allergy medications.
- Teach the patient about safety measures while taking barbiturates.
- Instruct the patient to avoid abrupt discontinuation of barbiturate therapy.
- Closely monitor respiratory function, CNS depression, and GI elimination.
- Warn the patient about the potentially addictive nature of long-term barbiturate use.

Do You UNDERSTAND?

DIRECTIONS: **Indicate in the space provided whether the statement is**
true **or** *false.*

_____ 1. Mephobarbital was the first widely effective antiepileptic drug.

_____ 2. Phenobarbital is a long-acting barbiturate that is indicated for long-term anticonvulsant therapy.

_____ 3. Older patients may react to barbiturate therapy with depression.

_____ 4. Medical approval is unnecessary for OTC cold or allergy medications.

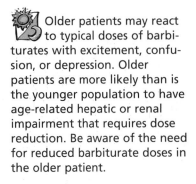

Older patients may react to typical doses of barbiturates with excitement, confusion, or depression. Older patients are more likely than is the younger population to have age-related hepatic or renal impairment that requires dose reduction. Be aware of the need for reduced barbiturate doses in the older patient.

TAKE HOME POINTS

- To ensure safe use of barbiturates for seizure management, the nurse must know which barbiturates have anticonvulsive actions at subhypnotic doses.
- Female patients who are taking estrogen-containing oral contraceptives should be advised to use an additional alternative method of birth control for the duration of barbiturate treatment.

 Barbiturates have an addictive nature with long-term use.

What IS a Benzodiazepine?

Benzodiazepine	Trade Names	Uses
lorazepam [lore-AZE-uh-pam]	Ativan	Treatment of status epilepticus
diazepam [DIE-aze-uh-pam]	Valium	Treatment of status epilepticus
clorazepate [klor-AZE-uh-PATE]	Tranxene	Treatment of partial seizures
clonazepam [kloe-NAY-ze-pam]	Klonopin	Treatment of absence, myoclonic, and akinetic seizures

Answers: 1. false; 2. true; 3. true; 4. false.

Action

Benzodiazepines act as CNS depressants that produce all levels of CNS depression, ranging from mild sedation to coma, depending on the dose. All benzodiazepines have both antiepileptic and anxiolytic properties that reduce seizures and anxiety.

Uses

Several of the benzodiazepines (e.g., diazepam, clonazepam, clorazepate, parenteral lorazepam) are used as anticonvulsants. Clorazepate and clonazepam are particularly useful in treating seizures that are difficult to control. Parenteral diazepam is the drug of choice in treating status epilepticus.

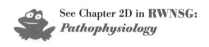

See Chapter 2D in **RWNSG:**
Pathophysiology

What You NEED TO KNOW

Contraindications/Precautions

Benzodiazepines are contraindicated for patients with acute narrow-angle glaucoma, coma, shock, and acute alcohol intoxication.

Drug Interactions

Concurrent use of antacids may delay the absorption of some benzodiazepines. Alcohol and other CNS depressants exacerbate benzodiazepines. Lorazepam and diazepam may increase the antiparkinsonism effects of levodopa. Benzodiazepines may increase phenytoin levels. Smoking decreases the antianxiety and sedative effects of lorazepam.

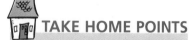 Benzodiazepines are contraindicated for pregnant and nursing women and for children under 12 years of age. Benzodiazepines should be used cautiously in older or debilitated patients.

Benzodiazepines should also be used cautiously in patients with renal or hepatic dysfunction, myasthenia gravis, GI disorders, and in those with suicidal tendencies.

Adverse Effects

The most common adverse effects include drowsiness, reduced mental and physical alertness, dizziness, visual disturbances, and cardiovascular irregularities. Constipation, nausea, and vomiting have also been noted. Prolonged use of benzodiazepines can cause physical dependency and result in withdrawal syndrome when they are discontinued. Symptoms of toxicity range from problems with short-term memory, confusion, and vertigo to bradycardia, ataxia, severe weakness, shortness of breath, and depression.

TAKE HOME POINTS

- Advise the patient to take antacids (when needed) at least 1 hour before or after the scheduled dose of benzodiazepines to ensure maximal drug absorption and effectiveness. Use of benzodiazepines results in reduced tolerance for alcohol, narcotics, antihistamines, MAOIs, analgesics, and other sedatives.
- All benzodiazepines have CNS depressant effects. Significant changes in BP and heart rate may indicate impending toxicity.

What You DO

Nursing Responsibilities

Diazepam and lorazepam may be given orally or parenterally. When giving diazepam by direct IV push, inject the drug slowly over at least 1 minute for every 5 milligrams. Because diazepam adheres to plastic infusion tubing, care must be taken during parenteral administration. Clorazepate and clonazepam are given orally. When administering benzodiazepines, the nurse should:

◆ Teach the patient the correct dose and administration schedule and the importance of taking the medication exactly as prescribed.

◆ Inform the patient of the potential for physical and psychologic dependence on benzodiazepines and the risk of withdrawal when these drugs are abruptly discontinued. Teach the patient to recognize signs and symptoms of benzodiazepine dependence and when to report them.

• Monitor renal and hepatic function periodically to assess adequate drug metabolism and excretion.

Do You UNDERSTAND?

DIRECTIONS: **Indicate in the space provided whether the statement is true or false.**

_____ 1. All benzodiazepines have either an antiepileptic or an anxiolytic property.

_____ 2. Parenteral diazepam is used for the treatment of status epilepticus.

_____ 3. The level of CNS depression with benzodiazepines is dose dependent.

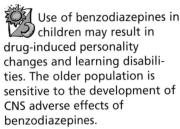 Use of benzodiazepines in children may result in drug-induced personality changes and learning disabilities. The older population is sensitive to the development of CNS adverse effects of benzodiazepines.

In the older population, lower-than-normal doses of benzodiazepines are required because of the development of CNS effects.

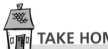 **TAKE HOME POINTS**

Administer IV diazepam as close as possible to the IV insertion site.

What IS a Succinimide?

Succinimides	Trade Names	Uses
ethosuximide [ETH-oh-SUX-ih-mide]	Zarontin	Treatment of petit mal seizures
methsuximide [meth-SUX-ih-mide]	Celontin	Treatment of petit mal seizures
phensuximide [fen-SUX-ih-mide]	Milontin	Treatment of petit mal seizures

Action

Succinimides depress nerve transmission in the motor cortex, thereby decreasing the frequency of petit mal seizures in children and adults. Succinimides also reduce the focal activity that produce spike and wave patterns on electroencephalograms (EEG) more effectively than does phenytoin. This action increases the seizure threshold and decreases seizure activity.

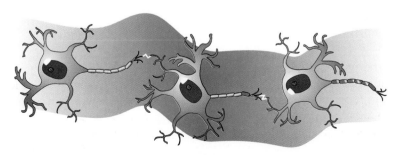

Answers: 1. true; 2. true; 3. true.

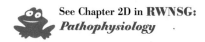
See Chapter 2D in **RWNSG:**
Pathophysiology

Uses

Succinimides are used in the treatment of petit mal seizures. Ethosuximide is the first drug of choice of the three succinimides. Methsuximide has a high risk of toxicity, and phensuximide is less effective than are the other succinimides.

What You NEED TO KNOW

Phensuximide should be used with caution in patients with acute intermittent porphyria.

Succinimides are contraindicated for women during pregnancy.

Contraindications/Precautions

Succinimides are contraindicated for patients with hypersensitivity, blood dyscrasias, severe renal and hepatic disease.

Drug Interactions

Only a few drug interactions are associated with the succinimides. When given concurrently with hydantoins, succinimides may increase hydantoin levels. Isoniazid may significantly increase ethosuximide levels when given together. Carbamazepine may decrease the concentration of a succinimide when given concurrently. When ethosuximide and phenobarbital are given together, the drug levels of both may be altered and may lead to increased seizure frequency. Valproic acid may increase or decrease succinimide levels when both drugs are given together.

Adverse Effects

Adverse effects following succinimide administration include GI effects of anorexia, nausea, vomiting, swollen tongue, weight loss, abdominal pain, constipation, and diarrhea. Neurologic adverse effects include alopecia, flushing, headache, inability to concentrate, drowsiness, dizziness, euphoria, restlessness, irritability, sleep disturbances, depression, night terrors, hyperactivity, aggressiveness, lethargy, confusion, and ataxia. Psychosis and suicidal ideation are rare adverse effects. GU adverse effects include vaginal bleeding, urinary frequency, hematuria, and albuminuria. Hematologic adverse effects involve leukopenia, thrombocytopenia, eosinophilia, agranulocytosis, aplastic anemia, and pancytopenia. Hypersensitivity reactions following succinimides include pruritic skin eruptions, exfoliative dermatitis, systemic lupus erythematosus (SLE), and Stevens-Johnson syndrome. Additional adverse effects from methsuximide therapy include renal and hepatic damage.

What You DO

Nursing Responsibilities

Liquid forms of succinimides should be stored at 59° to 86° F (15° to 30° C) in light-resistant containers. Capsules should be stored in air-tight containers. Suspensions should be shaken before administration. Adjustments in the succinimides dose must be made carefully and slowly. Succinimides are administered orally. Ethosuximide may be taken with food when GI distress occurs. When administering succinimides, the nurse should:

- Monitor serum succinimide drug level for a therapeutic effect. A normal serum level in adults ranges from 40 to 100 µ/cc.
- Monitor complete blood counts and signs of infection in patients who are taking succinimides to detect blood dyscrasias early.
- Instruct the patient to report any evidence of infection (e.g., sore throat) for early treatment of infection and detection of blood dyscrasias.
- Observe the patient who is taking succinimides closely for behavioral changes and report these changes to the health care provider. Succinimides should be withdrawn at the first signs of depression or aggression to prevent further psychosis.
- Instruct the patient to avoid abrupt discontinuation of the medication because abrupt withdrawal may precipitate seizures. A gradual dose-reduction schedule, designed by the health care provider, is required to maintain seizure control.
- Inform the patient that phensuximide may color the urine pink, red, or reddish-brown.
- Instruct the patient to avoid operating potentially hazardous machinery while undergoing succinimide therapy.
- Protect the patient who is taking succinimides when the mental status is altered through the use of safety precautions (e.g., side rails, low bed position, assistance with ambulation).

TAKE HOME POINTS

Instruct the patient to take succinimides with meals to reduce GI adverse effects.

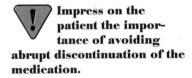

Impress on the patient the importance of avoiding abrupt discontinuation of the medication.

Do You UNDERSTAND?

DIRECTIONS: Indicate in the space provided whether the statement is *true* or *false*.

_____ 1. Mental depression is a common side effect of succinimide anticonvulsants.

_____ 2. When given together, succinimides increase the metabolism of hydantoin anticonvulsants.

_____ 3. Severe adverse effects following succinimides include Stevens-Johnson syndrome, SLE, and renal and hepatic damage.

What IS a Miscellaneous Anticonvulsant?

Miscellaneous Anticonvulsants	Trade Names	Uses
valproic acid [val-PROE-ic]	Depakote	Treatment of petit mal seizures
carbamazepine [kar-ba-MAZ-e-peen]	Tegretol	Treatment of grand mal or psychomotor seizures
gabapentin [GAB-uh-PEN-tin]	Neurontin	Adjunctive therapy in treatment of partial seizures

Answers: 1. false; euphoria is common; psychosis and suicidal ideation are rare; 2. false; succinimides may inhibit the metabolism of hydantoins; 3. true.

Action

A group of miscellaneous drugs, including valproic acid, carbamazepine, and gabapentin, are effective anticonvulsants and have different actions. Valproic acid inhibits the enzyme breakdown of gamma-aminobutyric acid (GABA) to a simpler form, thereby selectively increasing the concentration of GABA in the synapses, which reduces seizure activity. The increase of GABA decreases impulse transmission. Carbamazepine blocks sodium and calcium channels, which prevents the formation of repetitive action potentials in the abnormal focus, thereby reducing polysynaptic responses and blocking posttetanic potentiation. Gabapentin affects the transport of amino acids across neuronal membranes, which reduces seizure activity.

Uses

Valproic acid is approved for the treatment of simple and complex petit mal seizures. Effectiveness has also been demonstrated in mixed seizures, such as myoclonic and grand mal seizures. Carbamazepine is one of the drugs of choice that is used in the control of grand mal or focal seizures and trigeminal neuralgia. Carbamazepine is also effective in managing partial and mixed seizures. Gabapentin is used as adjunctive therapy for focal seizures.

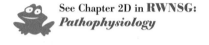

See Chapter 2D in **RWNSG:** *Pathophysiology*

Valproic acid is contraindicated for women during pregnancy and lactation. Valproic acid should be used with extreme caution in children under 2 years of age, particularly when they are undergoing multiple-combination anticonvulsant therapy. Additionally, caution should be used when administering valproic acid to patients who have congenital metabolic disorders, a history of severe seizures with accompanying mental retardation, or organic brain disease. This drug is strongly related to fatal hepatotoxicity, particularly in children under 2 years of age.

Gabapentin should be used cautiously in women during pregnancy and lactation and in children under 12 years of age. Carbamazepine and gabapentin should be given with caution to older patients.

What You NEED TO KNOW

Contraindications/Precautions

Valproic acid is contraindicated for patients with bleeding disorders and hepatic disease. Carbamazepine is contraindicated for patients with increased intraocular pressure, systemic lupus erythematosus (SLE), and hepatic or renal disease. These drugs are contraindicated for patients with hypersensitivity.

Drug Interactions

CNS depressants and alcohol increase the depressant effects when given concurrently with anticonvulsants. When these agents are administered with other anticonvulsants and barbiturates, anticonvulsant and barbiturate levels and the risk of toxicity are increased. When given with valproic acid, salicylates, chlorpromazine, erythromycin, felbamate, and cimetidine may increase valproic acid levels and toxicity. In addition to the anticonvulsant action, valproic acid inhibits the secondary phase of platelet aggregation. Therefore when valproic acid is administered concurrently with aspirin, dipyridamole, or warfarin, the risk of decreased clotting and spontaneous bleeding increases. When valproic acid is given with clonazepam, petit mal seizures may be exacerbated. Cholestyramine, rifampin, carbamazepine, topiramate, lamotrigine, and charcoal may decrease the absorption of valproic acid when given together.

When taken concurrently with oral contraceptives, carbamazepine increases the metabolism of estrogen, which decreases contraceptive effectiveness. When taken concurrently, other anticonvulsant serum concentrations may decrease because of increased metabolism. Carbamazepine decreases the hypoprothrombinemia effects of concurrent oral anticoagulants. Increased carbamazepine levels may result when this agent is taken with verapamil, erythromycin, ketoconazole, or nefazodone.

Gabapentin may cause an increase in phenytoin levels when given concurrently. Antacids reduce the absorption of gabapentin. Lamotrigine levels may be decreased when given with carbamazepine, phenytoin, phenobarbital, and primidone. Tiagabine levels may be decreased when given with carbamazepine, phenytoin, and phenobarbital. Increased CNS depression occurs when topiramate is taken together with alcohol and other CNS depressants. When given concurrently, carbamazepine, phenytoin, and valproic acid may decrease topiramate levels.

Adverse Effects

Common adverse effects of these agents include drowsiness, dizziness, weakness (asthenia), and incoordination (ataxia). Valproic acid appears to have a low incidence of adverse effects. Other adverse effects that may occur after valproic acid therapy include emotional upset, hallucinations, aggression, and prolonged bleeding. GI adverse effects from valproic acid include hypersalivation, anorexia or increased appetite, nausea, indigestion, vomiting, weight loss or gain, abdominal cramps, diarrhea, and constipation. Valproic acid may also cause skin rash, transient hair loss, curliness or waviness of hair, breakthrough seizures, tremors, amenorrhea, irregular menses, photosensitivity, hyperammonemia, and hepatic failure. Bone marrow depression may occur in the form of anemia, leukopenia, and thrombocytopenia.

When carbamazepine anticonvulsant drug therapy begins slowly and with gradually increasing dose increments, adverse effects are minor and tolerable. Adverse effects of carbamazepine include diplopia, nystagmus, increased intraocular pressure, headache, dry mouth, hives, tremors, urine retention, and constipation. Severe adverse effects include syncope, increased or decreased BP, dysrhythmias, MI, and congestive heart failure (CHF). Rare adverse effects involve hematologic toxicity with aplastic anemia, agranulocytosis, thrombocytopenia, leukopenia, Stevens-Johnson syndrome, hepatotoxicity, latent psychosis, and mental depression. In most patients, the adverse effects of carbamazepine usually disappear within 2 to 3 weeks after initiating therapy. Other adverse effects of gabapentin include blurred vision, slurred speech, headache, impaired concentration, weight gain, nystagmus, nausea, and vomiting.

What You DO

Nursing Responsibilities

These anticonvulsants are initially administered in small doses and gradually increased. Administration with meals enhances the absorption and decreases GI distress. Carbamazepine should be protected from heat and stored at 59° to 86° F (15° to 30° C). When administering miscellaneous anticonvulsants, the nurse should:

Valproic acid should be administered with caution to patients with renal disease or to those who are undergoing other anticonvulsant adjunctive therapy.

Carbamazepine should be administered with caution to patients with a history of cardiac disease.

Gabapentin should be given with caution to patients who are taking digoxin, other CNS depressants, or neuromuscular blocking agents, as well as to patients with impaired hepatic or renal function.

TAKE HOME POINTS

- Instruct the patient to avoid alcohol and OTC medications, particularly aspirin, sedatives, or allergy medications, to prevent exacerbating CNS depressant effects.
- Instruct women who are taking oral contraceptives to use an alternate form of birth control for the duration of their treatment with carbamazepine.

TAKE HOME POINTS

The patient may take anticonvulsants with food to decrease GI distress.

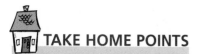

TAKE HOME POINTS

Emphasize the importance of avoiding abrupt discontinuation of the medication.

- Gradually initiate valproic acid therapy to minimize GI adverse effects. The therapeutic range for valproic acid is 50 to 100 μg/ml.
- Instruct the patient who is taking valproic acid to swallow capsules whole and to avoid chewing medication or taking the drug with carbonated drinks to avoid mouth and throat irritation.
- Frequently monitor the patient for early detection of neurologic toxicity.
- Monitor platelet counts, bleeding time, serum ammonia, and liver function tests at least every 2 months during the first 6 months of valproic acid therapy for the early detection of blood dyscrasias or hepatic dysfunction.
- Instruct the patient to report any fever, sore mouth or throat, unusual fatigue, spontaneous bleeding, bruising, nosebleeds, bleeding gums, rash, visual disturbances, jaundice, light-colored stools, vomiting, and diarrhea to the health care provider .
- Instruct the patient to avoid hazardous activities (e.g., driving) that require alertness until the drug response is known.
- Monitor laboratory test results for the patient taking carbamazepine for early detection of myelosuppression. The following results should be reported to the health care provider: hematocrit < 32%, hemoglobin < 11 g/dl, red blood cell count < 4 million/mm, reticulocyte count < 20,000/mm, white blood cell count < 4000/mm, platelet count < 100,000/mm, and serum iron > 150 μg/dl.
- Protect the patient when the mental status is altered through the use of safety precautions (e.g., side rails, low bed position, assistance with ambulation).
- Instruct the patient to avoid abrupt discontinuation of these drugs because this action may precipitate seizures, possibly status epilepticus. A gradual dose-reduction schedule designed by the health care provider is required to maintain seizure control.
- Instruct the patient to report signs of fluid retention, oliguria, and changes in BP or pulse patterns.
- Instruct the patient who is taking carbamazepine suspension to avoid taking the drug with any other liquid medication to prevent a precipitate forming in the stomach.
- Instruct the patient to avoid excessive sunlight or to use sunscreen with sun-protection-factor of 12 or above because photosensitivity reactions may occur.

Do You UNDERSTAND?

DIRECTIONS: Complete the following statements.

1. A _____ laboratory test should be initially monitored at least every 2 months when taking valproic acid.

2. Extra contraceptive precautions should be used to prevent pregnancy when taking _____.

3. Anticonvulsants should be discontinued _____.

Answers: 1. platelet counts; 2. carbamazepine; 3. gradually.

Section E
ANESTHETICS

This section reviews the pharmacologic agents that are used to produce anesthesia. Legally, only nurse anesthetists are permitted to administer anesthetic agents; however, other nurses should be aware of these agents and the effects on patients, primarily because these individuals will be providing nursing care in the perioperative period. Anesthetics are classified as local and general. Local anesthetics (**regional anesthesia**) block pain sensation in a limited region of the body but do not reduce consciousness. Local anesthetics are administered topically or by local infiltration into the tissues. A nerve block is a blockage of pain in a specific nerve of the body with local anesthetic agents. Blocking nerve transmission in the spinal cord is called epidural or spinal anesthesia.

General anesthetics block the body's response to painful stimuli. These blocked responses produce unconsciousness, muscle relaxation, and amnesia. General anesthetics can be administered IV, rectally, or by inhalation. This section includes local and IV anesthetic agents.

What IS a Local Anesthetic?

Local Anesthetics	Trade Names	Type	Uses
procaine HCl [PROE-kane]	Novocaine	Ester	Infiltration anesthesia, spinal anesthesia, epidural, peripheral nerve block
lidocaine [LYE-doe-kane]	Xylocaine	Amide	Nerve block or infiltration in dental procedures
bupivacaine [byoo-PIV-a-kane]	Marcaine	Amide	Local infiltration and sympathetic block; lumbar epidural; caudal block; peripheral nerve block; dental block

Action

Local anesthetics block pain at the injection site while allowing the continuation of consciousness. Local anesthetics inhibit ionic flux into nerve cells, slow nerve impulse production, and reduce the rate of electrical action potential of a nerve fiber, thereby preventing the conduction of nerve impulses. The order of nerve function loss proceeds in the following manner: pain, temperature, touch, proprioception, and skeletal muscle tone. When vasoconstrictors (e.g., epinephrine) are added to local anesthetics, they decrease systemic absorption, promote local hemostasis, and prolong the duration of action. The rate of absorption of local anesthetics depends on the dose and concentration of the drug, vascular supply, and the presence of vasoconstrictors.

To some extent, local anesthetics are distributed to all body tissues. Local anesthetics are classified into two types: esters and amides. Esters are derivatives of PABA and are metabolized by hydrolysis of the ester linkage by plasma cholinesterase. Hypersensitivities are more common with the ester type. Amides are derivatives of aniline and are metabolized in the liver and excreted in urine.

Uses

Local anesthetics are used in infiltration anesthesia and are used in spinal, epidural, caudal, brachial plexus, and peripheral nerve blocks.

What You NEED TO KNOW

Contraindications/Precautions

  Caution should be taken when administering local anesthetics to children, older adults, and pregnant or lactating women.

These local anesthetic agents are contraindicated for patients with hypersensitivity. Procaine is contraindicated for patients with cerebrospinal diseases, hypotension, hypertension, and heart block.

Drug Interactions

When different local anesthetic agents are mixed, the drug interaction produces an increased risk of toxicity. When sedatives are given concurrently, the drug interaction produces intensified CNS effects. Local anesthetics inhibit the action of sulfonamides when given together.

Caution should be taken when administering local anesthetics to patients with dysrhythmias, shock, and renal or hepatic dysfunction.

Adverse Effects

Adverse effects of local anesthetics are generally dose related. Most adverse effects involve CNS or cardiovascular depression. Adverse effects of local anesthetic agents include dizziness, fainting, blurred vision, double vision, tinnitus, euphoria, anxiety, restlessness, chills, nausea, vomiting, hypotension, bradycardia, convulsions, respiratory impairment, and ventricular dysrhythmias. Additionally, sensation of heat, cold or numbness, redness, itching, sneezing, excessive sweating, postspinal headache, and paralysis may occur. Some rare adverse effects include fecal or urinary incontinence, urinary retention, weakness, and loss of perineal sensation and sexual function.

What You DO

Nursing Responsibilities

An overdose of local anesthetics can occur with severe consequences (e.g., respiratory or cardiac arrest, dysrhythmias).

Acute emergencies from local anesthetics are usually a result of high concentrations in the plasma. Prevention of emergency situations is of major importance. The nursing responsibilities for caring for a patient who has received local anesthetic are to:
- Observe for evidence of an overdose (e.g., hypotension, bradycardia, convulsions, apnea, hypoxia, acidosis). Be prepared to provide respiratory support to patients who have experienced an overdose.

- Monitor the patient closely in the postoperative period.
- Inform patients who are receiving caudal or epidurals that they may experience temporary loss of sensation and motor activity, usually in the lower portion of the body.
- Caution patients who are having dental procedures to avoid eating food or hot liquids until sensation returns.

Do You UNDERSTAND?

DIRECTIONS: **Indicate in the space provided whether each statement is** *true* **or** *false.*

_____ 1. Local anesthetics are not systemically absorbed into the body.

_____ 2. The nurse should be prepared to provide respiratory support after local anesthetic use.

What IS an IV Nonbarbiturate Anesthetic Agent?

Nonbarbiturate Anesthetics	Trade Names	Uses
midazolam [MID-ah-ZOE-lam]	Versed	Anesthesia induction; conscious sedation
ketamine [KET-uh-MEEN]	Ketalar	Used in young children for minor surgical and diagnostic procedures that do not require skeletal muscle relaxation; because it causes immobility, it is ideal for burn cases
propofol [PRO-puh-fole]	Diprivan	Induction and maintenance of anesthesia; conscious sedation
fentanyl [FEN-tuh-nill]	Sublimaze	Short-acting neuroleptic analgesia and tranquilizer during operative and perioperative period of surgical or diagnostic procedures
droperidol [droe-PER-I-dahl]	Inapsine	Reduces nausea and vomiting; produces tranquilizing effect; adjunct drug during induction and maintenance of anesthesia

Action

Midazolam is a short-acting benzodiazepine that interferes with the reuptake of GABA and promotes its accumulation at nerve cell synapses, thereby intensifying GABA activity. Ketamine is a rapid-acting general anesthetic that selectively interrupts association pathways of the brain, producing somatesthetic sensory blockade. This action blocks consciousness of body sensations and is called dissociative anesthesia. Propofol acts as a sedative-hypnotic. Fentanyl is a short-acting neuroleptic analgesic and tranquilizer that blocks receptors for dopamine, which causes analgesia. Droperidol is a short-acting neuroleptic analgesic and tranquilizer that antagonizes emetic effects of drugs that act on the chemore-

Answers: 1. false; 2. true.

ceptor trigger zone (CTZ). This agent acts primarily at the subcortical level to produce sedative effects, reduce anxiety, and decrease motor activity.

Uses

IV nonbarbiturate anesthetics are CNS depressants that serve as supplements to anesthesia. These agents are used throughout the perioperative period for their desired effects. IV nonbarbiturate anesthetics are also used for the induction and maintenance of anesthesia, conscious sedation, reduction of nausea and vomiting, short-acting neuroleptic analgesia, and production of a tranquilizing effect.

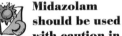 Midazolam, propofol, and fentanyl are contraindicated for women during pregnancy and lactation.

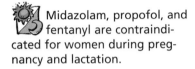 **Midazolam should be used with caution in patients with heart failure, COPD, renal failure, and in older adults. Fentanyl is contraindicated for children, patients with myasthenia gravis, or those who have received an MAOI within 14 days. Droperidol should be used with caution in older adults, pregnant and lactating women, children, and patients with renal or hepatic dysfunction.**

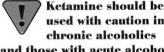 **Ketamine should be used with caution in chronic alcoholics and those with acute alcohol intoxication. Propofol should be used with caution in patients with severe cardiac or respiratory dysfunction and in those with a history of seizures. Fentanyl should be used with caution in older adults, debilitated patients, and individuals with COPD, head injuries, increased intracranial pressure, bradydysrhythmias, and renal or liver dysfunction.**

 # What You NEED TO KNOW

Contraindications/Precautions

Nonbarbiturate anesthetics are contraindicated for patients with hypersensitivity. Midazolam is contraindicated for acute narrow-angle glaucoma, acute alcohol intoxication, coma, and shock. Ketamine is contraindicated for patients with significant hypertension and a history of psychiatric illness. Propofol is contraindicated for patients with increased intracranial pressure and impaired cerebral circulation.

Drug Interactions

Drug interactions that may occur with droperidol include peripheral vasodilation and hypotension when given concurrently with other anesthetics. CNS depressants have an additive or intensifying effect when given together with IV nonbarbiturate anesthetics. When ketamine is given together with muscle relaxants, prolonged respiratory depression may develop. Administration of thyroid hormones and ketamine together may lead to hypertension and tachycardia. When halothane and ketamine are given concurrently, decreased cardiac output, BP, and heart rate may occur. The hypnotic effect of thiopental may be antagonized when given with ketamine.

Adverse Effects

Nonbarbiturates may cause respiratory depression. Midazolam may cause cardiac arrest. The adverse effects of ketamine include emergence delirium, hallucinations, confusion, excitement, irrational behavior, diplopia, nystagmus, elevated intraocular pressure, hypotension, hypertension, tachycardia, bradycardia, dysrhythmia, anorexia, nausea, vomiting, and laryngospasm. Adverse effects of propofol include cough, hiccups, headache, dizziness, hypotension, twitching, vomiting, abdominal cramping, jerking, decreased intraocular pressure, and ventricular asystole. Fentanyl may cause hypotension. Adverse effects of droperidol include drowsiness, tachycardia, hypotension, hypertension, muscular rigidity, chills, dizziness, shivering, laryngospasm, bronchospasm, hallucinations, restlessness, anxiety, hyperactivity, and extrapyramidal symptoms (e.g., dystonia, akathisia, oculogyric crisis).

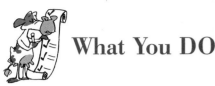

What You DO

Nursing Responsibilities

Slow administration over 2 or more minutes and allowing 2 or more minutes between injections can reduce the adverse effects of midazolam. Fentanyl and droperidol are available premixed and known as Innovar. When administering IV nonbarbiturate anesthetics, the nurse should:

- Monitor the cardiac and respiratory status of a patient who is receiving IV nonbarbiturate anesthetics.
- Monitor the patient for drug-induced excitation (e.g., twitching, tremors, spasmodic muscular contractions between antagonistic muscle groups).
- Advise the patient to avoid driving, operating hazardous machinery, or engaging in hazardous activity for 24 hours after anesthesia with ketamine.

Do You UNDERSTAND?

DIRECTIONS: Fill in the blanks with the appropriate responses.

1. The dissociative anesthetic agent is _____.
2. _____ is an IV nonbarbiturate anesthetic that is contraindicated when a patient has received an MAOI 1 week earlier.

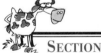

SECTION F

PSYCHOTHERAPEUTIC AGENTS

Thoughts, feelings, and actions are transmitted in the CNS as electrochemical impulses. When an impulse reaches the end of one neuron (**presynaptic neuron**), chemicals (**neurotransmitters**) are released that cross the synaptic cleft and bind to specific receptor sites on the next neuron (**postsynaptic neuron**). This binding action triggers electrical changes that either inhibit or continue the conduction of the impulse. After the neurotransmitter's function has been completed, the chemicals are either inactivated by enzymes or stored for future use (**reuptake**). The reuptake process is important in understanding the actions of certain psychotropic drugs. The availability or concentration of neurotransmitters at the postsynaptic receptors is significant. Any alteration or decrease is associated with some form of neuropathologic condition.

Answers: 1. ketamine; 2. fentanyl.

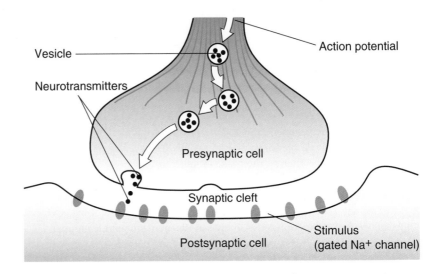

The major categories of neurotransmitters are cholinergics, monoamines, and neuropeptides. Each type of neurotransmitter is associated with the conduction of impulses in different areas of the CNS. For example, serotonin is a monoamine transmitter that innervates receptors in the pons, medulla, thalamus, and limbic system. A decrease in serotonin level is associated with clinical depression. Another important example is the amino acid inhibitory transmitter, which is a type of GABA. GABA innervates receptors in the hypothalamus, cortex, cerebellum, basil ganglia, and hippocampus. A decrease in GABA availability is associated with anxiety disorders and schizophrenia. The medications discussed in this section are anxiolytics, sedative-hypnotics, antidepressants, and antipsychotics.

Anxiolytic Agents

Antianxiety medications are nonspecific CNS depressants that alleviate symptoms of distress but do not affect underlying factors that cause the anxiety. Anxiolytic medications are dose dependent with increasing dose resulting in sedation and hypnosis. The actions of the anxiolytic medications are not well known. Anxiolytics may act to exacerbate the effects of the inhibitory neurotransmitter GABA, reduce serotonin turnover in cortical tissues, and depress the CNS at the limbic and subcortical levels of the brain. The anxiolytics can be divided into two subgroups: benzodiazepines and nonbenzodiazepines.

What IS a Benzodiazepine Anxiolytic Agent?

Benzodiazepines Anxiolytic Agents	Trade Names	Uses
diazepam [dye-AZ-eh-pam]	Valium	Treatment of anxiety disorders
alprazolam [al-PRAY-zoe-lam]	Xanax	Treatment of anxiety disorders

Action

Benzodiazepines (BZDs) are composed of a large group of chemically similar drugs that are believed to act on neural BZD receptors in the CNS. Stimulation of these receptors leads to stronger impulse inhibition at postsynaptic neurons by the neurotransmitter GABA. As a result, depression of the CNS is observed at the limbic and subcortical levels of the brain. In initial metabolism, many of the BZDs are converted into metabolites that are active CNS depressants. Chronic administration of BZDs that have long lasting, active metabolites can cause an accumulation of both the medication and the metabolite, resulting in oversedation and CNS depression.

The BZDs work quickly to reduce anxiety symptoms, with the most improvement occurring within the first week of treatment. The efficacy of BZD therapy decreases after 3 to 4 months of continuous use.

Uses

BZDs are used in the treatment of mild-to-severe anxiety (including panic disorder), seizure control in acute alcohol withdrawal, sleep induction, muscle relaxation, and as a preoperative medication. The BZDs are ineffective in treating severe psychotic disorders or severe clinical depression, although they may be used in conjunction with other medications when depression is accompanied by severe anxiety. Medications such as alprazolam, clorazepate, and diazepam are approved for treatment of anxiety and panic disorder. Estazolam, flurazepam, quazepam, and triazolam are used primarily for their hypnotic effect and are approved for the treatment of insomnia.

See Chapter 2C in **RWNSG:** *Pathophysiology*

What You NEED TO KNOW

Contraindications/Precautions

BZDs are contraindicated for patients with renal or hepatic dysfunction, unless no other options are available. Certain BZDs (e.g., alprazolam, clorazepate, lorazepam, midazolam) may aggravate acute angle-closure glaucoma and are contraindicated for these patients.

Short-acting BZDs (i.e., those with a short-acting plasma half-life), such as temazepam and lorazepam, are preferred for older adults or patients who are debilitated because these agents are less likely to accumulate in the body.

Because of altered metabolism that may allow BZDs or their metabolites to accumulate in the plasma and lead to excessive sedation and ataxia, caution must be used when BZDs are administered to older or debilitated patients.

BZDs are believed to cause fetal anomalies when taken during the early stages of pregnancy. BZDs may cause fetal dependence with resulting withdrawal symptoms in the neonate when taken at the end of the third trimester of pregnancy. BZDs taken at the time of labor will cause CNS depression in the neonate. Therefore BZDs are contraindicated for women during pregnancy and lactation, unless no other alternatives are available.

 Although overdose of BZDs is rarely fatal, combined use of BZDs and other CNS depressants is dangerous.

 Sedation and ataxia are the most common adverse effects of BZDs, with older adults being the most susceptible.

 The outcome of these common effects is an increased risk of falls and subsequent injuries.

TAKE HOME POINTS

Assess the patient for history of substance abuse and current use of CNS depressants (e.g., opioids, alcohol, or OTC sleep aids). BZDs should be given in the smallest dose possible for the shortest period possible.

Drug Interactions

Administering cimetidine with BZDs other than oxazepam or lorazepam results in increased serum levels of the BZD. This action results in prolonged sedation, drug hangover, and an increased likelihood of adverse effects. Concurrent use of BZDs and digoxin increases serum digoxin levels, decreases digoxin elimination, and increases the risk of digoxin toxicity.

The use of BZDs in combination with other CNS depressants (e.g., barbiturates, opioids, alcohol, antihistamines) results in additive effects. Additive effects include deepened and prolonged sedative effect, motor impairment, enhanced CNS and respiratory depression, and death.

Adverse Effects

Adverse effects from BZDs include GI disturbances (e.g., nausea, constipation), jaundice, headache, incontinence, urinary retention, hypotension, and rashes. Additional infrequent adverse effects include anterograde amnesia and paradoxical effects. Anterograde amnesia is an inability to remember events that occur after BZD administration.

Paradoxical effects are opposite of that expected. These effects are rare but can be serious. The paradoxical effects most likely to be observed include increased excitation, insomnia, anxiety, and hallucinations.

 # What You DO

Nursing Responsibilities

Chronic use of BZDs can produce physiologic dependence and cross-tolerance to other members of the benzodiazepine group. BZD use should be closely monitored and time limited. Therefore BZDs should be used at the lowest effective dose for the shortest time possible. BZDs are administered either orally or parenterally, with the oral route preferred. Absorption rates for IM administration are slower and vary according to the injection site used. For example, when diazepam is given IM, the preferred injection site is the deltoid because the rate of absorption from that area is more constant when compared with other areas.

The nurse's primary responsibility in administering BZDs is patient safety. To maintain patient safety:

- Review the patient's medical, medication, and substance abuse history. Excessive CNS depression may occur when the patient has history of hepatic or renal impairment and a likelihood of medication or active metabolite accumulation in the body.
- Review the actions, effects, administration routes, and the rationale for current drug therapy.
- Assess the patient for suicidal behaviors or suicidal ideation because BZDs (frequently in combination with other CNS depressants) have been used in attempted suicides.

🍎 Counsel patients who have taken BZDs for a long time to avoid abrupt discontinuation of the therapy. The abrupt discontinuation, particularly of the short-acting BZDs, may cause rebound CNS excitation (including seizures) or withdrawal symptoms.

Do You UNDERSTAND?

DIRECTIONS: **Indicate in the space provided whether each statement is**
true **or** *false.*

_____ 1. Because of their sedative, antispasmodic, and antiseizure effects, BZDs are appropriate medications for the treatment of acute alcohol withdrawal symptoms.

_____ 2. Chronic use of BZDs can produce physiologic dependence and cross-tolerance to other classifications of CNS depressants.

_____ 3. Caution must be used in administering BZDs to a patient who is concurrently taking digoxin because the interaction of the drugs can prolong the half-life of the BZD, allowing over sedation and CNS depression.

_____ 4. Concurrent administration of cimetidine with a BZD is contraindicated.

What IS a Nonbenzodiazepine Anxiolytic Agent?

Nonbenzodiazepine Anxiolytics	Trade Names	Uses
buspirone [byoo-SPY-rone]	BuSpar	Short-term treatment of anxiety disorders
meprobamate [meh-pro-BAM-ate]	Equanil, Miltown	Short-term treatment of anxiety disorders

Action

Nonbenzodiazepine anxiolytic agents produce CNS depression and a reduction in anxiety symptoms. Buspirone is a member of the azapirone classification of drugs. The exact action of buspirone is unknown, but it is believed to inhibit neuronal firing and to reduce serotonin turnover in certain CNS structures. Buspirone appears to stimulate the serotonin receptors of the CNS. Meprobamate is a general CNS depressant that affects multiple sites of the CNS, including the thalamus and limbic system.

Answers: 1. true; 2. false; chronic use of BZDs can produce physiologic dependence and cross-tolerance to other members of the BZD group; 3. false; concurrent BZD and digoxin leads to increased digoxin levels and predisposes the patient to digitalis toxicity; 4. true, because it raises BZD levels.

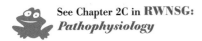

See Chapter 2C in **RWNSG:**
Pathophysiology

Uses

Buspirone is considered to be as efficient as the BZD group in treating chronic or generalized anxiety. This medication has a gradual onset of approximately 1 to 4 weeks. Therefore buspirone is inappropriate for acute anxiety or panic attacks. Meprobamate is used in the short-term management of anxiety disorders. The effectiveness of using meprobamate for greater than 4 months has not been determined.

What You NEED TO KNOW

Contraindications/Precautions

Nonbenzodiazepine anxiolytic agents are contraindicated for patients with hypersensitivity.

Nonbenzodiazepine anxiolytic agents are contraindicated for lactating and pregnant women. Buspirone is contraindicated for children under 18 years of age. Meprobamate is contraindicated for children under 6 years of age.

Drug Interactions

Although buspirone does not usually cause sedation, administration of this medication with other CNS depressants can increase the effects of the depressant and cause oversedation. Buspirone should not be given to anyone who has received an MAOI within the preceding 14 days. Concurrent use of these medications can cause a dangerous and possibly lethal elevation in BP.

Oversedation, CNS depression, and respiratory depression occur when hydroxyzine or meprobamate is administered in conjunction with other CNS depressants, such as alcohol, opioids, or barbiturates. Psychologic and physical dependence on meprobamate may occur with long-term use.

Meprobamate should be used with caution in patients with renal or hepatic dysfunction. Meprobamate should be used cautiously in patients with seizure disorders, suicidal tendencies, or a history of alcoholism or drug abuse.

Adverse Effects

Adverse effects that may occur with nonbenzodiazepines include dizziness, drowsiness, headache, nervousness, insomnia, nausea, dry mouth, and blurred vision. Buspirone may cause tremors, decreased concentration, mood changes, tachycardia, and palpitations. Meprobamate may cause ataxia, GI distress, slurred speech, hypotension, arrhythmias, and seizures. Thrombocytopenia and aplastic anemia have been noted but are rare. Unusual bleeding, bruising, fever, or sore throat can indicate toxicity.

What You DO

Nursing Responsibilities

Buspirone is administered orally. The onset of action from buspirone is gradual, and optimal results may not appear for 3 to 4 weeks.

Meprobamate is administered orally. When the medication has been used long-term, discontinuation of the therapy must be gradual over the period of at least 2 weeks. Rapid termination of meprobamate can result in severe seizure

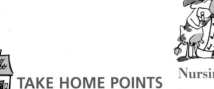
TAKE HOME POINTS

Buspirone should not be administered when the patient has taken an MAOI within the previous 14 days to avoid a lethal elevation of BP.

activity and withdrawal symptoms. The nursing responsibilities with regard to patients who are taking nonbenzodiazepine anxiolytics include the following:

- Monitor the patient who is taking nonbenzodiazepine anxiolytic agents for CNS and respiratory depression, particularly when the patient has a history of taking barbiturates, opioids, or BZDs.
- Assess patient for whom meprobamate is prescribed for a history of suicidal behaviors or ideation. Any patient who has a history of these behaviors must be monitored closely because the medication has a history of being used in attempted suicides.
- Instruct the patient to take buspirone with food for increased drug effectiveness.
- Warn the patient to avoid abrupt discontinuation of the BZD when buspirone is to be given to a patient who is already taking a benzodiazepine.
- Instruct the patient to taper buspirone when on other combination BZD therapy to prevent withdrawal symptoms and possible seizure activity.

Do You UNDERSTAND?

DIRECTIONS: **Match the the statements in Column A with the appropriate medication in Column B.**

Column A

_____ 1. Does not increase the effects of alcohol and is not associated with withdrawal symptoms when discontinued.

_____ 2. Is comparable to benzodiazepine anxiolytics but does not produce sedation or impair motor function.

_____ 3. Is appropriate for short-term management of acute anxiety, rather than management of chronic anxiety.

Column B

a. Meprobamate

b. Buspirone

Sedative-Hypnotic Agents

What IS a Sedative-Hypnotic Agent?

Sedative-Hypnotics	Trade Names	Uses
butabarbital [byoo-ta-BAR-bi-tal]	Butisol	Treatment of insomnia and anxiety
secobarbital [see-koe-BAR-bi-tal]	Seconal	Treatment of insomnia and acute agitation
zolpidem [ZOL-pi-dem]	Ambien	Treatment of insomnia

Answers: 1. b.; 2. b.; 3. a.

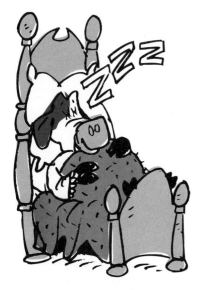

Action

The groups of medications that comprise the sedative-hypnotic classification include barbiturates, selected BZDs, and other miscellaneous CNS depressants. Sedative-hypnotic agents are nonspecific CNS depressants that act in a dose-dependent fashion. These agents produce drowsiness, a calming effect, activity reduction, and sleep induction. These drugs also alleviate symptoms of insomnia but do not affect underlying causative factors.

The precise action of barbiturates (butabarbital and secobarbital) has not been established, but they appear to decrease the excitability of the presynaptic and postsynaptic neurons in the cerebral cortex and the reticular formation of the CNS. Zolpidem tartrate is a general depressant that acts on the GABA receptor sites of the CNS. Dissimilar to barbiturates, zolpidem tartrate preserves all stages of sleep, including REM and deep sleep. This action is the result of its preference for the omega receptors in the GABA receptor complex.

Uses

Sedative-hypnotic agents should be used as aids to minimize distress that interrupts rest and sleep. These medications cannot take the place of natural sleep cycles, and long-term use can adversely affect or diminish necessary sleep and dreaming. Relatively low doses of barbiturates will depress the sensory cortex, depress motor activity, and produce sedation. Barbiturates suppress REM sleep and decrease stages III and IV of normal sleep. After discontinuing barbiturates, it is not unusual for a patient to experience sleep disturbances from REM rebound.

 Barbiturates have been associated with fetal abnormalities and are contraindicated for pregnant and lactating women. Zolpidem should be used with caution in children under 18 years of age.

What You NEED TO KNOW

Contraindications/Precautions

Sedative-hypnotics are contraindicated for patients with severe respiratory disorders. Butabarbital and secobarbital are contraindicated for patients with porphyria, a history of addiction, and uncontrolled pain.

Drug Interactions

The concurrent use of barbiturates may increase the metabolism and decrease drug effectiveness of corticosteroids, digoxin, estrogen, oral contraceptives, theophylline, verapamil, beta blockers, quinidine, tricyclic antidepressants, griseofulvin, and doxycycline. Administration of zolpidem tartrate with other CNS depressants can cause oversedation and respiratory depression.

Adverse Effects

When taken for a prolonged period, sedative-hypnotic agents may produce psychologic and physiologic dependence. The most common adverse effects of zolpidem tartrate include dizziness, drowsiness, and diarrhea. Other adverse effects include headache, hangover, vomiting, and amnesia.

 TAKE HOME POINTS

Sedative hypnotics are contraindicated for women during pregnancy and lactation.

 Sedative-hypnotics should be used with caution in patients with renal or hepatic impairment, as well as patients with depression, suicidal tendencies, and a history of drug dependence.

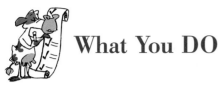

What You DO

Nursing Responsibilities

Barbiturates can be administered orally, rectally, IM, or IV. Zolpidem tartrate is administered orally. Short-term treatment (7 to 14 days) of insomnia is appropriate; long-term use is not recommended. Because of the respiratory depression from zolpidem tartrate, closely monitor any patient with a history of respiratory insufficiency. This medication should be administered in the lowest possible effective dose. The presence of food significantly reduces the absorption of zolpidem. Therefore zolpidem should be administered at bedtime.

When administering sedative-hypnotics, the nurse should:

- Instruct patient to take zolpidem immediately before bedtime.
- Closely monitor patients who are taking sedative hypnotics to prevent medication hoarding and self-administration of larger than prescribed doses.

Do You UNDERSTAND?

DIRECTIONS: Indicate in the space provided whether each statement is *true* or *false*.

_____ 1. Barbiturates that are given in conjunction with oral contraceptives will result in an in a lower serum barbiturate level and a decreased effectiveness of the sedative-hypnotic.

_____ 2. The best use of sedative-hypnotic medications is as a short-term therapy for insomnia.

_____ 3. Chloral hydrate is one of the sedative-hypnotics that is well tolerated by older patients.

_____ 4. Zolpidem tartrate is known to cause fetal abnormalities and must not be given during the first trimester of a pregnancy.

_____ 5. Patients with hepatic, renal or respiratory insufficiency have an increased risk for over sedation and CNS depression when given sedative-hypnotics.

Antidepressant Agents

Depressive symptoms are related to the sensitivity of catecholamine receptors in the presence of low serotonin levels. This alteration of chemicals allows changes in affective states that are governed by the neurotransmitter norepinephrine. Lowered norepinephrine levels cause depression. Increased norepinephrine levels cause mania. Antidepressants alter levels of serotonin and norepinephrine, which moderate the patient's depression.

Older patients are more likely than is the younger population to experience over-sedation and CNS depression because of aging changes, such as slowed metabolic rate and decreased renal function. Therefore when administering a barbiturate to an older patient, the initial dose should be reduced.

TAKE HOME POINTS

- Patients who are taking sedative-hypnotics and have a history of suicidal ideation or behaviors must be closely monitored because these drugs have a history of use in suicide attempts.
- Sedative-hypnotics that are taken in conjunction with other CNS depressants can cause oversedation and respiratory depression.

Answers: 1. false; barbiturates results in increased metabolism and decreased drug effectiveness of oral contraceptives, corticosteroids, digoxin, estrogen, theophylline, verapamil, tricyclic antidepressants, griseofulvin, and doxycycline; 2. true; 3. true; 4. false; barbiturates; 5. true.

Four categories of antidepressants have been identified: tricyclic antidepressants (TCAs), selective serotonin reuptake inhibitors (SSRIs), MAOIs, and miscellaneous antidepressants. Lithium is an antidepressant with only one specific use.

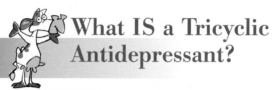

What IS a Tricyclic Antidepressant?

Tricyclic Antidepressants	Trade Names	Uses
amitriptyline [am-eh-TRIP-tih-leen]	Elavil	Treatment of depression
doxepin [DOX-uh-pin]	Sinequan	Treatment of depression and anxiety
imipramine [im-IPP-ruh-meen]	Tofranil	Treatment of depression

Action

TCAs decrease the reabsorption of norepinephrine and serotonin. The decreased rate of reabsorption at the nerve terminals allows more of the neurotransmitters to be available to the postsynaptic receptors. This action prolongs the stimulatory effects.

Uses

TCAs are most useful for treating major depressive episodes that reflect disturbances in sleep, hunger, appetite, sexual activity, and physical activity. Other indications for administration of a tricyclic medication include panic disorder, obsessive-compulsive disorders, enuresis, and idiopathic chronic pain.

TCAs were, at one time, the drug of choice for treating depression. Because of the possibility of multiple adverse effects and the strong potential for overdose, TCAs are no longer the preferred initial choice for treatment. TCAs are more likely to be reserved for patients who fail to respond well to other antidepressant medications.

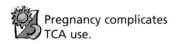
Pregnancy complicates TCA use.

What You NEED TO KNOW

Contraindications/Precautions

Precautions must be taken when TCAs are prescribed for a patient with a history of either suicidal behaviors or ideation.

TCAs are contraindicated for patients during the acute recovery phase following an MI or for those with severe coronary artery disease. Because of possible cardiotoxic effects, TCAs are contraindicated for patients with hyperthyroidism or those who are undergoing thyroid hormone therapy. Other medical conditions that complicate TCA use are benign prostatic hypertrophy, seizure disorders, narrow-angle glaucoma, and diabetes.

Drug Interactions

The use of other CNS depressants (e.g., barbiturates, opioids, alcohol) can increase CNS depression. Concurrent use of these medications with TCAs should be avoided. Smoking may lower the plasma concentration of the prescribed medication. When cimetidine, SSRIs, and oral contraceptives are given together with TCAs, TCA blood levels and the risk of adverse effects are increased. Concurrent administration of TCAs with clonidine, epinephrine, and norepinephrine leads to an increased risk of hypertensive effects or hypertensive crisis. Concurrent use of TCAs and MAOIs may cause extreme excitation, hyperpyrexia, and seizures.

Adverse Effects

Amitriptyline and doxepin have a slow onset of therapeutic antidepressant effects but strong anticholinergic effects that rapidly appear. These two drugs are the most sedating of the TCAs. Cholinergic effects include dry mouth and mucus membranes, urinary difficulty, blurred vision, and constipation. Other adverse effects include headache, migraine headache, orthostatic hypotension, tremor, weight gain, insomnia, and photosensitivity.

Older or debilitated patients who are taking TCAs are particularly susceptible to morning orthostatic hypotension.

TCAs are highly dangerous when taken in overdose amounts, causing cardiovascular effects (e.g., tachycardia, life-threatening dysrhythmias, CHF, CVA). TCA overdose can also produce respiratory depression, apnea, seizures, confusion, delirium, hallucinations, hyperpyrexia, bowel and bladder paralysis, and coma. Even at nontoxic levels, TCAs frequently cause orthostatic hypotension.

What You DO

Nursing Responsibilities

When TCA therapy is initiated, a prolonged period (2 to 4 weeks) may elapse before the therapeutic effects are noted. TCAs are administered either orally or IM. TCAs are easily absorbed through the GI tract, and the presence of food does not adversely affect the rate of absorption.

TCAs are extremely dangerous in overdose amounts. Any patient who is prone to overdose should be issued only a small number of pills, or another responsible person in the family should control the patient's access to the medication.

When administering TCAs, the nurse should:
- Administer these medications at bedtime, which helps alleviate daytime sedation.
- Monitor patients with a history of suicidal behaviors or suicidal ideation for attempted drug overdose.
- Warn patients of the possibility of morning orthostatic hypotension.
- Teach patient smoking cessation methods when needed.
- Monitor patients with heart disease for cardiotoxic symptoms.

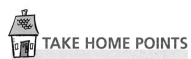

TAKE HOME POINTS

Advise patients who are taking TCAs against smoking.

Do You UNDERSTAND?

DIRECTIONS: Indicate in the space provided whether each statement is *true* or *false*.

_____ 1. Neurotoxicity or seizure activity is not associated with TCA overdose.

_____ 2. Because of the multiple side effects of the TCAs and the risk for overdose, these medications are no longer the initial drug of choice in dealing with depression.

_____ 3. Orthostatic hypertension is an early indicator of TCA toxicity in older or debilitated patients.

_____ 4. Because of the propensity for cardiac arrhythmias, TCA therapy is contraindicated for anyone who is recovering from a recent heart attack.

_____ 5. The interaction of thyroid hormone and TCAs can increase the danger of cardiotoxicity.

What IS a Selective Serotonin Reuptake Inhibitor?

Selective Serotonin Reuptake Inhibitors	Trade Names	Uses
fluoxetine [flew-OX-uh-teen]	Prozac	Treatment of depression and obsessive-compulsive disorders
paroxetine [puh-ROCKS-uh-teen]	Paxil	Treatment of depression and panic disorders
sertraline [SIR-truh-leen]	Zoloft	Treatment of depression and panic disorders

Action

SSRIs are a potent and widely prescribed class of antidepressants that decrease the reuptake of serotonin at selected nerve terminals in the CNS. These agents also have weak effects on the reuptake of norepinephrine and dopamine. The increased availability of serotonin prolongs the stimulatory potential of the receptors, resulting in mood elevation and reduced anxiety. The elevated mood follows a similar time course as do TCAs.

Uses

Because SSRIs are well tolerated, they are usually considered as a first line of therapy. SSRIs are the drugs of choice for treating mild-to-moderate depression. Fluoxetine is appropriate for the treatment of obsessive-compulsive disorder. Paroxetine and sertraline are used in the treatment of panic disorder.

Answers: 1. false; 2. true; 3. false; orthostatic hypertension occurs at nontoxic levels; 4. true; 5. true.

What You NEED TO KNOW

Contraindications/Precautions

SSRIs are contraindicated for patients with a hypersensitivity to these agents. Paroxetine is contraindicated for patients with concurrent use of MAOIs.

Drug Interactions

Fluoxetine and paroxetine cause inhibition of certain hepatic enzymes. This action can lead to increased plasma levels of medications, such as phenothiazines, BZD, and antidysrhythmics. Concurrent administration of cimetidine can decrease the rate of SSRI metabolism, allowing accumulation of the SSRI and an increased risk of adverse effects. Use of warfarin during SSRI therapy can result in an increased prothrombin time and possible bleeding.

Concurrent administration of lithium, TCAs, barbiturates (e.g., phenobarbital), or alcohol may increase the CNS effects of SSRIs. Concurrent use of SSRIs and phenytoin can increase the serum levels of phenytoin.

Adverse Effects

Because of selectivity, SSRIs are as efficient as are the TCAs and produce fewer anticholinergic effects. The common adverse effects of SSRIs are usually mild and dissipate within 4 to 6 weeks. Agitation, anxiousness, overstimulation, insomnia, and jitteriness are usually found in the beginning phase of SSRI therapy. Patients with a history of panic disorder are more likely to experience these adverse effects. Both male and female patients may experience some sexual dysfunction (usually occurring late in the course of therapy). Other adverse effects include headache, nausea, diarrhea, dry mouth, and anorexia.

SSRIs can stimulate manic activity with patients who have a history of mania. For patients who demonstrate anxiety as part of their disease process, overstimulation can exacerbate the patient's feelings of anxiety. Understanding that SSRIs may cause seizure activity is important.

Fluoxetine should be used cautiously in patients with diabetes mellitus, renal and hepatic dysfunction, suicidal ideations, and hyponatremia. Paroxetine should be used with caution in patients with renal or hepatic dysfunction.

Fluoxetine should not be used in patients who are pregnant and lactating. Paroxetine should be used with caution in patients who are pregnant and lactating. SSRI use in children has not been established and should be used cautiously in older adults.

Administration of an SSRI with an MAOI may lead to potentially lethal effects. When given concurrently, these drugs can cause hyperthermia, twitching, rigidity, rapid fluctuations in vital signs, mental status changes, delirium, coma, and death.

What You DO

Nursing Responsibilities

SSRIs are administered orally and are slowly absorbed into the system. Elimination of the medication from the body is slow, taking as long as 5 weeks for the medication to clear the system completely.

Before beginning SSRI therapy, an in depth history of past suicidal tendencies, depressive episodes, and previous antidepressant drug use should be obtained. When the patient has used an MAOI, a minimum of a 2-week

TAKE HOME POINTS

Limit the suicidal patient's access to SSRIs to prevent a suicide attempt. SSRIs should never be given together with an MAOI. When the MAOI is being discontinued, 14 days should elapse before starting the SSRI. Caution the patient against self-medication with OTC drugs.

washout period is required to clear the patient's system to prevent any drug interaction with the initiation of an SSRI. Conversely, when the patient is changing from SSRI therapy to the administration of an MAOI, the washout period must be 5 weeks.

When administering SSRIs, the nurse should:

- Monitor liver function studies before administering SSRIs and throughout therapy.
- Monitor patients with a history of seizure disorders because of the potential of a lowered seizure threshold.
- Teach the patient the importance of compliance with the prescribed regimen.
- Caution the patient against using other prescriptions, OTC medications, or herbal remedies to control depression (e.g., TCAs, MAOIs, or St. John's Wort) that might interfere with the action or metabolism of SSRIs or lead to toxicity.
- Advise the patient who is taking SSRIs to avoid alcohol and other CNS depressants.

Do You UNDERSTAND?

DIRECTIONS: **Indicate in the space provided whether each statement is** *true* **or** *false.*

_____ 1. Patients who have been prescribed an SSRI should be concerned when they experience insomnia because this is an early symptom of neurotoxicity.

_____ 2. A thorough knowledge of a patient's history of suicidal behavior or suicidal ideation is essential to prevent self-administered SSRI overdose.

_____ 3. When an SSRI is administered in conjunction with an MAOI, the patient may experience rapid fluctuations in vital signs that are difficult to control and potentially lethal.

What IS a Monoamine Oxidase Inhibitor?

Monoamine Oxidase Inhibitors	Trade Names	Uses
phenelzine [FEN-el-zeen]	Nardil	Treatment of depression
tranylcypromine [tran-ill-SIP-roe-meen]	Parnate	Treatment of severe depression

Action

MAOIs block the action of monoamine oxidase in the presynaptic nerves. Monoamine oxidase is an enzyme that is found in cells of the brain, liver, spleen, kidneys, and in blood cells. The primary action of monoamine oxidase is to metabolize amines that are found in the body, such as epinephrine, norepinephrine, tyramine, and serotonin. These enzymes then accumulate in the liver, brain, and sympathetic nerves. Inhibiting the metabolism of the neurotransmitters increases their availability for impulse conduction in the CNS. Current studies indicate that depression is partly a reflection of decreased levels of norepinephrine and dopamine. With the increase in transmitters, depressive effects are reduced.

Uses

MAOIs alleviate symptoms of clinical depression. Phenelzine is also used in the treatment of manic-depressive psychosis. Tranylcypromine is usually reserved for severe depression in patients who have failed to respond to other treatment.

What You NEED TO KNOW

Contraindications/Precautions

MAOIs are contraindicated for patients with impaired renal or hepatic function, coronary artery disease, CHF, hypertension, and cerebrovascular defects.

Drug Interactions

Most of the drug interactions affect the cardiovascular and hepatic systems and the CNS. These interactions can be severe. For example, MAOIs should not be administered concurrently with opioids, barbiturates, or alcohol, because marked exacerbating effects occur. Hypertensive crisis, convulsions, coma, and respiratory depression can result when MAOIs are given concurrently with meperidine. Drugs that interact with MAOIs to produce increased BP include diuretics, antihistamines, antihypertensives, and ephedrine (frequently found in OTC cold medications). General anesthetics also interact adversely with MAOIs.

MAOIs cross the placental barrier, causing fetal damage and are excreted in breast milk. MAOI therapy is contraindicated for pregnant or lactating women.

Adverse Effects

MAOIs have the potential for severe and unpredictable adverse effects. Primary adverse effects of the MAOIs include orthostatic hypotension, weight gain, sexual dysfunction, and edema. These effects are usually transitory and diminish as the patient adjusts to the medications. An interaction of MAOIs and foods that are high in tyramine and caffeine-containing beverages can lead to hypertensive crisis.

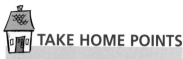

TAKE HOME POINTS

Closely monitor patients because MAOIs have the potential to cause severe and unpredictable adverse effects. Monitor liver function and a blood test to determine monoamine oxidase activity before initiating MAOIs. Repeat this procedure on a regular basis during the course of therapy. MAOI therapy should be discontinued at least 10 days before elective surgery.

MAOIs in combination with dietary tyramine will cause a dangerous hypertensive crisis. Overdose of MAOIs is a life-threatening event that can result in extensive organ damage.

What You DO

Nursing Responsibilities

At the beginning of MAOI therapy, a blood test to assess the monoamine oxidase activity of platelets is recommended. The patient should have this test repeated on a regular basis throughout the course of treatment to monitor toxicity levels. Before initiating MAOI therapy, obtaining a thorough history from the patient is also important, which includes information regarding cardiovascular, hepatic, and neurologic status. After a stable serum drug level is obtained, the dose is then decreased to a maintenance level.

After discontinuing MAOIs, resumption of normal monoamine oxidase metabolism is slow. Inactivation of monoamine oxidase by phenelzine is irreversible, and the enzymes must be redeveloped. A period of up to 2 weeks is needed to reestablish normal metabolism. The return to normal metabolism, after administration of tranylcypromine, is only slightly faster.

When administering MAOIs, the nurse should:

- Instruct the patient who is taking MAOIs to avoid foods that are high in tyramine and to limit caffeine intake as well. These foods and beverages include cheese, smoked meats, red wines, soy sauce, yeast extracts, sour cream, nuts, raisins, and yogurt. The dietary limitations can be one of the most difficult problems for the patient who is undergoing MAOI therapy. The patient may need considerable support and assistance to maintain compliance.
- Monitor the patient who is receiving MAOI therapy for signs of suicidal activity or ideation.
- Strictly limit access to MAOI medication to prevent a self-administered overdose.

Do You UNDERSTAND?

DIRECTIONS: Indicate in the space provided whether each statement is
          ***true* or *false*.**

_____ 1. Current literature associates depression with low levels of the neurotransmitters norepinephrine and dopamine.

_____ 2. Because of their unpredictable nature, MAOIs are usually prescribed only when the patient fails to respond to other less dangerous antidepressants.

_____ 3. Therapeutic effects of MAOIs appear between 1 and 4 weeks after initiating therapy.

_____ 4. MAOIs are contraindicated for patients with renal impairment.

Answers: 1. true; 2. true; 3. true; 4. true.

_____ 5. MAOIs must be discontinued 1 month before elective surgery to prevent complications during recovery.

_____ 6. Patients who are taking MAOIs need not decrease their coffee intake during the course of the therapy.

What IS a Miscellaneous Antidepressant?

Miscellaneous Antidepressants	Trade Names	Uses
bupropion [byoo-PRO-pee-ahn]	Wellbutrin	Treatment of depression
venlafaxine [VEN-luh-fax-een]	Effexor	Treatment of depression

Action

Miscellaneous antidepressants are also known as second-generation antidepressants. These antidepressants include a varied group of medications with different chemical properties but with the same mood-elevating effects.

Bupropion is an aminoketone that inhibits the reuptake of dopamine and blocks serotonin and norepinephrine reuptake. Venlafaxine is a phenylamine and a strong inhibitor of both norepinephrine and serotonin reuptake. Venlafaxine is also a weak blocker of dopamine reuptake.

Uses

These miscellaneous antidepressants are appropriate for the treatment of mild-to-moderate depression. These agents are also frequently used as alternative therapy when patients are unable to tolerate or respond to other antidepressants, such as SSRIs.

What You NEED TO KNOW

Contraindications/Precautions

Bupropion is contraindicated for patients with a history of head trauma, CNS tumor, seizure disorders, or with concurrent administration of drugs that lower seizure threshold. Bupropion is not recommended in patients with a history of a recent heart attack, unstable angina, and hepatic or renal insufficiency.

Miscellaneous antidepressants (with the exception of bupropion) are contraindicated for women during pregnancy because they present a risk for adverse fetal development.

Drug Interactions

Concurrent administration of bupropion with levodopa, phenothiazines, or TCAs is contraindicated because these drugs increase the risk of seizure activi-

Answers: 5. false; at least 10 days; 6. false; limits on beverages that are high in caffeine and foods that are high in tyramine are required.

ty. Administering bupropion concurrently with a rapid withdrawal of BZD is associated with an increased risk of seizure activity. Smoking cessation medications (e.g., Zyban) contain bupropion, thus concurrent administration of bupropion and smoking cessation medication can cause an overdose, leading to seizures. Concurrent administration of venlafaxine and MAOIs can lead to symptoms that are similar to those of neuroleptic malignant syndrome, including myoclonus, seizures, and hyperthermia; death may also occur.

Adverse Effects

Bupropion has a rapid onset that is frequently associated with nausea, agitation, and CNS stimulation. Bupropion is associated with dose-dependent seizure activity. Common adverse effects of bupropion include headache, anxiety, sedation, tremor, insomnia, decreased appetite, dry mouth, and weight loss.

Common adverse effects of venlafaxine include nausea, sleepiness, dizziness, dry mouth, sweating, and headaches. Venlafaxine is associated with a dose-dependent, sustained elevation in BP.

What You DO

Nursing Responsibilities

All miscellaneous antidepressants are administered orally. When giving miscellaneous antidepressants, the nurse should:

- Closely monitor patients who are taking any of the miscellaneous antidepressants for any suicidal activity or ideation. Patients should be given only the smallest possible amount of medication, or a reliable family member should be given responsibility for administering the medication.
- Monitor the patient who is taking venlafaxine with a history of hypertensive disease because venlafaxine is associated with sustained (dose-dependent) elevations in BP.
- Monitor patients who are taking bupropion for seizure activity.
- Instruct women who are taking one of the miscellaneous antidepressants to notify her health care provider when she is or becomes pregnant.

Do You UNDERSTAND?

DIRECTIONS: **Indicate in the space provided whether each statement is true or false.**

_____ 1. Concurrent administration of an MAOI and venlafaxine can result in effects that are similar to those of neuroleptic malignant syndrome.

_____ 2. Among the miscellaneous antidepressants, bupropion is the least likely to cause seizure activity.

TAKE HOME POINTS

- Teach patients that a 14-day hiatus must occur between the last dose of an MAOI and the initiation of venlafaxine.
- Monitor patients for overdose of these antidepressants because these agents may cause severe and possibly lethal effects.

Answers: 1. true; 2. false; bupropion is associated with dose-dependent seizure activity.

What IS Lithium?

Action

Lithium is a general term that is used to identify two medications: lithium carbonate and lithium citrate. Both drugs are alkali metals that change biochemical, electrolyte, and endocrine function in the body. The actions of lithium are thought to inhibit the release of both norepinephrine and dopamine, as well as increase the reuptake of catecholamines in the CNS. This action may be a result of lithium's ability to compete with or replace sodium ions in brain cells. Lithium provides the patient with a feeling of calmness and controls other manic symptoms, such as motor hyperactivity, elation, flight of ideas, restlessness, aggressiveness, hostility, insomnia, and poor judgment. When lithium is given in maintenance therapy, recurrent manic episodes are prevented or diminished in frequency and intensity.

Uses

Lithium is used specifically to treat bipolar disorder and is the medication of choice for individuals who are experiencing acute manic and hypomanic episodes.

What You NEED TO KNOW

Contraindications/Precautions

Lithium is contraindicated for patients with renal dysfunction, leukemia, CHF, organic brain disease, dehydration, and sodium depletion.

Lithium is contraindicated for patients who are pregnant and lactating.

Drug Interactions

Concurrent administration of aminophylline and sodium bicarbonate can cause an increased excretion rate of lithium and lower serum levels. Administering carbamazepine, fluoxetine, methyldopa, probenecid, spironolactone, thiazide diuretics, or nonsteroidal antiinflammatory drugs (NSAIDs) can increase the effects of lithium and toxicity. Concomitant use of neuroleptics (usually chlorpromazine and haloperidol) may cause encephalopathy and may result in acute extrapyramidal effects. Finally, when neuromuscular blockers are given in conjunction with lithium, prolonged paralysis or weakness may occur.

Lithium should be used with extreme caution in any patient who is on a sodium-restricted diet or receiving concurrent diuretics. Caution should also be used in patients with diabetes or a thyroid disorder.

Adverse Effects

Most patients experience some adverse effects from the administration of lithium, but toxicity usually depends on the dose given and the length of therapy.

Serum concentrations of lithium in excess of 2.5 mEq/L can cause coma, cardiovascular collapse, and death.

Monitor older patients who are taking lithium more frequently than younger patients.

Warn the female patient to use contraceptive measures during lithium therapy because of the risk to the fetus.

Slurred speech, drowsiness, vomiting, diarrhea, tremors, lack of coordination, and unsteady gait are evidence of mild-to-moderate toxicity or 1.5 to 2.0 mEq/L. Toxic lithium levels of 2.0 to 3.0 mEq/L usually cause giddiness, agitation or manic behavior, blurred vision, tinnitus, increasing confusion, twitching, and urinary or fecal incontinence. Toxic lithium levels above 3.0 mEq/L usually lead to hypotension, spasticity, seizures, dysrhythmias, and coma.

TAKE HOME POINTS

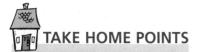

Lithium has an extremely narrow range between therapeutic and toxic levels.

Adverse effects include dizziness, headache, confusion, recent memory loss, dry mouth, metallic taste, drying and thinning hair, reversible leukocytosis (14,000 to 18,000/mm^3), and weight gain or loss. The margin between therapeutic and toxic lithium levels is extremely narrow. The development of toxic symptoms is gradual. These symptoms include nausea, gastric upset, fine tremors (particularly of the upper extremities), and urinary frequency. Without treatment, the tremors become coarse, the gastric distress intensifies, and the CNS effects increase.

What You DO

Nursing Responsibilities

Lithium is administered orally and is available in both liquid and tablet form. This agent is also available in a sustained-release formula. The serum lithium levels recommended are 1.5 mEq/L for acute mania, 0.6 to 1.2 mEq/L for maintenance therapy, and 2.0 mEq/L as a maximal serum level. Patients who are receiving lithium therapy require regularly repeated laboratory tests to determine serum levels of the medication. When administering lithium, the nurse should:

- Monitor regular lithium levels for patients who are receiving lithium therapy to determine serum levels of the medication.
- Instruct the patient to take lithium with meals or milk to prevent GI distress.
- Advise the patient who is taking lithium to withhold one dose and report to the health care provider when evidence of toxicity is present.
- Caution the patient to avoid performing tasks that require alertness, such as driving, until the drug response is known.
- Instruct the patient to maintain a normal diet, including salt and a fluid intake of 2000 to 3000 cc initially during the dose-stabilization period and 1500 cc per day afterward.
- Caution the patient that prolonged exposure to sunlight can lead to dehydration. Advise the patient to report continued thirst and dilute urine (signs of dehydration) to the health care provider.
- Monitor the complete blood count of the patient who is taking lithium for early detection of reversible leukocytosis.
- Monitor glucose in patients with diabetes who are taking lithium because transient hyperglycemia may occur.
- Teach the patient to monitor weight for early detection of weight loss or gain.
- Inform the patient that with normal renal function, 10 to 12 days may be required for lithium to be completely clear of the body.

Do You UNDERSTAND?

DIRECTIONS: **Indicate in the space provided whether each statement is** *true* **or** *false*.

_____ 1. The typical serum lithium level for acute mania is 2.0 mEq/L.

_____ 2. Concurrent administration of thiazide diuretics can increase the rate of lithium excretion and decrease the effectiveness of the medication.

_____ 3. Lithium crosses the placental barrier and, when given during the first trimester of pregnancy, can cause fetal cardiac anomalies.

_____ 4. Lithium undergoes significant metabolism in the liver before excretion via the kidneys.

_____ 5. Concurrent administration of lithium and haloperidol can cause cardiac arrhythmias and cardiovascular collapse.

> ⚠ **Patients should have lithium blood levels drawn 8 to 12 hours after the initial dose and again 2 to 3 times per week during the first month of therapy. Thereafter, the patient's serum levels should be checked weekly to monthly as indicated by the patient's response to the medication. Lithium decreases reabsorption of sodium in the kidneys, which may result in hyponatremia.**

Antipsychotic Agents

What IS an Antipsychotic Agent?

Antipsychotic Agents	Trade Names	Uses
Aliphatic chlorpromazine [klor-PROE-ma-zeen]	Thorazine	Treatment of manic-depression and hallucinations
Piperidine phenothiazine thioridazine [thigh-oh-RID-uh-zeen]	Mellaril	Treatment of psychotic disorders and severe depression
Piperazine phenothiazine trifluoperazine [tri-floo-oh-PER-uh-zeen]	Stelazine	Treatment of psychotic disorders and severe anxiety

Action

Antipsychotic agents are also referred to as neuroleptics. Antipsychotic drugs interfere with the transmission of dopamine in lower brain structures (e.g., midbrain, hypothalamus, limbic system, brainstem, basal ganglia). These drugs inhibit neuronal uptake of norepinephrine and serotonin, as well as suppress the release of ACh. These medications also improve mood and thought disorders, as well as cause hallucinations, delusions, and agitation. Prolonged use of these drugs is not associated with habituation or addiction.

Antipsychotics can be roughly divided into two groups: phenothiazines and nonphenothiazines. The phenothiazine group contains the majority of the neuroleptic medications. This group is divided into three subcategories: the aliphatic, piperidine, and piperazine phenothiazines. Each of these subcategories has special properties and differs from each other in the type and strength of its adverse effects. Selection of a specific phenothiazine neuroleptic may be based

Answers: 1. false; **1.5 mEq/L; 2.** false; increases effects of lithium and risk of toxicity; **3.** true; **4.** false; lithium is not metabolized and is excreted unchanged in kidneys; **5.** false; this combination may cause encephalopathy and result in acute extrapyramidal syndromes.

in part on the type and strength of the anticipated adverse effects. Piperazine phenothiazines have mild anticholinergic, hypotensive, and antiemetic effects.

Uses

 Piperidine phenothiazines are effective for organic brain disease (in older adults) and severe behavioral problems in children.

These drugs are a group of chemically different drugs that are effective in relieving the symptoms of acute and chronic psychoses. Although antipsychotic medications are not curative, they are able to suppress adverse symptoms and improve quality of life. The aliphatic group contains chlorpromazine and promazine, which are particularly effective in controlling hallucinations and delusions. Piperidine phenothiazines include thioridazine and mesoridazine, useful for short-term treatment of major depression and sleep disturbances. Piperazine phenothiazines include trifluoperazine, which is particularly useful in patients who are withdrawn or apathetic.

Nonphenothiazine antipsychotics may be selected when the patient is unable to tolerate phenothiazines. Thiothixene is frequently used in treating chronic schizophrenia when other medications have been ineffective. Loxapine is useful in treating patients with both psychosis and symptoms of a mood disorder.

What You NEED TO KNOW

Contraindications/Precautions

Because of the likelihood of orthostatic hypotension and tachycardia, phenothiazines are contraindicated for patients with known cardiovascular disease or a recent MI. These drugs are contraindicated for patients with a history of bone marrow depression because the effects can mask or exacerbate agranulocytosis. Phenothiazines are contraindicated for patients with renal or hepatic dysfunction, hypothyroidism, and Parkinson's disease. Because of the anticholinergic effects of phenothiazines, phenothiazines are contraindicated for patients with glaucoma or those with a history of peptic ulcer disease, prostatic hypertrophy, and urinary retention. Haloperidol is contraindicated for patients with Parkinson's disease or those who display symptoms similar to those of Parkinson's.

Phenothiazines are not recommended in women during pregnancy and lactation.

Drug Interactions

Concurrent administration of antacids with the antipsychotics can block the absorption of the antipsychotic from the GI tract. Concurrent administration of CNS depressants with antipsychotics can increase the depressive effects of both drugs and may produce severe respiratory depression. Concurrent administration of the antipsychotics and anticonvulsants may require an increase dose of the anticonvulsant because many phenothiazines and nonphenothiazines lower the seizure threshold.

Administering antihypertensives, diuretics, and epinephrine in conjunction with neuroleptics can exacerbate the potential for orthostatic hypotension. When phenothiazines are given with antiarrhythmics, this combination may produce problems for patients with known cardiovascular disease symptoms.

Adverse Effects

Chlorpromazine and promazine produce strong sedative effects, as well as moderate-to-strong extrapyramidal effects. Thioridazine and mesoridazine have moderate or strong anticholinergic effects, strong sedative effects, and mild extrapyramidal effects. Trifluoperazine and prochlorperazine produce less sedation than do the other phenothiazines. These agents have mild anticholinergic, hypotensive, and antiemetic effects but have extremely strong extrapyramidal effects.

The most prominent of the adverse effects of the phenothiazine neuroleptics are the extrapyramidal symptoms (EPS). Six reactions have been identified: acute dystonia, parkinsonism, akathisia, neuroleptic malignant syndrome, periorbital tremor, and tardive dyskinesia. Among the six reactions, the first four are usually present early in therapy (within the first 60 days). The remaining two (periorbital tremor and tardive dyskinesia) generally occur after prolonged therapy, which may be a result of delayed clearance of medication via the renal system or of an increased sensitivity to the drug's anticholinergic effects.

Other adverse effects of phenothiazines include a lowering seizure threshold, orthostatic hypotension, tachycardia, breast engorgement (in both men and women), and abnormal lactation.

Nonphenothiazine antipsychotics, similar to phenothiazines, have the ability to cause significant EPS, including malignant neuroleptic syndrome and tardive dyskinesia. Among all nonphenothiazines, haloperidol has the strongest EPS effects. Thiothixene causes strong EPS but weak anticholinergic, hypotensive, and sedative effects. This medication is frequently used in treating chronic schizophrenia when other medications have been ineffective.

Older patients (generally over age 60) experience an increased occurrence of adverse side effects.

Some individuals (particularly older patients) may experience difficulty in regulating body temperature (poikilothermia), and changes in room temperature may produce hypothermia or hyperthermia.

What You DO

Nursing Responsibilities

Antipsychotic medications are available for administration either orally or IM. The antipsychotic medications (particularly phenothiazines) tend to have erratic absorption patterns, particularly when administered orally. When administering antipsychotics, the nurse should:

- Administer antipsychotic medications IM to provide a more stable rate of absorption and up to ten times more active medication in the system. Most of these drugs are stored in the fatty tissues and may take weeks to be totally cleared from the body.
- Carefully monitor the patient who is taking antihypertensives, diuretics, or epinephrine together with the neuroleptics for orthostatic hypotension. Because of the quinidine-like effects of the neuroleptics (particularly some of the phenothiazines), care must be taken when the patient is concurrently taking an antiarrhythmic.

Do You UNDERSTAND?

DIRECTIONS: **Indicate in the space provided whether each statement is** *true* **or** *false.*

_____ 1. Phenothiazine neuroleptics may cause a patient (particularly a patient over age 60) to experience difficulty in maintaining normal body temperature.

_____ 2. Concurrent administration of CNS depressants with neuroleptics can result in exacerbation of depressant effects and may cause respiratory depression.

_____ 3. The normal slowing of hepatic and renal function as a result of age may be one of the factors that cause older patients to experience increased adverse effects from antipsychotic medications.

_____ 4. Among the EPS that can occur with the neuroleptic medications, only tardive dyskinesia may be anticipated to appear within the first 60 days of therapy.

_____ 5. Administering an antipsychotic to a patient with a known history of seizure may require a decrease of the patient's anticonvulsant dose because of the potential of anticonvulsants by neuroleptics.

Answers: 1. true; 2. true; 3. true; 4. false; acute dystonia, parkinsonism, akathisia, neuroleptic malignant syndrome usually occur within the first 60 days of treatment; other EPS (e.g., periorbital tremors, tardive dyskinesia) occur after prolonged therapy; 5. false; antipsychotics require an increase in dose.

3 Drugs Affecting the Hematologic System

Coagulation disorders can be treated pharmacologically by preventing intravascular blood clots (**thrombi**) formation or by dissolving existing thrombi. Antiplatelet, anticoagulant, and thrombolytic drugs are used in the treatment of coagulation disorders. These drugs inhibit platelet aggregation, suppress coagulation, or promote clot dissolution, thereby interfering with normal homeostasis.

Bleeding is stopped in two stages. In stage one, a platelet plug is formed, followed by coagulation with fibrin reinforcement. After detecting vessel injury, platelets adhere to the injured site. At this time, adenosine diphosphate (ADP) and thromboxane A_2 (TXA_2) are released, causing more platelets to stick to the injured site. Cyclooxygenase is an enzyme that is required for TXA_2 synthesis.

Coagulation occurs when the fragile platelet plug is reinforced with fibrin through a converging series of reactions called the intrinsic pathway and extrinsic pathway. The extrinsic pathway is thus named because a factor outside of the vascular system (**tissue thromboplastin**) is necessary for the reaction to occur. The extrinsic pathway is faster than is the intrinsic pathway and begins with tissue damage outside of the blood vessel. All necessary clotting factors for the intrinsic system are present within the blood vessel, and the cascade of reactions begins with vessel injury. The pathways converge at factor X.

Anemia is a decrease in red blood cell number, size, or hemoglobin. Anemia has several causes, including blood loss, hemolysis, and bone marrow dysfunction. Iron deficiency is the most common cause of anemia, but folic acid and vitamin B_{12} deficiencies can also be causative factors.

What IS an Antiplatelet?

Action

Antiplatelets are a class of hematologic drugs that interfere with platelet membrane function, prevent release of platelet constituents, and prolong bleeding time, thereby inhibiting platelet aggregation. Antiplatelet drugs affect the synthesis and release of cyclooxygenase, TXA_2, and ADP.

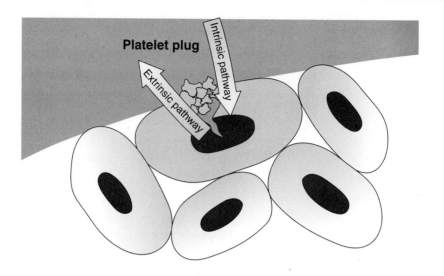

Aspirin is the most frequently used antiplatelet drug with an indirect mechanism of action. Aspirin inhibits cyclooxygenase, an enzyme that is needed by platelets to synthesize TXA_2. TXA_2 acts in two ways to promote hemostasis. TXA_2 acts on platelets to promote aggregation, and it acts on vascular smooth muscles to promote vasoconstriction. When suppression of TXA_2 synthesis occurs, platelet aggregation is inhibited.

Dipyridamole, similar to aspirin, inhibits the formation of TXA_2. Ticlopidine inhibits ADP-mediated platelet aggregation. A single dose of aspirin, ticlopidine, or dipyridamole causes suppression of platelet aggregation. This suppression persists for the life of the platelet, which is 7 to 10 days.

Clopidogrel acts by preventing ADP from binding to its platelet receptor. The action is irreversible, thus bleeding time is prolonged.

Antiplatelets	Trade Names	Uses
acetylsalicylic acid [ah-SEE-til-sal-ih-SILL-ick]	ASA or aspirin	Prevention of MI, TIA, and CVA
ticlopidine [ti-CLO-pi-deen]	Ticlid	Prevention of CVA
dipyridamole [dye-peer-ID-a-mole]	Persantine	Prevention of thromboembolism
clopidogrel [clo-PI-dro-grel]	Plavix	Prevention of MI, CVA, and vascular death

Uses

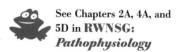

See Chapters 2A, 4A, and 5D in RWNSG: *Pathophysiology*

Antiplatelet drugs are used most frequently to prevent arterial thrombosis. Aspirin is indicated for thromboembolic disorders to prevent myocardial infarction (MI), reinfarction, and cerebrovascular accident (CVA) when a transient ischemic attack (TIA) history is present. Ticlopidine is approved only for prevention of thrombotic CVA in patients who are intolerant to aspirin. Dipyridamole is approved only for prevention of thromboembolism following heart valve replacement surgery and as an adjunct for thallium stress testing. Clopidogrel is used in the prevention of MI, CVA, and vascular death in patients with arterial disease.

 # What You NEED TO KNOW

Contraindications/Precautions

Antiplatelets are contraindicated for patients with drug hypersensitivity, pathologic bleeding disorders, and severe liver impairment.

Aspirin is contraindicated for patients with hypersensitivity to nonsteroidal antiinflammatory drugs (NSAIDs) or persons with "allergic triad" (i.e., nasal polyps, aspirin hypersensitivity, asthma). Patients with vitamin K deficiency, hemophilia, chronic rhinitis, chronic urticaria, or congestive heart failure (CHF) should not use aspirin.

Drug Interactions

Antiplatelets may increase the risk of bleeding when given with anticoagulants. When aspirin is given with ammonium chloride and other acidifying agents, renal elimination is decreased and the risk of salicylate toxicity is increased. With aspirin doses that are greater than 2 grams per day, increased hypoglycemia occurs. Carbonic anhydrase inhibitors enhance salicylate toxicity, and corticosteroids add to ulcerogenic effects. Low doses aspirin may antagonize the uric acid lowering effects of probenecid and sulfinpyrazone. When NSAIDs are given together with clopidrogrel, the risk of bleeding is increased.

Adverse Effects

Tolerability of antiplatelets is variable. Adverse effects of antiplatelet drugs include rash, purplish red spots (petechiae), bruising, nausea, vomiting, diarrhea, abdominal cramps, anorexia, or flatulence. Hypersensitivity adverse effects include anaphylactic shock, laryngeal edema, bronchospasm, and hives (urticaria). Additional adverse effects of aspirin include ulceration, occult blood, GI bleeding, hemolytic anemia, thrombocytopenia, dizziness, drowsiness, confusion, tinnitus, and hearing loss. Dipyridamole may also cause headache, weakness, fainting, white blood cell deficit or complete lack (agranulocytosis), reduction of all types of blood cells (pancytopenia), reduced amount of neutrophils (neutropenia), and reduced amount of white blood cells (leukopenia). Additional adverse effects of clopidrogrel include back pain, depression, and hypercholesterolemia.

Antiplatelets are contraindicated for women during pregnancy and lactation.

Safe and effective use of ticlopidine and dipyridamole in patients under 18 years of age is not established. The use of aspirin for children or adolescents with influenza-like symptoms or chickenpox is contraindicated because of possible association with Reye's syndrome. Use of aspirin with children under 2 years of age is contraindicated, except under the supervision of a health care provider.

Cautious use of aspirin is advised in patients with renal impairment, gastrointestinal (GI) bleeding, hypotension, and in patients who are at risk for bleeding from anticoagulation therapy, bleeding disorders, trauma, or surgery. Cautious use of aspirin is advised in patients with otic diseases, gout, hyperthyroidism, glucose-6-phosphate dehydrogenase (G6PD) deficiency, anemia, and Hodgkin's disease.

What You DO

TAKE HOME POINTS

- Administer antiplatelets with food to reduce gastric irritation of aspirin and improve absorption of ticlopidine.
- Monitor the patient for adverse conditions, such as salicylate toxicity.

 Salicylate toxicity is a primary concern with aspirin use, particularly in older adults because of a decline in serum protein to bind salicylate and a reduced ability to excrete it.

TAKE HOME POINTS

Antiplatelets may increase the risk of bleeding when given concurrently with anticoagulants.

Nursing Responsibilities

Antiplatelets are usually administered orally, but can also be given rectally or intravenously (IV), depending on the purpose of administration and the condition of the patient. Ticlopidine absorption from the GI tract is increased when taken with food.

Aspirin interferes with pregnancy test results, decreases serum cholesterol, potassium, protein-bound iodine (PBI), T_3 and T_4 concentrations, and falsely deceases plasma theophylline levels. Aspirin may increase serum T_3 resin uptake, uric acid, and urine vanillylmandelic acid (VMA) values. Aspirin may interfere with test results for urine glucose, urine 5-hydroxyindoleacetic acid (5-HIAA), and phenolsulfonphthalein (PSP) excretion. Liver function abnormalities may cause high plasma salicylate levels.

The nurse who is administering antiplatelets should:
- Monitor the patient's fluid intake and output.
- Monitor the patient who is taking aspirin for tinnitus and muffled hearing because these symptoms frequently indicate chronic salicylate overdose.
- Be aware that salicylate hypersensitivity is more common in patients with asthma, hay fever, chronic urticaria, nasal polyps, and perennial rhinitis.
- Observe the patient for bleeding, such as petechiae, ecchymoses, and bloody urine or stool. Bleeding time is prolonged, and 5 or more grams per day of aspirin prolongs prothrombin time.
- Discontinue antiplatelets 1 week before surgery to reduce the risk of bleeding.

Do You UNDERSTAND?

DIRECTIONS: Fill in the blanks with appropriate responses.

1. To ensure safety, the nurse should be aware of the increased risk of neurologic adverse effects with the use of aspirin. They are:

   _____

   _____

   _____

   _____

   _____

2. Both _____ and
   _____ age groups
   are at increased risk of salicylate should they become dehydrated.

3. To promote safe administration, the nurse should be aware that ticlopidine acts as an antiplatelet by inhibiting _____ release.

Answer: 1. tinnitus, hearing loss, dizziness, drowsiness, confusion; 2. children, older adults; 3. ADP.

What IS an Anticoagulant?

Anticoagulants	Trade Names	Uses
warfarin [WAR-far-in]	Coumadin	Prevention and treatment of thrombus or embolism
heparin [HEP-a-rin]	Heparin	Prevention and treatment of thrombus or embolism
enoxaparin [e-NOX-a-pa-rin]	Lovenox	Prevention and treatment of thrombus or embolism

Action

Anticoagulants are drugs that suppress the production of fibrin, thereby disrupting the coagulation cascade. Both anticoagulants and antiplatelets suppress thrombosis but through different mechanisms. Warfarin is thought to have an indirect effect on vitamin K–dependent coagulation factors. Warfarin depresses hepatic synthesis of vitamin K. Reducing the amount of vitamin K also reduces the dependent coagulation factors II, VII, IX, and X.

Heparin directly increases the action of antithrombin III. Thus the conversion of prothrombin to thrombin and the conversion of fibrinogen to fibrin are blocked.

Enoxaparin blocks factor IIa and factor Xa, thereby preventing clot formation. Enoxaparin inactivates Xa and does not bind to protein, tissues, or prothrombin as do the longer molecules in heparin.

Uses

Anticoagulants are used most frequently to prevent venous thrombosis. Warfarin is the drug of choice for long-term prevention of thrombosis. Warfarin is also approved for use in prophylaxis and treatment of pulmonary embolism (PE), atrial fibrillation, and MI.

Heparin is the drug of choice for prevention and treatment of deep vein thrombosis (DVT), PE, atrial fibrillation with embolization, and diagnosis and treatment of disseminated intravascular coagulation (DIC). Heparin is used to treat acute coronary occlusion and to prevent thromboembolic complications that arise from cardiac or vascular surgery. Heparin is approved for use in preventing the clotting of heparin locks, blood samples, and during dialysis. Heparin is also used to prevent cerebral thrombosis in evolving strokes and to prevent stroke or left ventricular thrombi after an MI.

Enoxaparin is a low–molecular-weight heparin prototype that is used to prevent DVT after abdominal surgery and after hip or knee surgery. Enoxaparin is also used for treatment of DVT, PE, and acute coronary syndrome.

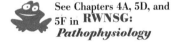

TAKE HOME POINTS

- Warfarin inhibits the formation of new clots but does not dissolve existing clots.
- Heparin inhibits the formation of new clots but does not dissolve existing clots.

See Chapters 4A, 5D, and 5F in **RWNSG:** *Pathophysiology*

What You NEED TO KNOW

Heparin may be used during pregnancy because the drug does not cross the placental barrier. Heparin is contraindicated for women during lactation and the postpartum period.

Low–molecular-weight heparin drugs are contraindicated for patients who are allergic to pork or those who may have religious objections to the consumption of pork products.

Cautious use of anticoagulants is advised in alcoholics, patients with hazardous occupations, and those with an indwelling catheter.

Contraindications/Precautions

Warfarin and heparin are contraindicated for patients with bleeding disorders, vitamin K deficiency, severe hypertension, and advanced renal, kidney, or liver disease. Heparin should also be avoided in patients with severe thrombocytopenia and those who are at risk for bleeding.

Drug Interactions

With the concurrent use of low–molecular-weight heparin and spinal-epidural anesthesia or spinal puncture, epidural or spinal hematomas may occur. Many of the hematomas cause neurologic injury, including long-term or permanent paralysis.

Adverse Effects

The principal adverse effect of anticoagulants is bleeding. The risk increases with higher doses and the addition of antiplatelet drugs. Hypersensitivity reactions are exhibited as dermatitis, urticaria pruritus, fever, and bronchospasm with anaphylactic reaction. Other adverse effects of warfarin include nausea, vomiting, diarrhea, abdominal cramps, or anorexia. Heparin has similar adverse effects, but these are frequently more severe. Injection site reactions may occur along with transient thrombocytopenia. Large doses of heparin for prolonged periods may suppress renal function, causing osteoporosis, hypoaldosteronism, or hyperkalemia.

What You DO

Nursing Responsibilities

Warfarin is given only by mouth. Heparin can be administered IV or subcutaneously (SC), depending on the speed of response desired and condition of the patient. The only route for administering enoxaparin is SC.

Anticoagulants begin to work within 10 to 15 minutes when given SC. IV administration has a rapid onset of 1 to 3 minutes. When warfarin is taken orally, the onset of action is approximately 2 to 7 days. The peak of drug action for oral medications is 12 hours to 3 days. The peak for IV heparin is within minutes and duration is 2 to 6 hours. When heparin is given SC, the onset occurs in 20 to 60 minutes and lasts 8 to 12 hours. Enoxaparin has an onset of action of 20 to 60 minutes and a duration of 12 hours. Enoxaparin has a peak action in 3 to 5 hours.

Monitor the patient's international normalized ratio (INR) values every week for the first month and then once a month to adjust drug dose. The warfarin dose must be adjusted based on each person's unique response. An INR in the target range of 2:3 is usually acceptable in reducing the risk of bleeding and providing therapeutic benefits. Higher INRs are associated with a greater risk of bleeding.

Monitor the partial thromboplastin time (PTT) or activated partial thromboplastin time (APTT) level of the patient who is taking heparin for dose determination. The therapeutic dose range is usually $1^{1}/_{2}$ to 2 times the normal.

The heparin dose is adjusted to achieve desired range of lab values. Dissimilar to heparin, low–molecular-weight heparins (e.g., enoxaparin) do not require APTT, PTT, or INR monitoring and can be given on a fixed schedule.

Other nursing responsibilities include the following:

- Monitor intake and output of the patient who is taking anticoagulants.
- Monitor the patient who is taking anticoagulants for any signs of overt or hidden bleeding.
- Instruct patients and family members to report signs of bleeding to the health care provider immediately.
- Monitor the patient for signs of toxicity and medication effectiveness.
- Be aware that anticoagulants may cause elevated results for alanine aminotransferase (ALT), aspartate aminotransferase (AST), and thyroid function. Heparin causes prolonged bromsulphalein (BSP) levels, decreased triglycerides and cholesterol, and an alteration in blood gases.
- Be aware that protamine sulfate is the antidote for heparin and low–molecular-weight heparin overdose. Protamine sulfate binds to heparin and keeps it from working. Vitamin K is the antidote for warfarin.

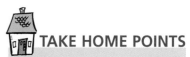

TAKE HOME POINTS

- An INR in the target range of 2:3 usually is acceptable.
- Heparin is given parentally based on the PTT or APTT. The therapeutic dose range of heparin is usually $1^{1}/_{2}$ to 2 times the normal.

Do You UNDERSTAND?

DIRECTIONS: Indicate in the space provided whether each statement is *true* or *false*.

_____ 1. Warfarin is the drug of choice for long-term prevention and prophylaxis of thrombosis.

_____ 2. Warfarin is used after abdominal surgery and to prevent DVT after hip or knee surgery.

_____ 3. Heparin blocks factor IIa and factor Xa, thereby preventing clot formation.

_____ 4. Enoxaparin depresses hepatic synthesis of vitamin K.

Answers: 1. true; 2. false; 3. false; 4. false.

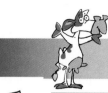

What IS a Thrombolytic?

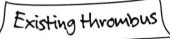

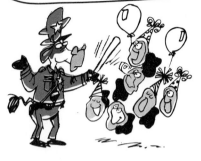

Thrombolytics	Trade Names	Uses
streptokinase [strep-toe-KYE-nase]	Streptase	Treatment of thrombosis and embolism
alteplase recombinant [AL-te-plase]	Activase tPA	Treatment of thrombosis and embolism

Action

Thrombolytics (**fibrinolytics**) break down existing thrombus, rather than preventing thrombi from forming. Thrombolytics work directly or indirectly to convert plasminogen to plastin, an enzyme that acts to digest the fibrin matrix of clots. Plastin is capable of degrading fibrin, fibrinogen, and factors V, VIII, and XII.

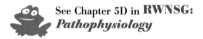

See Chapter 5D in **RWNSG:** *Pathophysiology*

Uses

Thrombolytic drugs are used to treat acute MI, massive PE, thrombotic strokes, and DVT. Thrombolytic therapy is most effective when started within 4 to 6 hours after an event. Streptokinase is extracted from cultures of streptococci and contains foreign protein, which contributes to allergic reactions and antibody production that neutralize drug effects. Recombinant deoxyribonucleic acid (DNA) technology is used with reteplase recombinant and alteplase recombinant. These thrombolytics are devoid of foreign proteins and are nonallergic.

What You NEED TO KNOW

Contraindications/Precautions

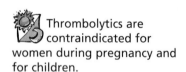

Thrombolytics are contraindicated for women during pregnancy and for children.

Thrombolytics are contraindicated for patients with known hypersensitivity, hemorrhagic disorders, severe uncontrolled hypertension, and an increased risk of bleeding.

Drug Interactions

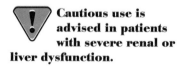

Cautious use is advised in patients with severe renal or liver dysfunction.

When thrombolytics are given concurrently with aspirin, abciximab, dipyridamole, and heparin, the risk of bleeding is increased. Coagulation and fibrinolytic tests are unreliable because of the decrease in plasminogen and fibrinogen. Aminocaproic acid reverses the action of streptokinase.

Adverse Effects

Adverse effects of thrombolytics include hemorrhage and anemia. Hypersensitivity is common (12%) with streptokinase use, urokinase, and anistreplase and may include bronchospasm and anaphylaxis or milder symptoms, such as urticaria, itching, and headache. Adverse effects reported with streptokinase include fever, hypotension, unstable blood pressure, and reperfusion-atrial or ventricular arrhythmias.

What You DO

Nursing Responsibilities

Thrombolytics are only administered IV or infused directly into the occlusion.

Drug effects develop within minutes of IV administration. The half-life of thrombolytics varies from 40 to 80 minutes for streptokinase and anistreplase to 5 to 20 minutes for alteplase, reteplase, and urokinase.

Additional nursing responsibilities include the following:
• Monitor intake and output in patients who are taking thrombolytics.
• Monitor patients for anaphylactic reactions and bleeding. Drug discontinuation may be indicated in the event of these adverse effects.

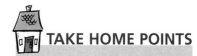

TAKE HOME POINTS

• Thrombolytics are only administered IV or infused directly into the occlusion.
• Thrombolytic therapy is most effective when started early, within 4 to 6 hours after an event.
• Drug discontinuation may be indicated for adverse effects, such as anaphylactic reactions and bleeding.

Do You UNDERSTAND?

DIRECTIONS: Match the terms in Column A with the appropriate terms in Column B.

Column A	Column B
_____ 1. Streptokinase	a. Increased risk of dysrhythmias
_____ 2. Alteplase recombinant	b. Devoid of foreign proteins or nonallergics

What IS an Antianemic Agent?

Refer to page 360 for a discussion of antianemic agents such as iron and vitamin B_{12} (cyanocobalamin) and on page 363 for a discussion of vitamin B_9 (folic acid).

CHAPTER 4

Drugs Affecting Blood Pressure and Blood Flow

SECTION A
ANTIHYPERTENSIVES

This chapter reviews pharmacologic methods that are used to control high blood pressure. Because blood pressure (BP) depends on cardiac output (CO) and peripheral vascular resistance (PVR), pharmacologic interference of either factor can lead to BP control. Body systems that control CO, PVR, and BP involve the vascular, cardiac, renal, and sympathetic nervous system. Antihypertensive drugs that act on these body systems to lower BP include angiotensin-converting enzyme (ACE) inhibitors, angiotensin II inhibitors, α-adrenergic blockers, β-adrenergic blockers, α-beta blockers, calcium channel blockers, central-acting agents, peripheral adrenergic neuron antagonists, and direct vasodilators. Diuretics decrease fluid volume, the action of which is also helpful in reducing BP. These drugs are discussed in Chapter 9, Section A, of this text.

What IS an ACE Inhibitor?

ACE Inhibitors	Trade Names	Uses
captopril [KAP-toe-prill]	Capoten	Treatment of hypertension and unresponsive CHF
benazepril [BEN-AZE-uh-prill]	Lotensin	Treatment of hypertension
enalapril [eh-NAL-uh-prill]	Vasotec	Treatment of hypertension and adjunct therapy in CHF
quinapril [KWIN-uh-prill]	Accupril	Treatment of hypertension and adjunct therapy in CHF
ramipril [RAM-uh-prill]	Altace	Treatment of hypertension and CHF post MI

Action

ACE inhibitors are a classification of antihypertensive medications that interfere with the renin-angiotensin-aldosterone system (RAAS), thereby decreasing BP. In the RAAS, an ACE converts angiotensin I to angiotensin II. Normally, angiotensin II is a potent vasoconstrictor and stimulator of aldosterone, which increases vasoconstriction and fluid volume, resulting in PVR. Through the process of blocking the ACE and its conversion of angiotensin I to angiotensin II, vasodilation, fluid volume reduction, and decreased PVR lead to a reduction in BP.

Uses

ACE inhibitors are indicated for early control of mild-to-severe hypertension in patients with normal renal function. Captopril is widely used to treat hypertension in patients with chronic renal failure (CRF).

ACE inhibitors are frequently used as the first drug of choice in the treatment of hypertensive patients with the following conditions: congestive heart failure (CHF), myocardial infarction (MI), peripheral vascular disease (PVD), and diabetes mellitus (DM). ACE inhibitors maintain their "first drug of choice" status because of their cardioprotective effects. ACE inhibitors are effective in monotherapy or in combination with other antihypertensives and thiazide diuretics.

 Because of efficiency and tolerability, ACE inhibitors may be used for all age groups.

See Chapter 4C in **RWNSG:** *Pathophysiology*

ACE inhibitors have greater effectiveness in young Caucasians than they do in African Americans. Combination therapy with low-dose diuretics can increase the effectiveness of ACE inhibitors in African Americans.

 # What You NEED TO KNOW

Contraindications/Precautions

ACE inhibitors are contraindicated for patients with hypersensitivity, renal artery stenosis, and hyperkalemia.

Drug Interactions

Several drugs affect the absorption of other drugs and interact adversely. Antacids decrease the absorption of ACE inhibitors. When tetracycline and ACE inhibitors are taken concurrently, the absorption of tetracycline is decreased. Nonsteroidal antiinflammatory drugs (NSAIDs) and rifampin decrease the ACE action when taken concurrently with ACE inhibitors. Concurrent drugs that increase the hypotensive action of ACE inhibitors include alcohol, nitrates, monamine oxidase inhibitors (MAOIs), benzodiazepines, probenecid, diuretics, and other antihypertensives. ACE inhibitors can increase the action of other drugs. For example, potassium supplements may cause hyperkalemia, lithium may cause lithium toxicity, and digoxin may cause digoxin toxicity when taken in combination with ACE inhibitors.

Adverse Effects

The most common adverse effect of an ACE inhibitor is the dry hacking cough, "ACE cough," which usually subsides within several days after drug discontinuation. The cough is related to an increased sensitivity of the cough reflex that

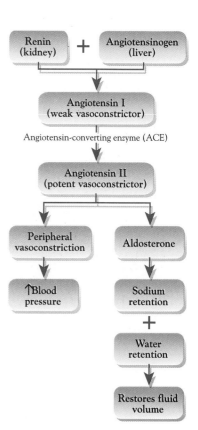

ACE inhibitors are con-traindicated for women during pregnancy.

 ACE inhibitors should be used with caution in lactating women.

 ACE inhibitors should be used cautiously in patients with CHF, aortic stenosis, and sodium and fluid volume depletion.

The life-threatening adverse effects of ACE inhibitors include fatal allergic reactions (e.g., anaphylaxis or angioedema of the face, lips, tongue, glottis, larynx, and the extremities), increased fetal mortality in the second and third trimester of pregnancy, and acute renal failure.

 Angioedema is a more common life-threatening adverse effect in African-American patients.

 TAKE HOME POINTS

Notify the health care provider when the BP reduction is considered significant (20 mm Hg). Instruct the patient to rise slowly from a lying position and dangle the legs for a few minutes before standing. Orthostatic hypotension is more common in patients with CHF.

bradykinin and prostaglandins induce. Adverse effects include rash, itching, fatigue, dry mouth, anorexia, nausea, vomiting, abdominal pain, diarrhea, insomnia, hyperkalemia, paresthesias, neutropenia, and agranulocytosis. Cardiovascular-related effects include headache, dizziness, tachycardia, palpitations, and first-dose phenomenon (first-dose syncope). This phenomenon involves severe hypotension and fainting that can occur within 1 to 4 hours after the initial dose or when the dose is rapidly increased. This severe hypotensive effect may occur with subsequent dosing but is less severe at that time. The phenomenon usually occurs in volume-depleted individuals and those with a sodium level that is less than 130 mmol/L.

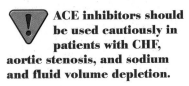 # What You DO

Nursing Responsibilities

ACE inhibitors are usually administered orally 1 hour before meals. In a hypertensive crisis in the acute care setting, ACE inhibitors are usually given intravenously (IV) for a fast response. Monitoring drug effectiveness in hypertensive crisis may be as frequently as every 5 to 15 minutes until the diastolic BP is less than 90 mm Hg. Monitoring usually continues every 30 minutes until the patient is stable. When administering ACE inhibitors, the nurse should:

- Monitor the BP hourly after the first dose or rapid dose increase for early detection of first-dose phenomenon. The patient may require IV volume expansion when BP reduction is excessive or too rapid.
- Instruct the patient to lie down for 3 to 4 hours after the first dose or a rapid dose increase.
- Adequately hydrate patients or discontinue diuretics 2 to 3 days before the initiation of ACE therapy to prevent first-dose phenomenon.
- Monitor the BP of stable patients in the acute care setting immediately before routine administration of antihypertensives and at least every 4 hours after administration. Patients who are experiencing orthostatic hypotension may require dose reduction or drug discontinuation. The health care provider frequently orders parameters that define an acceptable BP range. When the BP is lower than the parameter, the dose is withheld.
- Be certain of the correct drug name during administration because several drugs have similar names.
- Teach the patient about appropriate spacing between drug doses. Some medications require that a certain blood level be maintained for effectiveness. When an even blood level is required for a medication, the nurse should schedule the taking of medications at equally distant times (BID) (e.g., 9:00 AM and 9:00 PM).
- Instruct patients to refrain from activities that require mental alertness (e.g., driving) until the response to the drug is known.

 Inform the patient that if a dose is omitted, the next dose should not be doubled. A patient may take a missed dose of ACE inhibitor when the time before the next dose is greater than 4 hours.

 Instruct the patient to avoid substances that interfere with ACE inhibitors, such as caffeine-containing beverages (e.g., coffee, tea, cola) and over-the-counter (OTC) medications (e.g., cold remedies).

 Instruct the patient to report edema and weight gain greater than 3 pounds per day or 5 pounds per week.

• Monitor renal and liver function tests and complete blood count (CBC) throughout therapy with ACE inhibitors. A CBC should be monitored every 2 weeks for 3 months and then periodically because neutrophils, hemoglobin, and hematocrit levels may be reduced with ACE inhibitors.

• Monitor potassium levels for early detection of hyperkalemia.

• Monitor lithium and digoxin for potential toxicities.

Do You UNDERSTAND?

DIRECTIONS: **Complete the following statements with appropriate responses from the italicized terms listed below.**

1. When a patient is taking potassium concurrently with an ACE inhibitor, the nurse should monitor for potential ___Hyper Kelemia___ .
2. The most common adverse effect of ACE inhibitors is ___Cough___ .
3. ACE inhibitors have _____ effects and can safely be given to hypertensive patients with CHF, stable MI, PVD, and DM.

cardioprotective	hyperkalemia
detrimental	cough
hypokalemia	seizures

What IS an Angiotensin II Inhibitor?

Angiotensin II Antagonists	Trade Names	Uses
losartan [low-SAHR-tan]	Cozaar	Treatment of hypertension
valsartan [val-SAHR-tan]	Diovan	Treatment of hypertension
irbesartan [ir-be-SAHR-tan]	Avapro	Treatment of hypertension
candesartan cilexetil [kan-deh-SAHR-tan sigh-LEX-eh-till]	Atacand	Treatment of hypertension

Action

Angiotensin II inhibitors (angiotensin II antagonists or angiotensin receptor blockers) selectively block the binding of angiotensin II to specific AT₁-receptors found in vascular smooth muscle and adrenal glands. ACE inhibitors block the conversion of angiotensin I to angiotensin II, but other enzymes that ACE inhibitors fail to block can form angiotensin II. Therefore, by providing further blockage of the renin-angiotensin system and aldosterone release, angiotensin receptor blockers (ARBs) inhibit vasoconstriction. Blocking vasoconstriction allows vasodilation, which increases renal sodium and water excretion and decreases blood volume. With effective interference of PVR, BP is lowered. Maximal therapeutic reduction of BP from ARBs is usually noted within 3 to 6 weeks after initiating therapy.

Uses

ARBs are beneficial to patients who are unable to tolerate ACE inhibitors but require BP reduction. Losartan is particularly useful in decreasing BP in patients with renal insufficiency without diminishing renal function. ARBs are now recognized as a possible first drug of choice for hypertension.

See Chapter 4C in RWNSG: *Pathophysiology*

These drugs are effective in all age groups but are less effective in monotherapy for African Americans. For groups other than African Americans, ARBs are effective in monotherapy or combination therapy in the treatment of hypertension.

ARBs are contraindicated for women during pregnancy and lactation.

Caution should be taken when administering ARBs to patients with hepatic or renal dysfunction and hypovolemia.

What You NEED TO KNOW

Contraindications/Precautions

ARBs are contraindicated for patients with hypersensitivity.

Drug Interactions

The ARB serum level and efficacy are reduced when given concurrently with phenobarbital. When both drugs are necessary, dose adjustments may be required.

Adverse Effects

ARBs have few adverse effects. Adverse effects of ARBs are headache, dizziness, weakness, hypotension, rash, dry skin, alopecia, dry mouth, tooth pain, nausea, diarrhea, and abdominal pain. ARBs do not appear to induce cough, angioedema, or significant hyperkalemia as do ACE inhibitors.

What You DO

Nursing Responsibilities

When administering ARBs, the nurse should:
- Monitor the patient on initiation of ARB therapy for first-dose phenomenon, particularly in volume-depleted patients.
- Monitor electrolyte levels and hepatic and renal function studies.

Do You UNDERSTAND?

DIRECTIONS: Select the correct response from the italicized word to fill in the blanks.

1. ARBs cause _____.
   (*vasoconstriction, vasodilation*)
2. ARBs cause sodium and water _____.
   (*retention, excretion*)

What IS an α_1-Adrenergic Blocker?

Alpha-Adrenergic Blockers	Trade Names	Uses
prazosin [PRAY-zoe-sin]	Minipress	Treatment of hypertension
doxazosin mesylate [DOX-uh-zoe-sin MEH-suh-late]	Cardura	Treatment of hypertension
terazosin [ter-AZE-oh-sin]	Hytrin	Treatment of hypertension

Action

α_1-Adrenergic blockers (α_1-blockers, α-adrenergic antagonists, or sympatholytics) selectively block stimulation of postsynaptic α_1-receptors that regulate vasomotor tone. This action inhibits norepinephrine reuptake by smooth muscle cells and reduces vasoconstriction and PVR. The result is vasodilation in both arterioles and veins, leading to a decrease in supine and standing BP. α_1-Blockers trigger the baroreceptor reflex, which causes an increase in heart rate. During long-term therapy, increased renin leads to sodium and water retention in many patients, decreasing the typical postural hypotension.

Uses

α_1-Blockers are used effectively in mild-to-moderate hypertension with monotherapy or in combination therapy with a diuretic or BB. α_1-Blockers are more beneficial in reducing diastolic pressure than they are in reducing systolic pressure.

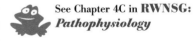

See Chapter 4C in RWNSG: *Pathophysiology*

Answers: 1. vasodilation; 2. excretion.

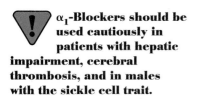

α_1-Blockers are contraindicated for children and for women during pregnancy and lactation.

α_1-**Blockers should be used cautiously in patients with hepatic impairment, cerebral thrombosis, and in males with the sickle cell trait.**

What You NEED TO KNOW

Contraindications/Precautions

α_1-Blockers are contraindicated for patients with hypersensitivity.

Drug Interactions

When α_1-blockers are taken concurrently with alcohol, the patient will experience increased hypotension. When taken together with epinephrine and ephedrine, vasoconstriction and hypertension are decreased.

Adverse Effects

Cardiovascular adverse effects of α_1-blockers include the first-dose phenomenon, flushing, headache, dizziness, fainting, edema, tachycardia, palpitations, and dysrhythmias. Gastrointestinal (GI) adverse effects include dry mouth, nausea, vomiting, abdominal pain, and diarrhea. Other adverse effects include visual disturbances, drowsiness, insomnia, nervousness, confusion, depression, fatigue, paresthesia, nasal congestion, urinary frequency, alopecia, priapism, impotence, and bronchospasm. An advantage of α_1-blockers is that no metabolic or lipid adverse effects are present.

What You DO

Nursing Responsibilities

α_1-Blockers can be taken with milk or meals to minimize GI distress. When administering α_1-blockers, the nurse should:

- Inform the patient that postural hypotension and palpitations usually disappear with continued therapy but may reappear when performing strenuous exercise, eating a large meal, drinking alcohol, or when other conditions that promote vasodilation are present.
- Instruct the patient to lie or sit down immediately when dizziness occurs.
- Advise the patient to avoid sudden changes in position.
- Instruct the recumbent patient to sit upright for a few minutes and dangle the legs before ambulating.
- Inform the patient that the therapeutic effect of α_1-blockers usually occurs within 2 weeks after initiating therapy.
- Instruct the patient to report any weight gain or ankle edema.
- Instruct the patient to avoid excess caffeine or OTC drugs, particularly cold remedies.

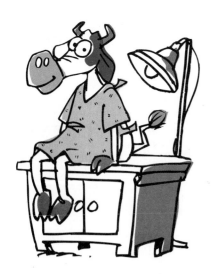

Do You UNDERSTAND?

DIRECTIONS: Indicate in the space provided whether each statement is *true* or *false*.

_____ 1. α_1-Blockers block α_1-receptors, causing vasoconstriction.
_____ 2. α_1-Blockers are used in treating mild-to-moderate hypertension.

What IS a β-Adrenergic Blocker?

Beta Blockers	Trade Names	Uses
propranolol [pro-PRAN-oh-lahl]	Inderal	Treatment of hypertension, angina, MI, and ventricular dysrhythmias
atenolol [ah-TEN-oh-lahl]	Tenormin	Treatment of hypertension, angina, and MI
metoprolol [meh-TOE-proe-lahl]	Lopressor	Treatment of hypertension, angina, and MI
nadolol [nay-DOE-lahl]	Corgard	Treatment of hypertension, angina, and MI

Action

β-Adrenergic blockers (**beta blockers, b-adrenergic antagonists, or sympatholytics**) block both cardiac and bronchial receptors or β-receptors, which compete with epinephrine and norepinephrine for available β-receptor sites. Blocking the sympathetic nervous system's catecholamines results in reduced renin and aldosterone release, and fluid volume. By inhibiting B_1-receptors, the heart rate, contractibility (negative inotrope), myocardial oxygen demand, automaticity, and conduction decrease. Blocking B_2-receptors causes vasodilation of the arterioles and a reduction of PVR and BP.

Uses

Beta blockers (BBs) are used in patients with normal PVR, normal blood volume, high plasma-renin levels, angina, and previous MI. These agents are also used in the initial treatment of uncomplicated hypertension. (BBs increase the tolerance of exercise for the patient with stable angina; they also decrease oxygen requirements.) Therefore BBs are used as antianginal agents in the long-term prevention of angina. These agents are not used in the immediate relief of an acute anginal attack. In recent years, BBs have also been used to preserve the myocardium and to reduce the cardiac workload that is associated with cardiac ischemia, MI, severe heart failure (particularly diastolic failure), and cardiomyopathy. BBs are also used to treat dysrhythmias, and acebutolol is used to treat ventricular tachycardia and PVCs. Propranolol and esmolol are used to suppress sinus and atrial tachydysrhythmias.

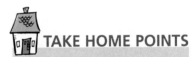

TAKE HOME POINTS

Blocking B_2-receptors causes bronchoconstriction, which is an adverse rather than a therapeutic effect.

See Chapter 4C in **RWNSG:** *Pathophysiology*

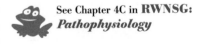

BBs are effective in reducing the BP in young Caucasian hypertensive patients with high CO.

Answers: 1. false; the action causes vasodilation; 2. true.

What You NEED TO KNOW

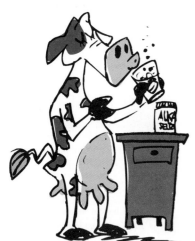

BBs should be used with caution in women during pregnancy and lactation.

Caution should be taken in patients with acute bronchospasm, chronic obstructive pulmonary disease (COPD), asthma, depression, PVD, sick sinus syndrome, bradycardia, heart block, valvular heart disease, and systolic heart failure.

Contraindications/Precautions

BBs should be used with caution in patients with DM, thyrotoxicosis, cerebrovascular insufficiency, and hepatic and renal dysfunction.

Drug Interactions

Administering BBs in combination with other drugs that have similar effects results in additive effects. For example, calcium channel blockers also decrease heart rate and BP, thus may result in bradydysrhythmias or hypotension. Antacids decrease absorption of BBs in the GI tract when given together. NSAIDs reduce the hypotensive effects of BBs, while cimetidine, prazosin, and terazosin may increase severe hypotensive effects of the first BB dose. When given concurrently with insulin and sulfonylureas, the signs of hypoglycemia and hyperglycemia may be masked. The use of BBs with high doses of tubocurarine may exacerbate neuromuscular blockade. Tricyclic antidepressants and atropine may block bradycardia when given concurrently with BBs. β-Adrenergic agonists increase the effect of BBs.

Adverse Effects

Common adverse effects that are associated with BBs include headache, flushing, dizziness, bradycardia, postural hypotension, fatigue, drowsiness, confusion, bronchospasm, and bronchoconstriction. GI adverse effects include taste alteration, nausea, vomiting, and diarrhea. Other adverse effects include insomnia, cough, wheezing, dyspnea, malaise, lethargy, hypoglycemia, impotence, peripheral vasoconstriction, dysrhythmias, and heart failure. Rare adverse effects include bizarre dreams, depression, and blood dyscrasias.

What You DO

Nursing Responsibilities

When administering BBs, the nurse should:

- Assess BP and heart rate before BB administration and monitor closely, particularly when administered with a calcium channel blocker or other similar agents.
- Instruct the patient to report any weakness, dizziness, or fainting because these may be indicative of hypotension and bradycardia.
- Delay the BB dose and notify the health care provider when the patient's systolic BP is less than 90 mm Hg or the apical pulse is less than 60 beats per minute.
- Instruct the patient to take BBs before meals because food delays peak effects.

- Frequently assess the breathing pattern of the patient who is taking BBs to detect bronchoconstriction and bronchospasms.
- Instruct the patient with diabetes who is taking BBs to monitor blood glucose levels regularly and to expect dose changes in the insulin or oral hypoglycemics.
- Instruct the patient to avoid substances that interfere with BBs, such as caffeine-containing beverages (e.g., coffee, tea, cola) and OTC medications (e.g., cold remedies).
- Instruct the patient to report edema and weight gain that is greater than 3 pounds per day or 5 pounds per week.
- Monitor CBC, potassium, renal and liver functions tests, and triglycerides. BBs may decrease high-density lipoprotein cholesterol and increase blood urea nitrogen (BUN) levels in patients with severe heart disease.
- Monitor the patient for acute heart failure (fine crackles in the posterior bases of the lungs) that is the result of excess myocardial depression, and immediately notify the health care provider.
- Teach the patient the proper way to gradually reduce the dose over a 1- to 2-week period when discontinuing BBs after long-term use.

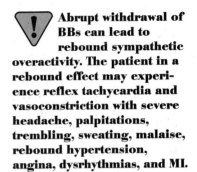

Abrupt withdrawal of BBs can lead to rebound sympathetic overactivity. The patient in a rebound effect may experience reflex tachycardia and vasoconstriction with severe headache, palpitations, trembling, sweating, malaise, rebound hypertension, angina, dysrhythmias, and MI.

TAKE HOME POINTS

- When treatment is being transferred to an alternative BB, weaning is unnecessary, because the patient may be transferred directly to comparable doses without treatment interruption.
- Administer BBs with equally distant spacing between doses to prevent hypotension and hypertension.

Do You UNDERSTAND?

DIRECTIONS: In the spaces provided, indicate the appropriate direction: increased (I) or decreased (D).

BBs cause:

_____ 1. renin release
_____ 2. fluid volume
_____ 3. BP
_____ 4. CO
_____ 5. bronchoconstriction

_____ 6. dizziness
_____ 7. pulse
_____ 8. myocardial contractility
_____ 9. vasodilation

What IS an α-Beta Blocker?

Alpha-Beta Blockers	Trade Names	Uses
labetalol [la-BET-uh-lahl]	Trandate	Treatment of hypertension
carvedilol [car-ve-DIE-lahl]	Coreg	Treatment of hypertension

Action

α-Beta antagonists (α-beta adrenergic antagonists, α- and β-adrenergic blocking agents, or α-beta blockers) combine the blocking of selective α-receptors and nonselective blocking of β-receptors. Blockage of α-receptors affects vasomotor

Answers: 1. D; 2. D; 3. D; 4. D; 5. I; 6. I; 7. D; 8. D; 9. I.

α-Beta blockers have greater effectiveness in African Americans than do BBs.

See Chapter 4C in **RWNSG:** *Pathophysiology*

α-Beta blockers are also contraindicated for women during pregnancy and lactation.

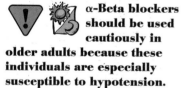α-Beta blockers **should be used with caution in patients with DM, PVD, COPD, pheo-chromocytoma, hepatic dysfunction, and bronchospasm.**

α-Beta blockers **should be used cautiously in older adults because these individuals are especially susceptible to hypotension.**

tone and results in vasodilation and decreased PVR. Blockage of β-receptors leads to a reduction of heart rate, a delay in atrioventricular (AV) conduction, and a depressed cardiac contractility. BP is reduced primarily because of a decrease in PVR.

Uses

α-Beta blockers are used in stage one or two of hypertension. These agents may be used alone or in combination with a thiazide or loop diuretic. Labetalol, when given IV, can decrease BP rapidly and is used in the treatment of hypertensive emergencies.

What You NEED TO KNOW

Contraindications/Precautions

α-Beta blockers are contraindicated for patients with severe bradycardia, heart block, asthma, shock, and uncontrolled CHF.

Drug Interactions

Drug interactions with α-beta blockers include increased effects when given with cimetidine and halothane. Decreased antihypertensive effects occur when given with glutethimide and rifampin. β-Agonists, MAOIs, phenothiazines, and tricyclic antidepressants antagonize the hypotensive effects of α-beta blockers. Carvedilol may increase digoxin levels and may enhance hypoglycemic effects of oral hypoglycemic agents and insulin. Alcohol intensifies the orthostatic hypotension and sedative effect of α-beta blockers.

Adverse Effects

Common adverse effects of α-beta blockers include headache, dizziness, fainting, orthostatic hypotension, drowsiness, dyspnea, fatigue, diarrhea, impaired ejaculation, and edema with weight gain. Other adverse effects include visual disturbances, confusion, cough, nasal congestion, rhinitis, rash, alopecia, hypoglycemia, insomnia, tremors, paresthesias, and depression. GI adverse effects include dry mouth, anorexia, nausea, vomiting, and flatulence. More serious effects include dysrhythmias, CHF, pulmonary edema, cerebral vascular accident (CVA), bronchospasm, and bronchial obstruction.

What You DO

Nursing Responsibilities

When IV administration of this drug is given, the patient should be lying supine. The position should be maintained for 3 hours after administration. The patient should return upright slowly. The peak of postural hypotension is 2 to 4 hours after therapy. When administering α-beta blockers, the nurse should:

- Take a baseline BP before α-beta blocker administration and monitor throughout therapy.
- Administer IV α-beta blockers over 2 minutes for a 20 mg dose.
- Monitor the patient who is receiving IV α-beta blockers carefully, q5m for 30 minutes, then q30m for 2 hours, and then q1h for 6 hours.
- Administer α-beta blockers with or immediately after meals because food decreases the risk of orthostatic hypotension. Monitor the patient's intake and output.
- Monitor the BP after the patient has been standing for 10 minutes because dose titration is based on the standing BP reading.
- α-Beta blockers should be withdrawn gradually over a 1- to 2-week period.
- Monitor the patient's glucose levels frequently because α-beta blockers mask the signs of hypoglycemia.
- Monitor hepatic and renal tests to determine adequate function of the related organs.
- Monitor digoxin levels when carvedilol is given concurrently because digoxin levels may increase.
- 🍎 Instruct the patient to use caution in operating hazardous equipment after receiving an α-beta blocker until the individual's response to the drug is known.
- 🍎 Instruct the patient to lie down or sit down immediately when feeling dizzy, weak, or faint.
- 🍎 Advise the patient to report a weight gain of 2 or more pounds in 24 hours.
- 🍎 Counsel the patient that prolonged standing, hot baths or showers, hot weather, alcohol consumption, and strenuous physical exercise intensify orthostatic hypotension.
- 🍎 Warn the patient that diarrhea may be explosive and embarrassing.

Edema with weight gain is a common adverse effect, particularly in older adults or those with limited cardiac reserve.

Do You UNDERSTAND?

DIRECTIONS: Provide answers to the following questions.

1. What is the best time to check a standing BP? *P stand 10 min*

   _____

2. In which patients are α-beta blockers used?

   _____

   _____

   _____

Answers: 1. after standing for 10 minutes; 2. patients with stage 1 or stage 2 hypertension, patients in hypertensive emergency, African Americans.

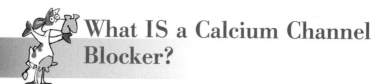

What IS a Calcium Channel Blocker?

Calcium Channel Blockers	Trade Names	Uses
diltiazem [dill-TYE-uh-zem]	Cardizem	Treatment of essential hypertension and angina
verapamil [veh-RAP-uh-mill]	Calan	Treatment of essential hypertension and angina
nifedipine [nye-FED-ih-peen]	Procardia	Treatment of mild-to-moderate hypertension and angina

Action

Calcium channel blockers (**calcium antagonists**) inhibit the influx of calcium into muscle cells through slow calcium channels during membrane depolarization. Calcium is blocked in intracellular sites of vascular smooth muscle, myocardium, and the cardiac conduction system. Extracellular calcium must move into the cell through calcium channels for the contraction of cardiac and smooth muscle to occur. Without this calcium influx coronary and peripheral vasoconstriction, myocardial contractility, automaticity, and conduction velocity are depressed in both cardiac and smooth muscle. The result is a relaxation of the smooth muscle of small arteries and a decrease in PVR. The normal adrenergic response to calcium channel blockers (CCBs) is a reflexive vasoconstriction, which decreases the hypotensive drug effect.

Uses

CCBs are effective in monotherapy for mild-to-moderate hypertension. When CCBs fail to reduce BP adequately, effectiveness is usually increased with BBs or diuretics. CCBs are beneficial and safe in patients with COPD, dysrhythmias, angina, hyperlipidemia, DM, and renal dysfunction. However, CCBs are not used in the immediate relief of an angina attack. Diltiazem and verapamil slow sinoatrial (SA) and AV conduction and are effective in decreasing the rate of paroxysmal atrial tachycardia, atrial flutter, and atrial fibrillation. Diltiazem and verapamil, as class IV antiarrhythmias, are occasionally effective in converting tachydysrhythmias to a normal sinus rhythm.

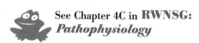 In older adults with diminished reflexes, this protective vasoconstriction is decreased and occasionally leads to excessive hypotension.

See Chapter 4C in RWNSG: *Pathophysiology*

CCB monotherapy is more effective compared with other antihypertensive classifications in older adults because these patients usually have low CO, decreased blood volume, high PVR, and high catecholamine or low renin levels.

CCBs monotherapy are beneficial and safe in African-American and Chinese populations, in whom renin levels are usually low.

What You NEED TO KNOW

Contraindications/Precautions

CCBs are contraindicated for patients with heart block, sick sinus syndrome, and hepatic or renal dysfunction. Diltiazem is contraindicated for patients with acute MI and pulmonary congestion. Verapamil is contraindicated for patients with severe left ventricular dysfunction and cardiogenic shock because of the profound vasodilation effect and its ability to compromise cardiac performance.

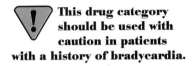
CCBs are also contra-indicated for women during pregnancy and lactation.

Drug Interactions

Serum digoxin levels are increased when digoxin is given concurrently with CCBs, which results in increased bradycardia and depression of the AV conduction. Cimetidine decreases the hepatic clearance of the CCB, which prolongs the action. Calcium and vitamin D decrease the action of CCBs. The interaction between CCBs and BBs causes myocardial depression and bradycardia. Similarly, quinidine may cause excess hypotension when given together with CCBs. The action of carbamazepine, cyclosporine, and nondepolarizing blockers is exacerbated when given with CCBs.

This drug category should be used with caution in patients with a history of bradycardia.

Adverse Effects

Common adverse effects that are associated with CCBs include primarily vasodilating effects, such as flushing, headache, dizziness, weakness, dysrhythmias, and bradycardia. Other adverse effects include photosensitivity, rash, itching, nasal congestion, nausea, vomiting, diarrhea, muscle fatigue and cramps, hyperglycemia, sexual dysfunction, mood changes, persistent peripheral edema, and orthostatic hypotension. More serious adverse effects include heart block hepatic damage, thrombocytopenia, and Stevens-Johnson syndrome.

What You DO

Nursing Responsibilities

When administering CCBs, the nurse should:
- Administer CCBs before meals. However, CCBs may be taken with food when GI distress occurs.
- Initially administer diltiazem IV with a bolus over 2 minutes, followed by a continuous infusion on a volumetric pump through microdrip tubing to ensure accurate dose administration. Before weaning and discontinuing administration, a regimen of oral diltiazem is usually initiated.

TAKE HOME POINTS

- Do not administer CCBs within a few hours of BBs because the result may cause depressed myocardial contractility and AV conduction, marked hemodynamic deterioration, and ventricular fibrillation.
- Keep the patient in the recumbent position for at least 1 hour after the first CCB dose.

Verapamil may cause hypotension, particularly in older patients, when given at a faster than normal rate.

- Monitor the BP and heart rate before CCB administration. When the heart rate is less than 60 beats per minute, systolic BP is less than 90 mm Hg, diastolic BP is less than 60 mm Hg, or the parameter ordered, the dose should be delayed and the health care provider should be contacted.
- Instruct the recumbent patient to sit upright for a few minutes and dangle the legs before ambulating. Patients should change positions slowly when taking CCBs. Supervise ambulation until the response is known.
- Monitor renal and hepatic function for early signs of impairment.
- Monitor glucose, electrolytes, and intake and output.
- CCBs should be tapered over a 2-week period because abrupt withdrawal may cause severe reactions.
- Counsel patients to avoid participating in activities that require alertness until response to the drug is known.
- Instruct the patient to check with the health care provider before taking any OTC medications because cold or allergy drugs interfere with CCBs.
- Instruct the patient to report edema and weight gain greater than 3 pounds per day or 5 pounds per week.
- Instruct the patient to avoid substances that interfere with CCBs, such as caffeine-containing beverages (e.g., coffee, tea, cola).

Do You UNDERSTAND?

DIRECTIONS: Complete the following statements appropriately.

1. _____ response weakens the hypotensive drug effect of CCBs.
2. When patients fail to respond to CCB monotherapy, _____ or _____ are usually added.

What IS a Central α-Adrenergic Agonist?

Central Alpha-Adrenergic Agonists	Trade Names	Uses
methyldopa [meth-ill-DOE-puh]	Aldomet	Treatment of hypertension
clonidine [KLOE-nih-DEEN]	Catapres	Treatment of hypertension
guanabenz [GWAHN-uh-benz]	Wytensin	Treatment of hypertension

Action

Central α-adrenergic agonists (**central agonists** or **sympatholytics**) stimulate central α_2-receptors. α_2-Stimulation decreases the sympathetic outflow from the central nervous system brainstem to the heart, kidneys, and peripheral vessels. The hemodynamic result is an inhibition of vasomotor and cardiac centers, causing a decrease in PVR and a slight decrease in CO. Decreased vascular resistance allows systolic and diastolic BP reduction while only slightly lowering the heart rate.

Uses

Central α-adrenergic agonists (CAAs) can be used for treating mild-to-moderate hypertension. Generally, CAAs are not used as a first-line drug option for hypertension. These agents have been used in monotherapy or in combination with other antihypertensive drugs.

What You NEED TO KNOW

Contraindications/Precautions

Methyldopa is contraindicated for patients with hypersensitivity to this drug and sulfites, mild hypertension, active hepatic disease, blood dyscrasias, pheochromocytoma, and concurrent use of MAOIs. Clonidine is contraindicated for patients with systemic lupus erythematosus (SLE), scleroderma, and polyarteritis.

Drug Interactions

CAAs exacerbate the action of other CNS depressants (e.g., analgesics, opiates, sedatives, barbiturates, anesthetics, alcohol). Tricyclic antidepressants inhibit the hypotensive effect of clonidine. When CAAs are given concurrently with other antihypertensives, the hypotensive effect is increased.

Adverse Effects

Common adverse effects from CAAs include nasal congestion, dry mouth, constipation, impotence, decreased libido, headache, dizziness, drowsiness, weakness, fatigue, and orthostatic hypotension. Sodium retention with weight gain usually occurs after initial administration but persists for only 3 to 4 days. Other adverse effects include rash, restlessness, nervousness, forgetfulness, vivid dreams, hallucinations, anorexia, vomiting, abdominal pain, depression, dyspnea, bradycardia, and rebound hypertension (with abrupt discontinuation). Potentially serious adverse effects include blood dyscrasias and hepatic dysfunction. Guanabenz may cause decreased fluid retention.

Methyldopa is typically preferred for hypertension during pregnancy.

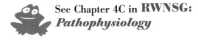 CAAs are used in African Americans, Caucasians, and those in all age groups.

See Chapter 4C in **RWNSG:** *Pathophysiology*

CAAs are contraindicated for women during pregnancy and lactation. Guanabenz is contraindicated for children under 12 years of age.

 CAAs should be used with caution in older adults because these patients are more prone to fainting and sedation.

Clonidine and guanabenz should be used with caution in patients with a recent MI, severe coronary insufficiency, and cerebrovascular disease. Methyldopa and clonidine should be used cautiously in patients with mental depression. Methyldopa should also be used with caution in patients with angina pectoris. Methyldopa and guanabenz should be given cautiously to patients with hepatic dysfunction. Caution should be used with clonidine administration in patients with Raynaud's disease and Berger's disease. This category should be used cautiously in patients with renal dysfunction.

What You DO

Nursing Responsibilities

When administering CAAs, the nurse should:

 Inform the patient that orthostatic hypotension is intensified with prolonged standing, hot baths or showers, hot weather, alcohol consumption, and strenuous physical exercise.

 Instruct the patient to avoid more than 4 cups of caffeinated coffee, tea, or cola per day.

 Inform the patient that CAAs should be taken at bedtime to avoid drowsiness or interference with driving or operating hazardous equipment.

• Withdraw slowly over 2 to 4 days when being discontinued to avoid rebound hypertension.

Do You UNDERSTAND?

DIRECTIONS: Complete the following statements appropriately by selecting the correct word from the italicized choices.

1. The best time of day to administer CAAs is _____.
   (*midmorning, bedtime*)
2. CAAs should be withdrawn over _____.
   (*2 to 4 days, 2 weeks*)
3. CAAs alter the heart rate by causing _____.
   (*bradycardia, tachycardia*)
4. The preferred antihypertensive during pregnancy is _____.
   (*methyldopa, clonidine*)

What IS a Peripheral Adrenergic Neuron Antagonist?

Peripheral Adrenergic Neuron Antagonists	Trade Names	Uses
reserpine [re-SER-peen]	Serpasil	Treatment of mild hypertension
guanadrel [GWAHN-uh-drell]	Hylorel	Treatment of hypertension
guanethidine [gwahn-ETH-ih-deen]	Ismelin	Treatment of moderate and severe hypertension

Action

Peripheral adrenergic neuron antagonists block the exit of norepinephrine (neurotransmitter) from storage granules, thereby inhibiting the activity of the sympathetic nervous system. These agents act in adrenergic neurons to deplete norepinephrine stores. Decreasing norepinephrine and vasoconstriction promotes vasodilation, which results in decreased PVR, CO, and BP.

Uses

Peripheral adrenergic neuron antagonists are used primarily to treat hypertension and are usually administered concurrently with other medications for efficacy. Reserpine is used as adjunctive therapy in severe hypertension. Guanadrel is used to treat hypertension when the patient is unresponsive to thiazide diuretics.

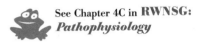 See Chapter 4C in **RWNSG:** *Pathophysiology*

 # What You NEED TO KNOW

Contraindications/Precautions

Peripheral adrenergic neuron antagonists are contraindicated for patients with hypersensitivity, depression, and pheochromocytoma.

> **Caution must be used in patients with DM, renal or hepatic impairment, peptic ulcer disease, asthma, recent MI, heart failure, and patients who are taking MAOIs.**

Drug Interactions

Other antihypertensives, diuretics, and alcohol increase the hypotensive effect. Tricyclic antidepressants, phenothiazines, and other sympathomimetics block the uptake of peripheral adrenergic neuron antagonists and block or reverse the hypotensive effect. Oral contraceptives may reduce the hypotensive effects. MAOIs antagonize the hypotensive effect when given concurrently. MAOIs should be discontinued at least 1 week before administering peripheral adrenergic neuron antagonists. When this drug category is given concurrently with cardiac glycosides, the patient requires careful monitoring because both drugs decrease heart rate.

Adverse Effects

Common adverse effects that are associated with peripheral adrenergic neuron antagonists include shortness of breath, fatigue, lethargy, headache, drowsiness, dizziness, diarrhea, impaired ejaculation, and profound orthostatic hypotension. Adverse effects that are related to the respiratory system include nasal congestion, bronchospasm, and respiratory depression. Psychologic and neurologic adverse effects include paresthesia, seizures, decreased libido, nightmares (with high doses), tardive dyskinesia, inability to perform complex tasks, and severe suicidal depression. Other adverse effects include insomnia, visual disturbances, weakness, GI distress, peripheral edema, leg cramps, hypothermia, bradycardia, and heart failure. Peptic ulcer disease may be exacerbated because reserpine may increase gastric acid secretion.

What You DO

Nursing Responsibilities

The full hypotensive effect of peripheral adrenergic neuron antagonists may take 3 weeks to achieve. An increased orthostatic hypotension risk exists with exposure to a hot environment, prolonged standing, and exercise. This drug should be discontinued at the first sign of depression. Periodic assessment of BP throughout the morning is useful to ensure that the BP surge that occurs when arising has been adequately eased. When administering peripheral adrenergic neuron antagonists, the nurse should:

- Monitor the patient for seizures and respiratory depression.
- Monitor the patient's BP and heart rate status. Following large IV doses of reserpine, a transient sympathomimetic effect with a small increase in BP may occur. When the patient is taking peripheral adrenergic neuron antagonists and cardiac glycosides together, heart rate is decreased.

Do You UNDERSTAND?

**DIRECTIONS: Indicate in the space provided whether each statement is
true or *false*.**

_____ 1. Depleting catecholamines increases norepinephrine and causes vasoconstriction.

_____ 2. Reserpine increases gastric acid secretion, which predisposes the patient to peptic ulcer disease.

What IS a Direct Vasodilator?

Direct Vasodilators	Trade Names	Uses
hydralazine [high-DRAL-uh-zeen]	Apresoline	Treatment of essential hypertension
minoxidil [min-OX-ih-dill]	Loniten	Treatment of severe hypertension

Action

Direct vasodilators relax vascular smooth muscles in the arterioles and decrease PVR. Some direct vasodilators affect both the arterial and venous systems, reducing both preload and afterload. As a result of arteriole dilation, decreased

Answers: 1. false; norepinephrine is a catecholamine that causes vasoconstriction; depleting norepinephrine catecholamine (a vasoconstrictor) promotes vasodilation; 2. true.

PVR, and reduced BP, the baroreceptors are stimulated to release cate-cholamines. This action leads to an increase in heart rate, fluid retention, CO, cardiac contractility, and cardiac workload. β-Adrenergic blocking agents may reduce increased cardiac workload.

Uses

Hydralazine is used in the treatment of moderate-to-severe hypertension. Minoxidil is used to manage severe hypertension that is associated with organ damage. Although direct vasodilators are highly effective antihypertensives, they are not used as initial monotherapy. Because minoxidil dilates renal arterioles, it can be used in cases of severe refractory hypertension or renal insufficiency.

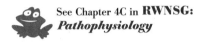

See Chapter 4C in **RWNSG:** *Pathophysiology*

What You NEED TO KNOW

Contraindications/Precautions

Direct vasodilators are contraindicated for patients with hypersensitivity, coronary artery disease, and mitral valve heart disease.

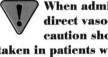

Direct vasodilators are also contraindicated for women during pregnancy.

Drug Interactions

NSAIDs decrease the therapeutic effects of direct vasodilators. BBs decrease tachycardia that results from hydralazine. The therapeutic effects of hydralazine are increased when given together with alcohol, other antihypertensives, MAOIs, nitrates, and general anesthetics. Diazoxide, when given with diuretics, increases hypotension and hyperuricemia. When direct vasodilators are taken concurrently with corticosteroids, estrogen, progesterone, and phenytoin, the risk for hyperglycemia is increased.

When administering direct vasodilators, caution should be taken in patients with renal impairment.

Adverse Effects

Common adverse effects that are associated with direct vasodilators include throbbing headache, profuse hirsutism on face and body, sodium and water retention, palpitations, and reflex tachycardia. Other adverse effects include nasal congestion, excess lacrimation, dizziness, flushing, anxiety, drowsiness, syncope, weakness, lethargy, restlessness, GI distress, constipation, tremors, euphoria, edema, weight gain, and impotence. More serious adverse effects include atrial and ventricular dysrhythmias, blood dyscrasias, leukopenia, agranulocytosis, temporary hearing loss, hyperglycemia, hematuria, nocturia, proteinuria, azotemia, severe rebound hypertension, pulmonary edema, and heart failure. Hydralazine (particularly with doses greater than 200 mg per day) can cause a syndrome resembling drug-induced SLE or rheumatoid arthritis, which involves fever, arthralgia, malaise, edema, myalgia, and the presence of antinuclear antibodies (ANAs). These drugs rarely cause orthostatic hypotension.

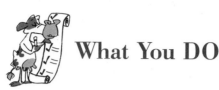

What You DO

Nursing Responsibilities

Hydralazine is usually administered orally. When a rapid decrease in BP is needed or the patient is unable to take an oral dose, hydralazine may be given intramuscularly (IM) or IV. The patient should remain recumbent for at least 1 hour after injection. Oral administration should replace parenteral therapy as soon as possible. Because of the excessive hair growth, minoxidil is not usually ordered for women, except in rare cases of severe hypertension that is resistant to multiple drug therapy. Additional nursing responsibilities include the following:

- Monitor intake and output, decreased urine output, edema, and weight gain for the patient who is taking direct vasodilators.
- Auscultate lungs frequently for early detection of pulmonary edema.
- Monitor renal and liver function tests, CBC, and ANA titer in patients throughout direct vasodilator therapy.
- Monitor BP in sitting and standing positions to determine orthostatic hypotension.

 Monitor BP in sitting and standing positions, particularly in older patients, to determine orthostatic hypotension.

Do You UNDERSTAND?

DIRECTIONS: Fill in the blanks with appropriate responses.

1. The most common adverse effects of minoxidil are _____ and _____.

2. In determining orthostatic hypotension, the position of the patient should be _____ when the nurse assesses his or her BP.

SECTION B
ANTIHYPERLIPIDEMICS

This section reviews the pharmacologic methods that are used to treat hyperlipidemia, which is an increase in lipids in the blood. Antihyperlipidemics are agents that lower lipids, including cholesterol, triglycerides, and low-density lipoproteins (LDLs). Cholesterol is a sterol lipid that is found in many body tissues, such as brain, spinal cord, kidneys, adrenal glands, and liver, and is important for metabolism and steroid hormones. Triglycerides constitute a large portion of lipids in the blood. LDLs deliver cholesterol to nonhepatic tissues and are responsible for the greatest contribution of cholesterol to coronary atherosclerosis.

Answers: 1. excessive hair growth, fluid retention; 2. sitting and standing after 10 minutes.

Investigations have established that cardiovascular morbidity and mortality is directly related to elevated total cholesterol, triglycerides, and LDL levels, in addition to inversely lowered high-density lipoprotein (HDL) levels. Therefore the primary goal of cholesterol-lowering drugs is to decrease total cholesterol and LDL levels and to increase HDL levels. Reducing LDL levels may arrest or reverse atherosclerosis, thereby reducing morbidity and mortality in cardiovascular disease. The selected antihyperlipidemic groups that are discussed include HMG-CoA reductase inhibitors, bile acid sequestrants, fibric acid derivatives, and other selected antihyperlipidemic agents.

What IS an HMG-CoA Reductase Inhibitor?

HMG-CoA Reductase Inhibitors	Trade Names	Uses
lovastatin [loe-vah-STAT-in]	Mevacor	Treatment of moderate hypercholesterolemia
simvastatin [sim-vah-STAT-in]	Zocor	Treatment of hypercholesterolemia
atorvastatin [a-tor-vah-STAT-in]	Lipitor	Treatment of elevated cholesterol, LDLs, and triglycerides
pravastatin [pra-vah-STAT-in]	Pravachol	Treatment of hypercholesterolemia

Action

HMG-CoA reductase inhibitors (**statins**) selectively inhibit the enzyme HMG-CoA reductase, which is the rate-limiting enzyme in cholesterol synthesis. HMG-CoA reductase inhibitors block the production of cholesterol, which decreases LDL cholesterol, total cholesterol, very low-density lipoprotein (VLDL) cholesterol, and triglycerides. These inhibitors also increase HDL cholesterol levels. The mechanism of the LDL-lowering effect leads to a decreased production or increased catabolism of LDLs.

Uses

HMG-CoA reductase inhibitors are used to treat hypercholesterolemia and dyslipidemia when dietary restrictions and other nonpharmacologic measures have been inadequate. These agents are also used to prevent atherosclerosis, coronary artery disease, and MI.

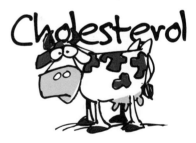

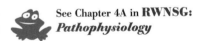

See Chapter 4A in **RWNSG:** *Pathophysiology*

What You NEED TO KNOW?

Contraindications/Precautions

HMG-CoA reductase inhibitors are contraindicated for patients with hypersensitivity, unexplained elevated liver function studies, and active liver disease.

HMG-CoA reductase inhibitors are contra-indicated for women during pregnancy and lactation.

 ## TAKE HOME POINTS

Instruct the patient who is taking HMG-CoA reductase inhibitors to discontinue these drugs immediately when becoming pregnant to avoid harmful effects to the fetus.

HMG-CoA reductase inhibitors should be used with caution in renal dysfunction, and doses may be decreased.

Rhabdomyolysis is a fatal disease involving skeletal muscle destruction.

 ## TAKE HOME POINTS

Instruct the patient who is taking HMG-CoA reductase inhibitors to report unexplained muscle pain, tenderness, or weakness, particularly when fever or malaise occurs.

Drug Interactions

Drug interactions of HMG-CoA reductase inhibitors include an increased risk of myopathy and rhabdomyolysis when given concurrently with cyclosporine, gemfibrozil, and erythromycin. Elevated creatine phosphokinase (CPK or CK) levels and renal dysfunction are usually associated with rhabdomyolysis.

Adverse Effects

The majority of adverse effects of HMG-CoA reductase inhibitors are usually mild and transient. Adverse effects include fever, malaise, dizziness, fainting, palpitations, migraine, photosensitivity, anxiety, orthostatic hypotension, hypertension, nosebleeds, and tinnitus. GI adverse effects of these agents include alteration in taste, anorexia, increased appetite, dry mouth, GI ulcerations, hepatitis, and pancreatitis. Other adverse effects include skin discoloration, sweating, hives, acne, petechiae, anemia, hyperglycemia, hypoglycemia, decreased libido, breast enlargement, gout, urinary frequency, urgency, retention, incontinence, and muscle pain. More serious adverse effects include facial paralysis, deafness, glaucoma, memory loss, depression, thrombocytopenia, renal calculi, angioedema, dyspnea, dysrhythmias, rhabdomyolysis, and Stevens-Johnson syndrome.

 # What You DO

Nursing Responsibilities

The peak therapeutic response of antihyperlipidemics occurs within 4 to 6 weeks and is maintained throughout therapy. HMG-CoA reductase inhibitors are more effective when taken in the evening compared with other times of the day because cholesterol is synthesized mostly at night. These agents may be taken without regard to meals. However, when combination therapy is used, HMG-CoA reductase inhibitors should be given at least 2 hours after a bile acid sequestrant. When administering HMG-CoA reductase inhibitors, the nurse should:

- Instruct patients to take HMG-CoA reductase inhibitors at bedtime for increased effectiveness.
- Instruct the patient to avoid prolonged sunlight and ultraviolet light exposure and to take safety measures of wearing protective clothing and using sunscreens.
- Instruct patients to report unexplained muscle pain or weakness, particularly when accompanied by fever or dark red-brown urine, which may indicate rhabdomyolysis.
- Monitor CPK levels carefully for early detection of rhabdomyolysis.
- Obtain baseline liver function studies before initiating therapy, again at 6 and 12 weeks, and at 6-month intervals thereafter.
- Reevaluate patients monthly to determine any dose adjustments.

Do You UNDERSTAND?

DIRECTIONS: Provide the appropriate responses to the following statements.

1. Rhabdomyolysis is an adverse effect of HMG-CoA reductase inhibitors characterized by what five symptoms?

   _____

   _____

   _____

   _____

   _____

2. What is the best time of day to take HMG-CoA reductase inhibitors?

   _____

3. Circle any of the following that are adverse effects of HMG-CoA reductase inhibitors.

Hypertension	Hyperglycemia
Hypotension	Hypoglycemia

What IS a Bile Acid Sequestrant?

Bile Acid Sequestrants	Trade Names	Uses
cholestyramine [koe-less-TEAR-a-meen]	Questran	Adjunct treatment of hypercholesterolemia
colestipol [koe-LESS-ti-pole]	Colestid	Adjunct treatment of hypercholesterolemia

Action

Bile acid sequestrants (**bile acid sequestering resins** or **bile acid-binding resins**) bind bile in the intestine to form an insoluble complex that is excreted in the feces. This action results in the partial removal of bile salts, preventing their reabsorption. The loss of bile salts leads to a decrease in LDL and serum cholesterol levels. These drugs increase hepatic synthesis of cholesterol but decrease plasma cholesterol levels resulting from an increased clearance rate of cholesterol lipoproteins.

Uses

Bile acid sequestrants agents are used to reduce elevated serum cholesterol in patients with hypercholesterolemia and elevated LDLs. These agents are usually initiated when other nonpharmacologic measures are inadequate.

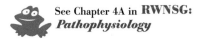

See Chapter 4A in **RWNSG:** *Pathophysiology*

Answers: 1. muscle pain, tenderness, weakness, fever, malaise; 2. evening; 3. all of the choices.

What You NEED TO KNOW

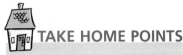

Caution should be used when administering bile acid sequestrants to children and to women who are pregnant or lactating.

Bile acid sequestrants should be used with caution in patients with bleeding disorders, GI disorders, and hemorrhoids.

Contraindications/Precautions

Bile acid sequestrants are contraindicated for patients with hypersensitivity and complete biliary obstruction.

Drug Interactions

Drug interactions that involve bile acid sequestrants include a decreased anticoagulant effect when given together with anticoagulants. Cholestyramine may enhance the elimination of piroxicam when given concurrently. Cholestyramine and colestipol may reduce the absorption of ursodiol. Malabsorption of fat-soluble vitamins A, D, E, and K may occur when given concurrently with bile acid sequestrants.

Adverse Effects

The most common adverse effect of bile acid sequestrants is constipation, leading to fecal impaction and the aggravation of hemorrhoids. Other less frequent adverse effects include headache, dizziness, anxiety, tinnitus, fainting, fatigue, drowsiness, insomnia, chest pain, tachycardia, anemia, increased prothrombin time, hypersensitivity, muscle and joint pain, dysuria, hematuria, weight loss or gain, increased libido, edema, and paresthesia. GI adverse effects include anorexia, abdominal pain, distention, flatulence, heartburn, nausea, vomiting, taste alteration, ulceration, and bleeding.

What You DO

Nursing Responsibilities

After initiating treatment with bile acid sequestrants, LDL levels decline in 4 to 7 days and serum cholesterol levels decrease in 1 month. When administering bile acid sequestrants, the nurse should:

- Advise patients to take bile acid sequestrants at mealtimes.
- Instruct the patient to mix powder forms with fluids and avoid taking the medicine dry. This process helps avoid accidental inhalation or esophageal distress.
- Monitor cholesterol and triglyceride levels frequently during the first few months of therapy and periodically thereafter to ascertain efficacy.
- Teach patients with coronary artery disease to take a laxative, stool softener, and increase fluid or fiber intake to avoid straining because these agents may cause constipation and fecal impaction.

TAKE HOME POINTS

Instruct the patient to increase daily fluid intake.

Do You UNDERSTAND?

DIRECTIONS: Indicate in the space provided whether each statement is
true **or** *false.*

_____ 1. During bile acid sequestrants therapy, malabsorption of vitamins B, C, and K may occur.

_____ 2. The most common adverse effect of bile acid sequestrants is diarrhea.

What IS a Fibric Acid Derivative?

Fibric Acid Derivatives	Trade Names	Uses
clofibrate [kloe-FY-brate]	Atromid-S	Adjunct therapy in hyperlipidemia
gemfibrozil [gem-FI-broe-zil]	Lopid	Treatment of very high triglyceride levels

Action

The action of fibric acid derivatives is unknown; however, the triglyceride-lowering effect seems to be a result of accelerated catabolism of VLDL to LDL and reduced hepatic synthesis of VLDL. Cholesterol formation is inhibited early in the process, and excretion of cholesterol is increased. Both of the fibric acid derivatives decrease serum triglycerides, cholesterol, LDLs, and VLDLs. Gemfibrozil also increases HDL levels.

> **Fibric acid derivatives should be used cautiously in patients with cholelithiasis, peptic ulcer disease, hypothyroidism, and cardiovascular disease. Gemfibrozil should be used with caution in patients with DM.**

Uses

Clofibrate is used to treat severe hyperlipidemia. Gemfibrozil is used to treat severe hypertriglyceridemia.

 See Chapter 4A in **RWNSG:** *Pathophysiology*

What You NEED TO KNOW

Contraindications/Precautions

These agents are contraindicated for patients with renal or hepatic dysfunction.

Drug Interactions

Clofibrate and gemfibrozil interact with oral anticoagulants, increasing the risk of bleeding. Probenecid increases the action of clofibrate when given together. When clofibrate is given concurrently with sulfonylureas, hypoglycemia is increased. When gemfibrozil and lovastatin are given together, the risk of myopathy and rhabdomyolysis are increased. When clofibrate is given concurrently with sulfonylureas, the hypoglycemic effects are enhanced.

> Fibric acid derivatives are contraindicated for children under 14 years of age and for women during pregnancy and lactation.

Answers: 1. false; vitamins A, D, E, and K; 2. false; constipation with fecal impaction.

Adverse Effects

The adverse effects of fibric acid derivatives include headache, dizziness, flatulence, nausea, vomiting, diarrhea, abdominal pain, rash, itching, hives, myalgia, muscle soreness, weakness, eosinophilia, anemia, neutropenia, leukopenia, agranulocytosis, renal dysfunction, elevated liver enzymes, or hepatic dysfunction. Additionally, clofibrate may cause drowsiness, gastritis, decreased libido, and impotence. Gemfibrozil may cause blurred vision, arthralgia, hypokalemia, and moderate hyperglycemia.

What You DO

Nursing Responsibilities

A therapeutic response usually occurs within 1 to 2 months. A rebound effect may occur in the second or third month, followed by a further decrease in lipids. When administering fibric acid derivatives, the nurse should:

- Instruct the patient who is taking gemfibrozil to take the drug 30 minutes before morning and evening meals, unless GI distress develops; gemfibrozil may then be taken with meals.
- Monitor patients for gastric pain, nausea, vomiting, and pulmonary edema.
- Evaluate baseline LDL, VLDL, triglyceride, and total cholesterol levels before therapy, again every 2 weeks during the first few months of therapy, and at monthly intervals thereafter.
- Monitor CBC, glucose, electrolytes, prothrombin time (PT), and renal and hepatic function studies frequently throughout fibric acid derivative therapy.
- Instruct the patient to report any bleeding, bruising, epistaxis, and hematuria.
- Counsel patients to avoid operating hazardous machinery until the drug effect is known.
- Warn patients to avoid self-dosing with OTC drugs without consulting the health care provider.

Do You UNDERSTAND?

DIRECTIONS: Indicate in the space provided whether each statement is *true* or *false*.

_____ 1. When gemfibrozil is combined with lovastatin, the risk of rhabdomyolysis is increased.

_____ 2. Fibric acid derivatives are ideal antihyperlipidemics for patients with renal and hepatic dysfunction.

TAKE HOME POINTS

Instruct the patient to report influenza-like symptoms of muscle soreness and weakness. This action facilitates differentiation of adverse effects from viral or bacterial disease.

Teach women of childbearing age about the importance of a birth control regimen. When clofibrate is given, the drug should be discontinued at least 2 months before conception.

Answers: 1. true; 2. false; fibric acid derivatives are contraindicated for patients with renal and hepatic dysfunction.

What IS a Miscellaneous Antihyperlipidemic Agent?

Nicotinic Acid Agents	Trade Names	Uses
niacin, nicotinic acid [NYE-a-sin]	Novo-Niacin	Treatment of hyperlipidemia
fenofibrate [fen-o-FI-brate]	Tricor	Treatment of elevated triglycerides

Action

The exact action of niacin (**nicotinic acid** or **vitamin B₃**) is unknown; however, niacin inhibits lipolysis in adipose tissue, decreases triglyceride esterification in the liver, and increases lipoprotein lipase activity. In summary, niacin reduces serum cholesterol, triglyceride, LDL, and VLDL levels and increases HDL levels. Fenofibrate inhibits triglyceride synthesis. This action lowers VLDL production, stimulates catabolism of triglycerides, and increases HDL cholesterol levels.

Uses

Niacin is used to treat hyperlipidemia. Fenofibrate is used to treat elevated triglyceride levels when patients fail to respond adequately to nonpharmacologic measures.

What You NEED TO KNOW

Contraindications/Precautions

Niacin is contraindicated for patients with hypersensitivity, hepatic dysfunction, severe hypotension, bleeding, and active peptic ulcers.

Fenofibrate is contraindicated for patients with hypersensitivity, hepatic or renal dysfunction, gallbladder disease, and thrombocytopenia.

Drug Interactions

Hypotension is increased when antihypertensives are given together with niacin. Absorption may be decreased when fenofibrate is given together with cholestyramine and colestipol. When combined with HMG-CoA reductase inhibitors, the risk of rhabdomyolysis or acute renal failure is increased. The combination of fenofibrate and cyclosporine may increase the risk of nephrotoxicity.

Adverse Effects

The adverse effects of niacin include flushing, warmth, headache, dizziness, hypotension, fatigue, tingling in extremities, fainting, nervousness, blurred vision, loss of central vision, dry skin, rash, itching, jaundice, flatulence, nausea, vomiting, peptic ulcers, hyperglycemia, hyperuricemia, hypoprothrombinemia,

 See Chapter 4A in **RWNSG:** *Pathophysiology*

Niacin should be used cautiously in patients with a history of gallbladder, liver, or coronary artery disease, peptic ulcers, glaucoma, DM, and gout.

Niacin and fenofibrate are contraindicated for women during pregnancy and lactation and for children.

Fenofibrate should be used cautiously in patients who are taking HMG-CoA reductase inhibitors and oral anticoagulants together.

Fenofibrate also should be used cautiously in patients with renal impairment, history of bleeding disorders, and myelosuppression (reduced bone marrow function), and in older adults.

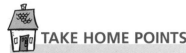

TAKE HOME POINTS

Assess the patient who is taking niacin and antihypertensives for hypotension.

TAKE HOME POINTS

Instruct the patient to take niacin agents with *cold* rather than hot beverages. Cold liquids will decrease the risk of persistent flushing. Inform the patient that taking aspirin 30 minutes before niacin may reduce the persistent flushing. Instruct the patient to report any visual disturbances.

and hypoalbuminemia. Dysrhythmias are rare adverse effects. Additional adverse effects of fenofibrate include arthralgia, paresthesia, insomnia, increased appetite, diarrhea, cough, rhinitis, sinusitis, decreased libido, and eye floaters.

What You DO

Nursing Responsibilities

This group of agents should not be given with hot beverages, but rather, with cold water to facilitate swallowing. The absorption is increased with food. However, when bile acid sequestrants are given concurrently, niacin should be separated and given 1 hour before or 4 to 6 hours after bile acid sequestrants. When administering nicotinic acid agents, the nurse should:

- Monitor lipid levels, liver function studies, and CBC periodically for patients who are taking niacin.
- Monitor patients with diabetes for necessary dose adjustments because of the risk of hyperglycemia.
- Monitor patients for hepatic dysfunction (e.g., itching, jaundice, dark urine, light-colored stools).
- Monitor the PT of patients who are taking niacin and Coumadin concurrently.
- Warn the patient who is taking niacin that transient flushing in the face, ears, and neck may occur within 2 hours after oral administration. Relief of transient flushing may be obtained with dose reduction or changing to a sustained-release form of niacin.
- Instruct the patient to report muscle pain, tenderness, and weakness. When muscle pain is present, the CPK should be monitored.
- Explain to the patient the importance of reporting any visual disturbances.

Do You UNDERSTAND?

DIRECTIONS: Fill in the blanks with appropriate responses.

1. Visual disturbances from niacin include _____.
2. The patient should be monitored for evidence of hepatic dysfunction, which includes _____.

Answers: 1. blurred vision, loss of central vision, or eye floaters; 2. itching, jaundice, dark urine, and light-colored stools.

5 Drugs Affecting the Cardiac System

AGENTS AFFECTING CARDIAC OUTPUT

This section reviews the pharmacologic methods that are used to affect cardiac output (CO). Antianginal medications that improve myocardial supply and decrease the demand for oxygen include nitrates, beta blockers, and calcium channel blockers. An inotropic agent that affects CO is a medication that increases the force of myocardial contractility. Inotropics that are discussed in this section include cardiac glycosides and phosphodiesterase inhibitors.

What IS a Nitrate?

Nitrate	Trade Names	Uses
nitroglycerin [nye-troe-GLIH-suh-rin]	Nitrobid	Treatment of acute angina
isosorbide dinitrate [EYE-sos-ORE-bide die-NYE-trate]	Isordil	Prevention and treatment of angina
isosorbide mononitrate [EYE-sos-ORE-bide MAH-no-NYE-trate]	ISMO, Imdur	Prevention and treatment of angina

Action

Nitrates are antianginal agents that use direct relaxation action on vascular smooth muscles to dilate coronary arteries that atherosclerotic plaque has not encompassed and to improve blood supply to the myocardium, thereby relieving chest pain. Although nitrates act on both arterial and venous smooth muscles, they act primarily on the venous system, causing considerable venous vasodilation. Because nitrates dilate veins, less blood is returned to the heart, which decreases preload (i.e., the amount of blood volume in the ventricles at the end

169

of diastole). Because diastole is the period during which the myocardial muscle fibers lengthen and the heart cavities fill with blood, nitrates reduce stretching and wall tension, thereby reducing the myocardial size and oxygen requirements that are required to pump blood out of the ventricles. The vasodilation effect of nitrates decreases the resistance of blood flow from each heart contraction or systole. Reducing the arterial resistance and the energy requirements for each myocardial contraction decreases myocardial oxygen requirements.

Uses

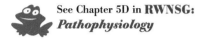

See Chapter 5D in **RWNSG:** *Pathophysiology*

Nitrates are indicated in the immediate relief or prevention of anginal pain. These agents are the drugs of choice in the treatment of acute chest pain and myocardial ischemia because of their ease of administration, rapid absorption, quick onset of action, and low cost. Nitrates can be used in monotherapy or multiple drug therapy with beta blockers or calcium channel blockers.

What You NEED TO KNOW

Contraindications/Precautions

Nitrates are contraindicated for patients with known hypersensitivity, severe anemia, acute myocardial infarction (MI), head trauma, cerebral hemorrhage, and cardiomyopathy.

> Nitrates are contraindicated for women during pregnancy and lactation.

Drug Interactions

Severe hypotension can result from drug interaction of nitrates with alcohol, calcium channel blockers, beta blockers, other antihypertensives, diuretics, haloperidol, phenothiazines, antihistamines, and tricyclic antidepressants. Antihistamines, antidepressants, and phenothiazines decrease the absorption of buccal and sublingual nitrate forms.

> **Nitrates should be given with caution to patients with hypotension, hypovolemia, tamponade, low pulmonary capillary wedge pressure, low ventricular filling pressure, or other conditions that limit CO to avoid an exacerbation of decreased CO. Caution should also be used in patients with hepatic or renal dysfunction because the metabolism or excretion may be affected.**

Adverse Effects

The most common adverse effects of nitrates involve vasodilation and include flushing, headache, dizziness, fainting, weakness, and orthostatic hypotension. Other adverse effects include nausea, vomiting, tachycardia, and palpitations. Most adverse effects following nitrate administration usually disappear when the dose is reduced. Large, continuous doses of nitrates may cause blurred vision, dry mouth, peripheral edema, and methemoglobinemia. Additionally, isosorbide mononitrate may cause anxiety, agitation, confusion, loss of coordination, insomnia, tremor, blurred vision, photophobia, and blood dyscrasias. Transdermal preparations of nitrates may cause local skin irritation. Alcohol intoxication can occur with large doses of intravenous (IV) nitroglycerin resulting from the alcohol preservative that is used in the ampule or vial storage of this drug. The most outstanding signs of alcohol intoxication following IV nitroglycerin are hypotension and reduced myocardial contractility. Other serious adverse effects include respiratory depression and cardiovascular collapse.

What You DO

Nursing Responsibilities

Because of the high vascularity of the oral mucosa, nitrates are absorbed rapidly and almost completely when given by sublingual, translingual spray, buccal, chewable tablets, or lingual aerosols. Oral capsules or sustained-release tablets are absorbed easily through the gastrointestinal (GI) tract. However, absorption is less predictable with topical ointment or transdermal patch because they depend on the amount of cutaneous circulation. When administering nitrates, the nurse should:

- 🍎 Instruct patients with angina pectoris to carry nitrates with them at all times for an unexpected anginal attack.
- 🍎 Teach patients the proper way to store nitrates: away from heat and in a light-protected, dark container. The cotton filler should be discarded because cotton can absorb the drug. The nitrate tablet supply should be replaced every 3 months for freshness.
- 🍎 Instruct the patient to avoid drinking alcoholic beverages during nitrate therapy to prevent excessive vasodilation, hypotension, and fainting.
- 🍎 Encourage the patient to avoid swallowing the sublingual nitrate tablet but allow it to absorb sublingually to ensure effectiveness in an emergency situation.
- 🍎 Inform the patient that the sustained release tablet should be swallowed and not chewed or crushed. This technique ensures that the capsule reaches the GI tract.
- 🍎 Inform patients that tolerance to nitrates may develop within 10 days to 2 weeks, particularly after high-dose, long-term therapy. Using the lowest effective dose and following an intermittent dose schedule can minimize nitrate tolerance.
- 🍎 Instruct the patient to observe safety precautions when rising from a lying to an upright position because of the nitrate's adverse effects of hypotension, dizziness, and fainting.
- Have the patient sit for a few minutes before standing to prevent orthostatic hypotension.
- 🍎 Instruct the patient to place a sublingual nitrate under the tongue or in the buccal pouch to relieve an acute anginal attack. The dose may be repeated twice at 5-minute intervals when chest pain is unrelieved.
- When pain persists after three nitrates, the health care provider should be notified.
- 🍎 Instruct the patient to use a plastic wrap cover over a transdermal patch to avoid clothing stains.
- 🍎 Instruct the patient to rotate the sites of topical nitrate to reduce the risk of skin abrasion and breakdown.
- Have the patient sit or lie down before administering the initial oral nitrate dose, and monitor the patient's pulse and blood pressure (BP).

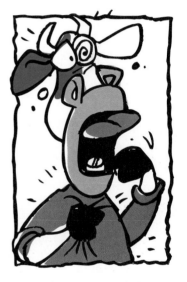

Inform the patient that nitrates should be gradually tapered on discontinuation of long-term therapy because abrupt withdrawal may cause an MI.

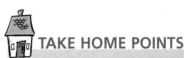

TAKE HOME POINTS

The normal sublingual dose range is 0.3 to 0.6 mg, with a maximum of three tablets given at 5-minute intervals over a 15-minute period.

- Monitor the patient's BP and pulse every 5 to 15 minutes while titrating the IV nitroglycerin dose, then every hour thereafter.
- Use the IV tubing that the manufacturer supplied when administering IV nitroglycerin to ensure efficacy because standard IV tubing absorbs nitroglycerin.
- Use an infusion pump when administering IV nitroglycerin and carefully calculate the dose according to manufacturer's tables.

Do You UNDERSTAND?

DIRECTIONS: **Indicate in the space provided whether the statement is** *true* **or** *false.*

_____ 1. Nitrates increase preload and afterload, thereby acting as antianginals.

_____ 2. Nitrates may be taken for immediate relief or prevention of anginal pain.

What IS a Calcium Channel Blocker?

Refer to page 152 for the discussion of calcium channel blockers.

What IS a Beta Blocker?

Refer to page 147 for the discussion of β-adrenergic antagonists.

What IS a Cardiac Glycoside?

Cardiac Glycoside	Trade Name	Uses
digoxin [dih-JOX-in]	Lanoxin	Treatment of CHF, atrial dysrhythmias, and cardiogenic shock

Action

Cardiac glycosides are naturally occurring substances that are found in foxglove plants and certain toads. These drugs affect the mechanical and electrical action of the heart. The mechanical effect increases myocardial contractility. Digitalis

Answers: 1. false; nitrates decrease preload and afterload; 2. true.

alters the electrical activity in noncontractile tissue and ventricular muscle, which includes the sinoatrial (SA) node, atrioventricular (AV) node, and the Purkinje fibers. Digitalis has the ability to alter automaticity, refractoriness, and impulse conduction. Automaticity refers to the automatic or involuntary functioning of cardiac muscle because the autonomic nervous system is responsible for controlling cardiac muscular activity. Refractoriness refers to the brief period of repolarization of neuron or muscle fibers when excitability is depressed. The cell may respond at this time when stimulated, but a stronger-than-normal stimulus is required. Impulse conduction refers to electrical impulses transmitted through the conduction system of the heart.

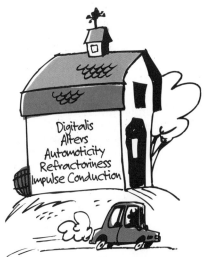

The mechanical effects of cardiac glycosides involve a positive inotropic action on the heart (i.e., an increase in the force of ventricular contractility). Digitalis inhibits an enzyme known as sodium-potassium-ATPase (**Na-K-ATPase**), thereby accomplishing a positive inotropic action. Inhibition of the Na-K-ATPase enzyme blocks the entry of potassium into a cardiac cell and forces sodium out. With each successive action after digitalis alteration, the cardiac cell level of potassium decreases and sodium increases. An increase in sodium leads to an increase in calcium. The calcium accumulation acts to increase the contractile force of the cardiac tissue via proteins, actin, and myosin. Mechanically increasing myocardial contractility increases CO. Results from digitalis-induced increase in CO include decreased sympathetic tone (reducing the heart rate and allowing more ventricular filling time), decreased arterial constriction (allowing greater ventricular emptying), and decreased venous constriction (allowing a reduction in pulmonary congestion and peripheral edema). Another result of a digitalis-induced increase in CO, which improves renal flow, is an increase in urine production, allowing a loss of water and blood volume. Finally, the third result of a digitalis-induced increase in CO is a decrease in renin release, allowing a decrease in the renin-angiotensin-aldosterone system (RAAS), a decrease of vasoconstriction, and a decrease of sodium and water retention.

The electrical effects of digitalis involve inhibiting the Na-K-ATPase enzyme and enhancing the vagal influence on the heart. Because inhibiting Na-K-ATPase decreases the potassium level and increases the sodium and calcium levels in cardiac cells, this ion redistribution alters electrical cell responsiveness. This digitalis-induced alteration in ion distribution and increase in central nervous system stimulation of vagal fibers innervating the heart cause decreased automaticity of the SA node, decreased conduction through the AV node (which prolongs the refractory period), and increased automaticity in the Purkinje fibers.

Uses

The use of cardiac glycosides is for treating heart failure (HF) because the actions of digitalis reverse its harmful effects. The reversal of harmful effects includes improving CO, decreasing heart rate and size, reducing vasoconstriction, and reducing water retention and blood volume, thereby reducing peripheral and pulmonary edema. Cardiac glycosides are also used in treating atrial fibrillation, atrial flutter, paroxysmal atrial tachycardia, supraventricular dysrhythmias, and cardiogenic shock.

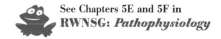

See Chapters 5E and 5F in
RWNSG: *Pathophysiology*

What You NEED TO KNOW

Cardiac glycosides are contraindicated for patients in ventricular fibrillation and for women during pregnancy and lactation.

Cardiac glycosides should also be used cautiously in premature infants, children, older adults, and debilitated patients.

Cardiac glycosides should be used cautiously in patients with hypokalemia, hypothyroidism, advanced heart disease, acute MI, and renal insufficiency.

Advanced age may also predispose an individual to digitalis toxicity.

Contraindications/Precautions

Digitalis is contraindicated for patients with a hypersensitivity or ventricular fibrillation.

Drug Interactions

The therapeutic effects of cardiac glycosides are decreased when taken concurrently with antacids, neomycin, sulfasalazine, barbiturates, phenytoin, rifampin, metoclopramide, kaolin, pectin, and cholestyramine. Giving BBs, succinylcholine, and thyroid preparations with cardiac glycosides may lead to excessive bradycardia and other dysrhythmias. Giving verapamil, amiodarone, anticholinergics, quinidine, spironolactone, hydroxychloroquine, erythromycin, itraconazole, omeprazole, and calcium preparations concurrently with cardiac glycosides may lead to digitalis toxicity. Additionally, when amphotericin B, steroids, and potassium-wasting diuretics are given with cardiac glycosides, hypokalemia and digitalis toxicity may occur.

Adverse Effects

The adverse effects of cardiac glycosides include dizziness, drowsiness, headache, confusion, mental depression, hallucinations, malaise, fatigue, muscle weakness, paresthesia, diaphoresis, agitation, visual disturbances, anorexia, nausea, vomiting, diarrhea, hypotension, and dysrhythmias. Cardiac glycosides have a narrow therapeutic range, thus they may lead to digitalis toxicity. Conditions that may predispose a patient to digitalis toxicity include hypokalemia, hypomagnesemia, hypothyroidism, hypoxemia, hypercalcemia, increased vagal tone, and myocardial ischemia.

The most frequent early signs of digitalis toxicity include anorexia, nausea, vomiting, and diarrhea. Typically, the subsequent signs of toxicity include visual disturbances of blurred vision, visual illusions (e.g., yellow-green halos around objects), blind spots, flashing lights, diplopia, and photophobia. Bradycardia (i.e., a pulse less than 60 per minute) is a common sign of digitalis toxicity, in addition to premature ventricular contraction and first-degree, second-degree, or complete heart block. The antidote for severe digitalis toxicity is digoxin immune Fab (Digibind). This agent binds with digoxin to form complex molecules that are excreted in the urine.

What You DO

Nursing Responsibilities

To avoid waiting for weeks for a desired therapeutic concentration, cardiac glycosides are initially begun with loading doses. After the loading dose raises the digitalis blood concentration level rapidly, a smaller dose that maintains the drug concentration in a therapeutic range is given on a regular schedule. When administering cardiac glycosides, the nurse should:

- Monitor digoxin serum levels throughout digitalis treatment.
- Ensure that the digitalis level has been drawn at least 8 hours after the last dose to avoid falsely elevated serum levels. Preferably, the blood should be drawn immediately before administering the daily dose, which allows 24 hours since the last dose. The normal therapeutic range is 0.8 to 2.0 ng/ml. A serum level of 2.0 ng/ml or more is considered toxic.
- Teach patients to take their own pulse and report a pulse rate that is less than 60 per minute, changes in regularity, or signs of digitalis toxicity.
- Encourage the patient to eat foods that are high in vitamin K, such as, orange juice, bananas, apples, prunes, raisins, dates, cantaloupe, watermelon, beans, potatoes, and squash, unless the patient is taking a vitamin K supplement.
- Instruct patients to consult with their health care provider before taking any other medication, including OTC drugs.
- Assess the apical heart rate and rhythm before administering digitalis. When the pulse is less than 60 beats per minute or a change in rhythm is noted, the nurse should withhold the drug and notify the health care provider.
- Administer an IV digitalis dose slowly over 5 minutes.
- Instruct patients who are taking digitalis to avoid taking an extra dose when a dose is missed, but rather, to notify their health care provider.

TAKE HOME POINTS

Drugs that reduce digitalis absorption (e.g., antacids, kaolin, pectin) should not be given concurrently.

Do You UNDERSTAND?

DIRECTIONS: Provide appropriate responses to the following questions.

1. What is the best time to draw digoxin blood level?

2. What is the normal therapeutic range for digoxin blood level?

3. What important nursing intervention should the nurse carry out before administering digoxin administration?

Answers: 1. immediately before the daily dose or at least 8 hours after the previous dose; 2. 0.8 to 2.0 ng/ml; 3. Check the heart rate to ensure that it is 60 or more beats per minute and that no change in rhythm has occurred.

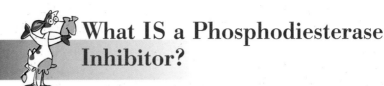

What IS a Phosphodiesterase Inhibitor?

Phosphodiesterase Inhibitors	Trade Names	Uses
amrinone lactate [AM-rih-nohn LAK-tate]	Inocor	Short-term treatment of congestive heart failure
milrinone lactate [MILL-rih-nohn LAK-tate]	Primacor	Short-term treatment of congestive heart failure

Action

Phosphodiesterase inhibitors exert an inotropic effect on the heart, thereby increasing the force of myocardial contractility. These agents also dilate arteries and veins, which decreases preload and afterload. Inhibiting cyclic adenosine monophosphate phosphodiesterase (cAMP) activity in cardiac and vascular muscle tissue helps accomplish this action. Because cAMP serves as a second control of intracellular calcium and myocardial contraction, interference of cAMP by phosphodiesterase inhibitors leads to the inhibition of cAMP degradation and resultant enhanced myocardial contractility. This action causes a rise in intracellular adenosine monophosphate, leading to an increased contractility, increased CO, decreased systemic vascular resistance, decreased venous return, reduced ventricular filling pressure, and reduced pulmonary capillary wedge pressure (PCWP).

Uses

See Chapter 5E in RWNSG: *Pathophysiology*

Phosphodiesterase inhibitors are indicated in short-term management of HF (up to a 48-hour infusion). Milrinone has been used to increase cardiac function before heart transplantation.

What You NEED TO KNOW

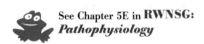
Phosphodiesterase inhibitors should be used with caution in patients with hepatic or renal dysfunction.

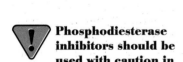
Caution should be used when administering phosphodiesterase inhibitors to women who are pregnant or lactating and to older adults.

Contraindications/Precautions

Phosphodiesterase inhibitors are contraindicated for patients with hypokalemia (until corrected) or hypersensitivity. Amrinone is also contraindicated for patients who are hypersensitive to bisulfites.

Drug Interactions

Few drug interactions occur with phosphodiesterase inhibitors. When phosphodiesterase inhibitors are given concurrently with disopyramide, excessive hypotension may result.

Adverse Effects

Adverse effects of phosphodiesterase inhibitors include headache, anorexia, nausea, vomiting, abdominal cramps, hypotension, and dysrhythmias. Amrinone also may cause thrombocytopenia. Other serious adverse effects include hepatotoxicity and nephrogenic diabetes insipidus.

What You DO

Nursing Responsibilities

Because phosphodiesterase inhibitors are administered IV, the patient must be monitored carefully. When giving phosphodiesterase inhibitors, the nurse should:

- Monitor the BP and cardiac rhythm frequently because of the potential risk for severe hypotension and dysrhythmias.
- Slow or cease the phosphodiesterase inhibitor IV solution immediately in the presence of significant hypotension and dysrhythmias. Doses should be titrated for maximal hemodynamic effect according to prescribed parameters.
- Monitor the patient's cardiac status, heart rate, rhythm, CO, PCWP, and respirations carefully during and for several hours after administration.
- Monitor the blood level of these drugs. The normal therapeutic amrinone level is 0.5 to 7.0 μg/ml.
- Monitor the platelet count before treatment for a baseline and frequently during treatment because of potential thrombocytopenia. When the platelet count drops below 150,000/mm, the nurse should immediately report this information to the health care provider.
- Be aware that the natural color of amrinone is a clear yellow. When amrinone is discolored or contains a precipitate, it should be discarded.
- Carefully monitor the patient's BP, cardiac rhythm, pulse, heart rate, CO, and PCWP during and for several hours after administering phosphodiesterase inhibitors.

Do You UNDERSTAND?

DIRECTIONS: Place a check next to the statements that correctly describe phosphodiesterase inhibitors.

_____ 1. Increased preload

_____ 2. Long-term therapy

_____ 3. Monitor cardiac status, rhythm, pulse, BP, CO, heart rate, and PCWP

_____ 4. Stop infusion for significant hypotension or dysrhythmias

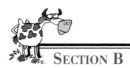

SECTION B
ANTIARRHYTHMICS

Antiarrhythmics suppress dysrhythmias typically using one or a combination of the following actions: depression of automaticity; decrease in conduction; or an increase in refractoriness to premature stimulation. Some agents are more effective than are others against atrial or ventricular dysrhythmias or both. Antiarrhythmics are classified according to their effect on the heart's electrical conduction. Class I is subdivided into three categories. The classes of antiarrhythmics are grouped as class I (A, B, and C), II, III, and IV. Miscellaneous antiarrhythmics are also discussed at the end of the chapter.

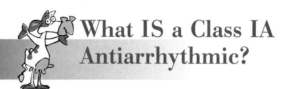

What IS a Class IA Antiarrhythmic?

Class IA Antiarrhythmics	Trade Names	Uses
moricizine [mor-I-ci-zeen]	Ethmozine	Treatment of ventricular tachycardia and PVCs
quinidine [KWIN-ih-deen]	Quinidex	Treatment of premature atrial and ventricular dysrhythmias
procainamide [pro-CANE- uh-mide]	Pronestyl	Treatment of life-threatening atrial and ventricular dysrhythmias
disopyramide [DIE-so-PIR-uh-mide]	Norpace	Treatment of life-threatening ventricular dysrhythmias

Action

Class IA antiarrhythmics (**class IAs**) suppress abnormal automaticity and prolong the P-R and Q-T intervals. Most class IAs reduce impulse conduction velocity and depress myocardial excitability, thereby decreasing myocardial contractility. Moricizine has local anesthetic activity and stabilizes the myocardial membrane. Moricizine also decreases the rapid current that is carried inward by sodium ions. Moricizine shortens repolarization, leading to decreased action potential and an effective refractory period.

Uses

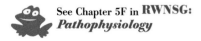

See Chapter 5F in RWNSG: *Pathophysiology*

Moricizine is used to suppress life-threatening ventricular dysrhythmias, particularly ventricular tachycardia. Quinidine sulfate is used primarily to treat atrial dysrhythmias and rarely is used for ventricular dysrhythmias, such as premature ventricular contractions (PVCs) and ventricular tachycardia. Procainamide is used to treat both atrial and ventricular dysrhythmias. Disopyramide is used to suppress PVCs and ventricular tachycardia but is used primarily for its unlabeled use of treating supraventricular tachycardias, such as paroxysmal atrial tachycardia (PAT), atrial flutter, and atrial fibrillation.

What You NEED TO KNOW

Contraindications/Precautions

Class IAs are contraindicated for patients with second- or third-degree AV block, bradycardia, cardiogenic shock, and bundle branch block, unless a pacemaker is present. Because the drug prolongs the P-R and Q-T intervals, heart blocks may be worsened. Procainamide and quinidine are contraindicated for patients with myasthenia gravis.

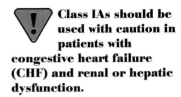

Class IAs should be used with caution in patients with congestive heart failure (CHF) and renal or hepatic dysfunction.

Drug Interactions

Cimetidine increases levels of class IAs. Moricizine decreases levels of theophylline. Additive anticholinergic effects may occur when class IAs are given with antihistamines and tricyclic antidepressants.

Disopyramide and quinidine sulfate can exacerbate the anticoagulation effects of warfarin. Rifampin, phenobarbital, and phenytoin decrease the blood levels of disopyramide and quinidine sulfate. Procainamide and quinidine can enhance neuromuscular blocking agents. Antihypertensives and nitrates may increase the hypotensive effect of procainamide and quinidine. Procainamide and quinidine may reduce the effects of cholinesterase inhibitors.

Disopyramide should not be given within 48 hours before or 24 hours after verapamil because this combination causes excessive prolonging of conduction and decreased CO. Procainamide can cause central nervous system (CNS) toxicity when given with lidocaine. Quinidine and trimethoprim increase the effects of procainamide. Quinidine increases digoxin levels, and amiodarone increases quinidine levels. Foods that alkalinize the urine may increase quinidine levels and cause toxicity.

Adverse Effects

CNS adverse effects of class IAs include dizziness, headache, fatigue, and nervousness. Common GI adverse effects of class IAs include nausea, vomiting, and diarrhea. Diarrhea is particularly common with quinidine, which is frequently the reason for which this antiarrhythmic is not used.

Moricizine may worsen dysrhythmias and actually cause ventricular tachycardia or PVCs. Other adverse effects of quinidine include hemolytic anemia and thrombocytopenia. Signs and symptoms of quinidine toxicity include tinnitus, hearing loss, visual disturbances, headache, nausea, and dizziness. Adverse effects of procainamide include seizures, confusion, leukopenia, agranulocytosis, and thrombocytopenia. Signs of procainamide toxicity include confusion, dizziness, drowsiness, nausea, vomiting, and tachydysrhythmias.

The most common and dangerous adverse effects of class IAs are the cardiovascular adverse effects. Class IAs may slow conduction excessively resulting in second- or third-degree AV block, asystole, widened QRS, and prolonged P-R or Q-T intervals. Procainamide, particularly when given IV, tends to widen the QRS complex, causes AV blocks, and produces hypotension in some patients.

A rare but serious cardiovascular adverse effect of class IAs is the occurrence of torsades de pointes.

Class IAs may depress the myocardium excessively and precipitate acute CHF. Torsades de pointes is an adverse effect that may occur when the serum level of class IAs becomes subtherapeutic (i.e., the level drops below the therapeutic range). This type of ventricular tachycardia is dangerous because it usually does not produce a pulse and has a twisting-type shape.

What You DO

Nursing Responsibilities

A loading dose is usually given followed by a continuous infusion. The loading dose should not be given at a rate that exceeds 20 mg/min, and the dose should not exceed 1 gram to prevent hypotension, heart blocks, and asystole. When administering class IAs, the nurse should:

- Administer class IAs either 1 hour before or 2 hours after meals because they are absorbed better on an empty stomach and are absorbed poorly with food.
- Instruct patients who are taking quinidine to avoid all fruits (except cranberries, prunes, and plums), all vegetables, and milk.
- Monitor renal and hepatic function studies for the patient who is taking class IAs. Doses of moricizine should be reduced in the presence of hepatic or renal failure.
- Monitor cardiac rhythm, particularly during the initial doses of class IAs to assess whether the drug is effective in terminating dysrhythmias, and report any dysrhythmias to the health care provider.
- Report any signs and symptoms of CHF (e.g., crackles in the lung bases) immediately to the health care provider.
- Instruct patients to take all doses as prescribed and to avoid trying to catch up on missed doses by doubling.
- Advise patients to carry identification that lists the medication.
- Teach patients to report any shortness of breath, irregular heartbeats, or palpitations.
- Be aware that procainamide is the only class IA antiarrhythmic that may be given IV.
- View of a cardiac monitor should be available while administering procainamide IV.
- Administer the loading dose and continuous infusion of procainamide on a volumetric pump through micro-drip tubing to ensure accurate dose administration. The loading dose should be diluted in either 50 or 100 ml of either D_5W or 0.9% normal saline. The dilution for the continuous infusion should be mixed as follows: 2 grams in 250 ml of either D_5W or 0.9% normal saline. The continuous infusion is usually given at a rate of 2 to 4 mg/min but may be given up to 6 mg/min.
- Discontinue procainamide immediately and notify the health care provider when the QRS complex widens by 50%, the P-R interval is prolonged, and hypotension develops.

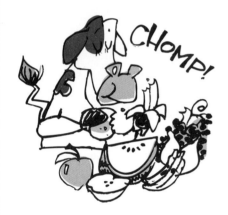

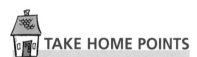

TAKE HOME POINTS

Report any worsening of ventricular arrhythmias or signs and symptoms of CHF immediately to the health care provider.

Discontinue procainamide and immediately report to the health care provider when the patient develops bradycardia, AV blocks, widening of QRS complex by 50%, prolonged P-R or Q-T interval, and hypotension.

- Be aware that procainamide infusions should not be weaned or discontinued until 1 to $1^1/_2$ hours after an oral dose of procainamide is given to prevent the recurrence of the dysrhythmia.
- Monitor N-acetylprocainamide (NAPA) and procainamide levels for patients who are taking procainamide. Procainamide is converted in the liver to NAPA, which is the active antiarrhythmic substance. The therapeutic range is 4 to 8 µg/ml. Toxicity occurs when the levels reach 8 to 16 µg/ml.
- Monitor quinidine levels for patients who are taking quinidine. The therapeutic range is 2 to 6 µg/ml. Toxicity results when levels exceed 8 µg/ml.
- Monitor CBCs and platelet counts for patients who are taking quinidine or procainamide.
- Warn patients to avoid participating in activities that require alertness until response to the medication is determined.
- Teach patients about the proper way to take their pulse and report when the pulse is less than 60 beats per minute.

Do You UNDERSTAND?

DIRECTIONS: **Complete the following statements with the appropriate terms from the italicized list provided.**

1. Foods that alkalinize the urine can increase the levels of

   _____.

2. _____ should not be given within 48 hours before or 24 hours after verapamil.

3. _____ can cause central nervous system toxicity with lidocaine.

4. _____ increases quinidine levels.

5. _____ is contraindicated for a patient with third degree AV block.

   amiodarone   *procainamide*   *moricizine*
   disopyramide   *quinidine*

 # What IS a Class IB Antiarrhythmic?

Class IB Antiarrhythmics	Trade Names	Uses
lidocaine [LIE-doe-cane]	Xylocaine	Treatment of acute ventricular dysrhythmias
mexiletine [MEX-ih-leh-teen]	Mexitil	Treatment of life-threatening ventricular dysrhythmias
phenytoin [FEN-ih-toe-in]	Dilantin	Treatment of dysrhythmias
tocainide [TOE-cane-ide]	Tonocard	Treatment of life-threatening ventricular dysrhythmias

Answers: 1. quinidine; 2. disopyramide; 3. procainamide; 4. amiodarone; 5. moricizine.

Action

Class IB antiarrhythmics (**class IBs**) decrease automaticity and the spontaneous depolarization of the ventricles during diastole, thereby suppressing ventricular dysrhythmias. These agents also decrease the duration of the action potential and the refractory period in the conduction system.

Uses

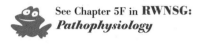

See Chapter 5F in **RWNSG:** *Pathophysiology*

Class IBs are used to treat ventricular dysrhythmias but are ineffective against atrial dysrhythmias. Lidocaine is used to treat emergency situations that involve ventricular dysrhythmias. Amiodarone, a class III antiarrhythmic, is the first-line antiarrhythmic drug that is used to treat ventricular fibrillation and ventricular tachycardia, according to the American Heart Association's (AHA) Advanced Cardiac Life Support (ACLS) guidelines.

http://www.american heart.org/heart_and_ stroke_A_Z_Guide

Phenytoin is primarily an anticonvulsant drug and, in rare cases, is used to treat ventricular dysrhythmias that are associated with digoxin toxicity. Mexiletine and tocainide are oral class IBs that are used to treat life-threatening ventricular dysrhythmias, such as ventricular tachycardia.

Class IBs are contra-indicated for women during pregnancy and lactation and for children.

What You NEED TO KNOW

Contraindications/Precautions

Lidocaine, phenytoin, and tocainide should be used with caution in patients with renal or hepatic dysfunction and CHF. Lidocaine and phenytoin should be given with caution to patients with respiratory depression. Lidocaine should be used cautiously in patients with shock and myasthenia gravis. Phenytoin should be given with caution to patients with hypotension, alcoholism, blood dyscrasias, brady-cardia, and diabetes mellitus. Tocainide should be given with caution to patients who are undergoing multiple drug therapy.

Lidocaine and tocainide are contraindicated for patients with hypersensitivity to amide anesthetics. Lidocaine is contraindicated for patients with blood dyscrasias, supraventricular dysrhythmias, severe SA and AV block, and Stokes-Adams syndrome. Mexiletine is contraindicated for patients with severe brady-dysrhythmias, severe ventricular CHF, and cardiogenic shock. Phenytoin is contraindicated for patients with bradycardia, complete or incomplete heart block, and Stokes-Adams syndrome. Tocainide is contraindicated for second- and third-degree AV block, hypokalemia, and myasthenia gravis.

Drug Interactions

Rifampin, phenobarbital, and phenytoin may decrease the blood level of mexiletine, and cimetidine may increase mexiletine blood level. Rifampin and cimetidine may decrease the blood level of tocainide. Phenytoin blood levels can increase when given with phenylbutazone, disulfiram, alcohol, amiodarone, isoniazid, chloramphenicol, sulfonamides, fluoxetine, benzodiazepines, omeprazole, metronidazole, ketoconazole, fluconazole, miconazole, estrogens, succinimides, halothane, salicylates, methylphenidate, phenothiazines, tolbutamide, trazodone, and felbamate. Phenytoin may cause excessive sedation when given with CNS depressants. Myocardial depression can result when phenytoin is given with lidocaine or BBs.

Foods that alkalinize the urine can increase levels of mexiletine and cause toxicity. Foods that alkalinize the urine include all fruits (except cranberries, prunes, and plums) all vegetables, and milk. Opioids, atropine, and antacids may slow the absorption of mexiletine, while metoclopramide increases its absorption.

Class IBs should be given with caution to older or debilitated patients.

Adverse Effects

CNS effects are the most common type of adverse effects that may occur with class IBs. Confusion, excitation, dizziness, and nervousness may occur with tocainide, mexiletine, and lidocaine. Adverse effects of phenytoin include ataxia, agitation, dizziness, drowsiness, and extrapyramidal symptoms. Seizures can result from tocainide and lidocaine. Signs and symptoms of lidocaine toxicity include confusion, excitation, blurred vision, nausea, vomiting, ringing of ears, tremors, twitching, convulsions, dizziness, and bradycardia.

Serious cardiovascular adverse effects from class IBs include hypotension, bradycardia, dysrhythmias, and cardiac arrest. Mexiletine may also cause palpitations and edema. Tachycardia can result from phenytoin, particularly when it is given IV at a rate that exceeds 50 mg/min. Other cardiovascular adverse effects of tocainide include palpitations, tachycardia, and CHF.

Mexiletine and tocainide can cause hepatic dysfunction. Hematologic adverse effects can occur with all class IBs (except lidocaine). Mexiletine, phenytoin, and tocainide can cause thrombocytopenia. Leukopenia can result from phenytoin and tocainide. Phenytoin can also cause aplastic anemia.

Older patients who are taking lidocaine are particularly sensitive to adverse effects involving the CNS.

What You DO

Nursing Responsibilities

When administering class IBs, the nurse should:

- Monitor cardiac rhythm, particularly during the initial doses to assess whether the drug is effective in terminating the dysrhythmia, and report any dysrhythmias and hypotensive episodes to the health care provider.
- View a cardiac monitor while administering lidocaine. Lidocaine is given IV. A loading dose is usually given, followed by continuous infusion. Some lidocaine preparations come in prefilled syringes for both the bolus and the continuous infusion. The bolus prefilled syringe contains 100 mg and the prefilled syringe that is used for the continuous infusion contains 2 grams. The loading dose is as follows: 1 mg/kg given IV at a rate of 25 to 50 mg/min. The dilution for the continuous infusion is mixed as follows: 2 grams in 250 ml of either D_5W or 0.9% normal saline. The continuous infusion is usually given at a rate of 2 to 4 mg/min.
- Administer continuous lidocaine infusion on a volumetric pump through micro-drip tubing to ensure accurate dose administration.
- Be aware that the earliest signs of lidocaine toxicity involve CNS effects (e.g., confusion).
- Administer IV phenytoin at a rate no faster than 50 mg/min to prevent CNS depression, hypotension, and cardiovascular collapse. IV phenytoin is compatible only with 0.9% normal saline solution.
- Monitor CBC and platelet count for patients who are taking mexiletine, phenytoin, or tocainide.

Lidocaine should be discontinued immediately and the health care provider notified when any heart blocks, bradycardia, or sinus arrest develop. The nurse must differentiate between the two types of prefilled lidocaine syringes because it can be lethal if the prefilled, 2 g of lidocaine is given to a patient as a bolus!

Patients who are older and those who have renal or hepatic dysfunction are particularly sensitive to lidocaine toxicity.

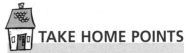

TAKE HOME POINTS

Administer IV phenytoin at a rate no faster than 50 mg/min.

- Monitor renal and hepatic function studies for patients who are receiving mexiletine or tocainide.
- Monitor phenytoin and mexiletine levels for early detection of toxicity.
- Instruct the patient to take all doses as prescribed and to avoid trying to catch up on missed doses by doubling.
- Caution patients to carry identification that lists the medication.
- Warn patients to avoid participating in activities that require alertness until response to the drug is known.
- Advise patients to report any shortness of breath, unusual bruising, and irregular heartbeats.
- Teach patients the proper way to take their pulse and report when the pulse is less than 60 beats per minute.
- Teach the patient who is taking mexiletine to avoid foods that alkalinize the urine.

Do You UNDERSTAND?

DIRECTIONS: Indicate in the space provided whether the statement is *true* or *false*.

_____ 1. Phenytoin is used primarily as an antiarrhythmic agent.

_____ 2. Tocainide is given IV for ventricular arrhythmias.

_____ 3. Class IBs decrease the action potential.

_____ 4. Class IBs are used to treat only ventricular arrhythmias.

What IS a Class IC Antiarrhythmic?

Class IC Antiarrhythmics	Trade Names	Uses
flecainide [fleh-CANE-ide]	Tambocor	Prevention of life-threatening ventricular dysrhythmias
propafanone [pro-PA-fan-one]	Rythmol	Treatment of ventricular dysrhythmias

Action

Class IC antiarrhythmics (**class ICs**) alter the transport of ions across cell membranes, thereby slowing conduction. Flecainide slows conduction velocity and increases ventricular refractoriness. Propafanone reduces spontaneous automaticity and suppresses ventricular tachycardia, which stabilizes action on myocardial membranes.

Uses

Class ICs are oral agents that are used to treat life-threatening ventricular dysrhythmias, particularly ventricular tachycardia. Flecainide is used to prevent paroxysmal atrial flutter or fibrillation (PAF) and paroxysmal supraventricular tachycardias (PAVTs).

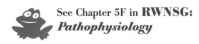 See Chapter 5F in **RWNSG:** *Pathophysiology*

What You NEED TO KNOW

Contraindications/Precautions

Class ICs are contraindicated for patients with cardiogenic shock. Flecainide is also contraindicated for patients with second- or third-degree AV block and severe hepatic dysfunction. Propafanone is contraindicated for patients with severe CHF, SA or AV block, severe hypotension, bradycardia, emphysema, and electrolyte imbalances.

Class ICs are contraindicated for mothers who are nursing. Flecainide is contraindicated for women during pregnancy and for children under 18 years of age. Propafanone should be used with caution in women during pregnancy and for children and older adults.

Drug Interactions

An increased risk of dysrhythmias is present when flecainide is taken with other antiarrhythmics (e.g., CCBs, disopyramide, BBs). Amiodarone increases the blood level of flecainide by 50%. Flecainide increases digoxin levels, thus the risk for digoxin toxicity increases.

Foods that alkalinize and acidify the urine affect the blood level of flecainide. Alkalinizing foods promote reabsorption increasing flecainide levels. Acidifying foods (e.g., cheese, cranberries, eggs, fish, grains, meat, plums, poultry, prunes) increase renal elimination of flecainide.

Propafanone increases the levels of propranolol and metoprolol. Propafanone increases the effects of warfarin and the levels of cyclosporine and digoxin. Rifampin decreases blood levels of propafanone.

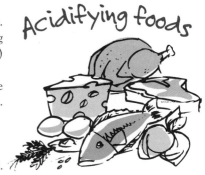

Acidifying foods

Adverse Effects

The adverse effects of class ICs primarily concern the cardiovascular and CNS. Flecainide can cause dysrhythmias, chest pain, and CHF. Propafanone can cause atrial and ventricular dysrhythmias, conduction disturbances, bradycardia, and hypotension. CNS adverse effects include dizziness, shaking, weakness, headache, depression, and tremors.

Class ICs should be used with caution in patients with renal dysfunction. Flecainide should be used with caution in patients with CHF. Propafanone should be given cautiously to patients with hepatic dysfunction.

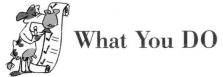

What You DO

Nursing Responsibilities

When administering class ICs, the nurse should:

- Monitor cardiac rhythm, particularly during the initial doses to assess whether the drug is effective in terminating the dysrhythmia, and report any

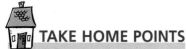

TAKE HOME POINTS

Notify the health care provider immediately of any adverse cardiovascular or CNS-related effects.

dysrhythmias, hypotension episodes, and any CNS adverse effects (e.g., dizziness, headache, depression, tremors) to the health care provider.

- Be aware that doses of class ICs should be decreased for patients with renal or hepatic dysfunction.
- Monitor blood levels of flecainide for early detection of toxicity.
- Instruct patients to take all doses as prescribed and to avoid trying to catch up on missed doses by doubling.
- Advise patients to carry identification that lists the medication.
- Instruct patients to avoid participating in activities that require alertness until response to the drug is known.
- Instruct patients to report any shortness of breath, irregular, fast, or slow heartbeats.
- Teach patients the proper way to take their pulse and report when the pulse is less than 60 beats per minute.
- Instruct patients who are taking flecainide to avoid foods that alkalinize or acidify the urine.

Do You UNDERSTAND?

DIRECTIONS: Complete the following statements with the appropriate terms from the list provided.

1. _____ increases the blood level of flecainide by 50%.
2. The renal elimination of _____ is increased by foods that acidify the urine.
3. _____ increases the effects of warfarin.
4. _____ increases the risk of arrhythmias when taken with flecainide.

   propafanone   *disopyramide*
   amiodarone   *flecainide*

What IS a Class II Antiarrhythmic?

Class II antiarrhythmics are β-adrenergic antagonists. Refer to page 147 for a discussion of β-adrenergic antagonists.

Answers: 1. amiodarone; 2. flecainide; 3. propafanone; 4. disopyramide.

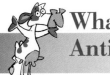

What IS a Class III Antiarrhythmic?

Class III Antiarrhythmics	Trade Names	Uses
amiodarone [A-MEE-oh-duh-rone]	Cordarone	Treatment of life-threatening ventricular dysrhythmias
bretylium [breh-TILL-ee-uhm]	Bretylol	Treatment of life-threatening ventricular dysrhythmias
ibutilide [ih-BYOO-tih-lide]	Corvert	Treatment of atrial flutter or atrial fibrillation
sotalol [SOTT-uh-lahl]	Betapace	Treatment of life-threatening ventricular dysrhythmias

Action

Amiodarone prolongs the action potential and the refractory period and inhibits adrenergic stimulation. Bretylium initially releases norepinephrine and then blocks its release. Bretylium increases the fibrillation threshold and therefore is effective in treating and preventing ventricular fibrillation. Ibutilide activates the slow inward current of sodium in cardiac tissue, resulting in delayed repolarization and prolonged action potential. Ibutilide also increases the refractory period. Sotalol is a BB that inhibits the β_1-receptors of the heart.

Uses

Amiodarone, bretylium, and sotalol are used to treat life-threatening ventricular dysrhythmias. Amiodarone is also frequently used for its unlabeled use of treating atrial tachydysrhythmias. Ibutilide is a unique drug that pharmacologically cardioverts patients and is effective in rapidly converting a recent onset of atrial fibrillation and atrial flutter to a normal sinus rhythm.

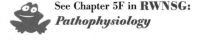

See Chapter 5F in **RWNSG:** *Pathophysiology*

The revisions of the AHA-developed ACLS guidelines in 2000 made several changes in the recommendations regarding antiarrhythmics. Amiodarone is the first drug that is preferred for the treatment of ventricular fibrillation and ventricular tachycardia. Bretylium was removed from the guidelines for treatment of ventricular fibrillation.

What You NEED TO KNOW

Contraindications/Precautions

Amiodarone and sotalol are contraindicated for patients with cardiogenic shock, bradycardia and heart block. Ibutilide is contraindicated for patients with hypokalemia and hypomagnesia. Sotalol is also contraindicated for patients with CHF.

Amiodarone, bretylium, and ibutilide are contraindicated for women during pregnancy and lactation and for children under 18 years of age.

Amiodarone should be given with caution to patients with thyroid dysfunction, CHF, lung disease, iodine hypersensitivity, and those who have had heart surgery. Bretylium should be used cautiously in patients who are taking digitalis or patients with angina, renal dysfunction, bradycardia, and fixed CO. Ibutilide should be used cautiously in patients with CHF, recent MI, hepatic dysfunction, and prolonged Q-T intervals. Sotalol should also be used cautiously within 14 days of administration of an MAOI to prevent acute hypertension. Ibutilide should not be given within 4 hours of administering amiodarone, disopyramide, procainamide, quinidine, and sotalol because excessive prolonging of the refractory period may occur.

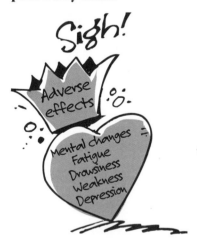

 Nurses should use caution and avoid confusing amiodarone with another drug that has the similar name of amrinone.

Drug Interactions

When digoxin is given with amiodarone, digoxin levels are increased by 50%. Amiodarone increases levels of cyclosporine, dextromethorphan, methotrexate, phenytoin, and theophylline when given concurrently. Amiodarone enhances the anticoagulation effects of warfarin. Bradydysrhythmias may occur when amiodarone is taken with BBs or CCBs. Cholestyramine decreases amiodarone levels, and cimetidine increases amiodarone levels.

Bretylium increases the actions of dopamine and norepinephrine. Digoxin toxicity can worsen dysrhythmias when bretylium is administered. Phenothiazines, tricyclic and tetracyclic antidepressants, antihistamines, and H_2-receptor blocking agents increase the risk for dysrhythmias with ibutilide.

Phenytoin and verapamil may cause further myocardial depression and resultant CHF when given with sotalol. Bradycardia may occur when sotalol is taken with digoxin. Antihypertensive agents, nitrates, and alcohol given with sotalol may cause hypotension. Sotalol and insulin may prolong hypoglycemia. Sotalol also decreases the effectiveness of theophylline.

Adverse Effects

Adverse effects of amiodarone include constipation, anorexia, hypotension, bradycardia, worsening of dysrhythmias, CHF, and hepatic dysfunction. Amiodarone can also cause CNS effects of dizziness, malaise, fatigue, headache, tremor, poor coordination, and paresthesia. Common adverse effects of bretylium include hypotension, dizziness, and fainting. Nausea and vomiting also are common when the bolus dose is given at a rate that exceeds 8 minutes.

Ibutilide can cause ventricular tachycardia during infusion or up to 4 hours after administration. The adverse effects of sotalol include fatigue, dizziness, drowsiness, weakness, depression, and mental changes. Cardiovascular adverse effects include bradycardia, hypotension, CHF, cardiogenic shock, bradycardia, and heart block. Impotence and decreased libido may also result.

What You DO

Nursing Responsibilities

When administering class III antiarrhythmics, the nurse should:
- Monitor cardiac rhythm, particularly during initial doses to assess whether the drug is effective in terminating the dysrhythmia, and report any dysrhythmias and hypotension episodes to the health care provider.
- Be aware that all class III antiarrhythmics must be administered on a volumetric pump through micro-drip tubing to ensure accurate dose administration.
- Be aware that doses of class III antiarrhythmics must be reduced in patients with hepatic or renal dysfunction.
- Dilute IV amiodarone in D_5W.

- Dilute infusions that exceed 2 hours in a glass bottle or a nonpolyvinyl chloride bag to prevent the drug from adhering to the plastic. Polyvinyl chloride tubing does not affect absorption.
- Avoid weaning or discontinuing IV amiodarone until after the oral dose is given to prevent recurrence of the dysrhythmia.
- Be aware that when defibrillation and lidocaine are ineffective in the treatment of ventricular fibrillation, bretylium is used. A bolus dose is given over a period of 10 minutes or more to decrease adverse effects, followed by a continuous infusion. The infusion is prepared with 2 grams of bretylium in 250 ml of either D_5W or 0.9% normal saline.
- Monitor the cardiac rhythm while ibutilide is administered and for 4 hours after administration because sustained ventricular tachycardia can develop. IV ibutilide is given over 10 minutes and is diluted in 50 ml of either D_5W or 0.9% normal saline. Because of the risk of sustained tachycardia, a defibrillator-cardioverter should be available at the bedside.
- Monitor BUN, potassium, triglyceride, lipoprotein, and uric acid levels for patients receiving sotalol.
- Monitor blood glucose levels of patients who are taking insulin and sotalol for detection of hypoglycemia.
- Monitor hepatic function tests for the patient who is taking amiodarone.
- Instruct patients to take all doses as prescribed and to avoid trying to catch up on missed doses by doubling.
- Advise patients to carry identification listing the medication.
- Instruct patients to avoid participating in activities that require alertness until response to the drug is known.
- Instruct patients to report any shortness of breath, weakness, and fainting.
- Teach patients about the proper way to take their pulse and report when the pulse is less than 60 beats per minute.
- Instruct patients who are taking sotalol to avoid consuming alcohol because hypotension may result.

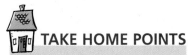

TAKE HOME POINTS

Nausea and vomiting are common when the bretylium bolus dose is given at a rate that exceeds 8 minutes.

Do You UNDERSTAND?

DIRECTIONS: Complete the following statements with the appropriate terms from the list of italicized words provided.

1. _____ is contraindicated for patients with CHF and cardiogenic shock.
2. The most common adverse effect of _____ is hypotension.
3. _____ increases digoxin levels by 50%.
4. _____ should not be given within 4 hours of administering procainamide.

   amiodarone   *ibutilide*
   bretylium   *sotalol*

Answers: 1. sotalol; 2. bretylium; 3. amiodarone; 4. ibutilide.

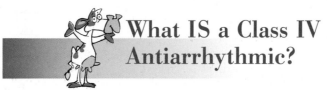

What IS a Class IV Antiarrhythmic?

Class IV antiarrhythmics are calcium channel blockers. Refer to page 152 for a discussion of these agents.

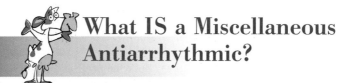

What IS a Miscellaneous Antiarrhythmic?

Miscellaneous Antiarrhythmics	Trade Names	Uses
adenosine [ah-DEN-oh-seen]	Adenocard	Treatment of paroxysmal supra-ventricular tachycardia
digoxin [dih-JOX-in]	Lanoxin	Treatment of atrial flutter and fibrillation, paroxysmal atrial tachycardia, and cardiogenic shock
isoproterenol [eye-so-pro-TER-uh-nahl]	Isuprel	Treatment of shock

Action

Each miscellaneous antiarrhythmic has a unique action that is effective in treating dysrhythmias. Adenosine restores a normal sinus rhythm from interrupting reentrant pathways in the AV node, which causes conduction to slow in the AV node and is thereby effective in suppressing atrial tachydysrhythmias. Because adenosine causes transient asystole, the SA node is allowed to take over and initiate a normal sinus rhythm. Digoxin prolongs the refractory period of the AV node and decreases conduction in the SA and AV nodes. Isoproterenol stimulates the β_1-receptors, causing an increase in the heart rate. The increase in heart rate shortens the Q-T interval, which suppresses the occurrence of torsades de pointes.

Uses

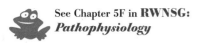

See Chapter 5F in **RWNSG:** *Pathophysiology*

Miscellaneous antiarrhythmics are used to treat dysrhythmias that are not identified in any of the standard antiarrhythmic classes. Adenosine and digoxin are used to treat atrial tachydysrhythmias. Adenosine is effective, but its duration is short (1 to 2 minutes), thus the dysrhythmia frequently returns. A longer-acting antiarrhythmic (e.g., digoxin) should also be used to prevent recurrence of the dysrhythmia. Isoproterenol (as an antiarrhythmic) is used only to treat the life-threatening ventricular tachycardia called torsades de pointes. This is a dangerous type of ventricular tachycardia because it does not usually produce a pulse. Torsades de pointes may occur when the serum level of a class IA becomes subtherapeutic.

What You NEED TO KNOW

Contraindications/Precautions

Adenosine is contraindicated for patients with AV block, second- or third-degree AV block, sick sinus syndrome, atrial flutter or fibrillation, and ventricular tachycardia. Digoxin is contraindicated for patients with ventricular tachycardia or fibrillation and digitalis toxicity. Isoproterenol is contraindicated for patients with tachycardias, ventricular dysrhythmias, digitalis toxicity, heart block, coronary artery disease, and cardiogenic shock.

Drug Interactions

Isoproterenol can have an additive effect on the cardiovascular system with adrenergic agonists, which may result in tachydysrhythmias, ventricular tachycardia, or ventricular fibrillation. Adenosine and corbamazine increases the risk of developing heart block. Dipyridamole increases the effect of adenosine. Theophylline and caffeine decreases the effect of adenosine. An increased risk of digoxin toxicity develops when digoxin is taken with thiazides, loop diuretics, mezlocillin, piperacillin, ticarcillin, amphotericin B, and glucocorticosteroids. Quinidine, cyclosporine, amiodarone, verapamil, diltiazem, propafanone, and diclofenac also increase digoxin levels in the blood. An increased risk for bradycardia is present when digoxin and BBs are taken together. Antacids, kaolin-pectin, cholestyramine, and a high-fiber diet decrease the absorption of digoxin.

Adverse Effects

When adenosine is given IV, a sudden onset of apprehension, dizziness, headache, shortness of breath, chest pain, flushing, transient arrhythmias, and hypotension may occur. Adverse effects that are associated with digoxin include fatigue, weakness, headache, dysrhythmias, bradycardia, and thrombocytopenia. Early signs of digitalis toxicity include nausea and vomiting. Common adverse effects of isoproterenol include tachydysrhythmias, sinus tachycardia, and chest pain.

 Adenosine should be used with caution in patients with renal or hepatic dysfunction and asthma. Digoxin should be used cautiously in patients with hypokalemia, hypothyroidism, lung disease, severe heart disease, incomplete AV block, and renal dysfunction. Isoproteranol should be used cautiously in patients with hypertension, cardiovascular disorders, tuberculosis, hyperthyroidism, glaucoma, diabetes mellitus, and renal dysfunction.

 Adenosine should be used with caution in women during pregnancy. Digoxin should be used with caution in women during pregnancy and lactation, as well as in children, older adults, and debilitated patients. Isoproterenol should be used cautiously in older adults and debilitated patients.

Isoproterenol is contraindicated for women during pregnancy and lactation.

What You DO

Nursing Responsibilities

When administering miscellaneous antiarrhythmics, the nurse should:

- Monitor cardiac rhythm, particularly during the initial dose to assess whether the drug is effective in terminating the dysrhythmia, and report any dysrhythmias to the health care provider.

TAKE HOME POINTS

Expect a short run (3 to 6 seconds) of asystole after administration of adenosine. Decrease the infusion rate or temporarily discontinue isoproterenol when heart rate is at or above 110 beats per minute.

Isoproterenol can be lethal when given by direct IV push!

- Administer adenosine as a rapid bolus IV over 1 to 2 seconds. Adenosine is ineffective when it is given at a slower rate. The nurse should prepare a 10 ml syringe with 10 ml of 0.9 % normal saline, and follow the bolus of adenosine with the normal saline immediately to facilitate the rapid bolus IV. Adenosine should be given in the port that is closest to the insertion site.
- Give IV digoxin (as an antiarrhythmic) in divided doses over 24 hours.
- Monitor digoxin levels to prevent toxicity. A level greater than 2.0 mg/ml indicates toxicity.
- Instruct the patient to take all doses as prescribed and to avoid trying to catch up on missed doses by doubling.
- Advise the patient to carry identification listing the medication.
- Teach patients the proper way to take their pulse and report when the pulse is less than 60 beats per minute.
- Administer isoproterenol only as a diluted infusion.
- Administer isoproterenol on a volumetric pump through micro-drip tubing to ensure accurate dose administration.
- Titrate isoproterenol slowly when treating torsades de pointes until a heart rate is achieved that will suppress the occurrence of the dysrhythmia. Isoproterenol can trigger ventricular dysrhythmias and tachycardia, which can cause myocardial ischemia and infarction.
- Discontinue isoproterenol and notify the health care provider immediately when other ventricular dysrhythmias occur or when the patient develops chest pain.

Do You UNDERSTAND?

DIRECTIONS: **Indicate in the space provided whether the statement is**
                 true **or** *false.*

_____ 1. Adenosine is used to treat torsades de pointes.

_____ 2. Digoxin is used to treat atrial tachydysrhythmias.

_____ 3. Isoproterenol inhibits β_1-receptors.

_____ 4. Isoproterenol shortens the Q-T interval.

Answers: 1. false; isoproterenol is used; 2. true; 3. false; isoproterenol stimulates β_1-receptors; 4. true.

CHAPTER 6

Drugs Affecting the Respiratory System

SECTION A

AGENTS AFFECTING UPPER RESPIRATORY DISORDERS

Antitussives, decongestants, expectorants and mucolytics are used to treat upper respiratory tract disorders. These pharmacologic agents are available as both prescription and over-the-counter (OTC) preparations.

When multiple symptoms are present, a combination form of these medications may be used. The medication that contains ingredients that are appropriate for relief of the patient's symptoms should be chosen when multiple symptoms exist. Most medications contain an analgesic (e.g., acetaminophen), antihistamine (e.g., diphenhydramine, chlorpheniramine), and a nasal decongestant (e.g., pseudoephedrine). Other medications may contain an expectorant (e.g., guaifenesin) or an antitussive (e.g., dextromethorphan). When only one symptom exists, using a single-ingredient preparation to individualize the action is best.

What IS an Antitussive?

Antitussives	Trade Names	Uses
Opioids		
codeine [KOE-deen]		Treatment of cough
hydrocodone bitartrate [HIGH-droe-KOE-done by-TAR-trate]	Vicodin	Treatment of cough
Nonopioids		
benzonatate [ben-ZOE-na-tate]	Tessalon Perles	Treatment of cough
dextromethorphan [DEX-troe-meth-OR-fan]	Robitussin DM	Treatment of cough

193

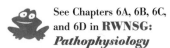 Opioid antitussives are contraindicated during pregnancy, in nursing mothers, and for children under 1 year of age.

See Chapters 6A, 6B, 6C, and 6D in **RWNSG:** *Pathophysiology*

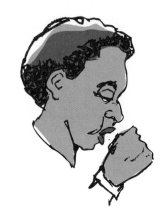

 Cautious use of opioid antitussives is indicated in patients with hepatic or renal dysfunction, history of drug abuse, prostatic hypertrophy, alcoholism, chronic pulmonary disease, hypothyroidism, head injury, and increased intracranial pressure.

Nonopioid antitussives are contraindicated for women during pregnancy and for nursing mothers. Dextromethorphan is contraindicated for children under 2 years of age and for women during the first trimester of pregnancy.

Action

Antitussives may act either centrally or locally to decrease the frequency and intensity of a cough. Centrally acting antitussives inhibit the cough response receptors in the cough center of the medulla of the brain, thereby suppressing the cough. A locally acting antitussive acts directly on the cough production at the site of irritation. Antitussives may be either opioid or nonopioid agents.

Uses

An antitussive is an agent that is generally used to suppress persistent, dry, or ineffective cough that prevents restful sleep. Benzonatate is frequently used in procedures (e.g., bronchoscopy, thoracentesis) when coughing should be avoided. In the treatment of coughs that are associated with the common cold or irritants, diphenhydramine (Benadryl), an antihistamine, may also be used.

What You NEED TO KNOW

Contraindications/Precautions

Opioid antitussives are contraindicated for patients with asthma or a hypersensitivity to codeine or morphine derivatives. Contraindications of nonopioid agents vary. Use of dextromethorphan is contraindicated for patients with asthma, productive or chronic cough, and hepatic dysfunction.

Drug Interactions

Concurrent use with central nervous system (CNS) depressant agents and alcohol may increase the action, causing further sedation. The opioid antitussives may increase the effects of MAOIs. Dextromethorphan may cause excitation, fever (**hyperpyrexia**), and hypotension when given concurrently with MAOIs. Dextromethorphan, the only antitussive with research-proven efficacy, is comparable to codeine but without addictive or respiratory depressive effects.

Adverse Effects

Opioid antitussives, given at high doses, have the adverse effects of CNS depression and dependency. At low doses, the risk of dependency and adverse effects are reduced. The adverse effects of antitussives range from common (e.g., dizziness, drowsiness, nausea, constipation, pruritus) to life threatening (e.g., respiratory depression, anaphylactic reaction).

Other CNS adverse effects include light-headedness, euphoria, sedation, and dysphoria. In addition to pruritus, hypersensitivity reactions may be manifested as diffuse erythema, rash, urticaria, excessive perspiration, facial flushing, or shortness of breath. Additional adverse effects that are observed with the use of opioid antitussives include palpitation, hypotension, orthostatic hypotension, bradycardia, tachycardia, circulatory collapse, vomiting, urinary retention, abnormal pupil constriction (**miosis**), lethargy, agitation, convulsions, and unconsciousness (**narcosis**).

The adverse effects of the nonopioid agents vary. Benzonatate has a low incidence of adverse effects that include drowsiness, sedation, headache, mild dizziness, constipation, nausea, skin rash, and pruritus. Adverse effects of dextromethorphan include dizziness, drowsiness, nausea, vomiting, and stomach pain.

What You DO

Nursing Responsibilities

When administering opioid antitussives, the nurse should:

- Monitor the patient's respiratory status. Antitussives should decrease the frequency and intensity of cough while the patient retains the protective cough reflex.
- Assess the respiratory rate and pattern before administering the medication and during treatment.
- Instruct the patient who is taking benzonatate perle to avoid breaking the soft capsule or allowing it to dissolve in the mouth to prevent an anesthetic or choking effect.
- Monitor bowel elimination and nausea accompanied by vomiting. When vomiting persists, the medication may need to be changed to another antitussive.
- Encourage the intake of fluids to prevent constipation when they are not contraindicated because of the patient's condition.
- Instruct the patient to take codeine with milk or food to decrease gastrointestinal (GI) upset.
- Instruct the patient to avoid driving or performing tasks that require mental alertness because of the sedative properties of opioid antitussives.
- Instruct patients to notify their health care provider of any cough that lasts longer than 1 week.

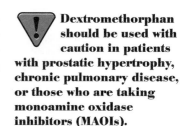

Dextromethorphan should be used with caution in patients with prostatic hypertrophy, chronic pulmonary disease, or those who are taking monoamine oxidase inhibitors (MAOIs).

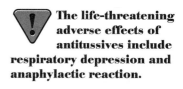

The life-threatening adverse effects of antitussives include respiratory depression and anaphylactic reaction.

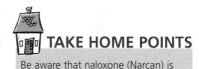

TAKE HOME POINTS

Be aware that naloxone (Narcan) is the antidote for overdose of opioids.

Do You UNDERSTAND?

DIRECTIONS: Match the statements in Column A with the appropriate descriptions in Column B.

Column A

_____ 1. An agent that is used to suppress coughs that interfere with sleep.

_____ 2. An adverse effect when a benzonatate perle breaks in the mouth.

_____ 3. Site of action of centrally acting antitussive.

_____ 4. The effect of opioid antitussives on the action of MAOIs.

Column B

a. Choking

b. Decrease

c. Increase

d. Medulla

e. Site of irritation

f. Antitussive

Answers: 1. f; 2. a; 3. d; 4. c.

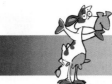

What IS a Decongestant?

Decongestants	Trade Names	Uses
ephedrine hydrochloride [eh-FED-rin]	Ephedsol Vantronol	Relief of nasal congestion
ipratropium bromide [eye-prah-TROE-pee-um]	Atrovent	Relief of nasal congestion
naphazoline [naf-AZ-oh-leen]	Allerest VasoClear	Relief of nasal congestion and minor eye irritation
phenylephrine HCl [fen-ill-EFF-rin]	Neo-Synephrine Sinex	Relief of nasal congestion and minor eye irritation
pseudoephedrine [SUE-doe-eh-FED-rin]	Sudafed Drixoral	Relief of nasal congestion

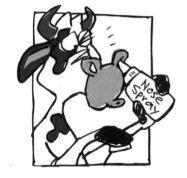

Action

Nasal decongestants in the form of topical sprays or drops are rapidly absorbed through the nasal mucosa. Decongestants act on the sympathetic nerve endings and the smooth muscle of the respiratory tract, causing vasoconstriction of arterioles. This vasoconstriction causes a decrease in blood flow, a reduction of fluid exudate, and shrinkage of edematous mucous membranes, resulting in decreased nasal congestion.

Uses

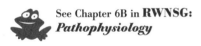

See Chapter 6B in **RWNSG:** *Pathophysiology*

Decongestants are agents that are used to relieve congestion in the nasal passages and eustachian tubes resulting from allergies, the common cold, rhinitis, and sinusitis. Phenylephrine is also used for pronounced dilation of pupil (**mydriasis**) in ophthalmoscopy examinations or surgery.

What You NEED TO KNOW

Contraindications/Precautions

Concomitant use of MAOIs and adrenergic decongestants are contraindicated. Adrenergic decongestants should be used with caution in patients with a history of hypertension, cardiac disease, diabetes mellitus, or hyperthyroidism.

Drug Interactions

Concurrent use of ephedrine with MAOIs, tricyclic antidepressants, guanethidine, and furazolidone may increase the α-adrenergic effects (e.g., fever, headache, hypertension). Epinephrine and norepinephrine increase the sympathomimetic effects of ephedrine. When ephedrine or phenylephrine is given together with α- and β-blockers, the effects of each are antagonized or counteracted. Tricyclic antidepressants, ergot alkaloids, reserpine, and guanethidine may elevate the blood pressure (BP) when taken with phenylephrine.

MAOIs may cause hypertensive crisis when given concurrently with phenylephrine or pseudoephedrine, and oxytocin may cause persistent hypertension when taken with phenylephrine. Concurrent use of pseudoephedrine with reserpine, methyldopa, and guanethidine increases the risk of hypertension. Urinary acidifiers cause a decrease in the decongestant effects. Urinary alkalinizer medications cause increased decongestant effects.

 Dysrhythmias may occur when phenylephrine is given together with digoxin or halothane.

Adverse Effects

Decongestants may cause mild CNS stimulation, such as restlessness, tremors, nervousness, headache, blurred vision, or insomnia. With higher doses, tachycardia, palpitations, dizziness, nausea, or vomiting may occur, particularly when the patient is hypersensitive to adrenergic drugs. Adverse effects following the use of adrenergic decongestants are less likely to occur with topical use.

The use of topical nasal decongestant drops or sprays may cause stinging, burning, or excessive drying of the nasal mucosa. Prolonged use of more than 3 to 5 days may cause rebound nasal congestion, chronic rhinitis, and possible ulceration of nasal mucosa. Rebound congestion is not observed with pseudoephedrine.

 # What You DO

Nursing Responsibilities

When administering decongestants, the nurse should:
- Monitor the patient's pulse and BP before administering adrenergic decongestants, particularly in patients with a history of cardiac disease.
- Advise the patient to avoid using nasal sprays for longer than 3 to 5 days to decrease the likelihood of rebound congestion.
- Instruct the patient in the use of topical nasal decongestants. The nurse should first instruct the patient to gently blow the nose before using nose drops or sprays to ensure open passages.
- For the instillation of nose drops, instruct the patient to position the head laterally with the head down to avoid the medication from entering the throat.
- For inhalation of nasal sprays, instruct the patient to bend the head slightly forward with the spray nozzle inserted in the nostril (being careful not to occlude the nostril) and to sniff briskly when sprayed. After use, rinse the dropper or spray tip with hot water to prevent contamination of the solution.

TAKE HOME POINTS

Because of the short duration and rapid effect, nasal decongestants may become habit forming.

Instruct patient to avoid chewing or crushing sustained release medications. Doing so will cause excessive absorption of the medication in the body at one time, rather than the steady dose over time as intended.

Do You UNDERSTAND?

DIRECTIONS: Match the statements in Column A with the correct answers in Column B.

Column A	Column B
_____ 1. The action whose result is decreased nasal congestion.	a. swallow
	b. take orally
_____ 2. Instruction to the patient taking sustained-release forms of medications.	c. do not chew
	d. topically
_____ 3. Adverse effect caused by prolonged use.	e. vasoconstriction
_____ 4. Route that may cause stinging or burning.	f. rebound congestion

What IS an Expectorant?

Expectorant	Trade Name	Uses
guaifenesin [GWHY-fen-ah-sin]	Robitussin	Treatment of dry, nonproductive cough

Action

An expectorant decreases the thickness (**viscosity**) of the sputum and stimulates productive coughing. The liquefied respiratory tract fluids are then easier to expel (**expectorate**) through coughing. Guaifenesin is a common ingredient of OTC cold medications.

Uses

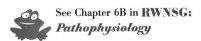

See Chapter 6B in RWNSG:
Pathophysiology

An expectorant is used in the treatment of dry coughs and when the patient is unable to expectorate mucus that is present in the respiratory tract. The cause of the cough may be a result of colds or minor upper respiratory tract infections.

What You NEED TO KNOW

Contraindications/Precautions

Guaifenesin is contraindicated in the treatment of chronic coughs, such as those resulting from asthma, emphysema, smoking, and copious or productive coughs.

Drug Interactions

Concurrent use of heparin may increase the risk of hemorrhage because guaifenesin inhibits platelet adhesiveness.

Answers: 1. e.; 2. c.; 3. f.; 4. d.

Adverse Effects

The use of guaifenesin presents a low incidence of adverse effects. However, GI upset, nausea, vomiting, drowsiness, urticaria, and rash may occur.

What You DO

Nursing Responsibilities

When administering expectorants, the nurse should:

- Advise the patient to increase fluid intake to 2 to 3 L per day to decrease mucus viscosity.
- Warn the patient to avoid driving or performing tasks that require mental alertness because drowsiness from guaifenesin may occur.
- Instruct patients to notify their health care provider when the cough lasts longer than 1 week or when a rash, fever, or persistent headache develops.
- Warn the patient that some OTC combination preparations may contain alcohol and should not be taken by individuals with a history of alcohol intolerance or abuse.

 TAKE HOME POINTS

Instruct the patient to follow each dose with a full glass of water to aid in thinning the secretions.

Do You UNDERSTAND?

DIRECTIONS: Indicate in the space provided whether the statement is *true* or *false*.

_____ 1. The patient's fluid intake should be increased to 2 to 3 liters per day.
_____ 2. Drowsiness is not an adverse reaction of guaifenesin.
_____ 3. Guaifenesin is a common ingredient of OTC cold medications.
_____ 4. An expectorant increases the viscosity of the sputum.

What IS a Mucolytic?

Mucolytic	Trade Name	Use
acetylcysteine [ass-cee-till-SIS-teen]	Mucomyst	Treatment of viscous mucous secretions

Action

Acetylcysteine, administered through inhalation or instillation, is rapidly absorbed through the mucosa of the respiratory tract. The action of a mucolytic involves the disruption of the chemical bonds between the muco-protein molecules of the respiratory secretions. The result is liquefaction of the mucus.

Answers: 1. true; 2. false; 3. true; 4. false.

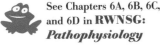

See Chapters 6A, 6B, 6C, and 6D in **RWNSG:** *Pathophysiology*

Uses

Mucolytics are used to facilitate the removal of viscous, tenacious mucus secretions in the respiratory tract. Sodium chloride solution also has mucolytic actions. Oral acetylcysteine is also used as the antidote for acetaminophen overdose.

What You NEED TO KNOW

Contraindications/Precautions

Hypersensitivity and risk of gastric hemorrhage contraindicates the use of mucolytics. Cautious use is recommended for patients with asthma.

Drug Interactions

Mucolytics are incompatible with antibiotics and must be administered separately, not in the same nebulizer. Charcoal decreases the antidote effect.

Adverse Effects

Adverse effects of acetylcysteine include nausea, vomiting, stomatitis, rhinorrhea, rash, fever, drowsiness, chest tightness, bronchoconstriction, respiratory tract irritation, and an increased amount of bronchial secretions. The likelihood of bronchospasm is increased in patients with asthma.

Caution should be used with mucolytic administration in debilitated or older patients.

Administer acetylcysteine with compressed air for nebulization, not with a hand nebulizer.

What You DO

Nursing Responsibilities

When administering mucolytics, the nurse should:
- Counsel the patient that mucolytics have a disagreeable odor that soon disappears.
- Be aware that acetylcysteine may cause stickiness on the face when administered by facemask or nebulizer.
- Instruct the patient to wash the face with water to remove stickiness.

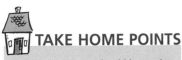

TAKE HOME POINTS

Suction equipment should be made available for the removal of excessive secretions to maintain an open airway when the patient is unable to expectorate.

Discontinue the mucolytic when bronchospasm occurs and notify the health care provider immediately.

Do You UNDERSTAND?

DIRECTIONS: Indicate in the space provided whether the statement is *true* or *false*.

_____ 1. Mucolytics are used to facilitate bronchodilation.

_____ 2. Oral acetylcysteine is given as the antidote for acetaminophen toxicity.

Answers: 1. false; 2. true.

_____ 3. Acetylcysteine given by inhalation may cause a stickiness on the face.

_____ 4. Patients who have asthma are likely to experience bronchospasm with acetylcysteine.

SECTION B
ANTIHISTAMINES

Two types of antihistamines have been classified: histamine H_1-receptor antagonists and histamine H_2-receptor antagonists. The H_1-antihistamines are used primarily to control symptoms that are associated with respiratory and allergic responses, particularly seasonal and allergic rhinitis. The H_2-receptor antagonists act primarily on the GI tract. Additionally, selected antihistamines are used as antiparkinsonism agents; other antihistamines are used as antiemetics for the treatment of vertigo and motion sickness.

The six subclasses of antihistamines are alkylamines, ethanolamines, ethylenediamines, phenothiazines, piperidines, and piperazines. Among the subclasses, varying degrees of sedative, antiemetic, anticholinergic, GI, or antipruritic effects are produced. First-generation antihistamines have more sedative effects and are referred to as _sedating_ antihistamines. The second-generation antihistamines produce less sedative effects, because they do not cross the blood-brain barrier. These agents are referred to as _nonsedating_ antihistamines.

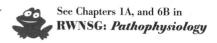

See Chapters 1A, and 6B in RWNSG: _Pathophysiology_

First-Generation Sedating Antihistamines

What IS a Sedating Antihistamine?

Sedating Antihistamines	Trade Names	Uses
Alkylamines		
brompheniramine [brome-fen-EAR-ah-meen]	Dimetane	Treatment of allergy and cough
chlorpheniramine [klor-fen-EAR-ah-meen]	Chlor Trimeton	Treatment of allergy and cough
Ethanolamines		
clemastine fumarate [kleh-MAS-teen]	Tavist	Treatment of allergic rhinitis
Ethylenediamines		
tripelennamine [try-pell-EN-ah-meen]	PBZ, Pelamine	Treatment of allergic conditions
Phenothiazines		
promethazine [proh-METH-ah-zeen]	Phenergan	Treatment of rhinitis and allergy conditions
Piperidines		
cyproheptadine [si-proh-HEP-tah-deen]	Periactin	Treatment of hypersensitivity reactions and allergic rhinitis

Answers: 3. true; 4. true.

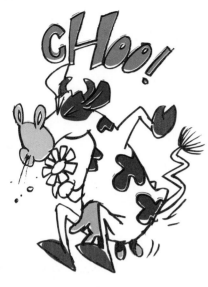

 See Chapters 1A and 13D in **RWNSG:** *Pathophysiology*

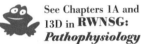 Tripelennamine is used in the treatment of children with herpetic gingivostomatitis for an analgesic effect on the oral mucous membranes.

Alkylamines, ethanolamines, and ethylenediamines are contraindicated for women during pregnancy and lactation. Promethazine is contraindicated during pregnancy and lactation, as well as for use in neonates and dehydrated or acutely ill children because of its potential for toxicity (e.g., dystonias). First-generation piperidines are contraindicated for use in children under 12 years of age.

Action

Alkylamines, ethanolamines, ethylenediamines, phenothiazines, and first-generation piperidines are first-generation antihistamines. Piperidines may be first- or second-generation antihistamines. Alkylamines, ethanolamines, and piperidines competitively block the H_1-receptor sites on effector cells and impede histamine-mediated responses. Ethylenediamines are H_1-receptor antagonists that compete with histamine at the receptor sites. Phenothiazines are antipsychotic drugs that block histamine effects at the H_1-receptor sites.

Uses

Sedating antihistamines are used for the treatment of symptoms that are associated with respiratory and allergic conditions (perennial and allergic rhinitis), transfusion reactions, and as an adjunct in anaphylactic reactions.

Ethanolamines and phenothiazines are used for the treatment of mild urticaria and angioedema. Diphenhydramine is used in the treatment of motion sickness, vertigo, parkinsonian conditions, and insomnia. Promethazine is also used in the treatment of motion sickness, nausea and vomiting, as a sedative, and as an adjunct to analgesics for pain control.

Unlabeled uses for cyproheptadine are as an appetite stimulant and as treatment of vascular headaches, Cushing's disease, and carcinoid syndrome.

What You NEED TO KNOW

Contraindications/Precautions

Alkylamines, ethanolamines, ethylenediamines, and phenathiazines are contraindicated for patients with narrow-angle glaucoma, sensitivity to antihistamines, GI obstruction, bladder neck obstruction, and prostatic hypertrophy. Alkylamines, ethanolamines, and ethylenediamines are also contraindicated for patients with asthma. Phenothiazines are also contraindicated for patients with bone marrow depression, severe CNS depression, and coma. First-generation piperidines are contraindicated for use in patients with hypersensitivity to H_1-receptor antagonists and those who are undergoing MAOI therapy.

Drug Interactions

Use of CNS depressants or alcohol with first-generation sedating antihistamines increases the sedative effects of when given together. Concurrent use of MAOIs may increase and prolong the drying (**anticholinergic**) effects of these agents. When promethazine is given with epinephrine, the result is a partial adrenergic blockade, leading to greater hypotension.

Adverse Effects

The most common adverse effects of sedating antihistamines are drowsiness and dry mouth. Alkylamines are potent antihistamines that have minimal sedative effects, moderate anticholinergic effects, and no antiemetic effects. Other adverse effects of alkylamines include dizziness, epigastric distress, thickening of bronchial secretions, and urinary retention.

Ethanolamines have moderate-to-high sedative effects, considerable anticholinergic and antiemetic effects, and a low rate of occurrence of GI effects. Adverse reactions of these agents include dizziness, epigastric distress, and the thickening of bronchial secretions. Blurred vision, hypotension, increased appetite, weight gain, urinary retention and rash are other adverse effects. Additional adverse effects of diphenhydramine include palpitations and tachycardia.

Ethylenediamines frequently cause more GI distress than do other antihistamines. Ethylenediamines also have moderate sedative effects and minimal anticholinergic and antiemetic effects. Other common adverse reactions of these agents include epigastric distress, anorexia, nausea, vomiting, and constipation. Blurred vision, headache, mild hypotension or hypertension, urinary hesitancy or retention, dizziness, nervousness, and rash are included as other adverse effects.

Phenothiazines have potent antihistamine actions, with strong sedative, anticholinergic, and antiemetic effects. Promethazine usually produces no extrapyramidal symptoms (EPS) as do the other phenothiazine derivatives. Other adverse CNS effects include blurred vision, confusion, dizziness, tremors, and impaired coordination. Mild hypotension or hypertension, anorexia, photosensitivity, urinary retention, and leukopenia are included as other adverse effects.

First-generation piperidines have moderate antihistamine activity, low-to-moderate sedative effects, moderate anticholinergic effects, and no antiemetic effects. Other adverse reactions to first-generation piperidines include epigastric distress, anorexia, nausea, vomiting, constipation, blurred vision, headache, mild hypotension, palpitations, tachycardia, urinary retention, dizziness, nervousness, rash, and thickening of respiratory secretions. Cyproheptadine has the adverse effect of appetite stimulation and may cause weight gain.

  Alkylamines and ethanolamines should be used with caution in women during pregnancy and in older patients. Safe use of ethylenediamines has not been determined for use in women during pregnancy, nursing mothers, or neonates. Cautious use of phenothiazines should be maintained in the treatment of older and debilitated patients. Caution with first-generation piperidines should be used for patients who are pregnant, nursing, older, or debilitated.

 Older patients may experience increased sedation, dizziness, and hypotension because an increased sensitivity to alkylamines and ethylenediamines.

Ethanolamines are to be used with caution for patients with a history of asthma, hypertension, hyperthyroidism, cardiovascular disease, and diabetes.

 # What You DO

Nursing Responsibilities

A major responsibility of the nurse, when administering sedating or first-generation antihistamines, is patient teaching. The nurse should:
- Encourage patients to increase their fluid intake to 2000 to 3000 ml per day.
- Teach the patient the importance of avoiding other CNS depressants and alcohol in any form when taking oral first-generation antihistamines.
- Instruct the patient to consult the health care provider before taking any OTC preparations to avoid adverse interactions. OTC allergy and cold preparations frequently contain alcohol.

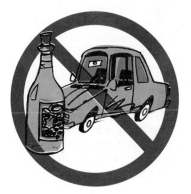

Diphenhydramine should be used with caution for patients with convulsive disorders. Use ethylenediamines with caution for patients with a history of asthma, cardiovascular disease, diabetes, hypertension, hyperthyroidism, or increased intraocular pressure. Use phenothiazines with caution in patients with impaired hepatic function, asthma, cardiovascular disease, hypertension, and respiratory impairment. Use first-generation piperidines with caution in patients with narrow-angle glaucoma, bladder neck obstruction, prostatic hypertrophy, history of asthma or chronic obstructive pulmonary disease (COPD), cardiovascular disease, and hypertension.

  Acute toxicity from an overdose of promethazine may cause paradoxical hyperexcitability and nightmares (in children), respiratory depression, coma, convulsions, and EPS.

Another life-threatening adverse effect that is observed with promethazine is agranulocytosis, particularly when it is used with cytotoxic agents.

Older patients commonly experience hypotension or sedation with antihistamine therapy and thus require assistance with ambulation to prevent falls.

- Instruct the patient to take first-generation antihistamines with food or milk to decrease GI adverse effects.
- Instruct the patient to chew gum or suck hard candy to relieve symptoms of dry mouth.
- Warn the patient to avoid driving or performing tasks that require mental alertness because of the sedative effects.
- Warn the patient to avoid prolonged exposure to sunlight and use sunscreen protection to decrease photosensitivity reactions.
- Instruct the patient to void before taking the ethanolamines to reduce urinary hesitancy.
- Be aware that tripelennamine should not be used within 14 days of MAOI therapy because of the adverse anticholinergic effects.
- Monitor the respiratory function of patients who are receiving promethazine because promethazine may thicken bronchial secretions and suppress the cough reflex.
- Assist the patient with ambulation as a prevention of falls because promethazine and piperidines frequently produces hypotension or sedation.
- Give IM promethazine injections deep into a large muscle with rotation of sites and daily observation.
- Instruct the patient in cyproheptadine therapy to notify the health care provider of any significant weight gain.
- Be aware that unless first-generation antihistamines are discontinued 4 days before allergy skin testing procedures, false negative results may occur. Promethazine may also produce false results in urine pregnancy tests.
- Be aware that respiratory depression is a life-threatening adverse effect of promethazine that is observed with acute toxicity.
- Be aware that subcutaneous administration of promethazine is contraindicated because irritation and necrosis may occur. Intraarterial injection of promethazine may cause arterial spasm and result in gangrene.

 # Do You UNDERSTAND?

DIRECTIONS: Complete the crossword puzzle.

Across

1. Antihistamines are mainly excreted in _____.
5. Antihistamines are metabolized by the _____.
7. An adverse GI reaction to ethylenediamines.
9. Administer at this time to lessen GI effects.
11. Days to stop antihistamines before allergy testing.
12. Use of these depressants will increase sedation.
13. Before meals.
16. Antihistamines are _____ in the GI tract.

Down

1. _____ of ethylenediamines is contraindicated during pregnancy.
2. This patient may be more sensitive to the normal dose.
3. Geriatric patients may experience more of this adverse effect.
4. H_1-receptor antagonists compete with histamine here.
6. Drowsiness is this type of reaction to antihistamines.
8. Increases CNS depressant effects and should be avoided.
10. An anticholinergic effect caused by antihistamines.
12. Overdose of PBZ-SR may cause this in children.
14. Instruct the patient not to _____ sustained-release formulations.
15. Route of most antihistamines.
17. This form of tripelennamine should not be given to children.

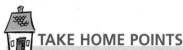

The sustained-release form of tripelennamine (PBZ-SR) is not recommended for use in children. Overdose may cause hallucinations, convulsions, coma, or cardiovascular collapse.

Instruct the patient to avoid chewing or crushing any sustained-release formulations.

TAKE HOME POINTS

Increased fluid intake helps thin respiratory secretions.

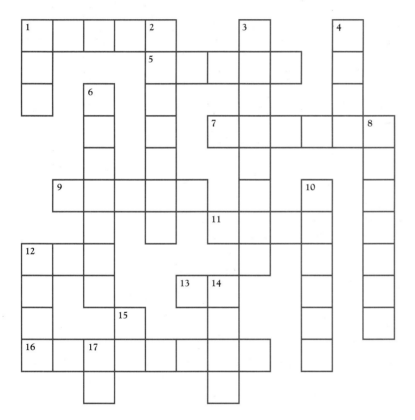

Answers: *Across:* 1. urine; 5. liver; 7. nausea; 9. meals; 11. four; 12. one; 13. ac; 16. absorbed. *Down:* 1. use; 2. elderly; 3. sedation; 4. site; 6. adverse; 8. alcohol; 10. drying; 12. coma; 14. chew; 15. PO; 17. SR.

Second-Generation Nonsedating Antihistamines

What IS a Nonsedating Antihistamine?

Nonsedating Antihistamines	Trade Names	Uses
Piperidines		
azatadine maleate [a-ZA-tah-deen]	Optimine	Treatment of allergic rhinitis
fexofenadine [fex-oh-FEN-ah-deen]	Allegra	Treatment of allergic rhinitis
loratadine [loh-RAH-tih-deen]	Claritin	Treatment of allergic rhinitis
Piperazines		
cetirizine [see-TIH-rah-zeen]	Zyrtec	Treatment of allergic rhinitis

Action

Piperidines may be first- or second-generation antihistamines. These agents competitively block the H_1-receptor sites on effector cells and impede histamine-mediated responses. A piperazine is a potent second-generation antihistamine (nonsedating) that blocks histamine at H_1-receptor sites.

Uses

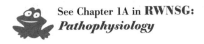

See Chapter 1A in RWNSG: *Pathophysiology*

Piperidines and piperazines are used primarily for the treatment of symptoms that are associated with allergic conditions, particularly perennial and allergic rhinitis and chronic urticaria.

What You NEED TO KNOW

Use piperidines and piperazines with caution in patients with impaired hepatic or renal function.

Second-generation piperidines and piperazines should be used with caution during pregnancy and lactation.

Contraindications/Precautions

Second-generation piperidines are contraindicated for patients hypersensitive to the drug. Piperazines are contraindicated for patients with hypersensitivity to H_1-receptor antihistamines or hydralazine.

Drug Interactions

Concurrent use of CNS depressants or alcohol with azatadine may increase sedation and drowsiness. MAOIs used concurrently with piperidines may prolong or increase anticholinergic effects of these agents. Tricyclic antidepressants will increase the anticholinergic effects when used with azatadine.

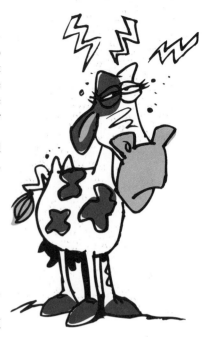

Adverse Effects

Piperazines and second-generation piperidines have moderate-to-high antihistamine activity, low to no sedative effects, low to no anticholinergic effects, no antiemetic effects, and fewer adverse effects. The most common adverse effect of fexofenadine is headache. Other adverse effects of fexofenadine include drowsiness, fatigue, nausea, dyspepsia, and throat irritation. Adverse effects are uncommon with loratadine; however, adverse effects that may occur are similar to those of the first-generation piperidines.

The most common adverse effects of piperazines include drowsiness and headache. Other adverse effects of piperazines include depression, constipation, diarrhea, and dry mouth.

What You DO

Nursing Responsibilities

When administering second-generation antihistamines, the nurse should:
- Administer azatadine with food, milk, or a full glass of water to lessen GI adverse effects.
- Give loratadine on an empty stomach, either 1 hour before or 2 hours after a meal.
- Instruct the patient to increase fluid intake, chew gum, or suck hard candy to help relieve dry mouth.
- Instruct the patient to avoid alcohol and the use of other CNS depressants because these substances may increase sedative effects.
- Instruct the patient to avoid taking piperazines concurrently with OTC antihistamines.
- Warn the patient to avoid driving or performing tasks that require mental alertness because drowsiness, dizziness, or blurred vision may occur with these agents.
- Be aware that H_1-receptor antagonists interfere with allergy skin testing when the tests are taken within 4 days of the last dose and may produce false results.
- Monitor the patient for paradoxical effects.
- Monitor the patient for sedation because of the possibility of sedative effects. Second-generation antihistamines produce few adverse reactions. However, the possibility of adverse effects may occur, as with all antihistamines, and the patient should therefore always be monitored for respiratory or cardiovascular effects.

TAKE HOME POINTS

Cetirizine should be taken orally once a day. Meals do not affect this medication.

The liquid form of cetirizine may be used for children when needed. Older patients are highly sensitive to the sedative effects of piperazines.

Do You UNDERSTAND?

DIRECTIONS: Match the statements in Column A with the appropriate word(s) in Column B.

Column A	Column B
_____ 1. Common side effect of first-generation piperidines.	a. Antiemetic
_____ 2. Action not observed with piperidine therapy.	b. Appetite stimulation
_____ 3. An adverse effect of cyproheptadine.	c. Drowsiness

SECTION C

ANTIASTHMATICS AND BRONCHODILATORS

Antiasthmatic and bronchodilator drugs are used for the treatment of obstructive respiratory disorders as a result primarily of inflammation and bronchoconstriction. These disorders include asthma, emphysema, and COPD. The medications that are used in the treatment and prevention of these disorders are primarily antiinflammatory agents and bronchodilators. The drug classes of antiinflammatory and bronchodilator agents that are discussed in this section include inhaled corticosteroids, β-agonists, leukotriene antagonists, xanthine derivatives, and anticholinergics.

What IS an Inhaled Corticosteroid?

Inhaled Corticosteroids	Trade Names	Uses
beclomethasone [be-kloh-METH-ah-zone]	Beclovent Vanceril	Treatment of seasonal or perennial rhinitis
dexamethasone [dex-ah-METH-ah-zone]	Decadron Decaspray	Treatment of allergic conditions
fluticasone [flu-TIH-kah-sone]	Flonase Flovent	Treatment of seasonal or perennial rhinitis; prevention and treatment of asthma
triamcinolone [try-am-SIN-oh-lone]	Azmacort	Treatment of allergic rhinitis and asthma

Answers: 1. c; 2. a; 3. b.

Action

Inhaled corticosteroids inhibit the inflammatory response in the airways and decrease edema of the airway mucosa. These agents also increase the number and sensitivity of bronchial β_2-receptors, promote smooth muscle relaxation, and decrease hyperresponsiveness of the airways, which combine to decrease the production of mucus.

Uses

Inhaled corticosteroids are used as prophylaxis and for treatment of asthma. These agents are also used in the treatment of steroid-dependent chronic bronchial asthma and as adjunctive treatment of asthma that nonsteroidal bronchodilators are unable to control. Inhaled corticosteroids should be avoided as treatment of an acute asthmatic attack because they do not provide immediate symptomatic relief. Intranasal inhaled corticosteroids are used in the treatment of seasonal and perennial rhinitis. Oral inhalation is used in the treatment of asthma. Beclomethasone and triamcinolone are also used intranasally to prevent recurrence of polyps after surgery for the removal of nasal polyps.

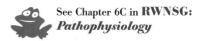

See Chapter 6C in **RWNSG:** *Pathophysiology*

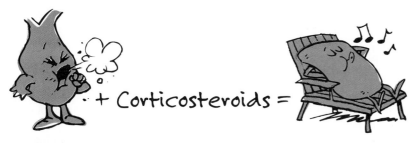

 What You NEED TO KNOW

Contraindications/Precautions

Contraindications for the use of inhaled corticosteroids are nonasthmatic bronchitis and primary treatment of status asthmaticus.

Drug Interactions

When inhaled corticosteroids are administered in the recommended doses, no significant interactions with other drugs occur. The concurrent use of corticosteroids and salicylates reduces salicylate effectiveness.

Adverse Effects

Inhaled corticosteroids have minimal systemic absorption, thus they decrease the risk of adverse effects. Common adverse reactions to the oral inhalant

Inhaled oral corticosteroids should be used with caution in patients who are undergoing systemic corticosteroid treatment and patients with ocular herpes simplex or active respiratory infections because serious illness may result because of the antiinflammatory effects. Nasal inhalant corticosteroids should be cautiously used in patients with nasal septal ulcers, nasal trauma, or surgery.

corticosteroids are fungal infections (e.g., *Candida albicans, Aspergillus niger*) of the oropharynx and larynx, hoarseness, dry mouth, and sore throat. Adverse effects of nasal inhalant corticosteroids include nasopharyngeal dryness, irritation, burning, itching, and ulceration. Other adverse effects include sneezing, epistaxis, headache, nausea, and vomiting. With the excessive administration of doses (overdosage), Cushing's syndrome or suppression of hypothalamic-pituitary-adrenal (HPA) function may occur as a result of systemic absorption.

What You DO

Nursing Responsibilities

Respiratory tissues rapidly absorb inhaled oral and nasal corticosteroids. Inhaled corticosteroids must be administered on a routine schedule to prevent asthma attacks. Inhaled corticosteroids are available as metered-dose inhalers (MDIs), which are hand-held canisters that deliver a measured dose of drug with each puff (inhalation). This action facilitates the opening of the airways and allows the corticosteroid to penetrate deeper into the lungs. When the prescribed dose is two puffs (inhalations), allow at least 1 minute between inhalations to allow absorption of the medication. When administering inhaled corticosteroids, the nurse should:

- Teach the patient the correct technique for using an MDI or nasal inhaler.
- Instruct the patient who is using intranasal inhalers to use decongestant nose drops first when nasal passages are blocked.
- Advise the patient to avoid using more doses than is prescribed and not to stop using the inhaler without consulting the health care provider.
- Counsel the patient to rinse the mouth with water after each use of a corticosteroid MDI to reduce or prevent the occurrence oropharyngeal fungal infections, hoarseness, or dry cough.
- Instruct the patient to rinse the mouthpiece and cap of the MDI (or the tip of the nasal inhaler) daily with warm, running water, and allow them to air dry before the next use. Instruct the patient to clean the mouthpiece and cap of the MDI weekly with warm water and mild dishwashing soap. Cleaning minimizes bacterial exposure and maintains patency.
- Instruct the patient to float the inhalant canister (MDI) in a bowl of water to determine whether the MDI is full or empty. When empty, the canister will float; when full, the canister will sink to the bottom of the bowl.

TAKE HOME POINTS

- Corticosteroids are not intended for emergency use because the medication takes 2 to 3 weeks to reach effective levels. Corticosteroids do not provide immediate symptomatic relief.
- Allow at least 1 minute between puffs or inhalations. When both a bronchodilator and corticosteroid inhaler are prescribed, administer the bronchodilator 5 minutes before using a corticosteroid inhaler to allow opening of airways and deeper lung penetration.

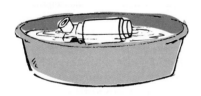

Do You UNDERSTAND?

DIRECTIONS: Complete the following statements with the appropriate terms from the italicized list provided.

1. Inhaled corticosteroids are used primarily for the treatment of
_____.

2. _____ is an intranasal corticosteroid that is used after a nasal polypectomy.

3. Excessive use of corticosteroids may result in _____.

4. A contraindication for the use of inhaled corticosteroids is _____.

   status asthmaticus   *flunisolide*
   asthma   *adrenal insufficiency*

What IS a β-Agonist?

β-Agonists	Trade Names	Uses
albuterol [al-BYOO-ter-ohl]	Proventil Ventolin	Prevention and treatment of asthma or bronchospasm
metaproterenol [met-ah-proh-TER-ih-nahl]	Alupent	Prevention and treatment of asthma or bronchospasm
terbutaline [ter-BYOO-tah-leen]	Brethine	Prevention and treatment of asthma or bronchospasm
salmeterol [sal-MET-er-ole]	Serevent	Prevention and treatment of asthma or bronchospasm

Action

β-Agonists ($β_2$-selective adrenergic agonists) are sympathomimetic agents that stimulate the $β_2$-receptors to relax the smooth muscles in the bronchioles of the lungs, thereby relaxing bronchospasms and producing bronchodilation. β-Agonists also inhibit histamine release from mast cells, decrease airway reaction to allergens, and increase ciliary motility, thereby facilitating expectoration of pulmonary secretions. Inhaled β-agonists are absorbed in the lungs; oral β-agonists are absorbed in the GI tract.

Uses

β-Agonists are available as oral, inhaled short-acting, and inhaled long-acting preparations. The oral and long-acting preparations are used for patients who have frequent asthma attacks. An increased response is achieved when the medication is taken on a fixed schedule. The short-acting preparations (e.g., albuterol, bitolterol, metaproterenol, pirbuterol, terbutaline) are used to treat acute exacerbation of asthma, for short-term relief of broncho-constriction that is associated with bronchitis and emphysema, and as a prophylaxis for exercise-

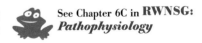
See Chapter 6C in **RWNSG:**
Pathophysiology

Answers: 1. asthma; 2. flunisolide; 3. adrenal insufficiency; 4. status asthmaticus.

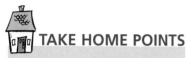

TAKE HOME POINTS

Salmeterol is not useful in the treatment of active bronchospasms.

Cautious use of β-agonists should be observed in patients with cardiovascular disease, hypertension, thyroid disease, diabetes mellitus, and sensitivity to sympathomimetics.

 β-Agonists are contraindicated for use during pregnancy and lactation. Bitolterol, metaproterenol, pirbuterol, salmeterol, and terbutaline are contraindicated for use in children under 12 years of age.

induced bronchospasm. The only long-acting β-agonist available is salmeterol, which is used for prophylaxis of bronchospasm and for the prevention of exercise-induced asthma.

What You NEED TO KNOW

Contraindications/Precautions

Cautious use of β-agonists should be observed in patients with cardiovascular disease, hypertension, thyroid disease, diabetes mellitus, and sensitivity to sympathomimetics.

Drug Interactions

Few drug interactions occur with the β-agonists, but those that occur are significant. Concurrent use of beta blockers and the β-agonists may negate the therapeutic effects of the β-agonist. The use of MAOIs or tricyclic antidepressants concurrently with β-agonists may exacerbate action on the vascular system. The use of other sympathomimetic bronchodilators may cause additive effects that may lead to hypertensive crisis.

Adverse Effects

Tremor is the most common adverse effect that is associated with oral administrations of β-agonists. Other adverse effects include anxiety, nervousness, restlessness, convulsions, weakness, dizziness, vertigo, headache, hallucinations, palpitations, hypertension, hypotension, bradycardia, reflex tachycardia, blurred vision, dilated pupils, nausea, vomiting, muscle cramps, hoarseness, and hypersensitivity reaction.

What You DO

Nursing Responsibilities

β-Agonists are available as oral medications, nasal sprays, and MDIs. Short-acting β-agonists provide immediate relief. When administering β-agonist agents, the nurse should:

- Monitor arterial blood gases and pulmonary function tests periodically during treatment with β-agonists.
- Monitor the patient's respiratory status and vital signs.
- Instruct the patient in the correct technique of using an MDI or nasal spray.
- Instruct the patient to rinse the mouthpiece and cap of the MDI (or the tip of the nasal spray container) daily with warm, running water, and allow to air

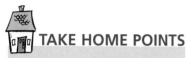

TAKE HOME POINTS

Oral preparations may be given with food to minimize GI adverse effects. Any palpitations, hypotension or hypertension, or any tachycardia should be reported to the health care provider.

dry before the next use. The mouthpiece and cap should be cleaned weekly with warm water and mild dishwashing soap. Cleaning minimizes bacterial exposure and maintains patency.

🍎 Advise the patient to avoid using more than the prescribed doses.

🍎 Instruct the patient to notify the health care provider immediately when no response to the usual dose occurs or when the symptoms worsen.

🍎 Instruct the patient to avoid using OTC medications without approval of the health care provider.

Do You UNDERSTAND?

DIRECTIONS: Complete the following statements with the appropriate terms from the italicized list provided.

1. _____ is the only long-acting β-agonist available.
2. _____ is an example of a short acting β-agonist.
3. β-Agonists are used for the treatment of _____.
4. Cautious use of β-agonists should be observed in patients with

_____

cardiovascular disease	*albuterol*
acute bronchospasms	*salmeterol*

What IS a Leukotriene Antagonist?

Leukotriene Antagonists	Trade Names	Uses
montelukast [mon-te-LOO-cast]	Singulair	Prevention and treatment of asthma
zafirlukast [zah-FIR-loo-cast]	Accolate	Prevention and treatment of asthma
zileuton [zye-LOO-ton]	Leutrol Zyflo	Prevention and treatment of asthma

Action

Leukotriene receptor antagonists are drugs that inhibit bronchoconstriction. Leukotrienes are inflammatory agents that induce bronchoconstriction and mucus production that are associated with the inflammatory process of asthma. Zileuton inhibits the enzyme that is required to start leukotriene synthesis, thereby blocking leukotriene formation. Zafirlukast selectively blocks leukotriene D_4 and E_4 receptors, components of slow-reacting substance of anaphylaxis (SRS-A); montelukast is the receptor antagonist of leukotriene D_4.

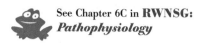

See Chapter 6C in **RWNSG:**
Pathophysiology

Uses

Leukotriene receptor antagonists are used for the prophylaxis and treatment of asthma.

What You NEED TO KNOW

 Zileuton and zafirlukast are contraindicated for use during lactation.

Contraindications/Precautions

Leukotriene antagonists are contraindicated for patients with hypersensitivity. Zileuton is contraindicated for use in patients with liver disease. Zafirlukast and montelukast are contraindicated during acute asthma attacks.

Drug Interactions

Montelukast, zileuton, and zafirlukast should be used with caution during pregnancy. Montelukast should be used with caution in children under 6 years of age. Zafirlukast should be used with caution in patients 65 years or older. Safe use of zafirlukast or zileuton has not been established for children under 12 years of age.

Concurrent use of zafirlukast or zileuton with warfarin may increase the prothrombin time (PT). Erythromycin decreases the bioavailability of zafirlukast. The theophylline levels may be doubled with increased toxicity when used with zileuton. Concurrent use of beta blockers (particularly propranolol) and zileuton may cause hypotension and bradycardia. Concurrent use of zileuton and terfenadine may cause prolonged Q-T intervals. Montelukast has decreased bioavailability and effects when taken concurrently with phenobarbital or rifampin.

Adverse Effects

The most common adverse effects of leukotriene antagonists include headache and dyspepsia. Other adverse effects include weakness (**asthenia**), fever, headache, dizziness, abdominal pain, dyspepsia, diarrhea, nausea, and liver dysfunction. Additional adverse effects of zileuton include pruritus, conjunctivitis, hypertonia, lymphadenopathy, vaginitis, urinary tract infection (UTI), and leukopenia. Other adverse effects of montelukast include nasal congestion, cough, influenza, laryngitis, pharyngitis, sinusitis, rash, and pyuria.

Montelukast and zafirlukast should be used with caution in patients with severe liver disease.

Children's chewable tablets of montelukast should not be swallowed whole.

What You DO

Nursing Responsibilities

Chewable montelukast tablets contain phenylalanine and should be administered with caution to patients with phenylketonuria.

Zafirlukast should be administered 1 hour before meals or 2 hours after meals because food decreases the bioavailability of zafirlukast. Montelukast should be administered in the evening for maximal effectiveness. Administer zileuton with meals and at bedtime. When administering leukotriene antagonist agents, the nurse should:

- Monitor the BP and heart rate for excessive beta blockage when the patient is taking propranolol and zileuton.

- Monitor the PT and international normalized ratio (INR) closely in patients who are concurrently taking zafirlukast or zileuton with warfarin.
- Monitor the complete blood count (CBC) and blood chemistries periodically while undergoing zileuton therapy.
- Monitor liver function tests monthly for the first 3 months of zileuton and zafirlukast therapy, then every 2 to 3 months for the first year, and periodically thereafter.
- Monitor the theophylline levels closely for patients who are taking concurrent zileuton and theophylline therapy for appropriate dosing.
- Monitor the phenytoin level with concurrent zafirlukast or zileuton and phenytoin therapy.
- 🍎 Warn the patient that leukotriene antagonists are not to be taken for acute asthma attacks.
- 🍎 Instruct the patient to take the medication regularly as prescribed and to avoid taking OTC medications without consulting the health care provider to avoid any adverse effects.
- 🍎 Advise patients to avoid any activities that require alertness and to use caution when driving when they experience any dizziness.
- 🍎 Instruct patients to notify their health care provider when they experience any acute asthma attacks or influenza-like symptoms.

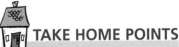

TAKE HOME POINTS

Theophylline levels may be doubled and increase toxicity when theophylline and zileuton are used concurrently.

Do You UNDERSTAND?

DIRECTIONS: Indicate in the space provided whether the statement is *true* or *false*.

_____ 1. Children's chewable montelukast tablets may be chewed or swallowed whole.

_____ 2. Patients taking warfarin and zileuton have an increased risk for bleeding.

_____ 3. Leukotriene antagonists are recommended for treatment of status asthmaticus.

What IS a Xanthine Derivative?

Xanthine Derivatives	Trade Names	Uses
theophylline [thee-OFF-ih-lin]	Theo-Dur	Prevention and treatment of asthma and bronchospasm
dyphylline [DYE-fi-lin]	Dilor	Prevention and treatment of asthma and bronchospasm
oxtriphylline [ox-TRYE-fi-lin]	Choledyl	Prevention and treatment of asthma and bronchospasm

Action

Xanthine derivatives or methylxanthine are agents that relax bronchial smooth muscle cells and suppress airway response to stimuli, thereby producing bronchodilation. The primary effects of methylxanthines are stimulation of the CNS and bronchodilation. Other effects of methylxanthines include cardiac stimulation, vasodilation, and diuresis.

Uses

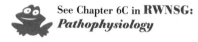

See Chapter 6C in **RWNSG:**
Pathophysiology

Xanthine derivatives are used for prophylaxis and the treatment of chronic asthma and for the treatment of bronchospasm that is related to chronic bronchitis and emphysema. Xanthine derivatives are used less frequently than they were in the past because more effective and safer medications (e.g., inhaled corticosteroids, β-agonists) are now available. In the treatment of asthma, theophylline is the primary xanthine derivative that is used.

What You NEED TO KNOW

Contraindications/Precautions

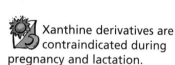

Xanthine derivatives are contraindicated during pregnancy and lactation.

Xanthine derivatives are contraindicated for patients with hypersensitivity to xanthines. Oxtriphylline is contraindicated for patients with coronary artery disease and renal and liver disease.

Drug Interactions

  Xanthine derivatives should be used with caution in neonates, young children, and older adults.

Concurrent use of xanthine derivatives with beta blockers, cimetidine, tacrine, zileuton, quinolones, macrolide antibiotics, high-dose allopurinol (more than 600 mg), and caffeine may increase theophylline levels. Concurrent use of theophylline or theophylline salts with lithium increases the excretion of lithium, thereby lowering lithium levels. Concurrent use of dyphylline and beta blockers may antagonize the bronchodilating effects. Use of halothane with dyphylline may increase the risk of cardiac dysrhythmias. Use of probenecid decreases the elimination of dyphylline.

Adverse Effects

Xanthine derivatives should be used with caution in patients with glaucoma and peptic ulcer disease. Theophylline and aminophylline should be used cautiously in patients with cardiac disease, cardiac dysrhythmias, hypertension, diabetes mellitus, prostatic hypertrophy, and hyperthyroidism.

Adverse effects that are associated with plasma theophylline levels less than 20 µg/ml are few. Levels of 20 to 25 µg/ml may cause nausea, vomiting, diarrhea, headache, insomnia, and restlessness, and levels greater than 30 µg/ml may cause severe dysrhythmias, convulsions, or death. Common adverse effects of xanthine derivatives include nervousness, nausea, and tachycardia. Other adverse effects include vomiting, anorexia, headache, flushing, insomnia, irritability, palpitations, hypotension, fever, and dehydration.

What You DO

Nursing Responsibilities

Xanthines should be administered routinely at the same times every day to maintain therapeutic levels. The dosing guidelines for aminophylline are the same as those for theophylline. When administering xanthine derivatives, the nurse should:

- Instruct the patient that the capsule may be swallowed or opened, with the contents sprinkled on a small amount of soft food (e.g., pudding, ice cream) before ingestion.
- Administer aminophylline and dyphylline 1 hour before or 2 hours after meals with a full glass of water to enhance absorption. When GI distress occurs, these agents may be given after meals to reduce GI adverse effects.
- Encourage the patient to drink at least 2000 ml of fluids daily to thin respiratory secretions.
- Advise the patient to avoid caffeine, colas, chocolate, and coffee to control cardiovascular and CNS adverse effects.
- Instruct the patient to avoid charbroiled foods because they decrease theophylline effectiveness. A high-protein, low-carbohydrate diet will increase theophylline elimination.
- Instruct the patient to take the medication only as prescribed, to avoid exceeding the prescribed dose, and to avoid using OTC drugs without the health care provider's approval. Many common OTC preparations for colds, allergies, and cough contain other sympathomimetics, caffeine, ephedrine, or other xanthines.
- Advise the patient to avoid smoking because cigarette and marijuana smoking decrease theophylline plasma concentration by 50%.
- Be aware that aminophylline is the only xanthine that can be administered IV and is rarely used orally.
- Examine the parenteral preparations for any precipitate before using, and avoid using these preparations when clumping occurs.
- Monitor vital signs and intake and output of urine when the patient is receiving IV aminophylline.
- Monitor theophylline drug levels routinely for evidence of toxicity (greater than 20 µg/ml) for patients who are receiving theophylline.
- Withhold theophylline and measure the theophylline level to rule out toxicity in any patient who develops nausea and vomiting. Theophylline levels are of no use in patients who are taking dyphylline because dyphylline is not metabolized to theophylline, as are the other xanthines. A therapeutic dyphylline blood level is 12 µg/ml.

 Theophylline should also be used with caution in patients with seizure disorders. Aminophylline should also be used with caution in patients with renal or hepatic dysfunction, fibrocystic breast disease, COPD, acute influenza, and in those who are receiving influenza vaccine. Dyphylline should be used with caution in patients with severe cardiac disease, hypertension, renal or hepatic dysfunction, and hyperthyroidism. Oxtriphylline should be used with caution in patients with prostatic hypertrophy and diabetes mellitus.

TAKE HOME POINTS

Instruct the patient to take medicine at the same time every day for maximal effectiveness. A dose of 156 mg of oxtriphylline is equivalent to 100 mg of theophylline. All doses should be based on ideal body weight. The rate of aminophylline infusion should not exceed 25/mg/min, diluted or undiluted. The therapeutic theophylline plasma level is 10 to 20 µg/ml.

Sustained-action capsules of theophylline should not be chewed or crushed. Rapid infusion of intravenous (IV) aminophylline may cause cardiac arrest. A sudden, sharp, unexpected rise in the heart rate is a clinical indicator of IV aminophylline toxicity.

Do you UNDERSTAND?

DIRECTIONS: Fill in the blanks with the appropriate responses to complete the following statements.

1. The therapeutic theophylline plasma level is _____.
2. Common adverse effects of xanthine derivatives are nervousness, _____, and tachycardia.

What IS an Anticholinergic?

Anticholinergic	Trade Name	Uses
ipratropium [eye-prah-TROH-pee-um]	Atrovent	Treatment of bronchitis and emphysema

Action

Anticholinergics are agents that block muscarinic cholinergic receptors in the bronchi and inhibit vagal-mediated responses (bronchospasms), thereby facilitating bronchodilation. The anticholinergic that affects the respiratory system is ipratropium.

Uses

See Chapter 6C in **RWNSG:** *Pathophysiology*

Ipratropium is used for the maintenance treatment of chronic asthma and bronchospasm that is associated with COPD, including emphysema and chronic bronchitis. The intranasal spray is used for the treatment of perennial rhinitis and rhinorrhea.

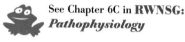
Ipratropium should be used cautiously for patients with narrow-angle glaucoma, bladder neck obstruction, and prostatic hypertrophy.

What You NEED TO KNOW

Contraindications/Precautions

Ipratropium is contraindicated for use as primary treatment in patients with hypersensitivity to atropine and acute bronchospasm episodes.

Ipratropium is contraindicated for use in children under 12 years of age.

Drug Interactions

No drug interactions are noted for anticholinergic agents.

Ipratropium should be used cautiously in women during pregnancy and lactation.

Answers: 1. 10 to 20 µg/ml; 2. nausea.

Adverse Effects

The most common adverse effects of ipratropium are cough and headache. Other adverse effects include blurred vision, eye pain, exacerbation of narrow-angle glaucoma, bitter taste, dry mouth, hoarseness, exacerbation of respiratory symptoms, nervousness, dizziness, fatigue, palpitations, nasal dryness, rash, urticaria, and urinary retention.

 # What You DO

Nursing Responsibilities

Ipratropium is available as nasal sprays and MDIs. When administering anti-cholinergics, the nurse should:

- Auscultate the patient's lungs before and after inhalations, and monitor the respiratory status.
- Instruct the patient to void before administration of the medication to avoid urinary retention.
- Instruct the patient to allow 1 minute between inhalations when the dose is two inhalations for maximal effectiveness. When the patient is taking other inhalants, instruct the patient to wait 5 minutes between inhalations.
- Teach the patient the correct technique for using an MDI or nasal spray.
- Instruct the patient to rinse the mouthpiece and cap of the MDI (or the tip of the nasal spray container) daily with warm, running water, and allow them to air dry before the next use. Instruct the patient to clean the mouthpiece and cap weekly with warm water and mild dishwashing soap. Cleaning minimizes bacterial exposure and maintains patency.
- Suggest to the patient who is using MDIs to rinse the mouth after use to decrease the bitter taste.
- Instruct patients to take medication as directed and to notify the health care provider when respiratory symptoms worsen.
- Warn the patient to avoid spraying the medication into the eyes. Blurred vision or eye pain may result.

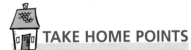 **TAKE HOME POINTS**

Ipratropium is not used for the treatment of an acute bronchospasm attack.

Do You UNDERSTAND?

DIRECTIONS: Complete the crossword puzzle.

Across

1. Oral inhalation may cause this to be bitter.
6. Minutes to wait between inhalations of ipratropium.
7. Ipratropium is a derivative of this drug.
8. Wait this many minutes before using another inhaler.
9. A 0.06% spray is treatment for the common one of these.
11. MDIs are this type of canister.
13. Ipratropium is excreted in this.
14. Hand-held canister for oral inhalation.

Down

2. Anticholinergic drug that is used for asthma.
3. After use of nasal spray, rinse this.
4. A common adverse reaction.
5. Route for treatment of asthma.
10. To avoid urinary retention, have the patient do this before taking the drug.
12. Painful when spray gets here.

Answers: Across: 1. taste; 6. one; 7. atropine; 8. five; 9. cold; 11. metered dose; 13. feces; 14. MDI. Down: 2. atrovent; 3. tip; 4. headache; 5. inhaled; 10. void; 12. eye.

Drugs Affecting the Endocrine System

SECTION A

PITUITARY AND ADRENAL HORMONES

This section discusses drugs that are used to treat patients with altered function of the anterior and posterior pituitary gland and the cortex of the adrenal gland. The pituitary gland is composed of the anterior and posterior lobes. The anterior lobe of the pituitary gland secretes hormones that regulate the growth, development, and proper functioning of other endocrine glands. Anterior pituitary hormone drugs are used to treat patients with conditions that are characterized by hormone deficiency. Nerve cells in the hypothalamus produce two hormones that the posterior pituitary gland secretes: antidiuretic hormone (**vasopressin**) and oxytocin. These two hormones are stored in the pituitary. Posterior pituitary hormone drugs are used to treat diabetes insipidus, a condition that results from a deficiency of antidiuretic hormone (ADH). Patients with diabetes insipidus are unable to control the amount of water lost in the urine and have a large urinary output (**polyuria**).

The adrenal cortex produces two classes of hormones: corticosteroids and androgenic steroids. All adrenal hormones are steroids that have similar chemical structures but different physiologic effects. Corticosteroids (**adrenocortical hormones** and **adrenocorticosteroids**) are divided into two groups: glucocorticosteroids (e.g., cortisol, cortisone, corticosterone) and mineralocorticoids (e.g., aldosterone, desoxycorticosterone). When adrenal cortex function is compromised, synthetic adrenal hormones can be used to replace those that are naturally produced. In rare cases, hormones from the adrenal cortex may exceed body requirements. When appropriate, adrenal hormone–inhibiting drugs are used to suppress the production of excess hormones.

What IS an Anterior Pituitary Hormone Replacement Agent?

Anterior Pituitary Hormone Replacements	Trade Names	Uses
somatropin [so-mah-TROH-pin]	Humatrope	Treatment of growth hormone deficiency
somatrem [SO-mah-trem]	Protropin	Treatment of growth hormone deficiency
corticotropin [kor-tih-koh-TROH-pin]	ACTH	Treatment of adrenal insufficiency
cosyntropin [koh-SIN-troh-pin]	Cortrosyn	Diagnostic of adrenocortical insufficiency

Action

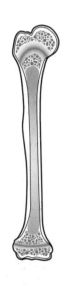

Somatropin and somatrem are human growth hormonelike drugs that facilitate the transport of amino acids across cell membranes. These agents increase cell size and encourage skeletal growth, particularly the ends of long bones (the epiphyseal plates). Somatropin and somatrem also decrease the transport of glucose into cells and reduce the amount of glucose that is used, thereby causing an increase in blood glucose levels. This action produces a diabeticlike state in the patient. Additionally, the movement of amino acids increases nitrogen balance and decreases urea production.

Somatropin and somatrem also prompt the release of free fatty acids from fat tissue, leading to increased fat storage in the liver and making more fatty acids available for energy. This action is referred to as *ketogenesis* because it results from fat breakdown and leads to the conversion of fatty acids to ketone bodies. When somatropin and somatrem are given to adults with adult-onset pituitary deficiency, a marked increase in high-density lipoproteins (HDL), known as "good" cholesterol, occurs. Low-density lipoprotein (LDL) levels, known as "bad" cholesterol, remain unchanged.

Corticotropin and cosyntropin stimulate the adrenal cortex to release glucocorticosteroids and mineralocorticoids. Corticotropin and cosyntropin are effective only when the adrenal cortex can respond to stimulation. The physiologic effects include increased energy levels and stabilized fluid and electrolyte balance.

Uses

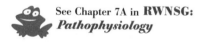

See Chapter 7A in **RWNSG:** *Pathophysiology*

Anterior pituitary agents are used to treat patients with a hormone deficit of the pituitary gland. Somatrem and somatropin promote anabolic tissue growth in patients with a deficiency of human growth hormone, a condition known as dwarfism.

Corticotropin and cosyntropin are used diagnostically to stimulate the synthesis of glucocorticosteroids, mineralocorticoids, and androgens. The corticotropin stimulation test helps differentiate primary from secondary adrenal cortex insufficiency. In patients with secondary insufficiency, plasma cortisol levels will rise after an injection of corticotropin. Corticotropin is also used as an anti-inflammatory or immunosuppressant drug when conventional glucocorticosteroid therapy fails. Additionally, corticotropin is occasionally used to help manage adrenal crisis.

What You NEED TO KNOW

TAKE HOME POINTS

Anterior pituitary hormone replacements are ineffective when impaired growth results from other causes or when used after puberty, during which the ends of long bones have closed.

Contraindications/Precautions

Corticotropin is contraindicated for patients with an excess production of adrenal cortex hormones. Because it exacerbates symptoms, corticotropin is also contraindicated for patients with psychoses. Corticotropin use should be avoided in patients with active tuberculosis or acquired immunodeficiency syndrome (AIDS) because immunity is decreased and the risk of gastrointestinal (GI) perforation and hemorrhage is increased. Corticotropin is also contraindicated for patients with peptic ulcer disease, scleroderma, osteoporosis, systemic fungal infections, and for those who are sensitive to pork and pork products.

Drug Interactions

When somatrem and somatropin are given concurrently with glucocorticosteroids or corticotropin, a decrease in growth response may result. Conversely, when these agents are given with anabolic steroids, estrogens, and thyroid hormones, an increase in growth may result. Corticotropin may increase metabolism of glucocorticosteroids when taken concurrently with barbiturates, phenytoin, and rifampin. Estrogens and oral contraceptives block the metabolism of corticotropin when given together. Salicylates increase the risk of GI bleeding when given with corticotropin. Insulin and oral hypoglycemics may require increased doses when given together with corticotropin. Amphotericin B, carbonic anhydrase inhibitors, mezlocillin, piperacillin, and ticarcillin increase the risk of hypokalemia and subsequent cardiac glycoside toxicity when given concurrently with corticotropin. Blood or blood products may render cosyntropin inactive when given together. Cosyntropin increases the metabolism of glucocorticosteroids when given concurrently.

Adverse Effects

Locally, somatrem and somatropin cause pain and swelling at the injection site. An additional adverse effect includes a slipped femoral epiphysis. Either drug can cause edema of the hands and feet. Somatrem depresses thyroid function and insulin production and may cause insulin resistance.

Generally, anterior pituitary agents cause an elevated serum glucose level (hyperglycemia) in susceptible individuals, thus these agents are used with caution in patients with a family history of diabetes. Somatropin and somatrem are used cautiously in patients with growth hormone deficiency resulting from lesions in the brain or those who have a coexisting adrenocorticotropic hormone (ACTH) deficiency. These agents are also used with caution in patients with thyroid dysfunction. Cautious use of corticotropin is warranted in patients with hypertension or heart failure resulting from sodium and water retention. Corticotropin should be used cautiously with patients with myasthenia gravis because muscle weakness is increased. Because of the risk of peptic ulcers, the drug should be used cautiously in patients who are taking salicylates and other nonsteroidal antiinflammatory drugs.

Safe use of anterior pituitary replacements during pregnancy and lactation has not been established.

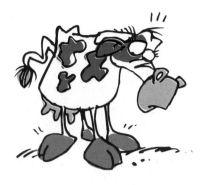

The adverse effects of corticotropin appear most frequently with chronic use of doses that exceed 40 units per day. The most common adverse effects of corticotropin include depression, nausea, superficial capillary bleeding (**petechiae**), sodium retention (**hypernatremia**), and adrenal suppression. Drug effects on the central nervous system (CNS) include seizure, vertigo, headache, personality changes, euphoria, mood swings, and psychosis. Impaired wound healing, thinning of the skin, bruising (**ecchymosis**), facial redness, increased sweating (**diaphoresis**), and hyperpigmentation may occur. Additionally, the patient may experience hypertension, fluid volume overload, heart failure, low serum calcium levels (**hypocalcemia**), low serum potassium levels (**hypokalemia**), alkalosis, and a negative nitrogen balance. Long-term use of corticotropin suppresses pituitary release of corticotropin, causing an overgrowth of adrenal cortex tissue (**adrenocortical hyperplasia**), decreased glucose tolerance, stunting of growth in children, and muscle weakness.

The adverse effect of cosyntropin is hypersensitivity, including anaphylaxis. Patients who are sensitive to pork or pork products may have an allergic response to corticotropin.

What You DO

Nursing Responsibilities

Somatropin and somatrem must be refrigerated before and after reconstitution with bacteriostatic water for injection. Reconstituted solutions should be clear and used within 14 days. When administering anterior pituitary replacements, the nurse should:

- Administer somatropin injections at least 48 hours apart. SC injections are preferred and most frequently given because they are less painful. Corticotropin is a protein substance that, when taken orally, proteolytic enzymes destroy in the GI tract.
- Reevaluate patients who continue to lose weight after the first 2 weeks of treatment.
- Conduct an evaluation of bone growth and growth rate, as well as height and weight every 3 to 6 months.
- Monitor thyroid function throughout therapy because these drugs may decrease thyroid hormone levels, iodine uptake, and thyroxine-binding capacity. When thyroid deficiency (**hypothyroidism**) becomes apparent, concurrent thyroid hormone replacement will be necessary for the growth hormone to be effective.
- Be aware that titrated doses are based on patient response because individual absorption rates vary widely.
- Monitor blood glucose levels periodically throughout therapy for patients who are taking somatrem, somatropin, or corticotropin for possible dose increase of insulin in patients with diabetes.

TAKE HOME POINTS

Do not shake the vial when reconstituting somatropin and somatrem, but rather, swirl gently. Serum growth hormone levels are greater after a subcutaneous (SC) abdominal injection when compared to an SC injection in the thigh. Growth hormone agents are useless for stimulating linear growth in adults because of the closure of the long bones.

- Stress routine monitoring of drug and hormone levels to the patient.
- Evaluate routine hematologic values and electrolytes for patients who are undergoing prolonged corticotropin therapy.
- Monitor inorganic phosphorous, alkaline phosphatase, and parathyroid hormone levels because somatropin may cause an increase in these levels.
- Inform the patient who is receiving anterior pituitary agents about the consequences of abruptly discontinuing treatment.
- Instruct the patient to report certain physical changes to the health care provider. Instruct the patient to report fever, sore throat, muscle weakness, sudden weight gain, and edema.
- Teach the patient about sodium-restricted diets that are high in vitamin D, protein, and potassium.
- Inform the patient that somatropin and somatrem have a great potential for misuse, primarily because of the real and perceived chance of increasing muscle mass and decreasing body fat. Enhanced athletic performance is the most commonly desired result.
- Advise patients who are taking anterior pituitary hormones to wear or carry MedicAlert identification and to check with the health care provider before using over-the-counter (OTC) drugs.
- Instruct patients who are taking anterior pituitary hormones to avoid immunizations that use live vaccines (e.g., mumps, measles, rubella) because this type of use decreases immunity.

Do You UNDERSTAND?

DIRECTIONS: Unscramble each of the following anagram phrases to find the pituitary drug name. Describe the drug's action and its effects or use.

1. Tricorn coop it:
   Action: _____
   Effects: _____
2. I am protons and toms mare:
   Action: _____
   Effects: _____
3. Onions crypt:
   Action: _____
   Use: _____

Answers: 1. corticotropin. *Action:* stimulates adrenal cortex to release glucocorticosteroids, mineralocorticoids, and androgens; *Effects:* increased energy levels and stabilized fluid and electrolyte balance; **2.** somatropin and somatrem. *Action:* stimulate growth via their effects on most body tissues, particularly on long bones; *Effects:* increased bone growth and rate; **3.** cosyntropin. *Action:* stimulates adrenal cortex to release glucocorticosteroids, mineralocorticoids, and androgens; *Use:* diagnosis of ACTH deficiency.

What IS a Posterior Pituitary Hormone Replacement Agent?

Posterior Pituitary Hormone Replacements	Trade Names	Uses
desmopressin acetate [des-moh-PRESS-in]	DDAVP	Prevention and treatment of diabetes insipidus
lypressin [lye-PRESS-in]	Diapid	Prevention and treatment of diabetes insipidus
vasopressin [vay-so-PRESS-in]	ADH, Pitressin	Treatment of diabetes insipidus

Action

Vasopressin and its analogs (desmopressin and lypressin) increase the reabsorption of water from the distal renal tubules, which decreases urine formation and controls water balance in the body. In large doses, desmopressin and lypressin stimulate smooth muscle contraction, particularly of the arterioles. The vasoconstriction decreases blood flow to the splenic, mesentery, coronary, GI, pancreatic, skin, and muscular systems and raises blood pressure. Importantly, the amount of drug that is necessary to promote water conservation is seldom sufficiently high to produce widespread effects on blood pressure. These drugs also increase peristalsis of the large bowel and contraction of the gall bladder and urinary bladder. Some oxytocic activity may also occur, causing uterine contractions. The mechanism by which desmopressin enhances platelet function is unknown. Vasopressin is prepared from the pituitary glands of cattle or pigs.

Uses

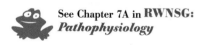

See Chapter 7A in **RWNSG:** *Pathophysiology*

With the exception of oxytocin, posterior pituitary hormones are used to treat diabetes insipidus, a condition characterized by thirst and the elimination of large amounts of extremely dilute urine. Vasopressin and lypressin are used primarily to control neurogenic diabetes insipidus. Desmopressin is used to treat nephrogenic diabetes insipidus and is useful in treating bedwetting (**enuresis**). Desmopressin is also indicated to control acute nosebleeds (**epistaxis**) when administered in the nose and GI hemorrhage when administered intravenously (IV).

Posterior pituitary hormone replacement agents should be used with caution in patients with angina pectoris and hypertension.

What You NEED TO KNOW

Contraindications/Precautions

Safe use of posterior pituitary replacements during pregnancy and lactation has not been established.

Vasopressin, desmopressin, and lypressin are contraindicated for patients with known hypersensitivity and type IIB or platelet-type von Willebrand's disease.

Drug Interactions

Chlorpropamide, clofibrate, carbamazepine, and fludrocortisone enhance the antidiuretic response to desmopressin when given concurrently. Lithium, norepinephrine, heparin, and alcohol reduce the antidiuretic response to desmopressin when given together. Ganglionic-blocking drugs, barbiturates, and cyclopropane increase the vasopressor effects of desmopressin.

Adverse Effects

The adverse effects of small doses of vasopressin are usually mild. The most common adverse effects include circumoral pallor, abdominal cramps, nausea, sweating, tremor, and severe headache. Uterine cramping and diarrhea may develop because of the stimulant effects of vasopressin. Shifts in fluid volume occur with initial therapy. Large doses of vasopressin can cause blood pressure elevations, anginal pain, dysrhythmias, and myocardial infarction (MI). The pressor effects of vasopressin are not usually evident with the dose used to manage diabetes insipidus. The adverse effects of desmopressin and lypressin, which are infrequent and mild, include conjunctivitis, runny nose, local irritation and congestion of nasal passages, headache, and heartburn.

  In patients with coronary artery disease, even small doses have been found to precipitate angina, particularly in older adults.

 # What You DO

  TAKE HOME POINTS

Should fluid overload develop, the drug should be withdrawn and the patient's fluid intake restricted until the urine specific gravity is at least 1.015 (normal: 1.010 to 1.030). Weigh the patient daily and assess for edema. Caution the patient to adhere to the prescribed dose of nasal spray.

Nursing Responsibilities

Posterior pituitary hormones, whether in natural or synthetic form, are proteins that, when the drug is taken orally, gastric enzymes will destroy. These drugs are therefore administered either parenterally or via nasal sprays. When administering posterior pituitary hormone replacement agents, the nurse should:

- Shake the oil formulation of vasopressin vigorously to disperse the ingredients before administration.
- Give the patient one or two glasses of water when the injection is given to minimize the GI adverse effects.
- Monitor for signs of fluid overload.
- Assess the patient for symptoms of dehydration (e.g., excessive thirst, dry skin and mucus membranes, tachycardia, poor skin turgor).
- Closely monitor older adults and patients who have difficulty tolerating fluid shifts that are associated with initial vasopressin therapy. The signs and symptoms of water toxicity include confusion, drowsiness, headache, weight gain, difficulty urinating, seizures, and coma.
- Administer desmopressin through a flexible nasal catheter (rhinyle) that is used to measure the medication. After the drug is drawn into the catheter, one end is placed in the patient's nose and the other end in the patient's mouth. The patient then blows into the catheter to deposit the drug in the nasal passages. The tube should be rinsed after each use.

 Owing to the age-related decline in hepatic and renal function, older adults are at an increased risk for drug overdose.

Because children are susceptible to fluid volume disturbances, drug therapies should be carefully chosen. An air-filled syringe may be attached to the rhinyle (flexible calibrated plastic tube) for children, infants, or obtunded patients.

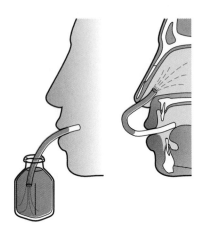

- Administer lypressin by holding the bottle upright with the patient sitting upright and the head tipped slightly backward. No more than three sprays should be taken at any one time.
- Instruct the patient that when a dose is missed, take the missed dose as soon as it is remembered, except when it is nearly time for the next dose. Doubling the dose and transferring any remaining medication to another bottle should be avoided.
- Contact the health care provider when the patient has increased urine output, runny nose, nasal irritation, or an upper respiratory infection for possible dose adjustment.
- Monitor hepatic and renal function tests for patients who are taking a posterior pituitary drug, particularly older patients.
- Monitor urine specific gravity, urine volume, and serum electrolytes throughout therapy.
- Advise patients to avoid using OTC drugs without checking with the health care provider and to wear or carry MedicAlert identification.

What IS a Glucocorticosteroid?

Glucocorticosteroids	Trade Names	Uses
cortisone [KOR-tih-zone]	Cortone	Treatment of adrenocortical insufficiency
dexamethasone [dex-ah-METH-ah-zone]	Decadron	Treatment of adrenocortical insufficiency
hydrocortisone [hye-droh-KOR-tih-zone]	Hydrocortone	Treatment of adrenocortical insufficiency
prednisone [PRED-nih-zone]	Deltasone	Treatment of adrenocortical insufficiency
triamcinolone [try-am-SIN-oh-lone]	Aristospan	Treatment of adrenocortical insufficiency

Action

A glucocorticosteroid is any substance that increases the synthesis of glucose from noncarbohydrate sources, such as amino acids and glycerol (**gluconeogenesis**). Glucocorticosteroids stimulate the formation of glucose, increase the breakdown of proteins to amino acids, and oxidize and mobilize fatty acids. These drugs mimic the activity of naturally occurring steroid hormones.

Corticotropin-releasing hormone (CRH) from the hypothalamus trigger the initial release of glucocorticosteroids from the adrenal cortex. The target organ for CRH is the anterior lobe of the pituitary gland. Reacting to the presence of CRH, the anterior lobe releases ACTH, which, in turn, stimulates the release of glucocorticosteroids from the adrenal cortex.

When present in large amounts, cortisol inhibits the release of histamine and counteracts potentially destructive activities of the immune system. Because the immune response can damage body cells, as well as those of foreign substances, the protective mechanisms of cortisol help preserve body cells at the site of the inflammatory response. Glucocorticosteroids decrease the migration and accumulation of white blood cells (**leukocytes**) at the site, thereby suppressing the inflammatory response. Additionally, glucocorticosteroids prevent the release of prostaglandins, leukotrienes, and macrophages, which are important to the inflammatory response. Other cellular factors that increase vascular permeability are inhibited. Glucocorticosteroids also reduce the number of T cells, while impairing the ability of antibodies (**immunoglobulins**) to bind with cell surface receptors, which reduces cell-mediated immune responses.

Uses

Glucocorticosteroids are used for many disorders and for the long-term management of numerous chronic inflammatory conditions, such as rheumatoid arthritis, systemic lupus erythematosus (SLE), asthma, and other chronic airway limitation (CAL) disorders. Glucocorticosteroids are helpful in managing idiopathic thrombocytopenic purpura (ITP), psoriasis, hemolytic anemia, multiple sclerosis, tuberculosis, ulcerative colitis, suppression of inflammatory responses during organ transplantation, and some neoplastic diseases.

Glucocorticosteroids are helpful in the short-term management of acute exacerbations of inflammation that are associated with the eye, dermatitis, urticaria, bronchitis, infectious diseases, sensitivity reactions, and Stevens-Johnson syndrome. Patients with head or spinal cord injuries may be helped because of the antiinflammatory effects of glucocorticoids. Glucocorticoids are also used in the treatment of adrenal insufficiency and other disorders when naturally occurring adrenal hormones are not present in sufficient quantities to sustain life.

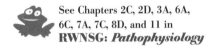

See Chapters 2C, 2D, 3A, 6A, 6C, 7A, 7C, 8D, and 11 in **RWNSG:** *Pathophysiology*

What You NEED TO KNOW

Contraindications/Precautions

Glucocorticosteroids are contraindicated in patients with systemic fungal infections because they may worsen.

Drug Interactions

Phenobarbital, phenytoin, rifampin, antidiabetics, isoniazid, and oral anticoagulants enhances elimination, thereby decreasing serum levels of glucocorticosteroid when given together. Ketoconazole, oral contraceptives, and salicylates increase serum levels of glucocorticosteroids when given concurrently. Glucocorticosteroids increase the effects of cyclosporin, digoxin, diuretics, amphotericin B, and theophylline and increase the risk of potassium loss when given together. Glucocorticosteroids may increase intraocular pressure when given with tricyclic antidepressants, anticholinergics, and adrenergics. Salicylates increase the risk of gastric ulcers when given concurrently with glucocorticosteroids.

Safe use of glucocorticosteroids during pregnancy and lactation has not been established. Safe use of cortisone, dexamethasone, hydrocortisone, and triamcinolone for children has not been established.

Caution is necessary when using glucocorticosteroids for long-term therapy because of the risk of adrenal suppression. Glucocorticosteroids are used with caution in patients with diabetes mellitus and peptic ulcers and those who are immunosuppressed, such as patients with cancer, kidney disease, or those who are infected with HIV.

An additional adverse effect of long-term glucocorticosteroid use is growth suppression in children.

A severe, life-threatening condition is treated through IV administration for quick action.

TAKE HOME POINTS

- Do not administer vaccinations that contain live viruses to patients who are taking glucocorticosteroids because the inflammatory response is suppressed.
- The normal adult adrenal gland secretes an average of 20 mg of cortisol per day. Administration of high-dose glucocorticosteroids turns off the normal negative-feedback loop that exists between the adrenal and pituitary glands. When the drug is suddenly discontinued, the patient's circulating levels of cortisol fall dramatically because the adrenal gland is unable to secrete sufficient quantities to sustain body needs. This action places the patient at risk for a life-threatening, permanent adrenal suppression (**Addison's disease**). Adrenal suppression is dose dependent and can last from months to years.

Adverse Effects

Muscle wasting and weakness, facial redness, impaired wound healing, hypertension, menstrual irregularities, Cushing's syndrome, cataract formation, GI bleeding, pancreatitis, peptic ulcer disease, psychosis, and osteoporosis are adverse effects that have been noted with the long-term use of glucocorticosteroids. Hypokalemia, alkalosis, negative nitrogen balance, weight gain, edema, abdominal distention, facial erythema, bruising, electrocardiogram (ECG) changes that are secondary to hypokalemia, headache, seizures, and candidiasis are also likely adverse effects.

 # What You DO

Nursing Responsibilities

Glucocorticosteroids are available in oral, IV, and topical formulations. The doses vary with the reason for use. The selected route varies with the severity of the patient's health. Oral and topical forms are used most frequently in patients with allergies or disorders that can be treated in a clinic or office. When administering glucocorticosteroids, the nurse should:

- Administer the lowest effective dose of glucocorticosteroids for the shortest period.
- Administer glucocorticosteroids in a pattern that mimics the natural hormone surges of the body. For example, two thirds of the daily dose may be administered in the morning with the remaining one third given in the late afternoon.
- Monitor the patient's fluids and electrolytes, particularly potassium, on a regular basis because these drugs cause sodium and fluid retention and potassium loss.
- Monitor glucose levels regularly because high-dose glucocorticosteroids increase serum levels.
- Instruct patients to take the medication with food to reduce gastric irritation and upset.
- Instruct patients to take their medication as prescribed and to avoid suddenly discontinuing therapy.
- Teach the patient the symptoms of glucocorticosteroid withdrawal syndrome (e.g., exhaustion, fever, diffuse musculoskeletal pain).
- Begin to taper therapy after the patient's condition stabilizes, meaning that the dose that is given on the first day of therapy is gradually reduced over a period of 1 to 2 weeks.
- Provide written instructions to the patient regarding the taper regimen.

Do You UNDERSTAND?

DIRECTIONS: Indicate in the space provided whether the statement is *true* or *false*. If the answer is false, then correct the statement to make it true using the margin space.

_____ 1. Physiologic doses of glucocorticosteroids help maintain normal nerve excitability.

_____ 2. Glucocorticosteroids cause excretion of sodium and increase the retention of calcium and potassium.

_____ 3. High doses of glucocorticosteroids decrease serum glucose levels.

_____ 4. Cortisol levels vary greatly throughout the day, with peak levels found at approximately 4:00 PM to 5:00 PM and the lowest levels at dawn.

_____ 5. Prednisone suppresses proliferation of lymphocytes and thus reduces the immune component of inflammation.

What IS an Adrenal Hormone Inhibiting Agent?

Adrenal Hormone Inhibiting Agents	Trade Names	Uses
aminoglutethimide [ah-mi-noe-glue-TETH-ih-mide]	Cytadren	Treatment of Cushing's syndrome
mitotane [MY-toe-tane]	Lysodren	Treatment of adrenocortical carcinoma
metyrapone [me-TIE-ra-pone]	Metopirone	Diagnostic of pituitary function

Action

Adrenal hormone inhibiting agents act primarily to inhibit activity of the adrenal cortex. In turn, the synthesis of all adrenal steroids is inhibited. Mitotane exerts a direct killing effect on the mitochondria of the adrenal cortex cells.

Uses

Adrenal hormone inhibiting agents are used as a temporary means of decreasing excessive glucocorticosteroid production in patients who are waiting for more definitive therapy (e.g., surgery). Aminoglutethimide has also been used to produce a so-called medical adrenalectomy in patients with advanced breast cancer and in those with metastatic cancer of the prostate gland. Mitotane is used in the treatment of inoperable adrenocortical cancer. Metyrapone is used in a test of pituitary activity.

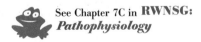

See Chapter 7C in RWNSG: *Pathophysiology*

Answers: 1. true; 2. false; sodium retention and calcium and potassium excretion; 3. false; increase serum glucose levels; 4. false; 6:00 PM to 8: 00 PM and midnight; 5. true.

What You NEED TO KNOW

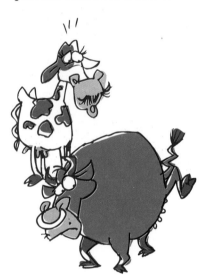

⚠ **Metyrapone and mitotane are used with caution in patients with liver disease.**

Contraindications/Precautions

Aminoglutethimide, metyrapone, and mitotane are contraindicated for patients with hypersensitivity. Metyrapone and mitotane should not be used for patients in shock or those who have experienced trauma.

Drug Interactions

Aminoglutethimide decreases the effect of the medroxyprogesterone, theophylline, oral anticoagulants, glucocorticosteroids, and digoxin when given together. The actions of aminoglutethimide, mitotane, and metyrapone are enhanced when given with alcohol. When given concurrently, phenytoin and estrogens increase the metabolism of metyrapone. When mitotane is given concurrently with barbiturates, oral anticoagulants, and phenytoin, the effects of the drugs are decreased. When mitotane is given with CNS depressants, additive CNS depression may occur. Spironolactone blocks the action of mitotane.

Adverse Effects

Adverse effects of adrenal hormone inhibiting drugs include nausea, abdominal distress, headaches, drowsiness, dizziness, and a measleslike rash (**morbilliform**). Additional adverse effects include hematologic abnormalities, hypothyroidism, muscle pain, and fever. Masculinization can occur in women and precocious sexual development may occur in men who are taking these drugs.

What You DO

Nursing Responsibilities

Adrenal inhibitor drug therapy requires multiple daily dosing. Doses vary depending on the drug that is used. Patients are started on small doses, with increases as necessary until vital signs stabilize, serum electrolytes and glucose levels return to normal, and emotional changes are less disruptive. When administering adrenal inhibitors, the nurse should:

 Inform patients about the signs and symptoms of adrenal insufficiency. Warn patients of the occasional erratic nature of the signs and symptoms and the possibility of recurrence of adrenal hormone excess.
• Monitor 24-hour urine samples of 17-hydroxyglucocorticosteroids and 17-ketogenic steroids, which reveal increased elimination of glucocorticosteroid byproducts to validate drug efficacy.

Do You UNDERSTAND?

DIRECTIONS: Fill in the blanks with the appropriate responses to complete the following statements.

1. Adrenal hormone inhibiting drugs inhibit or promote the metabolism of synthetic _____.

2. Aminoglutethimide is used as a temporary means of decreasing excessive _____ production in patients who are awaiting more _____.

3. Corticosteroid inhibiting drugs can produce signs and symptoms that are associated with adrenal _____.

What IS a Mineralocorticoid Agent?

Mineralocorticoids	Trade Names	Uses
fludrocortisone [flew-droh-KOR-tih-zone]	Florinef	Treatment of adrenocortical insufficiency
desoxycorticosterone [des-OX-e-kor-tih-co-steer-one]	DOCA	Treatment of adrenocortical insufficiency

Action

Mineralocorticoid agents are any of a group of hormones from the adrenal cortex, thus named because of their effects on sodium, chloride, and potassium concentrations in extracellular fluid. The primary mineralocorticoid hormone—aldosterone—is essential to the maintenance of extracellular and intracellular fluid volume, normal cardiac output, and adequate levels of blood pressure. Without mineralocorticoids, diminished cardiac output and fatal shock can quickly occur.

Desoxycorticosterone acetate and fludrocortisone (aldosterone-like drugs) promote the reabsorption of sodium and water and the excretion of potassium and hydrogen ions via the renal tubules. The secondary effects are related to the reabsorption of water, serum levels of sodium and potassium, anion reabsorption, and the secretion of hydrogen ions. The result is maintenance of fluid and electrolyte balance and therefore adequate cardiac output.

Uses

Mineralocorticoids are used primarily as replacement therapy for patients with adrenal insufficiency and with salt-losing forms of congenital adrenal hyperplasia. Fludrocortisone is the drug of choice for chronic mineralocorticoid therapy. However, in most cases, a glucocorticosteroid must also be administered for adequate control. Cortisone or hydrocortisone are the drugs of choice for replacement because they promote both mineralocorticoid and glucocorticosteroid activity.

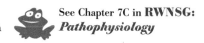

See Chapter 7C in **RWNSG:**
Pathophysiology

Answers: 1. adrenal hormones; 2. cortisol, definitive therapy; 3. insufficiency (Addison's disease).

What You NEED TO KNOW

Contraindications/Precautions

Mineralocorticoids are contraindicated for patients with systemic fungal infections or hypersensitivity to the drug.

 The medications should be used cautiously in patients with hypothyroidism, cirrhosis, ocular herpes simplex, emotional instability, psychotic tendencies, ulcerative colitis, diverticulitis, peptic ulcer disease, renal insufficiency, hypertension, osteoporosis, and myasthenia gravis.

Drug Interactions

Aminoglutethimide, carbamazepine, phenobarbital, phenytoin, and rifampin increase the metabolism of the mineralocorticoids when given concurrently. Fludrocortisone decreases the effectiveness of diuretics and potassium supplements when given concurrently. Fludrocortisone increases the metabolism of isoniazid and salicylates when given together.

Adverse Effects

At normal physiologic levels, the mineralocorticoids have no adverse effects or contraindications. When the dose is excessive, sodium and water are retained, and potassium is lost. The effects on water and sodium result in expansion of fluid volume, hypertension, edema, cardiac enlargement, and hypokalemia. Bruising, sweating, hives, and an allergic rash have been reported. Desoxycorticosterone (DOCA) may produce hypertensive changes in mental functioning and permanent brain damage in susceptible patients.

 Mineralocorticoids are used with caution in children because these drugs can cause suppression of the hypothalamic-pituitary-adrenal (HPA) axis.

What You DO

Nursing Responsibilities

Fludrocortisone is administered by mouth on a variable schedule, ranging from twice daily to three times weekly, depending on patient response. Supplemental doses may be required during physiologic stress resulting from serious illness, trauma, or surgery. When administering mineralocorticoids, the nurse should:

- Monitor the patient for significant weight gain, edema, hypertension, or severe headaches. Fludrocortisone therapy increases serum sodium levels and decreases potassium levels.
- Teach the patient to recognize the signs and symptoms of electrolyte imbalance (e.g., muscle weakness, paresthesia, numbness, fatigue, anorexia, nausea).
- Instruct the patient to report altered heart rhythm, mental status, increased urination, severe or continuing headaches, unusual weight gain, and swelling of the feet to the health care provider.

Do You UNDERSTAND?

**DIRECTIONS: Fill in the blanks with the appropriate responses to com-
plete the following statements.**

1. The net result of reabsorption of sodium and water and the excretion of
   potassium and hydrogen ions is the maintenance of
   _____ and therefore
   _____ output.

2. Monitor the patient who is taking fludrocortisone for significant
   _____, _____,
   _____, or severe _____.

SECTION B
THYROID AND PARATHYROID AGENTS

The endocrine system, which includes the hypothalamus, pituitary, thyroid,
parathyroids, pancreas, adrenals, ovaries, and testes, participates in the regulation of all essential activities. Hormones that are produced in each of these
glands are secreted and act as chemical influences on distant organs. This section will discuss specific antithyroid agents, thyroid hormones, hypocalcemic
agents, and hypercalcemic agents.

What IS an Antithyroid Agent?

Antithyroid Agents	Trade Names	Uses
propylthiouracil [pro-puhl-thigh-oh-YOU-rah-sill]	PTU	Treatment of hyperthyroidism and thyrotoxic crisis
methimazole [meth-IM-a-zole]	Tapazole	Treatment of hyperthyroidism
strong iodine solution	Lugol's Solution	Preparation for thyroidectomy
potassium iodide solution	SSKI	Short-term treatment of Grave's disease and thyrotoxic crisis

Action

Antithyroid drugs are pharmacologic preparations that are used to treat hyperthyroidism. Hyperthyroidism results when an over secretion of thyroid hormone
is present. The abundance of this hormone greatly increases metabolism and
may induce a toxic state. Antithyroid drugs decrease production or release of
thyroid hormones.

Answers: 1. fluid and electrolyte balance,
adequate cardiac; 2. weight gain, edema,
hypertension, headache.

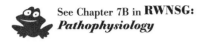

See Chapter 7B in **RWNSG:**
Pathophysiology

Uses

Thionamides (e.g., propylthiouracil, methimazole) and iodide solutions are drugs that are used to inhibit production or secretion of thyroid hormone. These agents are not chemically related but both help decrease the blood levels of thyroid hormone. Antithyroid drugs are used to treat the over secretion of thyroid hormone (**hyperthyroidism**), thus they may be given in preparation for a thyroidectomy, in conjunction with radioactive iodine therapy, and in the case of thyroid storm or thyrotoxic crisis.

What You NEED TO KNOW

 Thionamides and iodine preparations are contraindicated for women during pregnancy.

 Thionamides should be used cautiously during lactation because of the potential antithyroid effect on the infant.

Contraindications/Precautions

Contraindications for thionamides include any known sensitivity to antithyroid medication. The iodine preparations are contraindicated for patients with pulmonary edema and tuberculosis.

Drug Interactions

When potassium iodide solution is given with lithium, an increased hypothyroid action may result. Hyperkalemia may occur when potassium iodide solution is given with potassium supplements, potassium-sparing diuretics, and ACE inhibitors.

Adverse Effects

Adverse effects of antithyroid drugs are those that are associated with thyroid suppression (e.g., lethargy, bradycardia, nausea, skin rash). Propylthiouracil may be associated particularly with GI disturbances. Adverse effects of the iodine solutions, in addition to hypothyroidism, include iodism (e.g., metallic taste, stomach upset, diarrhea, discomfort of the mouth, teeth, and gums). Staining of the teeth, skin rash, and goiter may also occur.

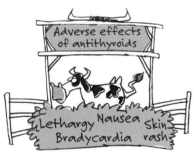

What You DO

Nursing Responsibilities

When administering antithyroid agents, the nurse should:
- Evaluate patients for allergy to any antithyroid medication.
- Instruct patients who are receiving propylthiouracil to divide the dose and take the medication around the clock to ensure consistent levels.
- Monitor patients who are receiving iodine solutions for signs of iodism, and immediately report these signs to the health care provider when they occur.

 TAKE HOME POINTS

Methimazole may cause bone marrow suppression. Propylthiouracil may be associated particularly with GI disturbances.

🐄 Teach patients who are undergoing iodine solution therapy to take the medicine orally through a straw to prevent staining of teeth.

🐄 Inform patients that they will undergo laboratory tests to evaluate the effectiveness of the antithyroid medication.

• Monitor patients for signs of adverse effects, such as anxiety, decreased cardiac output, ECG abnormalities, blood dyscrasias, and skin rash.

• Withdraw antithyroid medication gradually, and perform frequent evaluations to determine the likelihood of the patient remaining euthyroid.

TAKE HOME POINTS

Duration of therapy is usually until the patient is euthyroid for 6 to 12 months. Monitor frequent laboratory tests of patients who are taking methimazole for early detection of bone marrow suppression.

Do You UNDERSTAND?

DIRECTIONS: Fill in the blanks with the appropriate responses to complete the following statements.

1. Iodine solutions are contraindicated for _____.

2. Strong iodine solution is known as _____.

3. Hyperthyroidism is the result of _____
_____.

4. Antithyroid medications are used to treat hyperthyroidism by _____
_____.

5. Propylthiouracil should be taken _____
_____.

6. Iodine solutions should be taken _____
_____.

What IS a Thyroid Agent?

Thyroid Hormones	Trade Names	Uses
levothyroxine [lee-voe-thigh-ROX-een]	Synthroid	Treatment of hypothyroidism
liothyronine [lie-oh-THIGH-row-neen]	Cytomel	Treatment of hypothyroidism
liotrix [LYE-oh-trix]	Euthroid	Treatment of hypothyroidism

Action

Thyroid agents contain natural and synthetic thyroid hormones that control the rate of metabolism and thus significantly influence all bodily functions. Heart, skeletal muscle, liver, and kidneys are especially sensitive to the stimulating effects of these substances. These hormones are essential for normal growth and development. Thyroid hormones are also critical for brain and skeletal maturation. Thyroid hormones increase metabolic rate of body tissues, thereby increasing oxygen utilization.

Answer: 1. pregnancy; **2.** Lugol's solution; **3.** an over secretion of thyroid hormone occurs; **4.** decreasing production or release of thyroid hormone; **5.** in divided doses, usually three times a day, around the clock; **6.** through a straw to prevent staining of teeth.

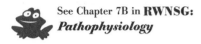

See Chapter 7B in **RWNSG:** *Pathophysiology*

Uses

Thyroid hormone agents are used for replacement therapy in hypothyroidism and in the treatment of myxedema, coma, goiters, and some thyroid cancers. These hormones are also used when thyroid hormone levels are low or absent and to control the pituitary gland's overproduction of the thyroid-stimulating hormone (TSH).

What You NEED TO KNOW

  During lactation, thyroid replacement hormones should be used with extreme caution.

Contraindications/Precautions

Thyroid replacement hormones are contraindicated for patients with a known allergy or sensitivity to the drugs or their binders. These hormones should not be used during an MI or in patients with hypoadrenal conditions.

Drug Interactions

Decreased absorption of thyroid hormones occurs when taken with cholestyramine. Thyroid hormones increase the potency of oral anticoagulants. These hormones may decrease the effectiveness of digitalis. Theophylline clearance is lowered in hypothyroid situations.

Loss of hair and skin reactions may occur, particularly in children during the first months of treatment.

Adverse Effects

With correct dosing for replacement therapy, adverse effects to thyroid hormones are few. Adverse effects of thyroid hormones included cardiac dysrhythmia, anxiety, headache, and sleeplessness.

What You DO

Nursing Responsibilities

Thyroid hormones are generally given in a single dose before breakfast. The initial dose is usually increased until desired effects are evident. When the patient is taking thyroid hormones and cholestyramine, these medications must be taken 2 hours apart. When administering thyroid replacement agents, the nurse should:

- Monitor the patient's response to thyroid agents and any adverse cardiac effect, hypertension, tachycardia, anxiety, or skin rash. The patient's metabolism should gradually increase to a more normal state.
- Instruct the patient to notify the health care provider immediately when any adverse signs appear.
- Evaluate specific drug interactions, particularly those related to cholestyramine, digitalis, and theophylline.
- Monitor periodic thyroid function blood tests to evaluate effectiveness.

Drug Groups and Mechanisms at a Glance

Drug Groups

1. Major Autonomic Nervous System Drug Classes
2. Major Cardiovascular System Drug Classes
3. Major Central Nervous System Drug Classes
4. Major Diuretic Drug Classes
5. Major Endocrine System Drug Classes
6. Major Gastrointestinal System Drug Classes
7. Major Immune System Drug Classes
8. Major Respiratory System Drug Classes

Drug Mechanisms

1. Sympathetic Drug Action
2. Parasympathetic Drug Action
3. Pharmacodynamics of Antidepressant Drugs
4. Site and Mechanism of Action of Antibiotics
5. Sites of Drug Action of the Renal System
6. Mechanism of Action of Laxatives
7. Insulin-Glucose Balance

PLATE 1

MAJOR AUTONOMIC NERVOUS SYSTEM DRUG CLASSES

SYMPATHETIC NERVOUS SYSTEM DRUGS
- Adrenergic agonists
- α-Adrenergic antagonists
- β-Adrenergic antagonists

PARASYMPATHETIC NERVOUS SYSTEM DRUGS
- Cholinergics
- Anticholinergics
- Cholinesterase inhibitors
- Dopaminergics

PLATE 2

MAJOR CARDIOVASCULAR SYSTEM DRUG CLASSES

THROMBOLYTICS

ANTIHYPERTENSIVES
- Angiotensin-converting enzyme inhibitors
- Angiotensin II antagonists
- α-Adrenergic blockers
- β-Blockers
- α-Beta blockers
- Calcium channel blockers
- Central-acting α-adrenergic agonists
- Direct-acting peripheral neuron antagonists
- Direct vasodilators

ANTIARRHYTHMICS

ANTIPLATELETS

ANTICOAGULANTS

INOTROPICS
- Cardiac glycosides
- Phosphodiasterase inhibitors

ANTIHYPERLIPIDEMICS
- HMG CoA reductase inhibitors
- Bile acid sequestrants
- Fibric acid derivatives

PLATE 3

MAJOR CENTRAL NERVOUS SYSTEM DRUG CLASSES

SKELETAL MUSCLE RELAXANTS
- Centrally acting
- Peripherally acting

CNS DEPRESSANTS

CNS STIMULANTS
- Psychomotor stimulates
- Anorexians
- Analeptics

PSYCHOTHERAPEUTIC DRUGS
- Benzodiazepine anxiolytics
- Nonbenzodiazepine anxiolytics
- Sedative-hypnotics
- Tricyclic antidepressants
- Selective serotonin reuptake inhibitors
- Monoamine oxidase inhibitors
- Antipsychotics
- Lithiums

ANTICONVULSANTS
- Hydantoins
- Barbituates
- Benzodiazepines
- Succinimides

ANALGESICS
- Opiates
- NSAIDs

ANESTHETICS
- Locals
- Nonbarbituates

PLATE 4

MAJOR DIURETIC DRUG CLASSES

- Thiazides
- Loop diuretics
- Osmotics

PLATE 5

MAJOR ENDOCRINE SYSTEM DRUG CLASSES

ADRENAL HORMONES
- Glucocorticoids
- Adrenal-inhibiting agents
- Mineralocorticoids

PITUITARY HORMONES
- Anterior pituitary
- Posterior pituitary

SEX HORMONES
- Estrogens
- Progestins
- Androgens

THYROID AND PARATHYROID HORMONES
- Antithyroids
- Thyroid hormones
- Hypercalcemics

ANTIDIABETICS
- Insulins
- Sulfonylureas
- α-Glucoside inhibitors
- Biguanides
- Thiazolidinediones
- Meglitinides

PLATE 6

MAJOR GASTROINTESTINAL SYSTEM DRUG CLASSES

- Antacids
- H_2-Antagonists
- Proton pump inhibitors
- Mucosal protectants
- Prostaglandins
- Antiflatulents
- Prokinetics
- Antiemetics
- Emetics
- Laxatives
- Antidiarrheal drugs

PLATE 7

MAJOR IMMUNE SYSTEM DRUG CLASSES

ANTIBIOTICS
- Penicillins
- Cephalosporins
- Sulfonamides
- Aminoglycosides
- Tetracyclines
- Macrolides
- Fluoroquinolones

ANTIFUNGAL DRUGS
- Polyenes
- Azoles

ANTIVIRAL DRUGS
- Protease inhibitors
- Nucleoside reverse transcriptase inhibitors
- Nonnucleoside reverse transcriptase inhibitors
- Nucleoside analogs

BIOLOGIC RESPONSE MODIFIERS
- Immunosuppressants
- Interferons
- Interleukins
- Colony-stimulating factors

ANTINEOPLASTICS
- Antimetabolites
- Mitotic inhibitors
- Alkylating agents
- Antitumor antibiotics

PLATE 8

MAJOR RESPIRATORY SYSTEM DRUG CLASSES

UPPER RESPIRATORY AGENTS
- Antitussives
- Decongestants
- Expectorants
- Mucolytics

BRONCHODILATORS
- Inhaled corticosteroids
- β-Agonists
- Leukotriene antagonists
- Xanthines
- Anticholinergics

ANTIHISTAMINES
- Sedating first-generation
- Nonsedating second-generation

PLATE 9

SYMPATHETIC DRUG ACTION

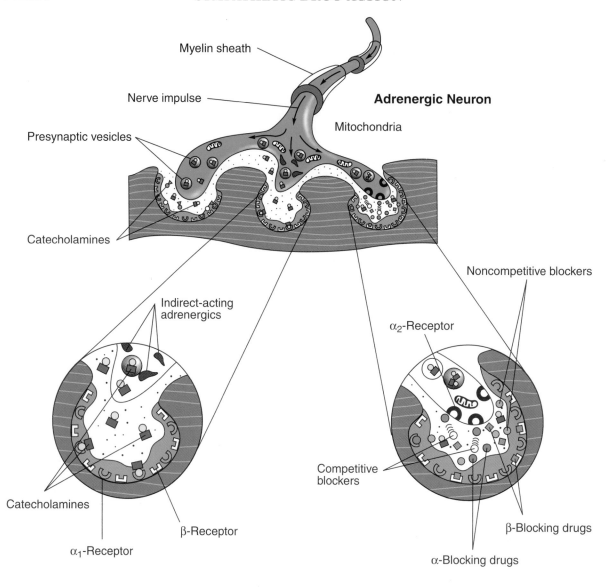

Myelin sheath

Nerve impulse

Adrenergic Neuron

Mitochondria

Presynaptic vesicles

Catecholamines

Noncompetitive blockers

α_2-Receptor

Indirect-acting
adrenergics

Competitive
blockers

β-Blocking drugs

Catecholamines

α-Blocking drugs

β-Receptor

α_1-Receptor

Adrenergic Agonist Drugs

Adrenergic Antagonist Drugs

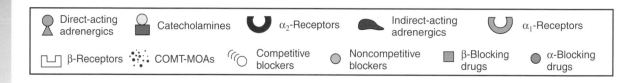

	Direct-acting adrenergics		Catecholamines		α_2-Receptors		Indirect-acting adrenergics		α_1-Receptors
	β-Receptors		COMT-MOAs		Competitive blockers		Noncompetitive blockers		β-Blocking drugs		α-Blocking drugs

PLATE 10

PARASYMPATHETIC DRUG ACTION

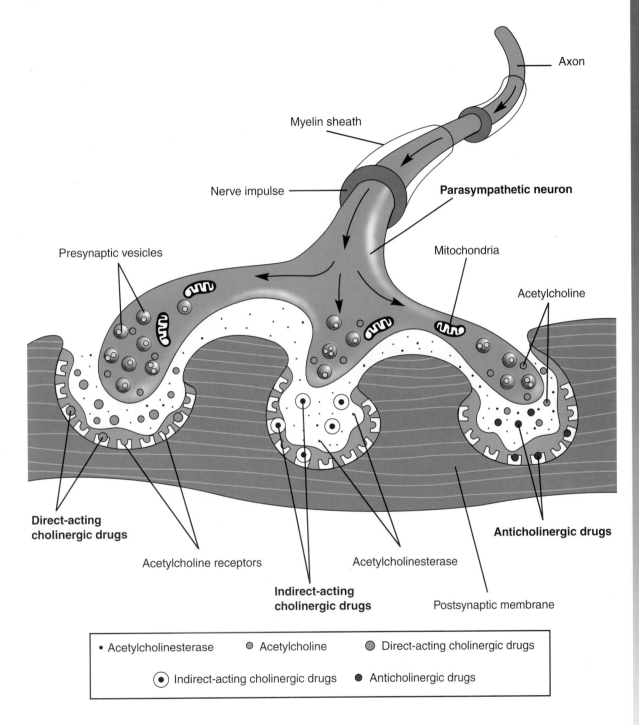

Axon

Myelin sheath

Nerve impulse

Parasympathetic neuron

Presynaptic vesicles

Mitochondria

Acetylcholine

Direct-acting cholinergic drugs

Anticholinergic drugs

Acetylcholine receptors

Acetylcholinesterase

Indirect-acting cholinergic drugs

Postsynaptic membrane

- Acetylcholinesterase
- Acetylcholine
- Direct-acting cholinergic drugs
- Indirect-acting cholinergic drugs
- Anticholinergic drugs

PLATE 11 PHARMACODYNAMICS OF ANTIDEPRESSANT DRUGS

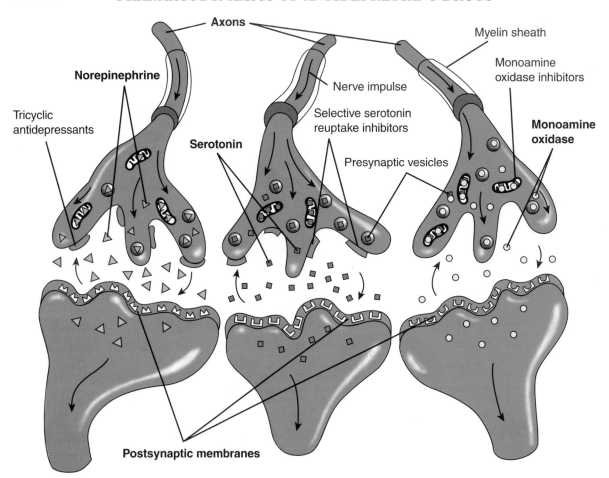

Axons

Norepinephrine

Tricyclic
antidepressants

Serotonin

Nerve impulse

Selective serotonin
reuptake inhibitors

Presynaptic vesicles

Myelin sheath

Monoamine
oxidase inhibitors

**Monoamine
oxidase**

Postsynaptic membranes

PLATE 12 SITE AND MECHANISM OF ACTION OF ANTIBIOTICS

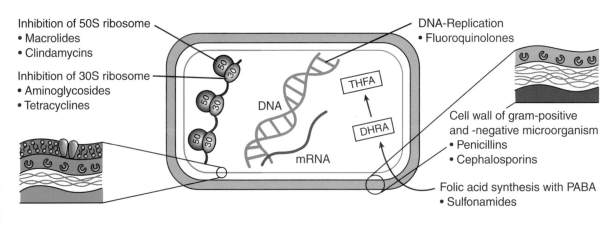

Inhibition of 50S ribosome
• Macrolides
• Clindamycins

Inhibition of 30S ribosome
• Aminoglycosides
• Tetracyclines

DNA-Replication
• Fluoroquinolones

THFA

DHRA

DNA

mRNA

Cell wall of gram-positive
and -negative microorganism
• Penicillins
• Cephalosporins

Folic acid synthesis with PABA
• Sulfonamides

PLATE 13 **SITES OF DRUG ACTION ON THE RENAL SYSTEM**

Distal tubule
• Potassium-sparing diuretics
• Thiazide diuretics (primary site)

Bowman's capsule

Renal cortical diluting tubule

Glomerular capillaries

Proximal tubule
• Thiazide diuretics (secondary site)

Collecting tubule

Ascending loop of Henle
• Loop diuretics

Thin descending loop of Henle

PLATE 14 **MECHANISM OF ACTION OF THE FOUR TYPES OF LAXATIVES**

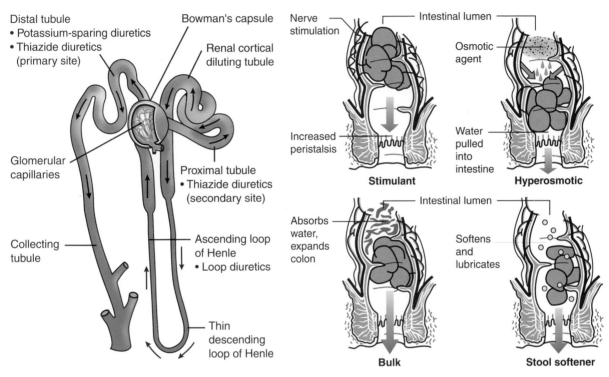

Nerve stimulation

Intestinal lumen

Osmotic agent

Increased peristalsis

Water pulled into intestine

Stimulant

Hyperosmotic

Absorbs water, expands colon

Intestinal lumen

Softens and lubricates

Bulk

Stool softener

PLATE 15 **INSULIN-GLUCOSE BALANCE**

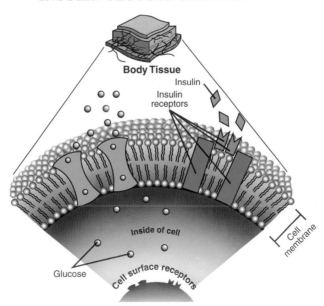

Body Tissue

Insulin

Insulin receptors

Inside of cell

Cell membrane

Glucose

Cell surface receptors

PLATE 16

RENIN-ANGIOTENSIN-ALDOSTERONE SYSTEM

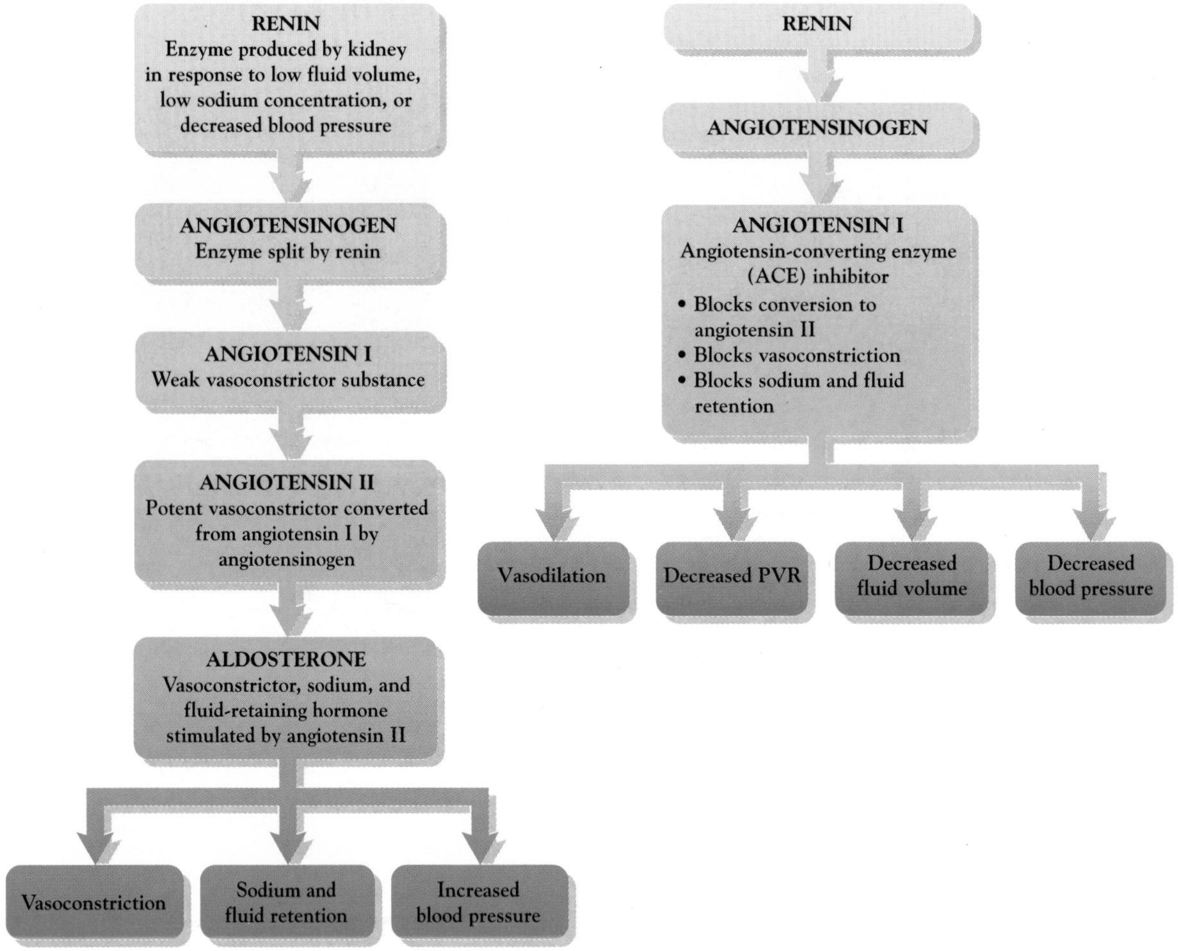

RENIN
Enzyme produced by kidney
in response to low fluid volume,
low sodium concentration, or
decreased blood pressure

↓

ANGIOTENSINOGEN
Enzyme split by renin

↓

ANGIOTENSIN I
Weak vasoconstrictor substance

↓

ANGIOTENSIN II
Potent vasoconstrictor converted
from angiotensin I by
angiotensinogen

↓

ALDOSTERONE
Vasoconstrictor, sodium, and
fluid-retaining hormone
stimulated by angiotensin II

↓

- Vasoconstriction
- Sodium and fluid retention
- Increased blood pressure

RENIN

↓

ANGIOTENSINOGEN

↓

ANGIOTENSIN I
Angiotensin-converting enzyme
(ACE) inhibitor
• Blocks conversion to
  angiotensin II
• Blocks vasoconstriction
• Blocks sodium and fluid
  retention

↓

- Vasodilation
- Decreased PVR
- Decreased fluid volume
- Decreased blood pressure

- Monitor bleeding times carefully.
- Monitor digitalis levels thus adjustments in the dose can be made appropriately.
- Be aware that as thyroid function returns to normal, the dose of theophylline should be altered accordingly when both drugs are taken concurrently.
- Realize that thyroid hormones increase cellular metabolism thus heat production. Carbohydrate and fat metabolism are increased under the influence of thyroid hormones.
- Warn the patient to avoid discontinuing thyroid hormones without checking with the health care provider.

 Stopping thyroid hormones without orders may lead to serious problems.

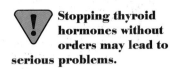 **TAKE HOME POINTS**

Liothyronine has an increased potential for cardiac problems and is therefore not recommended for patients with cardiac disease.

Do You UNDERSTAND?

DIRECTIONS: Fill in the blanks with the appropriate responses to complete the following statements.

1. Thyroid hormones _____ heart rate and cardiac output.
2. Thyroid hormones are critical for _____ and _____ maturation.
3. Decreased absorption of thyroid hormone occurs when taken with
   _____.
4. Thyroid hormones may cause decreased effectiveness of
   _____.
5. _____ are necessary to evaluate response to thyroid hormone therapy.
6. Thyroid replacement hormones are frequently taken
   _____

What IS a Hypocalcemic Agent?

Vitamin D compounds act therapeutically to regulate the absorption of phosphate and calcium. Vitamin D assists the parathyroid hormone (PTH) and calcitonin in regulating calcium.

Hypocalcemic agents are used to treat manifestations of hypocalcemia, such as neuromuscular irritability, which may progress to tetany. In acute severe hypocalcemia, calcium gluconate or calcium chloride may be prescribed. In long-term, less acute situations, oral calcium supplements and vitamin D may be indicated to maintain normal levels of calcium. Vitamin D is frequently used in chronic situations when calcium preparations alone are ineffective in maintaining normal calcium levels. Treatment of hypoparathyroidism consists primarily of vitamin D preparations and calcium supplements.

For the discussion of vitamin D and calcium, refer to pages 359 and 364, respectively.

Answers: 1. increase; 2. brain, skeletal; 3. cholestyramine; 4. digitalis glycosides; 5. laboratory tests; 6. before breakfast.

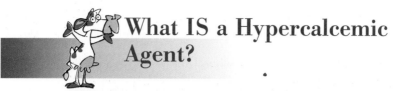

What IS a Hypercalcemic Agent?

Hypercalcemic Agents	Trade Names	Uses
calcitonin-human [kal-si-TOE-nin]	Cibacalcin	Treatment of Paget's disease and postmenopausal osteoporosis
calcitonin-salmon	Calcimar	Treatment of Paget's disease and postmenopausal osteoporosis
bisphosphonates-alendronate [a-LEN-dro-nate]	Fosamax	Treatment of Paget's disease and hypercalcemia associated with malignancy
bisphosphonates-etidronate [e-ti-DROE-nate]	Didronel	Treatment of Paget's disease and hypercalcemia associated with malignancy
gallium [GAL-lee-um]	Ganite	Treatment of hypercalcemia associated with malignancy

Action

Hypercalcemic agents lower serum calcium levels to normal or near-normal levels. These agents inhibit bone reabsorption, thus lowering calcium levels. However, hypercalcemic agents do not affect normal bone formation.

Hypercalcemia diminishes the ability of nerves and muscles to respond to stimuli. Problems that are associated with these elevated levels include GI disturbances, such as nausea, vomiting, constipation, abdominal discomfort, lethargy, syncope, hallucinations, and coma. Polyuria, polyphagia, and cardiac dysrhythmias may also occur. Calcium deposits in organs (e.g., kidneys, eyes) may lead to decreased function. Elevated levels of serum calcium may occur in hyperparathyroidism, malignancies, excessive ingestion of vitamin D, adrenal disorders, and immobilization. The ingestion of estrogen, thiazide diuretics, and lithium may also result in an elevated serum calcium.

Uses

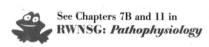

See Chapters 7B and 11 in
RWNSG: *Pathophysiology*

Calcitonin-salmon is used to decrease calcium levels. This agent may be used in prolonged immobilization and the treatment of hyperparathyroidism and osteoporosis. Calcitonin-human is a synthetic preparation that is used to treat Paget's disease. The bisphosphonates are used in the treatment of Paget's disease and hypercalcemia that is associated with some malignancies. Gallium also is used to treat hypercalcemia that is associated with malignancies.

What You NEED TO KNOW

Contraindications/Precautions

Bisphosphonates and gallium are contraindicated for patients with renal dysfunction. Bisphosphonates are also contraindicated for patients with acidosis, heart block, severe hypotension, hypertension, and spinal or epidural anesthesia. Calcitonins are contraindicated for patients with allergies to salmon and fish products.

Drug Interactions

The absorption of bisphosphonates is impaired when taken with multiple vitamins, iron, and antacids. When gallium is given concurrently with aminoglycosides, vancomycin, or amphotericin B, the risk of nephrotoxicity increases.

Adverse Effects

Common adverse effects of hypercalcemic agents include facial flushing and nausea. Other adverse effects include irritation at the insertion site, hand flushing, skin rash, eye pain, headache, anorexia, vomiting, abdominal pain, diarrhea, temporary increase in bone discomfort that is associated with Paget's disease, urinary frequency, nocturia, and renal failure. Additional adverse effects of etidronate include metallic or altered taste.

 # What You DO

Nursing Responsibilities

Hypercalcemics are given orally and IV. Because the absorption of bisphosphonates is impaired when taken with multiple vitamins, iron, and antacids, concurrent administration should be separated by at least 30 minutes. When treating osteoporosis, calcitonin-salmon is used primarily in the form of a nasal spray. When administering hypercalcemic agents, the nurse should:

- Instruct the patient to decrease intake of dairy products, as well as foods and medications that contain calcium.
- Administer calcitonin at bedtime to decrease discomfort.
- Encourage patients to drink 3000 to 4000 cc of fluids per day to minimize renal dysfunction.
- Observe for the signs of hypercalcemia, such as GI distress, lethargy, syncope, polyuria, and cardiac dysrhythmias.
- Monitor ECG changes, such as a shortened Q-T interval and inverted T wave.
- Evaluate the patient for signs of hypocalcemia with aggressive treatment of hypercalcemia.
- Monitor periodic calcium levels to determine effectiveness.
- Monitor renal function and fluid and electrolyte balance in patients who are receiving hypocalcemics for early detection of abnormalities.

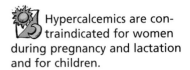 Hypercalcemics are contraindicated for women during pregnancy and lactation and for children.

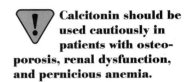 **Calcitonin should be used cautiously in patients with osteoporosis, renal dysfunction, and pernicious anemia.**

 Bisphosphonates should be used cautiously in older or debilitated patients.

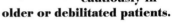 **TAKE HOME POINTS**

Rotate the injection sites when administering injections of calcitonin to decrease risk of inflammation. Aspirin should not be combined with bisphosphonates because of the increased risk of GI adverse effects.

 Because of the risk of renal failure, hypercalcemic agents must not be given with nephrotoxic drugs.

Do You UNDERSTAND?

DIRECTIONS: Provide the appropriate responses to the following statements or questions.

1. List three medications that may be associated with an elevated calcium level.

   _____

   _____

   _____

2. Bisphosphonates should not be given with what three medications?

   _____

   _____

   _____

3. Calcitonin-human (Cibacalcin) may cause what?

   _____

   _____

4. Gallium is contraindicated for patients with what?

   _____

Section C

ANTIDIABETICS

Antidiabetic drugs are medications that are used in managing diabetes mellitus. Insulins are used primarily in the treatment of type 1 diabetes. Insulins are also used in treating patients with type 2 diabetes who are unable to control their blood glucose levels by diet, exercise, and oral hypoglycemic agents. Insulins are also used in treating diabetic ketoacidosis (DKA) and hyperosmotic hyperglycemic nonketotic (HHNK) coma. Insulins are classified by their action times, concentration, and origin.

Oral hypoglycemic agents are used to treat type 2 diabetes. These agents are classified as sulfonylureas, α-glucosidase inhibitors, biguanides, thiazolidinediones and meglitinides. These agents may be used alone or in combination with other oral antidiabetics or insulin.

Answers: 1. lithium, thiazide diuretics, estrogen; **2.** antacids, iron supplements, multivitamins; **3.** nausea, facial and hand flushing; **4.** renal impairment.

What IS Insulin?

Classification	Onset	Peak	Duration
Rapid-acting insulin *Insulin Lispro* Humalog	< 15 min	0.5-1.0 hr	5-7 hr
Short-acting insulin *Insulin Injection (Regular)* Humulin R Novolin R Pork Regular Iletin II Purified Pork Regular Velosulin BR Velosulin Human	30-60 min	2-3 hr	5-7 hr
Insulin Zinc Suspension Prompt (Semilente) Semilente Insulin Semilente Purified Pork Insulin	30-60 min	4-7 hr	12-16 hr
Intermediate-acting insulin *Isophane Insulin Suspension (NPH)* Humulin N Ilene II Insulard NPH Mixtard Novolin 70/30 Novolin N	1.0-2.5 hr	7-15 hr	22 hr
Insulin Zinc Suspension (Lente) Humulin L Lente Iletin II Lente Purified Pork Novolin L	1-2 hr	8-12 hr	18-24 hr
Long-acting insulin *Insulin Protamine Zinc (IPZ)* Iletin II	4-8 hr	14-24 hr	36 hr
Insulin Zinc Suspension Extended (Ultralente) Humulin U	4-8 hr	16-18 hr	36 hr
Constant-acting insulin *Insulin Glargine* Lantus R	Immediate	Constant	24 hr

Doses are individualized and dose adjustments are made according to blood glucose levels.

Action

Insulin is a hormone that is secreted by the pancreas and is necessary for regulating the metabolism and storage of carbohydrates, fats, and proteins. Insulin binds to the insulin receptor sites of the cell membrane, thereby allowing the glucose molecules to cross the cell membrane and lowering the blood glucose concentration. Insulin is active in carbohydrate metabolism, facilitating the uptake and storage of glucose by the cells and promoting the conversion of glucose to glycogen. Insulin also promotes the normal cell's uptake and conversion of amino acids and fatty acids. Insulin is metabolized in the liver and kidneys and excreted in the urine.

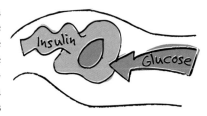

See Chapter 7D in **RWNSG:**
Pathophysiology

Uses

The wide variety of insulin types allows the health care provider to select the insulin that is best suited for the individual. Choice of insulin and the dose must be individualized according to the patient's needs and lifestyle. Insulins are classed by their action times (onset, peak, and duration) as rapid-acting, short-acting, intermediate-acting, long-acting, and constant-acting. Onset indicates the time after administration that the insulin begins to work. The peak is the time during which the maximal effect of the insulin occurs. Duration is the length of time that the insulin is active in the body.

Insulin is used to maintain normal or near-normal blood glucose levels in the treatment of type 1 and type 2 diabetes. Regular insulin is used in the emergency treatment of DKA and HHNK to regulate glucose levels and in the treatment of severe hyperkalemia to promote the intracellular shift of potassium. In psychiatry, insulin is used to induce hypoglycemic shock as therapy. Insulin is used IV as a secretion-stimulating test for the evaluation of pituitary growth hormone.

What You NEED TO KNOW

Contraindications/Precautions

Insulin is contraindicated for patients with a hypersensitivity to animal insulin protein.

Insulin should be used with caution during pregnancy.

Insulin glargine is contraindicated for children under 6 years of age.

Drug Interactions

Concurrent use of beta blockers, salicylates, anabolic steroids, alcohol, monoamine oxidase inhibitors (MAOIs), sulfinpyrazone, clofibrate, tetracyclines, guanethidine, and oxytetracycline may increase the hypoglycemic effects of insulin. Use of corticosteroids, dextrothyroxine, diltiazem, dobutamine, epinephrine, ethacrynic acid, and estrogens may decrease the hypoglycemic effects of insulin. Thiazide diuretics, furosemide, phenytoin, and thyroid preparations increase blood glucose levels and may require an increase in the insulin dose. Use of beta blockers may mask signs and symptoms of hypoglycemia.

Adverse Effects

Adverse effects of insulin include hypersensitivity, hypoglycemia, lipodystrophy of injection sites, and rebound hyperglycemia. Localized reactions (e.g., itching and erythema at the injection site) or systemic reactions (e.g., dyspnea, tachycardia, angioedema, anaphylaxis) are used to classify hypersensitivity. Evidence of an overdose (hypoglycemia) includes profuse perspiration, palpitations, tremulousness, and nausea. Other hypoglycemic adverse effects include tachycardia, hunger, confusion, incoherent speech, irritability, inability to concentrate, headache, blurred or double vision, convulsions, loss of consciousness, and coma.

What You DO

Nursing Responsibilities

Insulin is available in concentrations of 100 units/cc (U100) or 500 units/cc (U500). The origin of insulin preparations may be pork, beef, pork and beef, human, or an analog of human insulin. The most common form of insulin that is used is the biosynthetic human insulin. When administering insulin, the nurse should:

- Contact the health care provider for dose instructions when breakfast is delayed for diagnostic tests.
- Instruct the patient that insulin vials should be inspected for any clumping, discoloration, solid deposits, or a granular appearance before use and to discard when any of these are noted.
- Teach the patient the proper technique of mixing two insulins in one syringe. Instruct the patient to always withdraw the short-acting insulin into the syringe before the long-acting insulin (clear before cloudy). Rapid- and short-acting insulins are clear solutions. Intermediate- and long-acting insulin solutions appear cloudy. This distinction reduces the risk of the short-acting insulin accidentally being drawn into the long-acting insulin vial and causing an unexpected hypoglycemic reaction. Do not mix glargine with any other insulin.
- Inform the patient that insulin is to be injected at a 90-degree angle to prevent local reactions. Always use an insulin syringe.
- Rotate insulin injection sites to prevent tissue necrosis.
- Instruct the patient to apply gentle pressure to the injection site and to avoid massaging the site after injection.
- Check blood glucose levels at the time of the insulin's peak action to monitor for hypoglycemia. The frequency of blood glucose monitoring is determined according to the health status of the patient and the insulin regime.
- Administer insulin via a parenteral route (SC or IV) because insulin is a protein and is destroyed in the GI tract.
- Monitor the patient's blood pressure, intake and output, blood glucose level, and ketones every hour when administering IV insulin as a treatment for DKA.
- Instruct the patient to always carry some form of quick-acting complex carbohydrate, such as five to eight Lifesavers candies, other hard candies, or lump sugar, for the treatment of hypoglycemia.
- Teach patients and their family about signs of hypoglycemia and home emergency treatment.
- Advise patients to always carry identification, which identifies them as a person with diabetes who is undergoing insulin therapy.
- Counsel the patient to avoid taking OTC medications without consulting the health care provider.
- Inform the patient that blurred vision may occur at the beginning of therapy, but it will usually subside within 6 to 8 weeks.

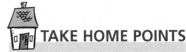

TAKE HOME POINTS

- U100 insulin is the most common concentration that is used in the United States. Always double check that the insulin that is being used is the insulin that was ordered. Rotate insulin injection sites systematically within one area, using all available sites, before moving to the next anatomic area. Massaging the site after insulin injection may alter the rate of absorption. Regular insulin is the only type of insulin that can be given IV.

- Food should be available before administering lispro administration. Glargine should be given at bedtime.

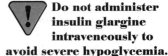 **Do not administer insulin glargine intravenously to avoid severe hypoglycemia.**

Do You UNDERSTAND?

DIRECTIONS: Complete the following crossword puzzle.

Down
1. Route of insulins
2. Short-acting insulin
3. Time that insulin is active in body

Across
4. Masks signs of hypoglycemia
5. Only regular insulin can be given this route.
6. Where insulin is excreted
7. Onset of this insulin is less than 15 minutes.

What IS a Sulfonylurea?

Sulfonylureas	Trade Names	Uses
First-generation		
acetohexamide [a-seat-oh-HEX-ah-mide]	Dymelor	Treatment of type 2 diabetes mellitus
chlorpropamide [klor-PROH-pah-mide]	Diabinese	Treatment of type 2 diabetes mellitus
tolazamide [toll-AZ-ah-mide]	Tolinase	Treatment of type 2 diabetes mellitus
tolbutamide [toll-BYOU-tah-mide]	Orinase	Treatment of type 2 diabetes mellitus
Second-generation		
glipizide [GLIP-ih-zide]	Glucotrol	Treatment of type 2 diabetes mellitus
glyburide [GLYE-byou-ride]	DiaBeta, Micronase	Treatment of type 2 diabetes mellitus
glimepiride [glye-MEH-pye-ride]	Amaryl	Treatment of type 2 diabetes mellitus

Action

Sulfonylureas are oral antidiabetic agents that decrease elevated blood glucose levels. Sulfonylureas bind to the potassium channels on the beta cells of the pancreas, thereby stimulating the pancreas to release insulin. These agents also increase the sensitivity of the peripheral insulin receptors, which increases insulin binding in the peripheral tissues. Sulfonylureas decrease the formation of glucose in the liver, reducing hepatic glucose release. The patient must have functional pancreatic beta cells that are able to produce insulin for sulfonylurea treatment to be effective.

Both generations of sulfonylureas lower blood glucose levels. The second-generation sulfonylureas are more potent than are the first-generation sulfonylureas. These agents lower the blood glucose levels with a smaller dose and longer duration of action compared with first-generation sulfonylureas.

Uses

Sulfonylureas are used in the treatment of mild to moderately severe type 2 diabetes mellitus when diet and exercise programs fail to maintain glycemic control. Sulfonylureas may be used alone, as an adjunct to diet and exercise, or in combination with other oral antidiabetics or insulin.

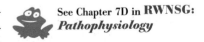

See Chapter 7D in **RWNSG:** *Pathophysiology*

What You NEED TO KNOW

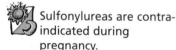

Use sulfonylureas with caution in patients with thyroid or endocrine impairment, glycosuria, and hyperglycemia resulting from primary renal disease. Sulfonylureas should be used with caution in nursing mothers.

Contraindications/Precautions

Contraindications for use of sulfonylureas include hypersensitivity, severe hepatic or renal impairment, type 1 diabetes mellitus, and complications of type 2 diabetes (e.g., HHNK, DKA, severe infections, major surgery, trauma, coma).

Drug Interactions

Use of sulfonylureas with insulin, sulfonamides, chloramphenicol, oxyphenbutazone, phenylbutazone, salicylates, probenecid, MAOIs, oral anticoagulants, alcohol, and clofibrate increases the risk of hypoglycemia. Beta blockers may mask signs of hypoglycemia. Concurrent use of diazoxide and sulfonylureas causes a decrease in effectiveness. An increased risk of hyperglycemia occurs when sulfonylureas are used with thiazides, other diuretics, nicotinic acid, glucocorticoids, thyroid hormone, rifampin, and oral contraceptives. Concurrent use of sulfonylureas and alcohol may produce a disulfiram-like reaction (e.g., facial flushing, sweating, tachycardia, headache, dyspnea), which may last up to 24 hours.

Sulfonylureas are contraindicated during pregnancy.

Adverse Effects

Common adverse effects of sulfonylureas include nausea, vomiting, anorexia, epigastric discomfort, heartburn, and hypoglycemia. Hypoglycemia is the primary adverse effect in patients with renal or liver impairment. Other adverse effects of sulfonylureas include diarrhea, jaundice, leukopenia, thrombocytopenia, agranulocytosis, hemolytic anemia, aplastic anemia, photosensitivity, rash, pruritus, and erythema. Chlorpropamide may also cause an antidiuretic adverse effect called the syndrome of inappropriate antidiuretic hormone (SIADH).

Hypoglycemia is the primary adverse effect in older adults.

What You DO

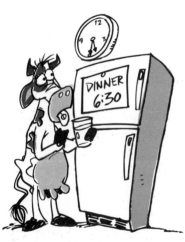

Nursing Responsibilities

When administering sulfonylureas, the nurse should:

- Instruct the patient of the exact times at which the oral antidiabetic should be taken (e.g., as a single morning dose, 30 minutes before breakfast and dinner, with breakfast) for the maximal effectiveness.
- Monitor laboratory values that are altered by sulfonylureas because these drugs may produce increased blood urea nitrogen (BUN) levels, increased creatinine levels, abnormal thyroid function tests, and reduced radioactive iodine (RAI) uptake.
- Monitor complete blood count (CBC), hemoglobin (HbA1c), electrolyte levels, and liver function tests.

- Instruct the patient to monitor and record blood glucose levels at the frequencies the health care provider prescribes when the patient experiences signs or symptoms of hypoglycemia and during illness.
- Stress to the patient the importance of diet and exercise in the control of diabetes.
- Warn the patient to avoid using OTC medications or discontinuing this medication without consulting with the health care provider.
- Be aware that acetohexamide is the sulfonylurea of choice to treat patients with diabetes who have gout because of its uricosuric properties.
- Be aware that second-generation sulfonylureas are more potent, produce fewer adverse reactions, and have longer duration times than do first-generation agents.

TAKE HOME POINTS

The health care provider individualizes the dose according to the blood glucose levels and the requirements of the patient. Instruct the patient to notify the health care provider of any hypoglycemic episodes or persistently low blood glucose levels.

Do You UNDERSTAND?

DIRECTIONS: Complete the following statements with the appropriate terms from the italicized list provided.

1. Sulfonylureas stimulate the pancreas to _____ insulin.
2. For sulfonylureas to be effective, pancreatic beta cells must be
   _____.
3. Use of alcohol when taking sulfonylureas may cause a
   _____ reaction.
4. The primary adverse effect of sulfonylureas is _____.

hypoglycemia	*metabolized*	*hyperglycemia*
functional	*excreted*	*inhibit*
stimulate	*disulfiram-like*	

What IS an α-Glucosidase Inhibitor?

Alpha-Glucosidase Inhibitors	Trade Names	Uses
acarbose [ah-CAR-bohs]	Precose	Treatment of type 2 diabetes mellitus
miglitol [MIG-lih-tohl]	Glyset	Treatment of type 2 diabetes mellitus

Action

An α-glucosidase inhibitor is an oral antidiabetic agent that lowers blood glucose levels after meals. α-Glucosidase enzyme inhibitors interfere with the digestion of carbohydrates to glucose.

TAKE HOME POINTS

α-Glucosidase inhibitors delay the absorption of glucose in the intestines, which lowers blood glucose and glycosylated hemoglobin levels.

Answers: 1. stimulate; 2. functional; 3. disulfiram-like; 4. hypoglycemia.

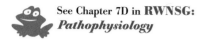

See Chapter 7D in **RWNSG:** *Pathophysiology*

Uses

Acarbose and miglitol are used to lower blood glucose levels in the treatment of type 2 diabetes. These agents may be used alone, as an adjunct to a diet and exercise regime, or in combination with a sulfonylurea to improve glycemic control.

What You NEED TO KNOW

Acarbose should be used with caution in patients with hepatic dysfunction.

Acarbose and miglitol are contraindicated for nursing mothers. Safe use of these agents during pregnancy has not been determined.

Contraindications/Precautions

Acarbose and miglitol are contraindicated for patients with inflammatory bowel disease, colon ulcers, partial bowel obstructions, renal dysfunction, and ketoacidosis.

Drug Interactions

Concurrent use of α-glucosidase inhibitors with sulfonylureas may increase the risk of hypoglycemia. Charcoal and digestive enzymes decrease the effectiveness of α-glucosidase inhibitors. Digoxin levels are lowered when taken with acarbose or miglitol. Pancreatin diminishes the effect of miglitol. Miglitol decreases the bioavailability of propranolol and ranitidine.

Adverse Effects

The most common adverse effects of α-glucosidase inhibitors include abdominal pain, diarrhea, flatulence, and hypoglycemia. Other adverse effects include anorexia, nausea, and vomiting. Acarbose may cause additional adverse effects of weakness, dizziness, sleepiness, headache, vertigo, anemia, and increased liver function levels. Miglitol may cause a transient skin rash.

What You DO

Nursing Responsibilities

Acarbose and miglitol should be given with the first bite of each meal. When administering α-glucosidase inhibitors, the nurse should:

- Monitor both fasting and postprandial blood glucose levels and glycosylated hemoglobin levels to evaluate the effectiveness of the medication.
- Monitor the hemoglobin, hematocrit, and liver function studies in patients who are taking acarbose for early detection of adverse effects.
- Warn the patient to avoid discontinuing the medication without consulting the health care provider.
- Instruct the patients to monitor their weight and to report any significant changes because these agents may cause weight loss.
- Advise the patient to notify the health care provider when any severe abdominal pain or distress develops for necessary dose adjustment.

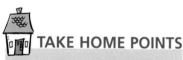

TAKE HOME POINTS

Teach the patient to take acarbose and miglitol with the first bite of each meal. Teach patients to take glucose tablets or gelatin caps for hypoglycemia for quicker action.

Instruct the patient that glucose tablets or gelatin caps should be given for hypoglycemia, not candy or sugar, because α-glucosidase inhibitors delay carbohydrate break down.

Do You UNDERSTAND?

DIRECTIONS: **Indicate in the space provided whether the statement is**
true or _false._

_____ 1. Miglitol therapy causes elevated glycosylated hemoglobin.
_____ 2. α-Glucosidase enzyme inhibitors delay the absorption of glucose.
_____ 3. Instruct the patient to take acarbose with the first bite of each meal.
_____ 4. Give candy for a hypoglycemic patient who is treated with miglitol.

What IS a Biguanide?

Biguanides	Trade Names	Uses
metformin [met-FOR-min]	Glucophage	Treatment of type 2 diabetes mellitus

Action

A biguanide is an oral antidiabetic agent that decreases blood glucose concentrations. Biguanides increase the binding of insulin at receptor sites, thereby enhancing the action of insulin. These agents inhibit hepatic glucose production and reduce glucose absorption in the intestines. Biguanides increase the glucose transport across the cell membrane, particularly in skeletal muscle cells, thus increasing glucose utilization. Biguanides have no effect on insulin secretion.

Uses

Biguanides are used in the treatment of type 2 diabetes mellitus when diet and exercise programs fail to maintain glycemic control. Metformin, the only biguanide that is approved for use in the United States, may be used alone or in combination with an oral sulfonylurea.

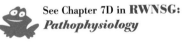

Metformin-Only Biguanide in U.S.

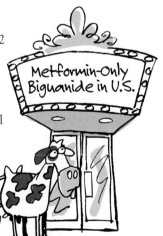

See Chapter 7D in **RWNSG:**
Pathophysiology

Answers: 1. false; 2. true; 3. true; 4. false.

What You NEED TO KNOW

 Biguanides are contraindicated during lactation.

 Biguanides should be used with caution during pregnancy.

Use of metformin with fluconazole, ketoconazole, itraconazole, and oral hypoglycemic drugs may cause severe hypoglycemia. Use of iodinated contrast material (e.g., dyes that are used in radiologic studies) can cause acute renal failure and lactic acidosis.

Contraindications/Precautions

Contraindications for use of biguanides include hypersensitivity, hepatic or renal impairment, alcoholism, metabolic acidosis, and DKA.

Drug Interactions

When biguanides are used concurrently with captopril, furosemide, or nifedipine, the risk of hypoglycemia is increased. Concurrent use of alcohol or glucocorticoids increases the risk of lactic acidosis. Concurrent use of cimetidine increases metformin peak levels.

Adverse Effects

The most common adverse effects of biguanides include nausea, vomiting, diarrhea, flatulence, abdominal pain or bloating, anorexia, and a bitter or metallic taste. Additional adverse effects include headache, dizziness, agitation, fatigue, decreased vitamin B_{12} level, and lactic acidosis.

What You DO

Nursing Responsibilities

When administering biguanide agents, the nurse should:
- Hold metformin for 48 hours before and after diagnostic studies in which the patient is administered iodinated contrast dye to prevent lactic acidosis or renal failure from occurring.
- Administer metformin with meals to reduce GI side effects.
- Expect the health care provider to reduce the doses of metformin when the patient is undergoing cimetidine therapy.
- Evaluate baseline renal and hepatic function tests because the use of metformin is contraindicated for patients with renal or hepatic insufficiency.
- Monitor CBC, HbA1c, and renal and hepatic function tests periodically.
- Instruct the patient to avoid using OTC drugs without consulting with the health care provider.
- Inform the patient that a bitter or metallic taste may occur but will subside.

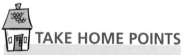 **TAKE HOME POINTS**

Monitor suspected or known alcoholics for decreased hepatic function.

Do You UNDERSTAND?

DIRECTIONS: Using the italicized words, fill in the blanks with the appropriate responses to complete the following statements.

1. When the patient is on cimetidine therapy, the nurse should expect the metformin dosage to be _____.
   (*increased, decreased, discontinued, not given*)
2. An adverse reaction of metformin is a _____ taste that usually subsides. (*sour, sweet, tangy, metallic*)
3. Administer metformin immediately before a diagnostic test using iodinated contrast dye. _____ (*true or false*)

What IS a Thiazolidinedione?

Thiazolidinediones	Trade Names	Uses
pioglitazone [PIE-oh-GLIT-ah-zone]	Actos	Treatment of type 2 diabetes mellitus
rosiglitazone [ROH-sih-GLIH-tah-zone]	Avandia	Treatment of type 2 diabetes mellitus

Action

Thiazolidinediones are oral antidiabetic agents that increase the effects of circulating insulin, thereby lowering the blood glucose concentration. Thiazolidinediones decrease insulin resistance of the tissues, which causes the skeletal muscles and adipose tissue to increase the uptake of glucose. Thiazolidinediones inhibit gluconeogenesis, thereby decreasing the liver's production of glucose. Thiazolidinediones require the presence of insulin to be effective; they do not stimulate the production of insulin.

Uses

Thiazolidinediones are used to lower blood glucose levels in the treatment of type 2 diabetes. These agents may be used alone, as an adjunct to diet and exercise, or in combination with sulfonylurea, insulin, or metformin to improve glycemic control.

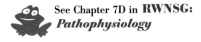

See Chapter 7D in RWNSG:
Pathophysiology

Answer: 1. decreased; 2. metallic; 3. false.

What You NEED TO KNOW

Contraindications/Precautions

Thiazolidinediones are contraindicated for patients with hypersensitivity, type 1 diabetes, DKA, and hepatic dysfunction.

Drug Interactions

Pioglitazone may reduce the effectiveness of oral contraceptives. Ketoconazole may increase pioglitazone levels.

Adverse Effects

The common adverse effects of thiazolidinediones include headache, pain, myalgia, infections, and fatigue. Other adverse effects include rhinitis, diarrhea, liver injury, upper respiratory infections, hypoglycemia, hyperglycemia, fluid retention, and weight gain.

 Thiazolidinediones are contraindicated for nursing mothers.

Thiazolidinediones should be used with caution during pregnancy.

Women who are premenopausal and anovulatory may be at risk for conception because ovulation may resume with thiazolidinedione therapy.

What You DO

Nursing Responsibilities

Thiazolidinediones may be administered without regard for meals. When administering thiazolidinediones, the nurse should:

- Expect the health care provider to consider a higher dose of oral contraceptives or to suggest an alternative method of contraception for women of childbearing age who are taking thiazolidinediones or both.
- Evaluate baseline and periodic liver function tests because thiazolidinediones are contraindicated for patients with liver failure.
- Evaluate frequent blood glucose levels to monitor the effectiveness of thiazolidinedione therapy.
- Teach the patient to avoid discontinuing this medication without consulting the health care provider.
- Advise the patient to maintain the prescribed diet and exercise program.

TAKE HOME POINTS

Teach the patient who is taking oral contraceptives to use barrier contraceptives because thiazolidinediones reduce the effectiveness of oral contraceptives.

Do You UNDERSTAND?

DIRECTIONS: Indicate in the space provided whether the statement is *true* or *false.*

_____ 1. Rosiglitazone is a second-generation sulfonylurea.
_____ 2. Thiazolidinediones must be taken with the first bite of the meal.
_____ 3. Thiazolidinediones may be used in combination with other oral antidiabetic agents.
_____ 4. A common adverse effect of thiazolidinediones is headache.

What IS a Meglitinide?

Meglitinides	Trade Names	Uses
repaglinide [re-PAY-gli-nide]	Prandin	Treatment of type 2 diabetes mellitus
nateglinide [nah-TE-gli-nide]	Starlix	Treatment of type 2 diabetes mellitus

Action

A meglitinide is an oral antidiabetic agent that stimulates endogenous insulin production to reduce postprandial glucose levels. This agent stimulates the beta cells of the pancreas to release insulin on demand, thus functioning beta cells must exist for this action to occur. Neteglimide, an α-phenylalanine derivative, stimulates maximal insulin secretion when taken with a meal, exerting a synergistic interaction with blood glucose levels.

Uses

Meglitinides are used to maintain glycemic control in the treatment of type 2 diabetes as an adjunct to diet and exercise. Meglitinides may also be used in combination with metformin.

What You NEED TO KNOW

Contraindications/Precautions

Contraindications for use of meglitinides include hypersensitivity, type 1 diabetes, and ketoacidosis.

Drug Interactions

No noted drug interactions occur with meglitinides.

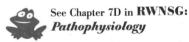

See Chapter 7D in **RWNSG:**
Pathophysiology

Meglitinides are contraindicated during pregnancy and lactation.

Caution should be maintained in patients with hypoglycemia or hepatic impairment.

Answers: 1. false; 2. false; 3. true; 4. true.

Adverse Effects

The most common adverse effect of meglitinides is hypoglycemia. Other adverse effects include nausea, vomiting, diarrhea, rhinitis, bronchitis, headache, chest pain, tooth disorder, allergy, arthralgia, back pain, and paresthesia.

What You DO

TAKE HOME POINTS

Meglitinides significantly lower post-prandial blood glucose levels. Meglitinides have a rapid onset and short half-life, which prevents hyperinsulinemias and decreases hypoglycemic episodes.

Nursing Responsibilities

Meglitinides should be administered within 30 minutes before meals. When the patient skips a meal, the dose that is scheduled before that meal should also be skipped to decrease the risk of hypoglycemia. When administering meglitinides, the nurse should:

- Monitor the glycosylated HbA1c and blood glucose tests to evaluate the efficacy of meglitinide treatment.
- Monitor liver function tests periodically.
- Instruct the patient that when meglitinide is replacing another oral antidiabetic, it may be started the morning after the last dose of the previous drug.
- Teach the patient to monitor capillary blood glucose routinely and record results for the health care provider for review.
- Advise the patient to maintain the prescribed diet and exercise program to control blood glucose levels.
- Discuss the signs and symptoms of hypoglycemia, and instruct the patient to notify the health care provider of any hypoglycemic occurrences.

Do You UNDERSTAND?

DIRECTIONS: **Indicate in the space provided whether the statement is** *true* **or** *false.*

_____ 1. Meglitinides may be given safely during pregnancy.

_____ 2. Meglitinides may be administered without regard to meal times.

_____ 3. Type 1 diabetics are treated with meglitinide to maintain glycemic control.

_____ 4. Meglitinides should be administered within 30 minutes before meals.

Drugs Affecting the Gastrointestinal System

SECTION A
AGENTS AFFECTING HYPERACIDITY, GASTRIC MUCOSA, MOTILITY, AND FLATULENCE

This chapter reviews the pharmacologic preparations used to treat hyperacidity, gastric mucosa, motility, and flatulence. The nurse must provide more consumer education with these gastrointestinal (GI) preparations than they do with any other over-the-counter (OTC) drugs because large quantities of these nonprescription or OTC drugs are purchased for self-medication. This section discusses nonsystemic antacids, histamine H_2-antagonists, proton pump inhibitors, mucosal protectants, prostaglandins, antiflatulents, GI stimulants, and prokinetics.

What IS a Nonsystemic Antacid?

Nonsystemic Antacids	Trade Names	Uses
Aluminum hydroxide	Amphojel	Treatment of hyperacidity
Calcium carbonate	Tums	Treatment of hyperacidity
Magaldrate [MAG-al-drate]	Riopan	Treatment of hyperacidity

Action

Antacids are alkaline drugs that directly neutralize hydrochloric acid that the stomach secretes. Antacids reduce the corrosive effect of hydrochloric acid on GI mucosa, thus they have a protective and restorative effect. Because the absorption is minimal, the residue of salts from the chemical neutralization of acid is subjected to the normal digestive process. Nonsystemic antacids are eliminated in GI tract via feces.

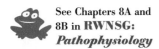

See Chapters 8A and 8B in **RWNSG:** *Pathophysiology*

TAKE HOME POINTS

Antacids neutralize hydrochloric acid through direct chemical reaction in the mid-portion of the stomach and provide a demulcent or soothing effect on GI mucosa.

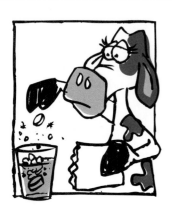

Caution should be used when administering antacids to patients with any conditions that electrolyte or acid-base imbalance, GI obstruction, or renal dysfunction may exacerbate.

TAKE HOME POINTS

Headache, irritability, nausea, vomiting, neuromuscular changes, muscle twitching, and coma are evidence of encephalopathy from systemic aluminum absorption.

Uses

Antacids are used to treat peptic ulcers and gastric hyperacidity. Examples of hyperacidity include heartburn, acid indigestion, and gastroesophageal reflux disease (GERD).

What You NEED TO KNOW

Contraindications/Precautions

Antacids are contraindicated for patients with any known allergy to any antacid component.

Drug Interactions

When antacids are taken with enteric-coated medications, antacids tend to disintegrate the coating and release the drug prematurely in the stomach. When antacids are taken with tetracycline and fluoroquinolone antibiotics, both drugs combine chemically and decrease absorption. This activity may indicate a needed change in dose requirements of tetracycline. Calcium and magnesium preparations exacerbate the action of digitalis, which also may require dose adjustments.

Adverse Effects

The most common adverse effects of antacids are associated with acid-base and electrolyte levels. Rebound acidity is a major concern with antacid administration. When the antacid changes the stomach contents to an alkaline environment, the stomach produces additional acid in response.

Systemic alkaline absorption (particularly aluminum) may result in encephalopathy. With systemic absorption of antacids, severe electrolyte disorders may occur. Some adverse effects of antacids may vary with the preparation that has been administered. Aluminum forms of antacids may cause constipation, delayed gastric emptying, and hypophosphatemia. Calcium forms of antacids may cause constipation, hypercalcemia, milk-alkali syndrome or severe alkalosis, and renal calculi. Magnesium preparations may lead to diarrhea, with resultant hypokalemia, iron deficiency, and hypermagnesemia. The adverse effects of hypermagnesemia following magnesium antacid administration include drowsiness, weakness, and cardiac dysrhythmias, all of which occur more frequently in patients with renal impairment. Sodium antacid preparations may cause a reduction of iron absorption and water retention.

What You DO

Nursing Responsibilities

Antacids are administered orally for their acid-neutralizing capacity (ANC) in liquid or chewable tablet form. The onset of drug action is within 5 to 15 minutes, and the duration is usually 2 hours. When giving antacids, the nurse should:

- Administer antacids at least 1 hour before or 2 hours after any other oral drugs to ensure adequate absorption.
- Monitor electrolytes of the patient who is taking antacids for early detection of an electrolyte imbalance.
- Instruct the patient to chew antacid tablets thoroughly and follow with one glass of water to ensure that the medication reaches the stomach for direct action and to avoid the development of intestinal concretions calculi.
- Inform patients that antacids should be stored in a tightly closed container at 15° to 30° C (59° to 86° F).
- Instruct the patient to report any shortness of breath, chest pain, darkened or tarry stools, sweating, or recurrent symptoms to the health care provider.
- Teach patients about acid rebound and that repeated use for 1 to 2 weeks might cause a rebound acid stimulation action, quickly leading to the development of a chronic antacid user.

Patients who receive large quantities of antacids over a prolonged period or those who are on a diet that is low in phosphorus (while taking antacids continuously) may develop hypophosphatemia within 2 weeks.

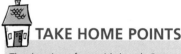

TAKE HOME POINTS

The duration of antacids is only 2 hours, thus they need to be taken frequently.

Do You UNDERSTAND?

DIRECTIONS: Fill in the blanks with the appropriate responses to complete the following statements.

1. _____ is a concurrent drug that is administered with antacids that poses a risk of decreased absorption.
2. Two of the most common adverse effects of antacids include _____ and _____.
3. _____ is the substance that antacids neutralize in the stomach.
4. List five conditions that antacids treat.
   _____
   _____
   _____
   _____
   _____
5. _____ and _____ are the acceptable timeframes during which an antacid may be administered before and after another drug to avoid absorption interference.

Answers: 1. tetracycline, digitalis; 2. acid-base, electrolyte imbalance; 3. hydrochloric acid; 4. upset stomach, peptic esophagitis, gastritis, hiatal hernia, peptic ulcer; 5. 1 hour before and 2 hours after.

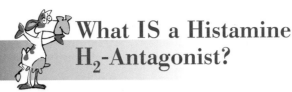

What IS a Histamine H$_2$-Antagonist?

Histamine H$_2$-Antagonists	Trade Names	Uses
cimetidine [sigh-MET-ih-deen]	Tagamet	Treatment of duodenal ulcers, GERD, and pathologic hypersecretion
ranitidine [ran-EYE-tih-deen]	Zantac	Treatment of duodenal ulcers, GERD, and pathologic hypersecretion
famotidine [fuh-MOE-tih-deen]	Pepcid	Treatment of duodenal ulcers, GERD, and pathologic hypersecretion
nizatidine [nigh-ZAT-ih-deen]	Axid	Treatment of duodenal ulcers, GERD, and prevention of heartburn

Action

Histamine H$_2$-antagonists directly inhibit histamine action on H$_2$-receptors to decrease acid production. This classification of GI agents selectively blocks histamine H$_2$-receptors, which are located on the gastric parietal cells. The blockage of histamine receptors prevents gastrin secretion. Because gastrin is responsible for local release of histamine, stimulation of hydrochloric acid and pepsin production is decreased.

Uses

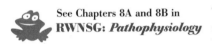

See Chapters 8A and 8B in RWNSG: *Pathophysiology*

This drug classification is used in the treatment of active gastric or duodenal ulcer maintenance therapy. Stress reduces the production of protective mucus. Histamine H$_2$-antagonists reduce the overall acid level, thereby alleviating discomfort and promoting healing. These agents are also used in the treatment of hypersecretory conditions, such as Zollinger-Ellison syndrome. By blocking the overproduction of hydrochloric acid, the condition is relieved. Histamine H$_2$-antagonists alleviate the discomfort of heartburn, acid indigestion, and GERD. These drugs are also used prophylactically to prevent stress-induced ulcers and acute upper GI bleeding.

What You NEED TO KNOW

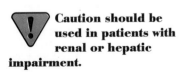

Cimetidine is contraindicated for women who are pregnant and lactating and for children.

Caution should be used in patients with renal or hepatic impairment.

Contraindications/Precautions

Cimetidine is contraindicated for patients with a known allergy and hepatic dysfunction.

Drug Interactions

When histamine H_2-antagonists are taken concurrently with warfarin, phenytoin, β-adrenergic blockers, quinidine, theophylline, chloroquine, benzodiazepines, nifedipine, pentoxifylline, tricyclic antidepressants, procainamide, triamterene, carbamazepine, and alcohol, metabolism is slowed and toxic serum levels may be reached. Nizatidine increases the serum levels of aspirin. Cimetidine may decrease the absorption of iron, tetracyclines, and lidocaine. When administered concurrently with morphine, cimetidine has been known to cause apnea. Antacids decrease the absorption of histamine H_2-antagonists.

Adverse Effects

The most common adverse effects of histamine H_2-antagonists include diarrhea, constipation, blurred vision, headaches, dizziness, fatigue, somnolence, confusion, hallucinations, bradycardia, hypotension, and dysrhythmias. Additional adverse effects that are related to histamine H_2-antagonists include musculoskeletal pain, arthralgia, myalgia, rash, allergic reaction, gynecomastia, breast tenderness, renal impairment, bone marrow depression, and leukocytosis. Famotidine may cause flushing, palpitations, hypertension, and tinnitus. Ranitidine has been known to cause vomiting and abdominal discomfort. Nizatidine may lead to hyperuricemia and hepatic damage.

 # What You DO

Nursing Responsibilities

Histamine H_2-antagonists may be administered orally. All but nizatidine are available for intravenous (IV) use. When administering histamine H_2-antagonists, the nurse should:

- Administer oral drug preparations before or with meals and at bedtime to ensure adequate protection when needed.
- Monitor renal and hepatic function tests for early detection of any organ damage.
- Monitor drug levels for potential drug interaction with concurrent administration of histamine H_2-antagonists that might lead to drug toxicity.
- Teach the patient about the medication to enhance compliance.

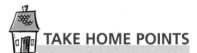

TAKE HOME POINTS

Nizatidine is the only histamine H_2-antagonist that is unavailable in an IV form.

Do You UNDERSTAND?

DIRECTIONS: When the following drugs are given concurrently with histamine H_2-antagonists, indicate a concern of increased or decreased absorption and increased metabolism or increased toxic serum levels.

1. Tetracyclines: _____
   (increased or decreased absorption)
2. Alcohol: _____
   (increased metabolism or increased toxic serum levels)
3. Theophylline: _____
   (increased metabolism or increased toxic serum levels)
4. Antacids: _____
   (increased or decreased absorption)
5. Nifedipine: _____
   (increased metabolism or increased toxic serum levels)

What IS a Proton Pump Inhibitor?

Proton Pump Inhibitors	Trade Names	Uses
omeprazole [oh-MEH-pruh-zohl]	Prilosec	Treatment of duodenal ulcers, GERD, and pathologic hypersecretion
lansoprazole [lan-SO-pruh-zohl]	Prevacid	Treatment of duodenal ulcers, esophagitis, and pathologic hypersecretion

Action

Proton pump inhibitors (**antisecretory agents**) act directly on the secretory surface of the gastric parietal cells at the final step of acid production to decrease acid levels in the stomach. These agents inhibit the hydrogen-potassium-ATPase gastric enzyme system, which catalyzes the final step. Proton pump inhibitors are absorbed rapidly when given orally. Their antisecretory effects last up to 72 hours.

Uses

Proton pump inhibitors are used in the treatment of esophagitis, GERD, peptic ulcers, duodenal ulcers, Zollinger-Ellison syndrome, and other hypersecretory syndromes.

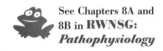

See Chapters 8A and 8B in **RWNSG:** *Pathophysiology*

Answers: 1. decreased absorption; 2. increased serum levels; 3. increased serum levels; 4. decreased absorption; 5. increased serum levels.

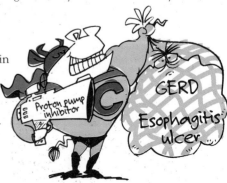

What You NEED TO KNOW

Contraindications/Precautions

Proton pump inhibitors are contraindicated for patients with a known allergy to the medication.

Drug Interactions

The absorption of concurrent drugs may be decreased because of the alteration of gastric pH by proton pump inhibitors, such as iron, digoxin, ampicillin, and ketoconazole. Omeprazole inhibits the metabolism and increases the drug level of diazepam, phenytoin, and warfarin, requiring dose adjustments for efficacy.

Adverse Effects

The incidence of adverse effects after administering proton pump inhibitors is low, and those that occur are relatively mild. Common adverse effects from proton pump inhibitors include headache, dizziness, cough, stuffy nose, hoarseness, and epistaxis. Other reported adverse effects include dry mouth, nausea, vomiting, flatulence, diarrhea, constipation, abdominal pain, weakness, vertigo, dream abnormalities, and insomnia. Adverse effects that are less common include rash, dry skin, fever, alopecia, and back pain.

What You DO

Nursing Responsibilities

When administering proton pump inhibitors, the nurse should:
- Instruct the patient to avoid opening, chewing, or crushing capsules. These medications should be swallowed whole for therapeutic effect.
- Instruct the patient to return for follow-up medical treatment when the symptoms are unresolved after 4 to 8 weeks of therapy.

Do You UNDERSTAND?

DIRECTIONS: Fill in the blanks with the appropriate response.

1. Is the incidence of adverse effects following proton pump inhibitors high or low? _____
2. List six common adverse effects of proton pump inhibitors.

_____   _____

_____   _____

_____   _____

 Proton pump inhibitors should be given with caution to patients who are pregnant or lactating.

 Caution should be used when giving proton pump inhibitors to patients with hepatic impairment because dose adjustments may be required.

 TAKE HOME POINTS

Proton pump inhibitors should be administered before meals to ensure drug efficacy.

 The patient should avoid opening, chewing, or crushing proton pump inhibitor capsules.

Answers: 1. low; 2. headache, dizziness, cough, stuffy nose, hoarseness, epistaxis.

3. List four conditions that proton pump inhibitors are used to treat.

_____   _____

_____   _____

4. Which time of day is best to administer proton pump inhibitors for better efficacy? _____

5. What instructions regarding ingestion of proton pump inhibitor capsules should the nurse teach the patient? _____

_____

What IS a Mucosal Protectant?

Mucosal Protectant	Trade Name	Use
sucralfate [soo-CRAWL-fate]	Carafate	Treatment of duodenal ulcer

Action

Mucosal protectants (**cytoprotective agents**) react with gastric acid and proteins at the ulcer site to form a thick paste that covers and sticks to the ulcer site. The paste helps protect the ulcer from gastric acid, pepsin, and bile; its action is local rather than systemic. Sucralfate contains an aluminum complex. The small amount that is absorbed through the GI tract is excreted in the urine of patients with normal kidney function. Ninety percent of the paste is excreted in the feces.

Uses

Mucosal protectants are drugs that are given to protect the wall of the GI tract from ulceration or injury from excess acid (**hyperacidity**). Sucralfate is given to prevent or treat ulcer disease and is used for short-term treatment (up to 8 weeks) of duodenal and gastric ulcers.

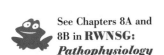

See Chapters 8A and 8B in **RWNSG:** *Pathophysiology*

Sucralfate should be used with caution in patients with chronic kidney failure or those on dialysis.

  Sucralfate should be used with caution in women who are pregnant and nursing and in children.

What You NEED TO KNOW

Contraindications/Precautions

Aluminum blood levels may be extremely elevated because aluminum is not removed via the impaired kidneys or dialysis of patients who may be receiving other drugs with aluminum (e.g., antacids).

Drug Interactions

Sucralfate may decrease the absorption and action of tetracyclines, fluoroquinolones, phenytoin, digoxin, and fat-soluble vitamins.

Answers: 3. esophagitis, GERD, peptic or duodenal ulcers, Zollinger-Ellison syndrome; 4. before meals; 5. avoid opening, chewing, or crushing capsules; rather, swallow them whole.

Adverse Effects

The most commonly reported adverse effect following mucosal protectant administration is constipation. Less frequent side effects include nausea, gastric discomfort, and diarrhea.

What You DO

Nursing Responsibilities

Sucralfate is given orally in either tablet or suspension form. When administering mucosal protectants, the nurse should:

- Administer sucralfate on an empty stomach (1 hour before meals and at bedtime). Schedule medication administration times to avoid giving sucralfate with other oral medications. Give other oral medications 2 hours before sucralfate.
- Administer other oral medications 2 hours before giving sucralfate to prevent drug interactions. Because sucralfate provides a protective barrier to the GI mucosa, administration with other oral medications may interfere with absorption and decrease the action of the other drugs.
- Consult the pharmacist to obtain the correct diluent to prevent clogging of the tube when giving sucralfate through a nasogastric tube. Mucosal protectant therapy should continue for 4 to 8 weeks, even when symptoms of the ulcer disappear, unless healing can be confirmed by endoscopy or x-ray film.
- Advise the patient to avoid smoking and spicy foods that might aggravate the ulcer.
- Monitor patients with chronic renal failure for increasing signs and symptoms of aluminum toxicity, such as acute dementia, osteomalacia, and bone pain, with or without fractures.
- Administer antacids 30 minutes before or after sucralfate.

TAKE HOME POINTS

Administer sucralfate 1 hour before meals and at bedtime.

Do You UNDERSTAND?

DIRECTIONS: **Indicate in the space provided whether the statement is** *true* **or** *false***. If false, then correct the statement to make it true using the space in the margin.**

_____ 1. Sucralfate form a thick coating that sticks to the ulcer, thereby protecting the mucosa.

_____ 2. Sucralfate can be administered either orally or IV.

_____ 3. Sucralfate can be given with oral antibiotics.

_____ 4. Administration of sucralfate and other oral medications together may reduce the bioavailability of the medications.

_____ 5. The most common side effects of nausea and vomiting occur in approximately 50% of patients who are taking sucralfate.

Answers: 1. true; 2. false; sucralfate can only be given orally; 3. false; sucralfate should be given 2 hours after oral medications to prevent drug interactions and possible decreased action of the oral antibiotic or other oral medication; 4. true; 5. false; constipation is the most common side effect of sucralfate, although all side effects are infrequent.

What IS a Prostaglandin?

Prostaglandin	Trade Name	Use
misoprostol [MY-so-PRAHST-ole]	Cytotec	Prevention of gastric ulcers

Action

Misoprostol is a synthetic prostaglandin E1 that decreases gastric acid secretion and helps protect the GI mucosa. Misoprostol may be used in patients who are taking nonsteroidal antiinflammatory drugs (NSAIDs), including aspirin, and in those who are at risk for NSAID-induced gastric ulcers. NSAIDs inhibit prostaglandin production, which leads to a decrease in bicarbonate and mucus production. The decrease in bicarbonate and mucus increases the risk of gastric mucosal injury from the NSAIDs. In contrast, misoprostol increases bicarbonate and mucus production, thereby having a protectant effect. Misoprostol also produces uterine contractions.

Uses

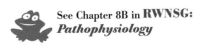

See Chapter 8B in **RWNSG:** *Pathophysiology*

Misoprostol is used to prevent NSAID-induced gastric ulcers in patients who are at a high risk for developing ulcers, such as patients with a history of gastric ulcers. The drug is usually used concurrently, as long as the patient is on NSAID therapy. The unlabeled use involves preventing and treating duodenal ulcers.

Misoprostol is used to prevent NSAID-induced gastric ulcers in older adults.

What You NEED TO KNOW

Contraindications/Precautions

Misoprostol is contraindicated for patients with hypersensitivity to prostaglandins.

Misoprostol is contraindicated during pregnancy because partial or complete abortion and uterine bleeding may result. Misoprostol is also contraindicated for nursing mothers and for children.

Drug Interactions

Antacids may reduce the action of misoprostol.

Adverse Effects

The most common adverse effects are diarrhea and abdominal pain. Diarrhea is usually dose related, mild, and self-limiting (resolving in approximately 8 days).

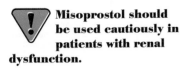

Misoprostol should be used cautiously in patients with renal dysfunction.

What You DO

Nursing Responsibilities

Misoprostol is an oral medication. No dose reduction is routinely suggested for patients with renal impairment or for older patients, unless the dose is not tolerated. When administering prostaglandins, the nurse should:

- Monitor for GI distress, the number and consistency of stools, and signs and symptoms of dehydration.
- Administer misoprostol at mealtime and at bedtime with food to prevent GI discomfort and medication-induced diarrhea.
- Avoid administering misoprostol with magnesium-containing antacids, which may increase the incidence and severity of diarrhea.

Advise the patient with childbearing potential to avoid pregnancy and to use an effective contraceptive method. When pregnancy occurs, discontinue the therapy and contact the health care provider immediately.

Do You UNDERSTAND?

DIRECTIONS: Fill in the blanks with the appropriate response.

1. Misoprostol is indicated for the prevention of _____ ulcers.
2. Misoprostol prevents ulcers by _____.
3. High-risk patients who are using _____ may be candidates for concurrent use of misoprostol.
4. The most common side effect of misoprostol is _____.
5. Misoprostol is contraindicated for use in patients who are

   _____.

What IS an Antiflatulent?

Antiflatulent	Trade Name	Use
simethicone [sigh-METH-ih-cone]	Mylicon	Treatment of flatulence

Action

Simethicone changes the surface tension of gas bubbles in the stomach and intestines. The changed surface tension allows gas bubbles to stick together to form larger bubbles. The larger bubbles are easier than are smaller bubbles to pass via peristaltic movement and motility in the GI tract through the mouth by belching or through the anus as flatus.

Answers: 1. gastric; 2. increasing bicarbonate and mucus; 3. NSAIDs; 4. diarrhea; 5. pregnant.

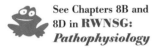
See Chapters 8B and 8D in RWNSG: *Pathophysiology*

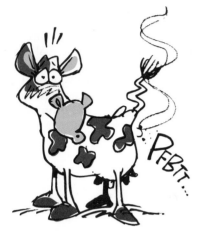

Uses

Antiflatulents are drugs that are given to treat the discomfort of excessive gas in the GI tract. Gas is introduced into the body by (1) swallowing air, (2) bacterial action leading to gas as a byproduct, and (3) diffusion of gas from the blood stream into the GI tract. Most of the gas in the stomach comes from swallowing air. Intestinal gas results primarily from bacterial action. An average of 7 to 10 liters of gas pass through the GI tract each day, most of which is reabsorbed. The use of simethicone is indicated for the symptoms of excess gas and discomfort particularly in patients who swallow air and cannot expel it or in postoperative patients with gaseous distention.

What You NEED TO KNOW

Contraindications/Precautions

No contraindications are listed.

Drug Interactions

No interactions are listed.

Adverse Effects

No adverse effects are listed.

What You DO

Nursing Responsibilities

Simethicone is given orally and is marketed under several different trade names, each with different amounts of the active ingredient. Some of the forms are combination drugs that may include an antacid or antidiarrheal medication. When administering antiflatulents, the nurse should:

- Mix the liquid forms of simethicone with water, infant formula, or other suitable liquids.
- Shake suspensions thoroughly before pouring.
- Teach the patient that tablets must be chewed thoroughly before swallowing. Gelatin caps should not be chewed.
- Assess bowel sounds for the presence of peristaltic activity, particularly in postsurgical patients before simethicone administration.
- Counsel the patient that activity (e.g., walking) will increase peristalsis.
- Instruct the patient that eating in an upright position and avoiding gas-producing foods or carbonated beverages may help decrease the swallowing of air and encourage gas movement through the GI tract.

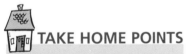

TAKE HOME POINTS

Teach patient that chewable tablets must be chewed and that suspensions should be thoroughly shaken before pouring.

Do You UNDERSTAND?

DIRECTIONS: **Indicate in the space provided whether the statement is *true* or *false*. If false, then correct the statement to make it true using the space in the margin at right.**

_____ 1. Simethicone liquid may be mixed with water, infant formula, or other liquids before administration.

_____ 2. Antiflatulents break up bubbles into smaller bubbles that can be expelled.

_____ 3. Simethicone tablets must be chewed before swallowing.

_____ 4. Simethicone suspension must be thoroughly shaken before pouring.

_____ 5. Adverse effects of simethicone include diarrhea.

What IS a Prokinetic Gastrointestinal Agent?

Prokinetic Gastrointestinal Agent	Trade Name	Use
metoclopramide [MET-oh-KLOE-pra-mide]	Reglan	Treatment of gastric stasis

Action

Prokinetic GI drugs increase the motion or movement through the GI tract. Metoclopramide is a cholinergic drug that stimulates motility of the upper GI tract without increasing gastric, biliary, or pancreatic secretions. Metoclopramide also increases the tone and force of gastric contractions, relaxes the pyloric sphincter, and increases peristalsis of the duodenum and jejunum. The result is increased transit time and decreased gastric emptying time. Metoclopramide also increases esophageal sphincter tone but has little effect on peristaltic movement in the colon. The exact mechanism of action is unknown, but metoclopramide appears to sensitize the GI smooth muscle to acetylcholine. Metoclopramide also has an antiemetic effect that is thought to be a result of blocking stimulation of dopamine receptors in the chemoreceptor trigger zone (CTZ) in the medulla.

Uses

Metoclopramide is indicated in short-term treatment (4 to 12 weeks) of adults with GERD who fail to respond to conventional treatment. Other indications are in patients who require radiographic examinations during which gastric emptying is important, those with symptomatic diabetes with gastric stasis, and postoperative patients with GI hypomotility. Metoclopramide also facilitates small bowel intubation when the tube will not pass the pylorus. Prokinetic GI

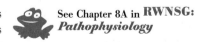

See Chapter 8A in **RWNSG:** *Pathophysiology*

Answers: 1. true; 2. false; antiflatulents cause smaller bubbles to stick together, producing larger bubbles; larger bubbles are easier to expel; 3. true; 4. true; 5. false; simethicone has few if any adverse effects.

agents are also useful in patients who are receiving cancer chemotherapy and in the prevention of postoperative nausea and vomiting when gastric intubation and suction is undesirable.

What You NEED TO KNOW

Contraindications/Precautions

Metoclopramide is contraindicated for patients with GI obstruction, hemorrhage, or perforation when stimulation of the GI tract may be dangerous. This agent is also contraindicated for patients with a known hypersensitivity, pheochromocytoma (because of the risk for a hypertensive crisis), epilepsy, and those who are receiving other drugs that are likely to cause extrapyramidal symptoms (EPS).

Drug Interactions

When metoclopramide is given concurrently with alcohol and CNS depressants, sedation may be increased. Phenothiazines may increase the risk of EPS when given with metoclopramide. Anticholinergics and opiate analgesics may antagonize the therapeutic effect of metoclopramide, thereby decreasing GI motility.

Adverse Effects

Adverse effects of metoclopramide increase with higher doses or with prolonged administration. The most common adverse effects include drowsiness, restlessness, fatigue, diarrhea, and EPS, particularly acute dystonic reactions. Other adverse effects include dizziness, visual disturbances, irritability, confusion, depression, bradycardia, insomnia, and suicidal ideation. Galactorrhea, gynecomastia, and menstrual disorders are adverse effects that resolve weeks after drug discontinuation. EPS effects usually subside within 2 to 3 months after discontinuation. Methemoglobinemia in neonates may occur with overdosing.

What You DO

Nursing Responsibilities

Metoclopramide is available in tablets and liquid form for oral administration and as an injectable for intramuscular (IM) or IV use. In diabetic gastroparesis, symptom severity determines the route of administration. Relief from nausea, vomiting, and anorexia indicate improvement in symptoms. The dose should be decreased by one half in patients with reduced renal function. Metoclopramide may be mixed with parenteral IV solutions. When administering prokinetic GI agents, the nurse should:

- Administer the oral dose 30 minutes before meals and at bedtime.

 Caution should be used in patients with a history of congestive heart failure, hypertension, renal impairment, mental depression, or Parkinson's disease.

 Metoclopramide is contraindicated for women during pregnancy and for children, with the exception of pediatric use in aiding small bowel intubation.

Caution should be used with nursing mothers who are receiving metoclopramide.

Methemoglobinemia in neonates may occur with overdosing.

 http://www.gerd.com/ http://www.rxmed.com/ prescribe.html

- Dilute IV doses above 10 mg or more in 50 ml of a parenteral solution and give slowly over 15 minutes or longer; 10 mg or less may be given over 1 to 2 minutes.
- Protect IV metoclopramide from light with aluminum foil or other protective covering.
- Monitor for EPS, which are most likely to occur early in the treatment, at high doses, in patients who are dehydrated, or in pediatric and young patients. Diphenhydramine HCL (Benadryl) or benztropine mesylate (Cogentin) may be given IM to reverse EPS.
- Monitor for tardive dyskinesia symptoms, including involuntary movements of the tongue, mouth or jaw, face, or extremities. Tardive dyskinesia is potentially irreversible. Metoclopramide may mask symptoms, which may make recognition of tardive dyskinesia more difficult. When symptoms occur, withhold metoclopramide and notify the health care provider.
- Encourage patients who are taking prokinetics to have adequate fluid intake.
- Advise the patient to avoid hazardous tasks (e.g., driving) for a few hours after taking metoclopramide because the agent may cause sedation and impair mental and physical abilities.
- Counsel the patient to avoid alcohol and other central nervous system (CNS) depressants, such as sedatives, hypnotics, narcotics, and tranquilizers, all of which may increase sedation.
- Monitor blood sugar and signs and symptoms of hypoglycemia. Insulin dose or administration schedule may require changing when hypoglycemia that is related to rapid transit of food through the GI tract occurs.

Do You UNDERSTAND?

DIRECTIONS: Fill in the blanks with the appropriate response.
1. Metoclopramide increases the tone in the _____.
2. Metoclopramide exerts an effect in the _____, thereby preventing nausea and vomiting.
3. EPS occur most frequently with the use of metoclopramide in
   _____.
4. Diphenhydramine HCL (Benadryl) given IM counteracts the symptoms of _____.

SECTION B
ANTIEMETICS, EMETICS, AND AGENTS USED FOR DIGESTIVE PROBLEMS

Antiemetic drugs are used to treat gastric mobility disorders, as well as nausea and vomiting. These drugs include phenothiazines, prokinetics, , serotonin antagonists, emetics, and acidifiers or digestive enzymes. The goal of treatment is to relieve symptoms and prevent serious nutritional and fluid-electrolyte deficits.

Answers: 1. esophageal sphincter; 2. CTZ; 3. first days of therapy; 4. EPS.

What IS a Phenothiazine?

Phenothiazines	Trade Name	Uses
prochlorperazine [pro-klor-PAIR-ah-zeen]	Compazine	Treatment of severe nausea and vomiting
promethazine [pro-METH-uh-zeen]	Phenergan	Treatment of motion sickness and nausea

Action

Phenothiazines block dopamine receptors in the CTZ. The CTZ is responsible for activating the vomiting reflex. Stimulation of the vomiting center produces reflex contraction of abdominal and respiratory muscles, relaxation of the cardiac sphincter in the stomach, and glottis closure. Dopamine, a potent neurotransmitter, is required for the conduction of impulses from excited afferent nerves to stimulate the medullary-vomiting center. Blocking dopamine receptors inhibits the stimulation of the vomiting center and an antiemetic effect results.

Phenothiazine drugs also block (to varying degrees) the neurotransmitters acetylcholine, histamine, and norepinephrine. Blocking a neurotransmitter or its receptor interrupts conduction of the nerve impulse across the synapse. Blocking acetylcholine, histamine, and norepinephrine receptors and the conduction of central and peripheral nerves across the synapse interrupts the impulse to vomit, resulting in an antiemetic effect.

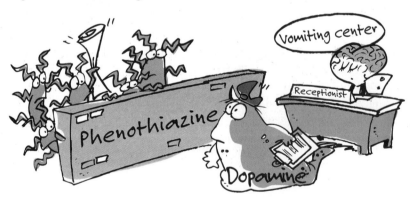

Uses

Phenothiazines are indicated for suppression of nausea and vomiting that is associated with varied noxious stimuli. Drugs in this classification are frequently considered first in the prevention and treatment of nausea and vomiting that are associated with anesthesia, antineoplastic therapy, radiation therapy, and motion sickness.

What You NEED TO KNOW

Contraindications/Precautions

Phenothiazines are contraindicated for patients with known hypersensitivity, depression, glaucoma, GI or genitourinary (GU) obstruction, and coma. Phenothiazines are also contraindicated for acutely ill and dehydrated patients.

Drug Interactions

Alcohol, nitrates, and antihypertensives cause increased hypotension when given with phenothiazines. CNS depressants (e.g., alcohol) produce additive CNS depression when given concurrently with phenothiazines. Antacids and antidiarrheal drugs reduce absorption of phenothiazines from the GI tract. The risk of granulocytosis is increased when phenothiazines are given with antithyroid drugs. Phenothiazines with lithium may present an increased risk of lithium toxicity. Beta blockers may increase the response to prochlorperazine. Phenobarbital increases the metabolism of prochlorperazine, thereby reducing its action. Prochlorperazine antagonizes the antihypertensive action of guanethidine.

Adverse Effects

Common adverse effects of phenothiazines include drowsiness, hypotension, and anticholinergic effects. Anticholinergic effects include dry mouth, flushing, blurred vision, tachycardia, photosensitivity, and constipation. Other adverse effects of phenothiazines include urine retention, darkened urine (pink to brown), anorexia, hypotension, hypertension, incoordination, respiratory depression, jaundice, leukopenia, agranulocytosis, and thrombocytopenia. Major adverse effects of phenothiazines include EPS, particularly with prolonged therapy. When phenothiazines block dopamine receptors, EPS that occur include prolonged muscle contraction, causing twisting, repetitive movements, or abnormal posture (**dystonia**), slow rhythmical movements (**tardive dyskinesia**), restlessness (**akathisia**), periorbital tremor, and tremors and rigidity (**pseudoparkinsonism**).

What You DO

Nursing Responsibilities

Phenothiazines may be administered orally, rectally, IV, or IM, depending on the desired speed of response and the condition of the patient. When administering phenothiazines, the nurse should:

- Mix oral prochlorperazine with 60 cc of fluids or soft food (e.g., tomato or fruit juice, milk, pudding) to disguise the taste and decrease GI distress.
- Monitor the patient for drug adverse effects, such as respiratory distress.

!   **Caution should be taken when phenothiazines are given to patients with cardiovascular disease, hypertension, asthma, breast cancer, and hepatic dysfunction.**

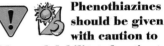 Phenothiazines are contraindicated for women during pregnancy and lactation and for children under 2 years of age.

!   **Phenothiazines should be given with caution to older and debilitated patients.**

Children under 12 are at increased risk for EPS, particularly when they become dehydrated, have chickenpox, or have a CNS infection.

!   **Although rare, agranulocytosis is an extremely serious adverse effect of phenothiazines. Extended use of chlorpromazine may lead to opacity of the lens of the eye.**

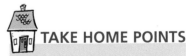 **TAKE HOME POINTS**

Tablets of prochlorperazine may be crushed to mix with food or liquids.

When skin comes in contact with prochlorperazine, wash hands immediately with soap and water.

Children and older adults are at an increased risk and should have ongoing assessment for EPS. Provide safety measures in assisting patients with ambulation, particularly older adults.

- Be aware that phenothiazines may depress the cough reflex and cause thickened secretions, placing the patient at risk for aspiration.
- Be aware that dehydrated persons are more likely to experience EPS.
- Teach patients to rise and change positions slowly to prevent orthostatic hypotension.
- Encourage adequate fluid intake for patients who are taking phenothiazines.
- Warn patients to report EPS (e.g., tremors, abnormal body movements).
- Evaluate complete blood count (CBC) periodically for ongoing phenothiazine therapy because blood dyscrasias may occur.
- Inform patients that an additive hypotensive effect occurs when taking phenothiazines concurrently with alcohol, antihypertensives, CNS depressants, or nitrates.
- Encourage patients to have an eye examination every 6 months for early detection of cataracts.
- Auscultate bowel sounds and monitor elimination patterns to prevent constipation.
- Avoid contact of prochlorperazine with the skin to prevent a rash and irritation.
- Instruct the patient to rinse the mouth frequently with water and suck on sugarless candy or ice chips to prevent drying of the oral mucosa.
- Encourage the patient to avoid driving or performing hazardous tasks until the response is known because prochlorperazine has a sedative effect.
- Instruct the patient to use sunscreen as protection against sunlight and to avoid prolonged exposure to prevent photosensitivity.
- Instruct patients to avoid altering the dose, changing the schedule, or discontinuing phenothiazine therapy without consulting the health care provider.

Do You UNDERSTAND?

DIRECTIONS: **Fill in the blanks with the appropriate response.**

1. An increased risk of what neurologic problem occurs with the use of phenothiazine?

2. What age groups are at increased risk of EPS should they become dehydrated?

3. To promote safe administration, what do phenothiazines block, thereby acting as antiemetics?

Answers: 1. EPS, tardive dyskinesia; 2. children and older adults; 3. dopamine and, to a varying degree, acetylcholine, histamine, and norepinephrine receptors.

What IS a Prokinetic?

Refer to page 269 for the discussion of prokinetics.

What IS a Serotonin Antagonist?

Serotonin Antagonists	Trade Names	Uses
granisetron [gran-ISS-eh-tron]	Kytril	Prevention of emetogenic chemotherapy
ondansetron [on-DAN-sih-tron]	Zofran	Prevention of emetogenic chemotherapy

Action

Antiemetics act as an antagonist of a selective serotonin receptor (5-HT3). Serotonin 5-HT3 receptors are located centrally in the CTZ and peripherally in the GI tract. When central serotonin receptors in the CTZ are blocked, the vomiting center is not activated, producing an antiemetic effect. Peripheral serotonin 5-HT3 receptors are located on the vagal nerve terminals in the upper GI tract. When serotonin is released from the walls of the small intestine, serotonin receptors transmit impulses on the vagal afferent nerve to initiate the vomiting reflex. Peripheral serotonin-receptor antagonists interrupt vagal impulse transmission, resulting in an antiemetic effect.

Uses

Serotonin antagonists are used to prevent nausea and vomiting that are associated with emetogenic cancer therapy. These agents are effective for initial and repeated courses of chemotherapy, including high-dose cisplatin. Serotonin antagonists are the most effective antiemetics for highly emetogenic anticancer drugs. Serotonin antagonists can also be used for postoperative nausea and vomiting.

What You NEED TO KNOW

Contraindications/Precautions

Serotonin antagonists are contraindicated for those with known hypersensitivity.

Drug Interactions

An increased risk of EPS is present when serotonin antagonists are taken with phenothiazines. Rifampin decreases ondansetron drug levels when given together.

 Granisetron requires cautious use for patients with liver disease.

 Cautious use of serotonin antagonists is advised during pregnancy and lactation. Ondansetron requires cautious use in children 2 years of age and younger.

Adverse Effects

Adverse effects of serotonin antagonists include headaches, drowsiness, fatigue, dizziness, agitation, insomnia, diarrhea, and constipation. Other adverse effects include rash, blurred vision, flushing, tachycardia, hypotension, hypertension, chest pain, dysrhythmias, and EPS. Granisetron may cause elevated liver enzymes. Additional adverse effects of ondansetron include seizures and bronchospasms.

What You DO

Nursing Responsibilities

Oral serotonin antagonist drugs have an onset of action in approximately 30 minutes, and IV has a rapid onset of 1 to 3 minutes. Duration of drug action for oral medications is 4 to 24 hours; the peak is 30 to 90 minutes. The granisetron IV dose regimen is initiated before chemotherapy to prevent the onset of nausea and vomiting. Similarly, orally administered drugs are given 30 to 60 minutes before chemotherapy. When administering serotonin antagonists, the nurse should:

- Monitor the patient's cardiovascular status for early detection of adverse effects of angina and tachycardia.
- Monitor fluid and electrolyte status resulting from the adverse effect of diarrhea.
- Monitor intake and output.
- Discuss methods of managing constipation with patients.
- Inform the patient that headache is a common adverse effect, which may require an analgesic for relief.
- Monitor liver function tests periodically. Elevated aspartate aminotransferase, alanine aminotransferase, or bilirubin levels return to normal within 2 weeks of serotonin antagonist withdrawal.

Do You UNDERSTAND?

DIRECTIONS: Indicate in the space provided whether the statement is *true* or *false*.

_____ 1. Serotonin antagonists rarely act as an effective antiemetic for highly emetogenic anticancer treatments.

_____ 2. Serotonin receptors of the 5-HT3 type are located centrally in the CTZ and peripherally in the GI tract.

_____ 3. Serotonin antagonists interrupt vagal impulse transmissions to the vomiting center, resulting in an antiemetic effect.

Answers: 1. false; 2. true; 3. true.

What IS a Miscellaneous Antiemetic?

Miscellaneous Antiemetics	Trade Names	Uses
dimenhydrinate [dye-men-HYE-dri-nate]	Dramamine	Treatment of motion sickness
diphenhydramine [dye-fen-HIGH-drah-meen]	Benadryl	Treatment of motion sickness
hydroxyzine [hye-DROX-ih-zeen]	Vistaril	Treatment of nausea and vomiting
droperidol [droh-PAIR-ih-dol]	Inapsine	Treatment of emetogenic chemotherapy
scopolamine [scoh-POLL-ah-meen]	Transderm-Scop	Treatment of motion sickness, preoperative nausea, and vomiting

Action

Dimenhydrinate depresses the labyrinth and vestibular function to decrease nausea and vomiting. Diphenhydramine competes for H_1-receptor sites, thereby blocking histamine release, prolonging dopamine action, and decreasing cholinergic activity. Hydroxyzine causes CNS depression and anticholinergic effects, the action of which controls emesis. Droperidol is classified as a butyrophenone that blocks dopamine-2 receptors in the CTZ, thereby suppressing emesis. The action of butyrophenones is similar to that of phenothiazines. Scopolamine exerts an anticholinergic effect to stop nausea and vomiting.

Uses

Several antihistamines are used for motion sickness and nausea control. Droperidol is a potent drug that is used for the control of chemotherapy-induced vomiting. Scopolamine, an anticholinergic drug, is also used for motion sickness and as a preanesthesia antiemetic.

What You NEED TO KNOW

Contraindications/Precautions

These antiemetics are generally contraindicated for patients with severe hypotension, glaucoma, prostatic hypertrophy, asthma, and GI obstruction.

Drug Interactions

Increased CNS depression may result when alcohol, CNS depressants, and monoamine oxidase inhibitors (MAOIs) are taken concurrently with dimenhydrinate and diphenhydramine. The anticholinergic effect is enhanced when tricyclic antidepressants are given together with dimenhydrinate, diphenhydramine, and hydroxyzine.

 These antiemetics are contraindicated for women during pregnancy and lactation and for children under 12 years of age.

 These antiemetics should be used with caution in older adults.

Antiemetics should be used with caution in patients with hypertension, hyperthyroidism, increased intraocular pressure, diabetes mellitus, cardiovascular disease, and seizure disorders.

Concurrent administration of dimenhydrinate and diphenhydramine may alter the results of skin tests.

Adverse Effects

These drugs may lead to adverse effects of drowsiness, dizziness, dry mouth, fatigue, headache, incoordination, blurred vision, restlessness, insomnia, tachycardia, hypotension, hypertension, and urinary frequency. Adverse effects of dimenhydrinate also include euphoria, confusion, anorexia, diarrhea, and constipation. Diphenhydramine may cause thickened secretions. Hydroxyzine may lead to wheezing. Droperidol may cause adverse effects that include EPS, respiratory depression, and bronchospasms.

What You DO

Nursing Responsibilities

When administering miscellaneous antiemetics, the nurse should:

- Provide safety for the patient who is taking these drugs because they cause sedation. Assist the patient with bed rails, and supervise ambulation for safety.
- Instruct the patient to avoid driving or performing hazardous activities because of the sedative effect.
- Advise the patient to avoid alcohol when taking these drugs to prevent oversedation.
- Instruct the patient and family to report EPS effects immediately (e.g., restlessness, facial grimacing, rigidity, tremors, involuntary movements).
- Monitor the patient's vital signs because of the adverse effects affecting blood pressure and heart rate.
- Instruct the patient that when a dose is missed, take the missed dose as soon as possible, except when it is nearly time for the next dose.
- Inform the patient that tablets may be crushed and capsules may be emptied and mixed with food or fluids.
- Warn the patient to check with the health care provider before taking OTC medications.
- Instruct the patient to report anorexia, persistent nausea, diarrhea, excess weight loss, aggression, and suicidal ideation.

TAKE HOME POINTS

Be prepared to treat EPS with anticholinergic drugs. Be prepared to treat hypotension with fluid therapy. The patient should avoid taking a doubled dose.

Do You UNDERSTAND?

DIRECTIONS: Complete the following statements with the appropriate terms from the italicized list provided.

1. Diphenhydramine is used as an antiemetic primarily for

_____.

2. Droperidol is used as an antiemetic primarily for

_____.

3. EPS may be an adverse effect of

_____.

emetogenic chemotherapy   *diphenhydramine*
motion sickness   *scopolamine*
preoperative nausea and vomiting   *hydroxyzine*
droperidol

What IS an Emetic?

Emetic	Trade Name	Use
ipecac [IP-eh-kak]	Ipecac Syrup	Treatment of oral poisoning or overdose

Action

Ipecac syrup, taken by mouth, is an OTC drug that stimulates the CTZ and acts directly on the gastric mucosa to stimulate vomiting.

Uses

Emetic drugs are used to expel toxic substances that may have been consumed by accident or overdose. The goal is to expel the toxic substance from the body before material is absorbed from the GI tract.

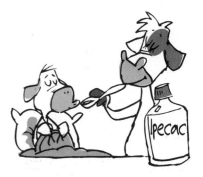

What You NEED TO KNOW

Contraindications/Precautions

Emetics are contraindicated for patients with cardiac dysfunction, hypersensitivity, severe inebriation, depressed gag reflex, and deep sedation, as well as those in shock and in a coma.

TAKE HOME POINTS

Vomiting should not be induced when caustic substances (e.g., ammonia, bleach, drain opener, lye, battery acid, gasoline, kerosene, lighter fluid) have been ingested.

The safe use of emetics in women during pregnancy and nursing mothers has not been established. The use of ipecac in infants under 6 months of age has not been established.

 Caution is advised when using an emetic in an anticonvulsant drug overdose victim because convulsions may be precipitated.

CNS stimulation, severe CNS depression, fatal respiratory depression, and circulatory collapse may occur with larger-than-normal doses.

TAKE HOME POINTS

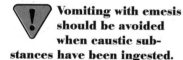
Follow ipecac with one to two glasses of water. Monitor vital signs, use side rails, and caution the patient to avoid ambulating without assistance.

Vomiting with emesis should be avoided when caustic substances have been ingested.

Drug Interactions

Milk and activated charcoal may inactivate ipecac. When ipecac is given together with carbonated beverages, abdominal distention may occur. Vegetable oil may delay the absorption of ipecac.

Adverse Effects

Adverse effects of ipecac include diarrhea, drowsiness, and mild GI upset. Adverse effects that may occur when ipecac is not vomited and is absorbed or when ipecac is overdosed include persistent vomiting, severe myopathy, tremors, cardiotoxicity, dysrhythmias, chest pain, bradycardia, tachycardia, hypotension, fatal myocarditis, depression, and coma.

What You DO

Nursing Responsibilities

The adult dose of ipecac should be followed with 8 to 16 oz of water. The dose may be repeated in 20 minutes as needed. Children over the age of 1 year should follow an oral dose with 6 to 8 oz of water. Children under 1 year of age should follow the dose with 4 to 8 oz of water. The dose may be repeated in 20 minutes in children. Regurgitating caustic substances may cause additional injury to the esophagus. When emesis is contraindicated, activated charcoal may be given. When administering emetics, the nurse should:

- Avoid storing ipecac syrup and ipecac fluid extract together. Ipecac fluid extract is 14 times stronger compared with ipecac syrup and has caused death when mistakenly given at the same dose as ipecac syrup. When the ipecac dose is not vomited and allowed to absorb, cardiotoxicity may occur. Activated charcoal may inactivate the ipecac.
- Caution parents and patients to be careful about confusing ipecac syrup with ipecac fluid extract.
- Teach families about the proper storage of ipecac, such as keeping it in a safe location and making it inaccessible to children.
- Counsel the patient to phone the emergency department or poison control center before using ipecac. Ipecac should be available in the home.
- Give ipecac before activated charcoal, not after.
- Prevent aspiration following emesis by positioning patients on their side.
- Use motion by gently bouncing the child patient to begin emesis. Emesis is reduced when lying still in a recumbent position.
- Teach parents about the proper procedure after ipecac has been given. When vomiting does not occur within 15 to 20 minutes, the health care provider should be contacted immediately and the dose of ipecac that was given should be recovered using gastric lavage and activated charcoal as needed.

Do You UNDERSTAND?

DIRECTIONS: Fill in the blanks with the appropriate responses.

1. List four CNS depression safety precautions.

_____

_____

_____

_____

2. Instruction on the proper storage of ipecac includes _____

_____

_____.

3. Before using ipecac, instruct the patient to phone the emergency department or _____.

What IS Acidifier-Digestive Enzyme?

Acidifier-Digestive Enzymes	Trade Names	Uses
pancreatin	Pancreatin	Replacement therapy for malabsorption syndrome
pancrelipase	Pancrease	Replacement therapy for malabsorption syndrome

Action

The action of pancreatic enzymes aids in the digestion of carbohydrate (CHO), fat, and proteins. The pancreas produces four digestive enzymes: lipase, amylase, trypsin, and chymotrypsin.

Pancrelipase is made from hog-porcine protein and is the preferred preparation because its enzyme activity is far greater than that of pancreatin. For example, the pancrelipase lipolytic enzyme activity is 12 times greater than that of pancreatin. Pancrelipase trypsin and amylase enzyme activities are four times greater than that of pancreatin. Enteric-coated preparations are preferred over conventional powders or tablets. Gastric pepsin and acid in the stomach may destroy conventional tablets. Enteric-coated preparations have an increased likelihood of dissolving in the duodenum, where pancreatic enzyme action is needed and most effective.

Uses

Pancreatic enzymes are used as replacement therapy when the body is producing and secreting insufficient amounts of pancreatic enzymes. Causes of deficiencies include disorders of the pancreas, such as pancreatitis, pancreatectomy, obstruction of the pancreatic duct, and cystic fibrosis.

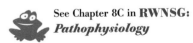

See Chapter 8C in RWNSG:
Pathophysiology

1. monitor vital signs, use side rails, caution the patient to avoid ambulating without assistance, have emergency equipment readily available; 2. placing the medication in a safe location (e.g., a locked cabinet) that is inaccessible to children; 3. poison control center.

What You NEED TO KNOW

Contraindications/Precautions

Pancrelipase is contraindicated for patients with acute pancreatitis.

Drug Interactions

The activity of pancreatic enzymes is decreased when given with H_2-blockers and calcium and magnesium antacids. Pancreatic enzymes decrease the absorption of iron when given concurrently.

Adverse Effects

Adverse effects of pancreatic enzymes that can occur with high doses include anorexia, ulcerative stomatitis, nausea, cramping, vomiting, diarrhea, and perianal irritation. Hyperuricemia and hyperuricosuria may also develop with high doses because of increased serum uric acid.

What You DO

Nursing Responsibilities

The dose of pancreatic enzyme is individualized and adjusted based on the degree of enzyme deficiency and the enzyme preparation that is selected. Pancreatic enzymes can be taken orally 1 to 2 hours before meals, with meals, 1 hour after meals, or with food eaten between meals. The amount of fat content in the diet determines the dose. Comparing fat intake with the amount of fat that is excreted in a 24-hour period indicates the effectiveness of treatment. When administering acidifiers, the nurse should:

- Educate patients on the proper use of pancreatic enzymes.
- Caution patients to avoid crushing or chewing enteric-coated preparations. Stomach acid or gastric pepsin may destroy pancreatic enzymes, thus an antacid or histamine-receptor blocker may be given before the enzyme to reduce gastric pH and protect the pancreatic enzyme from inactivation.
- Instruct the patient to follow pancreatic enzymes with a glass of water to ensure complete effectiveness.
- Counsel the patient to monitor weight loss and weight gain, intake and output, and quality of stools. Fatty stools indicate insufficiency of pancreatic enzyme. Adequate replacement decreases the number of bowel movements and improves stool consistency.
- Store pancreatic enzyme medication away from heat and light to protect the medication.
- Instruct patients to avoid changing brands without approval from their health care provider.

Cautious use of pancreatic enzymes is advised for persons with an allergy to hog protein or enzymes.

Safe use of pancreatic enzymes during pregnancy is not established.

Caution should be used with pancreatic enzymes during lactation.

Instruct patients to avoid crushing or chewing enteric-coated preparations of pancreatic enzymes.

Do You UNDERSTAND?

DIRECTIONS: Fill in the blanks with the appropriate response.

1. Instruct patients that enteric-coated preparations are not to be

_____.

2. _____ may be given
   before the enzyme to reduce gastric acid pH.

3. _____ indicate insufficiency
   of pancreatic enzyme.

SECTION C
LAXATIVE AND ANTIDIARRHEAL AGENTS

This section reviews the pharmacologic preparations that are used to treat constipation and diarrhea, thereby influencing GI motility. Many of these agents are nonprescription or OTC drugs that are purchased for self-medication, frequently requiring pharmacologic teaching from the nurse. This section explains stimulant, bulk, lubricant, and hyperosmotic laxatives, as well as stool softeners, antidiarrheals, and intestinal flora modifiers.

What IS a Stimulant Laxative?

Stimulant Laxatives	Trade Names	Uses
bisacodyl [BISS-uh-KOE-dill]	Dulcolax	Treatment of constipation and colon evacuation
cascara sagrada [cass-CARE-uh]	Cascara	Treatment of constipation and prevention of straining
senna [SEN-ah]	Senokot	Treatment of constipation and colon evacuation
castor oil	Neolid	Treatment of constipation
phenolphthalein [fee-nahl-THAY-leen]	Ex-Lax, Correctol	Treatment of constipation

Action

Stimulant laxatives irritate or stimulate the nerve plexus in the mucosa of the small intestine and colon to stimulate peristalsis and increase motility of the intestinal contents. The resulting stools of bisacodyl, phenolphthalein, cascara, and senna tend to be semi-soft, whereas castor oil produces a stool of watery consistency. Certain foods in the diet naturally contain organic acids that cause irritation of the intestinal mucosa and stimulation of peristalsis. These foods include prunes, raisins, figs, rhubarb, and pears.

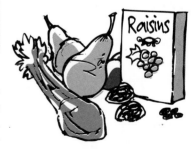

Answers: 1. crushed or chewed; 2. antacid or histamine-receptor blocker; 3. fatty stools.

Uses

Because stimulant laxatives produce defecation, they are used to treat constipation or to evacuate the bowel before radiologic examination or surgery. These drugs are frequently used for bowel retraining to reestablish normal elimination patterns in patients with spinal cord injury (SCI) or neurologic disorders. Stimulant laxatives may also be given to prevent straining after a myocardial infarction (MI) or GI surgery.

 # What You NEED TO KNOW

Contraindications/Precautions

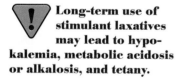
Stimulant laxatives are contraindicated for patients who are pregnant and lactating.

Stimulant laxatives are contraindicated for patients with hypersensitivity, undiagnosed abdominal pain, rectal fissures, ulcerated hemorrhoids, colon spasticity, Crohn's disease, ulcerative colitis, and other chronic inflammatory bowel diseases.

Because cascara sagrada contains alcohol, it should be avoided in patients with a known intolerance to alcohol.

Drug Interactions

The increased intestinal motility of stimulant laxatives allows quick passage and elimination from the GI tract. Increased GI motility reduces the absorption of other concurrently administered drugs, particularly sustained-release drugs.

Adverse Effects

Long-term use of stimulant laxatives may lead to hypokalemia, metabolic acidosis or alkalosis, and tetany.

Adverse effects to stimulant laxatives include nausea, vomiting, abdominal cramping, weakness, diarrhea, dehydration, and electrolyte imbalances. A burning sensation may occur after rectal administration of bisacodyl. After intestinal evacuation, a period may follow without bowel movements. This time lapse occurs to allow sufficient accumulation of fecal matter that is required for another evacuation. When large amounts of stimulant laxatives are taken, a potential for toxic absorption exists. The most common adverse effect after administering a stimulant laxative is abdominal cramping resulting from the increased peristalsis. Senokot may color urine and feces to a reddish or yellow-brown.

 # What You DO

Nursing Responsibilities

All stimulant laxatives can be given orally, although bisacodyl may also be given as a rectal suppository. The quick onset after rectal administration makes bisacodyl the drug of choice when surgery or procedures that require bowel cleansing need to be scheduled immediately. When administering stimulant laxatives, the nurse should:

 Inform patients that laxatives are to be taken as a short-term treatment, which avoids the development of laxative dependence.

 Counsel patients about appropriate dietary measures, environmental control, and exercise to encourage the return of normal bowel function.

 Inform patients that to promote optimal therapeutic action of oral laxatives, these drugs should be taken with a full glass of water and that tablets should not be chewed, but rather, swallowed whole to ensure reaching the GI tract for contact stimulation.

 Instruct the patient to report dizziness, confusion, sweating, or laxative dependence.

• Provide ready access to bathroom facilities and any necessary assistance with ambulation after laxative administration.

• Mix castor oil with fruit juice or carbonated drink to increase palatability.

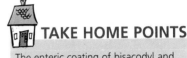

TAKE HOME POINTS

The enteric coating of bisacodyl and phenolphthalein is prematurely removed when taken concurrently within 1 hour of antacids or dairy products.

Do You UNDERSTAND?

DIRECTIONS: Fill in the blanks with the appropriate response.

1. What is the expected time frame of action of bisacodyl when given via rectal suppository?

2. What is the expected time frame of action of oral cascara?

3. Stimulant laxatives produce stools through what action?

4. Stimulant laxatives are used to treat patients with what?

What IS a Bulk Laxative?

Bulk Laxatives	Trade Names	Uses
psyllium [SILL-i-um]	Metamucil	Treatment of chronic constipation
polycarbophil [pol-i-CAR-boe-fill]	FiberCon	Prevention of straining and treatment of diarrhea

Action

Bulk laxatives combine with water in the intestine to form a gelatinous or viscous stool. The stool expansion causes the colon to distend and stimulate peri-

Answers: 1. 15 to 60 minutes; 2. 6 to 10 hours; 3. stimulating peristalsis; 4. constipation, bowel evacuation before surgery or studies, or bowel training regimen in patients with SCI or neurologic disorders.

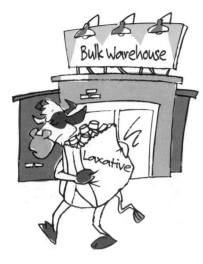

stalsis. This action increases intestinal motility and decreases stool transit time. Because the resultant stools are soft, they pass through the GI tract with ease with no trauma to rectal or anal tissues.

Bulk laxatives are indigestible, mild, and less apt to be habit-forming than are other laxatives. Because bulk laxatives evacuate only the descending colon, sigmoid colon, and rectum, the risk of laxative dependence is greatly reduced. This classification of laxatives does not interfere with the absorption of nutrients.

Uses

Bulk laxatives are useful in short-term treatment of constipation and long-term chronic constipation. Additionally, these agents are used to prevent constipation and straining, particularly after MI or rectal surgery.

What You NEED TO KNOW

Contraindications/Precautions

Bulk laxatives are contraindicated for patients with GI obstruction, acute abdominal pain, fecal impaction, rectal bleeding, and appendicitis, or those who have had bowel surgery or poisoning.

Drug Interactions

When taken concurrently with bulk laxatives, absorption of antibiotics, salicylates, warfarin, nitrofurantoin, and cardiac glycosides may be decreased.

Adverse Effects

Bulk forming laxatives may produce adverse effects of abdominal fullness, flatulence, and cramps. Hypersensitivity rarely occurs with administration of bulk natural laxatives. Excessive use of bulk laxatives may cause nausea, vomiting, and severe diarrhea. Serious adverse effects from bulk laxatives involve esophageal or intestinal obstruction.

What You DO

Nursing Responsibilities

Bulk laxatives, usually considered as the safest laxative, produce the same natural action as do 6 to 10 grams of dietary fiber per day. Fiber foods include cereals, bran, fresh fruits, and vegetables. When administering bulk laxatives, the nurse should:

- Monitor the patient for diarrhea because adequate hydration should be maintained.

Psyllium and poly-carbophil are contraindicated for women during pregnancy and lactation and for children under 3 years of age.

TAKE HOME POINTS

Bulk laxative administration must be accompanied with at least an 8-ounce glass of water to prevent esophageal or intestinal obstruction. Bulk laxative preparations contain sugar and may lead to elevated blood glucose levels with prolonged use.

Inform the patient that the laxative effect usually occurs in 12 to 24 hours and that 2 to 3 days may be required to establish regularity.

• Monitor blood glucose levels in patients with diabetes who take bulk laxatives.

Do You UNDERSTAND?

DIRECTIONS: Indicate in the space provided whether the statement is *true* or *false*.

_____ 1. Bulk laxatives irritate the intestinal mucosa.

_____ 2. Bulk laxatives should be avoided in patients following an MI.

_____ 3. Bulk laxatives should not be administered with water.

What IS a Lubricant Laxative?

Lubricant Laxative	Trade Name	Uses
Mineral oil	Kondremul Plain	Treatment of constipation and fecal impaction; prevention of straining

Action

Lubricant laxatives coat fecal material with a film, which prevents the reabsorption of water through the colon, and they soften the stool and lubricate the intestinal wall, which facilitates the smooth passage of feces. Mineral oil produces semi-soft stools.

Uses

These laxatives are used in the treatment of constipation or fecal impaction and to prevent straining following rectal surgery or an MI.

What You NEED TO KNOW

Contraindications/Precautions

Lubricant laxatives are contraindicated for patients with abdominal pain and intestinal obstruction.

Drug Interactions

Few drug interactions occur with mineral oil and concurrent medications. The absorption of food and fat-soluble vitamins (vitamins A, D, E, and K) may be reduced when administered with a lubricant laxative, which may necessitate

  Caution should be taken with mineral oil use in older and debilitated patients to avoid lipid pneumonia. Because of the decrease in fat-soluble absorption, mineral oil should be used cautiously during pregnancy.

Answers: 1. false; bulk laxatives expand intestinal feces with water, thereby distending the colon and stimulating peristalsis, which decreases transit time; **2.** false; bulk laxatives are used in patients after an MI to prevent straining; **3.** false; bulk laxatives should be given with an 8-ounce glass of water.

vitamin supplements. When stool softeners are given concurrently, the absorption of mineral oil may be increased.

Adverse Effects

The potential adverse effects following mineral oil include anorexia, nausea, vomiting, and nutritional deficiencies. When mineral oil droplets are aspirated, lipid pneumonia can occur. Repeated rectal administration can cause anal irritation from leakage. Prolonged use of mineral oil may lead to bowel-elimination dependence.

What You DO

Nursing Responsibilities

When administering lubricant laxatives, the nurse should:

- Administer mineral oil after the evening meal and before bedtime to avoid the loss of fat-soluble vitamins. When mineral oil is administered in the evening, it should be given at least 2 hours after meals to avoid interference with digestion of food. Because aspiration of mineral oil appears to be greatest during sleep, it should be given well before bedtime to prevent aspiration and resultant lipid pneumonia.
- Administer mineral oil to older and debilitated patients after placement in an upright position.
- Warn patients who are taking mineral oil that excessive use (longer than 2 weeks) can decrease absorption of fat-soluble vitamins, such as vitamins A, D, E, and K, and may require supplemental vitamins.
- Advise patients who take repeated rectal enemas of mineral oil that anal leakage can cause pruritus and soiling.

Instruct older and debilitated patients to maintain an upright position for at least 2 hours after administration.

Do You UNDERSTAND?

DIRECTIONS: Fill in the blanks with the appropriate response.

1. The action of a lubricant laxative involves _____ _____.

2. The best time to administer mineral oil is _____ _____.

3. The most serious adverse effect of mineral oil is _____ _____.

Answers: 1. coating feces with film, which softens stool and lubricates intestinal wall, facilitating stool passage; 2. 2 hours after the evening meal and well before bedtime; 3. aspiration with resultant lipid pneumonia.

What IS a Hyperosmotic Laxative?

Hyperosmotic Laxatives	Trade Names	Uses
magnesium hydroxide	Milk of Magnesia	Short-term treatment of occasional constipation
glycerin [GLI-ser-in]	Glycerol	Treatment of constipation
polyethylene glycol-electrolyte solution	GoLYTELY	Bowel evacuation
lactulose [LAK-tyoo-lose]	Cephulac	Treatment of chronic constipation and reduced ammonia

Action

Hyperosmotic laxatives are hypertonic drugs that draw water from surrounding tissues into the intestine, thereby creating an increased osmotic pressure in the bowel. The fluid moves from extracellular fluid compartments through the intestinal mucosa into the bowel. This additional fluid in the bowel changes stool consistency to liquid, which distends the bowel, stimulates stretch receptors, and stimulates peristalsis. As an osmotic agent, glycerin suppositories soften and lubricate feces and stimulate rectal contraction. Lactulose also promotes outward diffusion and elimination of ammonia in the feces, which promotes the reduction of blood ammonia levels. Lactulose also inhibits absorption of amines and acidifies bowel contents. Glycerin is not absorbed systemically. Lactulose is absorbed only slightly. Polyethylene glycol is nonabsorbable and does not alter electrolyte balance. Hyperosmotic laxatives that are absorbed include the magnesium preparations.

Uses

Hyperosmotic laxatives are used to treat constipation and cleanse the GI tract before surgery or examinations. Glycerin is used in bowel retraining to reestablish normal bowel function. Because of the increased transit time, saline laxatives are used as an adjunct treatment for poisoning and to treat parasitic infestations. Lactulose is also used to reduce high blood ammonia levels that are associated with portal system encephalopathy.

What You NEED TO KNOW

Contraindications/Precautions

Hyperosmotic laxatives are contraindicated for patients with nausea, vomiting, or undiagnosed abdominal pain. Magnesium preparations are contraindicated for patients with renal impairment. Sodium preparations are contraindicated for those who require sodium restriction (e.g., patients with edema and heart failure).

 Glycerin is contraindicated for women during pregnancy and lactation and for children.

 Glycerin should be given cautiously to older and dehydrated patients.

Glycerin should be given cautiously to patients with diabetes mellitus and cardiac, renal, or hepatic disease.

Drug Interactions

Hyperosmotic laxatives do not interact significantly with other concurrent drugs. Absorption of fluoroquinolones is decreased when given concurrently with magnesium preparations.

Adverse Effects

Adverse effects of glycerin include abdominal cramping, rectal irritation or burning, and hyperemia of rectal mucosa. Lactulose may cause nausea, vomiting, abdominal distention, flatulence, abdominal cramping, diarrhea, hypokalemia, hypovolemia, hyperglycemia, and increased hepatic encephalopathy. Adverse effects from hyperosmotic (**saline**) laxatives include weakness, lethargy, dehydration, hypernatremia, hypovolemia, hypermagnesemia, hyperphosphatemia, hypocalcemia, with resulting cardiac dysrhythmias and hypovolemic shock.

What You DO

Nursing Responsibilities

Oral hyperosmotic laxatives should not be given within 1 hour of other oral medications because the increased transit time of the laxatives will interfere with the absorption of other drugs. Glycerin is given via rectal suppository or enema when treating constipation. When administering hyperosmotic laxatives, the nurse should:

- Administer oral hyperosmotic laxatives with at least 8 ounces of water to prevent nausea.
- Administer polyethylene glycol electrolyte solutions orally over a 3-hour period and may be administered in 240 cc every 10 minutes. This administration should begin approximately 4 to 5 hours before the examination or procedure. When the patient is unable to take the polyethylene glycol orally, it may be administered through a nasogastric tube at a rate of 20 to 30 cc per minute.
- Monitor the patient's hydration carefully because of the potential risk of fluid and electrolyte imbalances. Fluids should be replaced as necessary.
- Instruct the patient to avoid activities that require mental alertness when drowsiness, weakness, or lethargy occurs.
- Advise the patient with diabetes who is taking lactulose to be aware of signs of hyperglycemia, which include polydipsia, polyphagia, polyuria, weakness, and drowsiness.
- Dilute lactulose with water or unsweetened juice before administration to decrease the sweetness and prevent nausea.
- Instruct the patient who is taking hyperosmotic laxatives to drink 8 to 13 glasses of fluid per day, unless contraindicated.
- Monitor the patient for hypermagnesemia (e.g., weakness, confusion, sedation).

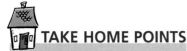

TAKE HOME POINTS

Polyethylene glycol is more palatable when given as a chilled solution. However, because of the large volume of a 4-liter dose, the patient should be monitored for hypothermia.

Do You UNDERSTAND?

DIRECTIONS: Complete the following statements with the appropriate terms from the italicized list provided.

1. The hyperosmotic laxative used primarily for GI cleansing before tests is
_____.

2. _____ is absorbed more than any other hyperosmotic laxative.

3. The most common adverse effect of continued use of hyperosmotic laxatives is _____.

glycerin	*magnesium preparations*
Golytely	*fluid overload*
lactulose	*electrolyte imbalance*

What IS a Stool Softener?

Stool Softeners	Trade Names	Uses
docusate sodium [DOK-yoo-sate]	Colace	Prevention of straining
docusate calcium [DOK-yoo-sate]	Surfak	Prevention of straining
docusate potassium [DOK-yoo-sate]	Dialose	Prevention of straining

Action

Docusate stool softeners are surface-active agents that emulsify and wet the stool by permitting water to penetrate and soften the stool for easier passage. As a surface-active agent, the effect of docusate is local (in the jejunum and colon) rather than systemic. Docusate softens the stool only and does not act as a laxative.

Uses

Stool softeners are drugs that are given to soften the stool to help in elimination. Docusate is indicated for constipation, painful anorectal conditions, cardiac, other conditions in which it is desirable to avoid straining and when laxatives are contraindicated.

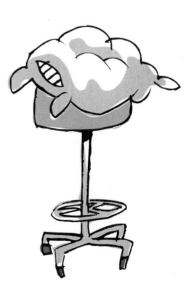

Answers: 1. Golytely; 2. magnesium preparations; 3. electrolyte imbalance.

What You NEED TO KNOW

Stool softeners are contraindicated during pregnancy.

Contraindications/Precautions

Stool softeners are contraindicated for patients with abdominal pain, fecal impaction, and intestinal obstruction. Docusate sodium is contraindicated for patients who are on sodium restriction. Docusate potassium is contraindicated for patients who have renal dysfunction.

Drug Interactions

Docusate may increase the systemic absorption of mineral oil when given together.

Adverse Effects

Few adverse effects occur following stool softener administration. A bitter taste, nausea, mild abdominal cramping, and diarrhea infrequently occur.

What You DO

Nursing Responsibilities

Docusate is available in capsules, tablets, syrup, and liquid. The dose should be adjusted to individual response. Liquid or syrup forms may be mixed with mild juice or infant's formula. Capsules and tablets must be given whole and not chewed or crushed. When administering stool softeners, the nurse should:

- Instruct patient that capsules and tablets should be swallowed whole and not chewed or crushed.
- Instruct patient to take the oral dose with a full glass of water, unless contraindicated.
- Monitor stools because the effect of the drug may take up to 3 days.
- Avoid concurrent use of mineral oil with docusate because systemic absorption of mineral oil may be increased.

Do You UNDERSTAND?

DIRECTIONS: Indicate in the space provided whether the statement is *true* or *false*. If false, then correct the statement to make it true using the margin at right.

_____ 1. Docusate acts by increasing bulk in the stool and increasing peristalsis.
_____ 2. The onset of action of docusate is 15 minutes when given orally.

Answers: 1. false; docusate increases the amount of water that is mixed in the stool thus making the stool softener and easier to pass; 2. false; the onset of oral docusate is 24 to 72 hours and 15 minutes when given as an enema.

_____ 3. Docusate may be indicated for the patient after rectal surgery.

_____ 4. Docusate tablets may be crushed and mixed with water to administer via a nasogastric tube.

What IS an Absorbent Antidiarrheal?

Absorbent Antidiarrheals	Trade Names	Uses
bismuth subsalicylate	Pepto-Bismol	Prevention and treatment of traveler's diarrhea
activated charcoal attapulgite	Kaopectate	Prevention of diarrhea
polycarbophil [pol-i-CAR-boe-fill]	FiberCon	Treatment of diarrhea and prevention of straining

Action

Absorbent antidiarrheals act by coating the GI mucosa, which absorbs water and toxic substances that cause diarrhea. Bismuth subsalicylate has two additional actions: (1) an added antiinflammatory action that is believed to decrease motility and the secretion of fluid and mucus into the colon by decreasing prostaglandin production and (2) an antimicrobial effect. The absorbent antidiarrheals have a local action with little or none being absorbed systemically, except bismuth subsalicylate, which is absorbed systemically.

Uses

Antidiarrheals are used for diarrhea, a common GI symptom characterized by frequent, watery stools. Diarrhea results from rapid transit of fecal material through the intestines and increased fluid in the stool. Causes of diarrhea include bacterial or viral enteritis, ulcerative colitis, psychogenic diarrhea, overuse of laxatives, Crohn's disease, irritable bowel disease, superinfections, bowel radiation, dietary intolerance, enteral feedings, and short-gut syndrome. Enteritis is the most frequent cause of diarrhea and can lead to fluid loss, dehydration, and electrolyte imbalance.

Absorbents are indicated for the adjunct treatment of diarrhea, in addition to identifying and eliminating the cause of the diarrhea. Bismuth subsalicylate may also be used in combination with antibiotics to treat ulcer disease caused by Helicobacter pylori. Indications for use of polycarbophil in diarrhea include patients with acute bowel syndrome, diverticulosis, irritable bowel, diarrhea caused by cholera, or following small-bowel surgery in which diarrhea may be a problem.

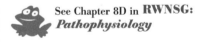

See Chapter 8D in **RWNSG:** *Pathophysiology*

Answers: 3. true; 4. false; docusate capsules and tablets should not be crushed or chewed; liquid docusate may be used.

What You NEED TO KNOW

Contraindications/Precautions

Use bismuth subsalicylate with caution in patients who are taking anticoagulant, diabetic, or gout medications. Cautious use of all antidiarrheals is indicated when diarrhea continues more than 2 days despite treatment or when a high fever is present with diarrhea.

Drug Interactions

Bismuth subsalicylate may decrease absorption when taken together with tetracyclines and quinolones. Serum salicylate levels are increased when taken with aspirin. Bismuth subsalicylate may increase the risk of bleeding when taken with heparin, warfarin, and thrombolytics. Activated charcoal and attapulgite may decrease absorption when given concurrently with oral medications. Polycarbophil may decrease absorption when given concurrently with oral antibiotics, warfarin, digoxin, nitrofurantoin, and salicylates.

Adverse Effects

Adverse effects are rare and mild, with abdominal fullness, diarrhea, and vomiting being the most common. Bismuth may cause temporary darkening of the stool.

What You DO

Nursing Responsibilities

Onset of action for the absorbent antidiarrheal agents varies but is generally approximately 1 day. Bismuth may be used prophylactically to prevent traveler's diarrhea in patients who are traveling to areas with poor sanitation. However, prophylactic use should be limited to 3 weeks. When administering absorbent antidiarrheals, the nurse should:

- Administer absorbent antidiarrheal agents at least 2 hours before or after other oral drugs.
- Instruct the patient to avoid using antidiarrheals for longer than 2 days or in the presence of high fever.
- Encourage fluid intake when taking absorbents to prevent dehydration.
- Monitor and record the number and consistency of stools, intake and output, and bowel sounds. Bismuth may cause temporary darkening of stools and mouth. However, darkened stools should not be confused with melena.
- Thoroughly shake bismuth suspensions before administration. Tablets should be chewed or allowed to dissolve in the mouth before swallowing. Caplets

  Bismuth subsalicylate and polycarbophil are contraindicated for pregnant and lactating women. Because bismuth subsalicylate contains salicylate, it is contraindicated for children and adolescents who have or are recovering from viral infections (because of the danger of Reye's syndrome) or in patients with an allergy to aspirin or other salicylates.

 The use of bismuth should be made cautiously in children under 3 years of age.

Use bismuth subsalicylate with caution in patients who are taking anticoagulant, diabetic, or gout medications. Cautious use of all antidiarrheals is indicated when diarrhea continues longer than 2 days despite treatment or when a high fever is present with diarrhea.

TAKE HOME POINTS

When diarrhea persists longer than 2 days, the health care provider should be consulted. Inform the patient that stools will be black when using charcoal. Bismuth may interfere with radiographic examinations of the GI tract because bismuth is radiopaque.

should be swallowed whole. Regular- and extra-strength attapulgite tablets must be swallowed whole. Polycarbophil tablets should be crushed or chewed before swallowing. Charcoal can be mixed with fruit juice or chocolate powder to improve the taste.

🍎 Instruct patient to avoid other salicylates unless directed by the health care provider because many OTC medications contain salicylates.

 http://www.nlm.hih.gov/ medlineplus/pepticulcer. html

http://niddk.nih.gov/health/ digest/pubs/hpylori/hpylori. htm#7

http://www.mayohealth.org/mayo/ 9909/htm/peptic.htm

http://pharminfo.com/pubs/msb/ tritec.html

Do You UNDERSTAND?

DIRECTIONS: Match each description in Column A with the correct drug in Column B. You may use an answer more than once.

Column A

_____ 1. A bulk laxative that is also used for the treatment of diarrhea.

_____ 2. A GI absorbent that is similar to kaolin and pectin combinations.

_____ 3. Contains subsalicylate.

_____ 4. Is frequently used in combination with other drugs to treat *Helicobacter pylori* infection.

_____ 5. An absorbent that is most commonly used in poisonings.

Column B

a. Attapulgite (Kaopectate)
b. Bismuth (Pepto-Bismol)
c. Activated charcoal
d. Polycarbophil (FiberCon)

 # What IS an Opioid and Opioid-Derivative Antidiarrheal?

Opioid and Opioid-Derivative Antidiarrheals	Trade Names	Uses
paregoric (opium tincture) [par-ih-GOR-ik]	Paregoric	Short-term treatment of diarrhea
diphenoxylate with atropine [dye-fen-OX-ih-late]	Lomotil	Treatment of diarrhea
loperamide [low-PER-a-mide]	Imodium	Treatment of diarrhea

Action

Opioid and opioid-derivative antidiarrheals are systemic drugs that decrease GI motility, prolong transit time, decrease fluid secretion into the bowel, and allow fluid and electrolytes to be reabsorbed because of the increased time that the stool remains in the colon. Most of the opioid and opioid-derivative antidiarrheals are rapidly and thoroughly absorbed after oral administration, except tincture of opium and loperamide hydrochloride, which have variable absorption. Peak plasma levels occur within 40 minutes to 5 hours, depending on the drug.

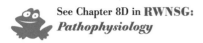

See Chapter 8D in **RWNSG:** *Pathophysiology*

Uses

Opioid and opioid-derivative antidiarrheals are the mainstay of treatment for moderate to severe diarrhea. Indications for use include acute diarrhea, acute exacerbations of chronic diarrhea, and for reduction of fecal volume from ileostomies.

What You NEED TO KNOW

 Opioid and opioid-derivative antidiarrheals are contraindicated for children under 2 years of age.

Contraindications/Precautions

Contraindications for all types of opioid antidiarrheals are a known sensitivity to the drug, obstructive jaundice, diarrhea in pseudomembranous colitis, and diarrhea that is associated with microorganisms that penetrate intestinal mucosa, such as Escherichia coli, Salmonella, or Shigella; chronic ulcerative colitis; and acute dysentery.

Drug Interactions

When diphenoxylate is given together with MAOIs, hypertensive crisis may occur. Diphenoxylate may increase the effects of barbiturates, tranquilizers, narcotics, and alcohol when taken together with these drug classifications.

Adverse Effects

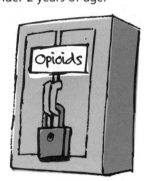

Adverse effects of the opioids include nausea, vomiting, dry mouth, dizziness, drowsiness, and headache. Overdosing effects include CNS depression, dryness of the skin and mucous membranes, nystagmus, pinpoint pupils, and respiratory depression. Respiratory depression may not be apparent initially but may occur up to 30 hours after overdose. Nearly all of the opioid and opioid derivatives are controlled substances, with the exception of loperamide. Camphorated opium tincture and tincture of opium remain available for clinical use but are not recommended and are less commonly used than are the synthetic opium derivatives.

Caution should be used in women during pregnancy and lactation.

Caution should be used in patients with prostatic hypertrophy, narrow-angle glaucoma, and liver disease.

What You DO

Nursing Responsibilities

The response to opioid antidiarrheals should be noticeable 48 hours after treatment begins. Opioid antidiarrheal agents are not innocuous drugs and are not intended for prolonged use. When administering opioid antidiarrheals, the nurse should:

🍎 Instruct the patient to reduce the dose after initial control of diarrhea. When no response is apparent, these agents will likely be ineffective and should be discontinued.

 TAKE HOME POINTS

Opioid antidiarrheal agents, with the exception of loperamide, are controlled substances and may have abuse potential that leads to dependence.

- Warn patients to follow dose recommendations and to avoid exceeding the maximal daily dose.
- Inform patient that drowsiness may be an adverse effect and that hazardous activities should be avoided.
- Monitor and record the patient's intake and output, number and consistency of stools, and bowel sounds.
- Instruct patient to notify the health care provider when a high fever develops, diarrhea persists, or when blood is noted in the stool.
- Warn the patient to avoid exceeding the recommended daily dose.
- Inform patients that diphenoxylate hydrochloride with atropine sulfate tablet may be crushed.
- Closely monitor patient with ulcerative colitis for abdominal distention and other GI symptoms, which may indicate toxic megacolon.
- Avoid confusing the two preparations of opium. Deodorized opium tincture contains 25 times more anhydrous morphine than does camphorated opium tincture. Similar to large doses of any narcotic, the respiratory depressant effects of an overdose may last longer than does an antagonist that is given to reverse effects. Monitor the patient for respiratory depression!

Avoid diphenoxylate hydrochloride with atropine sulfate use in patients who are taking MAOIs. This combination may cause a hypertensive crisis.

Do You UNDERSTAND?

DIRECTIONS: Fill in the blanks with the appropriate response.

1. _____ and _____ cross the placenta, causing an effect on the fetus.
2. Some of the adverse effects of diphenoxylate HCl (Lomotil) and difenoxin (Motofen) are a result of the addition of _____ sulfate to discourage abuse.
3. Opioid antidiarrheals _____ GI motility and _____ water reabsorption in the colon.
4. Adverse effects of opioid antidiarrheals include _____.
5. Opioid antidiarrheals should be discontinued after _____ when no improvement in diarrhea is noted.

What IS an Intestinal Flora Modifier?

Intestinal Flora Modifier	Trade Names	Uses
Lactobacillus acidophilus [LACK-tol-bah-SILL-us AS-id-off-ill-us]	Acidophilus Lactobacillus Lactinex	Prevent and treat superinfections

Answers: 1. camphorated opium tincture (Paregoric), tincture of opium; 2. atropine; 3. decrease; increase; 4. nausea, vomiting, drowsiness, sedation, headache, and dry mouth; 5. 2 days.

Action

Intestinal flora modifiers are bacterial cultures that contain lactobacillus acidophilus or lactobacillus bulgaricus. These agents are given to help augment or to replace the usual normal flora and to reestablish intestinal flora balance.

Numerous bacteria are normally present in the GI tract, particularly in the colon. Bacteria in the colon help to digest small amounts of cellulose and help form vitamin K, vitamin B_{12}, thiamin, and riboflavin. An additional byproduct is the production of gases in the bowel. The presence of favorable bacteria helps prevent an overgrowth of unfavorable bacteria in the colon. Following administration of antibiotics or after diarrhea, the normal flora of the intestine may be altered, leading to additional diarrhea and gas.

Uses

Indications for use are to assist in the restoration and maintenance of the normal flora of the oral and intestinal tracts. Unlabeled uses include the treatment of uncomplicated diarrhea, small ulcers of the mouth resulting from antibiotic use or other causes, and herpetic stomatitis.

 # What You NEED TO KNOW

Contraindications/Precautions

Contraindications include an allergy to milk and sensitivity to lactose.

Drug Interactions

No drug interactions have been notes for *Lactobacillus acidophilus*.

Adverse Effects

Adverse effects with *Lactobacillus acidophilus* are few. In patients with milk product allergies or intolerance, administration of *Lactobacillus acidophilus* may cause similar symptoms of bloating, cramps, diarrhea, and flatulence. Because *Lactobacillus acidophilus* may cause the same symptoms as those found in lactose-intolerant patients, genetic and cultural differences may be present in adverse effects that are associated with the administration of the supplement.

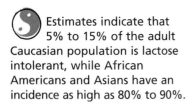 Safe and effective use in children under 3 years of age has not been established.

Estimates indicate that 5% to 15% of the adult Caucasian population is lactose intolerant, while African Americans and Asians have an incidence as high as 80% to 90%.

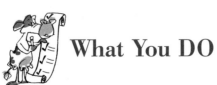 # What You DO

Nursing Responsibilities

Lactobacillus is an OTC oral nutritional supplement and is available in capsules, granules, chewable tablets, or powder. Recommended frequency of administration is one to four times daily. These agents should not be used for more than 2 days or in the presence of high fever, unless directed by health care provider. When administering miscellaneous antidiarrheal agents, the nurse should:

- Mix granules with cereal, food, milk, fruit juice, or water to increase palatability.
- Check the label or with the pharmacy to determine storage requirements. Most forms must be refrigerated to prevent contamination.
- Instruct the patient to notify the health care provider when bloating, cramps, flatulence, or diarrhea occur.

Do You UNDERSTAND?

DIRECTIONS: Match the following statements in Column A with the correct responses in Column B.

Column A

_____ 1. Lactobacillus may cause this adverse effect in lactose intolerant patients.

_____ 2. Lactose intolerance occurs frequently in patients of this racial or ethnic group.

_____ 3. *Lactobacillus acidophilus* is indicated for use with patients with this condition.

_____ 4. Prolonged antibiotic therapy may have this effect.

Column B

a. Constipation
b. European
c. Flatulence
d. Decrease of bacteria in the colon
e. Vomiting
f. African American
g. Sore mouth

Answers: 1. c; 2. f; 3. g; 4. d.

CHAPTER

9

Drugs Affecting the Genitourinary Tract and Renal Disorders

Urinary tract problems:

Antimicrobials
Antiseptic agents,
Antispasmodics,
Analgesics

SECTION A

AGENTS USED IN URINARY TRACT DISORDERS AND TO IMPROVE RENAL OUTPUT

This chapter reviews the use of pharmacologic methods that are used for urinary tract disorders, including the use of diuretic agents. Diuretics are classified according to their chemical structure and their site of action. Diuretics that are classified based on their chemical structure include thiazides, thiazide-like diuretics, and potassium-sparing diuretics. Diuretics that act on the proximal tubules include thiazides. Loop diuretics act primarily on the ascending loop of Henle. Diuretics that act on the distal tubules include potassium-sparing diuretics. Drugs that are used to treat urinary tract (UT) disorders (e.g., UT infections, neurogenic bladder) include antimicrobial antiseptics and antispasmodic analgesics.

What IS a Urinary Tract Antimicrobial Antiseptic?

Urinary Tract Antimicrobial Antiseptics	Trade Names	Uses
Fluoroquinolones		
ciprofloxacin *[sip-row-FLOX-ah-sin]*	Cipro	Treatment of urinary tract infection
ofloxacin *[oh-FLOX-ah-sin]*	Floxin	Treatment of urinary tract infection, prostatitis
Sulfonamides		
sulfisoxazole *[sul-fih-SOX-ah-zole]*	Gantrisin	Treatment of severe urinary tract infection

Continued

Urinary Tract Antimicrobial Antiseptics—cont'd	Trade Names	Uses
trimethoprim-sulfamethoxazole [tri-METH-oh-prim sul-fa-meth-ox-ah-zole]	Bactrim	Treatment of severe urinary tract infection
Urinary tract antiseptics methenamine [meh-THEEN-ah-meen]	Urised	Prevention of urinary tract infection
nalidixic acid [nah-lih-DIX-ik]	NegGram	Treatment of urinary tract infection
nitrofurantoin [NYE-troh-FYOOR-an-toyn]	Macrodantin	Treatment of urinary tract infection

Action

UT antimicrobial antiseptic agents act in various ways and are effective against different organisms. Fluoroquinolones are potent, broad-spectrum bactericidal drugs that inhibit deoxyribonucleic acid (DNA) gyrase (an enzyme that is needed for bacterial replication and protein synthesis). These drugs also exhibit postantibiotic effects, indicating that bacterial growth does not occur for several hours after drug exposure and a shorter dose regimen can be used for treating a urinary tract infection (UTI).

Sulfonamides are broad-spectrum antiinfectives that have a bacteriostatic effect. These agents interfere with the synthesis of purines and DNA in the organism. As broad-spectrum antimicrobials, sulfonamides are clinically effective against several pathogens.

UT antiseptics are bactericidal agents that inhibit primarily DNA replication and protein synthesis. Methenamine decomposes into ammonia and formaldehyde within the urine. High levels of formaldehyde kill the bacteria that are present in the urine. Although UT antiseptics exert antibacterial action on the urine, they have little or no systemic antibacterial action.

Uses

Selection of a UT antimicrobial antiseptic agent depends primarily on results of a urinalysis in addition to a culture and a sensitivity test. The primary UT antimicrobial agents that are used to treat UTIs are fluoroquinolones and sulfonamides. Additionally, fluoroquinolones are used for the treatment of lower respiratory tract, skin, bone, joint, and gastrointestinal (GI) infections, as well as gonorrhea.

Sulfonamides are frequently used for treatment of UTIs resulting from community-acquired microorganisms (e.g., *Escherichia coli*, *Klebsiella*, *Enterobacter*). Sulfonamides are ideal for patients with a first-time UTI because of their ease of administration, effectiveness, low cost, and safety. When sulfamethoxazole is combined with trimethoprim (a synthetic antiinfective), it is used to treat severe UTIs. The combined drug is also more effective in delaying drug resistance than when they are given separately.

The antiseptics are clinically effective with several microorganisms and are frequently used to treat UTIs.

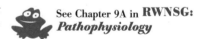

See Chapter 9A in RWNSG: *Pathophysiology*

What You NEED TO KNOW

 Antimicrobial antiseptics should be avoided in women during pregnancy and lactation and in children.

Cautious use of antimicrobial antiseptics is advised for patients with hepatic or renal impairment. Caution should be used with fluoroquinolones for patients with seizures, psychosis, and increased intracranial pressure (ICP). Sulfonamides should be used with caution for patients with asthma and blood dyscrasias. UT antiseptics should be used cautiously for patients with diabetes mellitus, electrolyte imbalances, vitamin B deficiency, and debilitation.

Hematologic life-threatening adverse effects include aplastic and hemolytic anemia, hypoprothrombinemia, thrombocytopenia, and agranulocytosis. Hypersensitivity adverse effects range from mild skin reactions of rash, itching, and burning to severe anaphylactic shock.

Contraindications/Precautions

Antimicrobial antiseptics are contraindicated for patients with hypersensitivity. Sulfonamides are also contraindicated for patients with porphyria and GI and genitourinary (GU) obstruction.

Drug Interactions

Theophylline levels are elevated 15% to 30% when administered with ciprofloxacin. When ciprofloxacin is given with warfarin, the prothrombin time (PT) level is increased, and when given with phenytoin, the phenytoin level is decreased. Sulfonamides increase the risk of hypoprothrombinemia when given with oral anticoagulants. The risk of hypoglycemia is increased when sulfisoxazole and sulfonylureas are given together. The absorption of nitrofurantoin and ciprofloxacin is decreased when given with antacids, sucralfate, and iron. When methenamine is given with acetazolamide and sodium bicarbonate, the conversion into formaldehyde may be prevented, thereby decreasing its action.

Adverse Effects

Adverse effects for most antimicrobial antiseptics include nausea, vomiting, diarrhea, constipation, gastric distress, and crystalluria. Other adverse effects include headache, dizziness, drowsiness, photosensitivity, fatigue, seizures, stomatitis, and hepatitis.

Insomnia, chest pain, edema, hypertension, euphoria, hallucinations, extrapyramidal symptoms (EPS), such as repetitive and abnormal movements, restlessness, rigidity, and neuroleptic malignant syndrome (NMS), which is a potentially fatal condition, with altered mental status, muscle rigidity, irregular pulse, tachycardia, blood pressure (BP) fluctuations, and sweating, have occurred from ofloxacin. Other sulfisoxazole adverse effects include pancreatitis, acute psychosis, and Stevens-Johnson syndrome. Pseudomembranous enterocolitis may be an adverse effect of trimethoprim-sulfamethoxazole. Seizures have been noted following nalidixic acid therapy.

What You DO

Nursing Responsibilities

Primarily, antimicrobial antiseptics are administered orally, but several of these agents can also be given intravenously (IV), depending on the purpose of administration and the condition of the patient. When administering antimicrobial antiseptics, the nurse should:

- Dilute IV ciprofloxacin adequately (1 to 2 mg/ml) and infuse slowly over 60 minutes. Ofloxacin should also be diluted (4 mg/ml).
- Administer antacids, sucralfate, and iron at least 4 hours apart from fluoroquinolones to ensure absorption.
- Assess fluid intake, urine output, and urine pH.
- Administer nitrofurantoin with food to decrease GI distress.
- Dilute nitrofurantoin in water or juice and instruct the patient to rinse the mouth thoroughly after taking medication.
- Monitor theophylline levels for patients who are taking theophylline and ciprofloxacin.
- Monitor renal and hepatic function studies for necessary dose adjustment.
- Assist the susceptible female patient in planning alternative contraception because oral contraceptives may be unreliable when taking sulfonamides.
- Monitor blood glucose in patients with diabetes who are taking sulfonamides for detection of hypoglycemia.
- Encourage patients to avoid driving or performing hazardous tasks until the response is known because these drugs have a sedative effect.
- Teach the patient to use sunscreen protection against sunlight and avoid prolonged exposure to sunlight to prevent photosensitivity.
- Instruct the patient who is taking nalidixic acid to report visual disturbances, particularly during the first few days of therapy. This adverse effect usually disappears with dose reduction or discontinuation.
- Monitor the complete blood count (CBC) for patients who are taking antimicrobial antiseptic drugs for early detection of blood dyscrasias.
- Advise the patient to report sore throat, fatigue, joint pains, pallor, bleeding, and jaundice for early detection of blood dyscrasias.
- Monitor the patient who is taking ofloxacin for early detection of EPS and NMS adverse effects and report these to the health care provider.
- Counsel the patient who is taking nalidixic acid to report vomiting, irritability, headache, insomnia, excitement, drowsiness, and mental depression.
- Instruct the patient who is taking antibiotics to report milky urine, foulsmelling urine, and perineal irritation for early detection of superinfections.
- Warn the patient to avoid alcohol with these drugs.

Do You UNDERSTAND?

DIRECTIONS: Provide the appropriate responses to the following questions.

1. To ensure safety, the nurse should be aware of the increased risk of what neurologic problem with the use of nalidixic acid?

2. Absorption of nitrofurantoin and ciprofloxacin is decreased when taken with what?

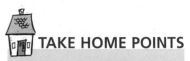

TAKE HOME POINTS

Do not administer IV ciprofloxacin with other concurrent IV medications. Monitor urine pH daily because crystalluria may occur with an altered pH.

⚠️ Do not crush nitrofurantoin tablets to prevent staining of teeth. Do not give theophylline and caffeine within at least 2 to 4 hours of ciprofloxacin because this drug combination may lead to central nervous system (CNS) stimulation (e.g., tachycardia, anxiety, nervousness, insomnia).

Provide safety measures in assisting patients with ambulation, particularly older adults.

Answers: 1. seizure, dizziness, drowsiness; 2. antacids.

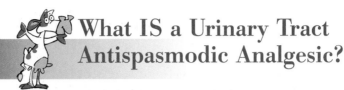

What IS a Urinary Tract Antispasmodic Analgesic?

Urinary Tract Antispasmodic Analgesics	Trade Names	Uses
Urinary tract antispasmodics		
flavoxate [fla-VOX-ate]	Urispas	Treatment of dysuria, nocturia, and incontinence
oxybutynin [ox-ee-BYOO-tih-nin]	Ditropan	Treatment of neurogenic bladder
Urinary tract analgesic		
phenazopyridine [fen-az-oh-PEER-ih-deen]	Pyridium	Treatment of cystitis

Action

Flavoxate acts as a parasympatholytic agent with papaverine-like activity on the detrusor muscles in the bladder. This antispasmodic effect increases bladder capacity in patients with spastic bladder. Oxybutynin acts as a parasympatholytic agent. This drug, classified as a synthetic amine with a prominent antispasmodic effect, directly inhibits the muscarinic effects of acetylcholine on smooth muscles of the bladder.

The analgesic action for phenazopyridine is unclear. The Azo dye of phenazopyridine has a direct anesthetic effect on the urinary mucosa with little or no antiinfective action.

Uses

UT antispasmodic drugs are used to treat a variety of symptoms, such as dysuria, urgency, nocturia, suprapubic pain, frequency, and incontinence. Oxybutynin is used to relieve symptoms that are associated with neurogenic bladder and to provide relief after transurethral surgery. UT analgesics are used to relieve discomfort that is associated with UTIs. The primary UT analgesic drug is phenazopyridine, which is also used in the treatment of cystitis.

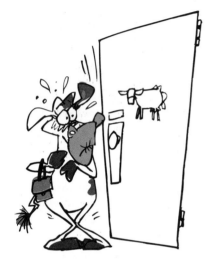

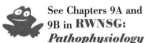

See Chapters 9A and 9B in **RWNSG:** *Pathophysiology*

What You NEED TO KNOW

Contraindications/Precautions

Antispasmodic analgesics are contraindicated for patients with glaucoma, GI or GU obstruction, and ileus. Flavoxate is contraindicated for patients with GI bleeding. Oxybutynin is contraindicated for patients with glaucoma, myasthenia gravis, severe colitis, megacolon, and cardiovascular disorders. Phenazopyridine is contraindicated for patients with GI inflammation or bleeding, renal impairment, and severe hepatitis.

Antispasmodic analgesics are contraindicated for women during pregnancy and lactation and for children under 12 years of age.

Drug Interactions

No drug interactions have been noted for flavoxate, oxybutynin, and phenazopyridine.

Adverse Effects

Adverse effects of UT antispasmodic analgesic drugs include headache, dizziness, drowsiness, mental confusion, insomnia, restlessness, nausea, vomiting, dry mouth, constipation, dysuria, hyperpyrexia, heart palpitations, blurred vision, and tachycardia. Hypersensitivity reactions, urinary hesitancy, retention, and impotence may also occur. Flavoxate and oxybutynin may lead to the adverse effects of jaundice and increased intraocular pressure. Eosinophilia has occurred from flavoxate. Other adverse effects from oxybutynin are fatigue, fever, decreased sweating, psychotic behavior, and suppression of lactation. Hemolytic anemia, renal stones, and acute renal failure may result from prolonged use of phenazopyridine.

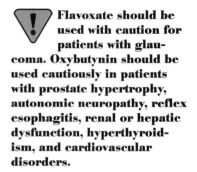

Cautious use is advised when treating older adults.

Flavoxate should be used with caution for patients with glaucoma. Oxybutynin should be used cautiously in patients with prostate hypertrophy, autonomic neuropathy, reflex esophagitis, renal or hepatic dysfunction, hyperthyroidism, and cardiovascular disorders.

What You DO

Nursing Responsibilities

Antispasmodic analgesics are only given orally. Flavoxate may be taken without regard to meals. Phenazopyridine may be taken with meals or after meals to decrease the GI distress. When administering antispasmodic analgesics, the nurse should:

- Confirm a diagnosis of neurogenic bladder before initiating oxybutynin treatment.
- Monitor vital signs of the patient who is taking flavoxate and oxybutynin for early detection of adverse effects and alert the health care provider.
- Caution the patient who is taking flavoxate to avoid activities requiring alertness (e.g., driving) until the response is known.
- Discontinue antispasmodic analgesic drugs when dysuria subsides, which is generally 3 to 15 days.
- Instruct the patient to report to health care provider immediately when jaundice (i.e., yellow skin discoloration) develops, which indicates liver impairment.
- Instruct the patient to wear protective clothing because phenazopyridine may change urine to an orange-red color and stain fabrics.
- Monitor the patient's CBC for early detection of blood dyscrasias.
- Assess the patient for adequate intake and output.
- Warn the patient who is taking oxybutynin to avoid hot environments.

 TAKE HOME POINTS

Teach patients who are taking flavoxate to take their apical pulse for 1 full minute and report tachycardia to the health care provider. Inform the patient that phenazopyridine may cause staining of contact lenses. Because of the decreased sweating adverse effect of oxybutynin, fever or heat stroke may occur in a hot environment.

Do You UNDERSTAND?

DIRECTIONS: Match the following statements in Column A with the appropriate responses in Column B.

Column A	Column B
_____ 1. Route of administration of antispasmodics	a. Orally
_____ 2. Side effect of oxybutynin	b. Subcutaneously
_____ 3. Side effect of pyridium	c. UT obstruction
_____ 4. Contraindication of flavoxate	d. Orange-red urine
	e. Abdominal pain

What IS a Loop Diuretic?

Loop Diuretics	Trade Names	Uses
furosemide [fur-OH-see-mide]	Lasix	Treatment of edema
bumetanide [byoo-MET-ah-nide]	Bumex	Treatment of edema

Action

Loop diuretics are classified based on their site of action in the nephrons of the kidneys. Loop diuretics inhibit sodium and chloride reabsorption through direct action primarily in the ascending loop of Henle but also in the proximal and distal tubules. Inhibiting sodium and chloride reabsorption causes potassium and magnesium loss. Phosphate and bicarbonate reabsorption is also inhibited. At the usual diuretic doses, loop diuretics produce only mild antihypertensive effects. The bumetanide diuretic action is 40 times greater than the action of furosemide.

Uses

Loop diuretics are used to treat edema that involves fluid volume excess resulting from a number of disorders of the heart, liver, or kidney (e.g., pulmonary edema, CHF, nephrotic syndrome, hepatic cirrhosis).

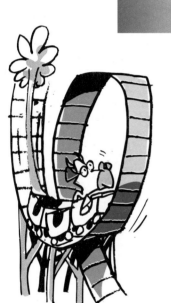

See Chapter 5E in RWNSG:
Pathophysiology

What You NEED TO KNOW

Contraindications/Precautions

Loop diuretics are contraindicated for patients with hypersensitivity to the specific drug or sulfonamides, severe adrenocortical impairment, anuria, progressive oliguria, fluid and electrolyte depletion, and hepatic coma.

 Furosemide and bumetanide are contra-indicated during pregnancy.

Drug Interactions

Digitalis toxicity may result when loop diuretics are given concurrently with digoxin and other potassium-depleting drugs (e.g., corticosteroids, amphotericin B). Lithium toxicity may result from its decreased elimination when given together with loop diuretics. When bumetanide is given with cisplatin and aminoglycosides, the risk of ototoxicity increases. Nonsteroidal antiinflammatory drugs (NSAIDs) reduce the diuretic and hypotensive activity of bumetanide.

 Cautious use is advised for older adults and infants.

Adverse Effects

The adverse effects of loop diuretics include ototoxicity, tinnitus, dizziness, hearing loss, muscle spasms, hyperglycemia, hypokalemia, hypotension, weakness, photosensitivity, blurred vision, paresthesias, nausea, vomiting, anorexia, constipation, and severe diarrhea. Hematologic effects include agranulocytosis, aplastic anemia, leukopenia, and thrombocytopenia. Renal changes include fluid and electrolyte imbalance, frequency, polyuria, hyperuricemia, irreversible renal failure, and allergic nephritis. Other adverse effects of furosemide include diuresis, circulatory collapse, acute pancreatitis, and SLE.

 Cautious use of loop diuretics is advised in patients with gout, severe renal or liver dysfunction, cardiogenic shock, and systemic lupus erythematosus (SLE). These drugs should also be used with caution in patients who are taking digoxin, potassium-depleting steroids, or those who are at risk for hypokalemia.

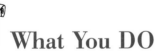

What You DO

Nursing Responsibilities

Furosemide may be administered orally, intramuscular (IM), and IV, preferably with meals to decrease gastric distress. When administering loop diuretics, the nurse should:

- Monitor adequate intake and output for effectiveness and adverse effects. Report severe diarrhea because the drug will usually be discontinued after occurrence of this adverse effect.
- Teach the patient and family to report evidence of ototoxicity (e.g., dizziness, tinnitus, hearing loss).
- Check the patient's weight and vital signs.
- Monitor potassium levels for the patient who is taking loop diuretics. Potassium supplements are usually given for patients who are undergoing long-term loop diuretic treatment.

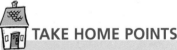 TAKE HOME POINTS

Hearing loss usually lasts a short time (1 to 24 hours). When diuresis is excessively vigorous, the patient may develop rapid and excessive weight loss or acute hypotension. The patient who is taking loop diuretics and digoxin is particularly prone to hypokalemia, and the patient who is taking loop diuretics while on a sodium-restricted diet is particularly prone to hyponatremia. Hypokalemia may result from loop diuretics, particularly in patients with ventricular dysrhythmias.

Excessive diuresis may lead to thromboembolic conditions (e.g., pulmonary emboli, cerebral vascular thrombosis), particularly in older adults.

- Monitor the patient who is taking loop diuretics for tachycardia, hypotension, and dysrhythmias for early detection of hypokalemia.
- Instruct the patient to report dry mouth, thirst, anorexia, weakness, drowsiness, restlessness, muscle cramps, oliguria, nausea, and vomiting.
- Monitor renal and hepatic function studies frequently during the first few months and periodically, thereafter for potential damage to these organs.
- Monitor the patient's uric acid levels because hyperuricemia is an adverse effect that may precipitate gout.
- Evaluate initial and ongoing CBC for potential blood dyscrasia development.
- Monitor glucose levels closely for patients with diabetes who are taking loop diuretics because these drugs may cause hyperglycemia.
- Advise the patient to use protection (e.g., sunscreen, protective clothing) when exposed to sunlight.

Do You UNDERSTAND?

DIRECTIONS: **Provide appropriate responses for the following questions.**

1. For patients on long-term treatment, what type of diet may be ordered?

2. What can hematologic problems include?

3. What is caused by Lasix and the other loop diuretics that requires close monitoring of glucose levels in patients with diabetes?

What IS a Thiazide and a Thiazide-Like Diuretic?

Thiazides and Thiazide-Like Diuretics	Trade Names	Uses
Thiazide diuretics **hydrochlorothiazide** [HY-droh-klor-ah-THIGH-ah-zide]	Diuril	Treatment of edema and hypertension
chlorothiazide [klor-ah-THIGH-ah-zide]	Esidrix	Treatment of edema and hypertension
Thiazide-like diuretic metolazone [meh-TOH-lah-zone]	Zaroxolyn	Treatment of hypertension

Answers: 1. potassium supplement diet; 2. agranulocytosis and anemia (aplastic); 3. hyperglycemia.

Action

Thiazide-like diuretics differ chemically from thiazides in the site of action but share similar use, contraindications, drug actions, precautions, adverse effects, and drug interactions. Although thiazides have some carbonic anhydrase inhibitory action, metolazone has none.

Thiazide and thiazide-like diuretics, acting primarily on the distal collecting tubules and on the proximal tubules as a secondary site, inhibit sodium and chloride reabsorption through direct action on the proximal tubules. Inhibiting sodium and chloride reabsorption causes potassium, magnesium, phosphate, and bicarbonate loss. These diuretics also produce elevated plasma renin activity, antihypertensive effect, uric acid retention, and precipitate diabetes onset in prediabetes patients. Thiazides and thiazide-like diuretics are chemically related to the sulfonamides.

Uses

Thiazide and thiazide-like diuretics are used to treat edema and hypertension. Thiazides are used in the treatment of CHF, hepatic cirrhosis, renal dysfunction, and during corticosteroid and estrogen therapy. Thiazide-like diuretics (e.g., metolazone) are used to treat hypertension. Metolazone is effective in patients with impaired renal function.

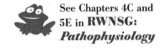

See Chapters 4C and 5E in **RWNSG:** *Pathophysiology*

What you NEED TO KNOW

Contraindications/Precautions

Thiazides and thiazide-like drugs are contraindicated for patients with hypersensitivity to sulfonamides and thiazides, hypokalemia, anuria, and concurrent administration of blood or blood products.

Thiazides and thiazide-like drugs are contraindicated for women during pregnancy and lactation and for children.

Drug Interactions

Alcohol and other CNS depressants exacerbate the sedative effects when taken with thiazide and thiazide-like diuretics. Corticosteroids and amphotericin B may increase hypokalemia when given with chlorothiazide. Because of hypokalemia and hypomagnesemia, the risk of digitalis toxicity is increased when digoxin is taken with thiazide and thiazide-like diuretics. The decreased lithium elimination may increase the risk of lithium toxicity when given with this drug classification. When thiazide and thiazide-like diuretics are given with diazoxide, hypoglycemia is increased.

Cimetidine, oral contraceptives, propylthiouracil, and methimazole increase the action of metolazone. Conversely, barbiturates and rifampin decrease the action of metolazone. Metolazone and verapamil taken concurrently increases the risk of heart block. When metolazone is given with verapamil and digoxin, bradycardia may occur.

 Hydrochlorothiazide should be used cautiously in older adults.

 Thiazides and thiazide-like drugs should be used cautiously in patients with asthma, gout, diabetes mellitus, SLE, renal and hepatic dysfunction, and those who are undergoing concurrent digoxin therapy.

Adverse Effects

Adverse effects with thiazide and thiazide-like diuretics include fluid and electrolyte imbalance, dehydration, photosensitivity, hypersensitivity, mood changes, drowsiness, weakness, dizziness, renal or hepatic damage, and SLE. GI adverse effects include dry mouth, nausea, vomiting, anorexia, and diarrhea. Hematologic effects include aplastic anemia, agranulocytosis, and leukopenia. Cardiovascular adverse effects include irregular heart rate, weak pulse, and orthostatic hypotension. Hyperglycemia and hyperuricemia are metabolic adverse effects.

What You DO

TAKE HOME POINTS

Adverse effects of thiazides and the thiazide-like diuretics include irregular pulse rate, weakened pulse, and acute hypotension.

Nursing Responsibilities

Thiazide and thiazide-like diuretics are given orally, except for chlorothiazide, which can also be given IV. When administering thiazide and thiazide-like diuretics, the nurse should:

- Assess adequate intake and output. Drug discontinuation may be needed when adverse effects develop.
- Assess the patient's weight and vital signs.
- Evaluate initial and ongoing CBC for early detection of blood dyscrasias.
- Monitor electrolytes for drug effectiveness and electrolyte imbalance. Patients are usually taking potassium supplements when undergoing long-term treatment.
- Monitor renal and hepatic function studies for early detection of organ damage.
- Monitor glucose levels closely in patients with diabetes because these drugs may cause hyperglycemia.
- Monitor serum uric acid for early detection of hyperuricemia, which may precipitate gout.
- Discontinue thiazides before parathyroid function tests are performed because they tend to decrease calcium excretion.

Do You UNDERSTAND?

DIRECTIONS: Indicate in the space provided whether the statement is *true* or *false*.

_____ 1. Thiazide diuretics are classified based on their chemical composition.

_____ 2. Inhibiting sodium and chloride reabsorption causes both potassium and magnesium loss.

_____ 3. Thiazides do not produce antihypertensive effects.

Answers: 1. true; 2. true; 3. false.

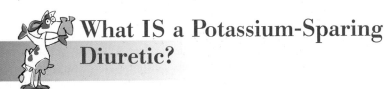

What IS a Potassium-Sparing Diuretic?

Potassium-Sparing Diuretics	Trade Names	Uses
amiloride [ah-MILL-oh-ride]	Midamor	Treatment of edema and hypertension
spironolactone [speer-on-oh-LAK-tone]	Aldactone	Treatment of edema and hypertension
triamterene [try-AM-ter-een]	Dyrenium	Treatment of edema

Action

Potassium-sparing diuretics have a mild diuretic and antihypertensive effect. Amiloride and triamterene have a direct effect on the distal tubules in the kidney. Presumably, spironolactone competes with aldosterone for cell receptor sites in the distal tubules. Potassium-sparing diuretics induce urinary excretion of sodium and reduce excretion of potassium and hydrogen ions, and they lower BP through an unknown mechanism.

Uses

Potassium-sparing diuretics are effective in preventing or treating diuretic-induced hypokalemia in patients with disorders of the heart, liver, kidney, and those with hypertension. These agents are also useful in reducing edema in patients with CHF, significant dysrhythmias, and those who are undergoing digoxin therapy, and they are used in managing primary aldosteronism. Potassium-sparing diuretics are usually combined with a thiazide or loop diuretic.

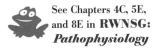

See Chapters 4C, 5E, and 8E in **RWNSG:** *Pathophysiology*

What You NEED TO KNOW

Contraindications/Precautions

Potassium-sparing diuretics are contraindicated for patients with hypersensitivity, anuria, severe renal dysfunction, hyperkalemia (potassium level above 5.5 mEq/L), and those who are taking another potassium-sparing diuretic.

Drug Interactions

When potassium-sparing diuretics are given concurrently with potassium supplements or angiotensin-converting enzyme (ACE) inhibitors, severe hyperkalemia with dysrhythmias or cardiac arrest may occur. NSAIDs decrease the amiloride action when given together. Salicylates decrease the diuretic action of spironolactone. Triamterene increases amantadine and cimetidine levels resulting from decreased urine elimination when given together. The drug combination of indomethacin and potassium-sparing diuretics increases the risk of acute renal failure.

 Potassium-sparing diuretics are contraindicated during pregnancy.

 Caution should be used for older adults and infants. Use of spironolactone is controversial during lactation because the drug label states that it is contraindicated during lactation, but the American Academy of Pediatrics considers spironolactone appropriate with breast-feeding.

⚠️ **Caution should be used for patients who are taking digoxin or those who are at risk for hyperkalemia. Cautious use of diuretics is also advised in patients with renal or liver impairment, gout, and diabetes.**

⚠️ **Avoid concurrent use of potassium-sparing diuretics with potassium supplements or ACE inhibitors.**

Adverse Effects

Potassium-sparing diuretic adverse effects include hyperkalemia, particularly in patients who have diabetes mellitus or renal impairment. Other adverse effects for the potassium-sparing drugs include weakness, dizziness, tinnitus, confusion, depression, headache, drowsiness, insomnia, tremors, paresthesia, and photophobia. Muscle cramps, hyperglycemia, hyperuremia, impotence, blurred vision, nausea, vomiting, anorexia, diarrhea, and constipation have been reported. Dissimilar to other diuretics, amiloride is not associated with hyperuricemia or hyperglycemia, but some association exists with triamterene and spironolactone. Other amiloride adverse effects include chest pain, palpitations, orthostatic hypotension, and dysrhythmias. Hematologic adverse effects of spironolactone and triamterene include agranulocytosis and mild acidosis, while amiloride may cause aplastic anemia and neutropenia.

What You DO

Nursing Responsibilities

Potassium-sparing diuretics are given orally. When administering potassium-sparing diuretics, the nurse should:
- Assess for adequate intake and output.
- Evaluate initial and ongoing levels of electrolytes for hyperkalemia.
- 🍎 Counsel the patient to avoid large amounts of potassium-rich foods (e.g., bananas, apricots, potatoes, squash, lima beans, tomatoes, oranges, avocados, milk).
- 🍎 Instruct the patient to report muscle cramps, weakness, fatigue, severe headache, dry mouth, nausea, and vomiting for early detection of electrolyte imbalances.
- Monitor the patient's weight and vital signs.
- Monitor uric acid levels for early detection of hyperuricemia, which may precipitate gout.
- Monitor blood glucose levels in patients with diabetes who are taking potassium-sparing diuretics because hyperglycemia may require dose adjustment.
- 🍎 Warn the patient to avoid tasks that require alertness or coordination until the response to the drug is known.
- 🍎 Inform the patient who is taking a single daily dose to take the drug in the morning to decrease interruption of nighttime sleep.
- 🍎 Advise the patient to use sun protection and limit exposure to sunlight.
- 🍎 Instruct the patient to report mouth soreness, sore throat, fever, bruising, or unusual bleeding for early detection of blood dyscrasias.

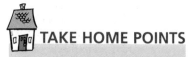

TAKE HOME POINTS

When a dose is missed, instruct the patient to avoid taking an extra dose. Take the regularly prescribed dose at the next dose interval.

Do You UNDERSTAND?

DIRECTIONS: **Indicate in the space provided whether the statement is**
true or _false_.

_____ 1. Potassium-sparing diuretics have a strong diuretic and antihypertensive effect.

_____ 2. Amiloride and triamterene have a direct effect on the distal tubules in the kidney.

_____ 3. Spironolactone compete with aldosterone for cell receptor sites in the distal tubules.

_____ 4. Potassium-sparing diuretics induce urinary excretion of sodium and increase excretion of potassium and hydrogen ions.

SECTION B
AGENTS USED IN RENAL FAILURE

For renal failure, several drug classifications are used to maintain adequate body function. As the patient's condition deteriorates, dose adjustments may be required. The drug classifications discussed in this section include ACE inhibitors, antianemic agents, iron and vitamin D supplements, phosphate-binding agents, cation exchange resins, heavy metal antagonists, and systemic antacids.

What IS an ACE Inhibitor?

Action

Approximately 80% to 90% of chronic renal failure patients have hypertension, which may be either the cause or the result of chronic renal failure. Elevated BP is usually a result of sodium and fluid overload, which leads to circulatory overload in a cyclic process, further elevating the BP. Elevated BP may also be a result of a malfunction in the renin-angiotensin-aldosterone system (RAAS), in which failing kidneys do not detect the BP increase and continue to produce renin. Additional renin furthers the vasoconstriction of vessels from angiotensin and reabsorption of more sodium and fluid from aldosterone stimulation, further elevating BP.

Refer to page 140 for the discussion of ACE inhibitors.

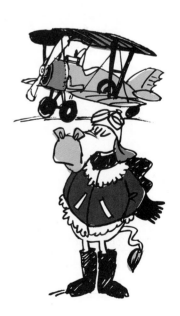

Answers: 1. false; 2. true; 3. true; 4. false.

What IS an Antianemic Agent?

Action

Anemia is the major hematologic abnormality in patients with CRF resulting from the decreased erythropoietin level. Erythropoietin, a hormone produced primarily in the kidneys in response to hypoxia, stimulates red blood cell production. Lowered levels of erythropoietin decrease red blood cell production. Erythropoietin elevates the hematocrit of patients with anemia that is secondary to CRF.

Refer to page 46 for the discussion of erythropoietin, an antianemic agent.

What IS an Iron Supplement?

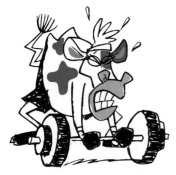

Action

Iron, a mineral that is essential for life, is transported to the bone marrow and used for the production of hemoglobin and red blood cells. Normally, iron is absorbed from food in the small intestine and travels in the blood to the bone marrow where 60% to 70% of body iron is used to produce hemoglobin. After forming hemoglobin, iron is used for red blood cell production. After the red blood cell circulates in blood for approximately 120 days, it is destroyed and the iron is used over again.

Refer to page 364 for the discussion of iron supplements.

What IS a Vitamin D Supplement?

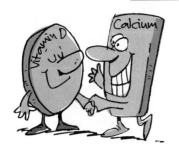

Action

Vitamin D is a fat-soluble vitamin that is usually deficient in the body that has nonfunctioning kidneys. This vitamin promotes intestinal absorption of dietary calcium. Vitamin D elevates serum calcium levels, decreases phosphatase and parathyroid hormone levels, and decreases bone resorption and mineralization defects, which improves bone density.

Refer to page 359 for the discussion of vitamin D.

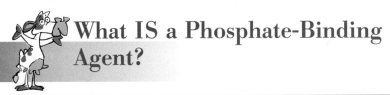

What IS a Phosphate-Binding Agent?

Phosphate-Binding Agents	Trade Names	Uses
calcium acetate	Phos-Ex PhosLo	Treatment of hypocalcemia and hyperphosphatemia
calcium carbonate	Caltrate Os-Cal Tums	Treatment of hypocalcemia and hyperphosphatemia
aluminum hydroxide	Amphojel	Treatment of hypocalcemia and hyperphosphatemia
aluminum carbonate	Basaljel	Treatment of hypocalcemia and hyperphosphatemia

Action

Hypocalcemia that results from hyperphosphatemia and decreased production of active vitamin D always accompanies renal insufficiency. Phosphate binding agents decrease serum phosphate levels, which decreases the incidence and severity of bone disease. These agents bind with phosphorus in the GI system to form calcium or aluminum phosphate, thereby preventing absorption of dietary phosphorus.

Uses

Phosphate-binding agents are used to prevent and treat hypocalcemia and hyperphosphatemia resulting from renal failure.

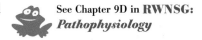

See Chapter 9D in RWNSG: *Pathophysiology*

What You NEED TO KNOW

Contraindications/Precautions

Phosphate-binding agents are contraindicated for patients with hypersensitivity, hypercalcemia, hypophosphatemia, or ventricular fibrillation. These agents should be used with caution in patients who are taking digitalis and those with cardiac, respiratory, or renal disease.

Drug Interactions

Drug interactions with phosphate-binding agents include reduced absorption of iron, thyroid hormone, salicylates, antimuscarinics, phenothiazines, anticoagulants, diazepam, isoniazid, vitamin A, tetracyclines, and fluoroquinolones. In contrast, glucocorticoids reduce absorption of oral calcium. Thiazide diuretics decrease the excretion of calcium and may lead to hypercalcemia. Additionally, when calcium compounds are given concurrently with digitalis, the actions of each are intensified, leading to toxic effects and dysrhythmias. This drug interaction is increased particularly when calcium is administered IV.

A large intake of dietary fiber may decrease calcium absorption because of increased GI transit time and formation of calcium-fiber complexes. Calcium acetate may also increase the effects of quinidine. Foods such as rhubarb, spinach, and cereals may decrease calcium absorption.

Adverse Effects

The adverse effects of phosphate-binding agents include flatulence, diarrhea, hypercalcemia, confusion, and renal calculi. As phosphate levels decrease, calcium levels increase. Therefore, in the presence of excess calcium, hypophosphatemia, aluminum toxicity, dysrhythmias, osteoporosis, and osteomalacia may occur. Rapid IV administration may lead to hypotension, bradycardia, dysrhythmias, fainting, and cardiac arrest.

What You DO

Nursing Responsibilities

Phosphate-binding agents are administered orally with meals or within 20 minutes of a meal. Tablets should be chewed thoroughly before they are swallowed with water. When given in liquid form, the solution should be diluted in water or juice and thoroughly shaken. The patient should avoid taking other oral drugs, antacids, large amounts of fiber-rich foods and drinking large amounts of alcohol or caffeine-containing beverages within 2 hours of taking phosphate-binding agents. When administering phosphate-binding agents, the nurse should:

- Monitor the serum calcium and phosphorus levels in the patient who is taking phosphate-binding agents. Ideally, the calcium level is maintained between 9.0 and 10.4 mg/dl (4.5 and 5.2 mEq/L) and the phosphorus level is maintained between 3.5 and 6.0 mg/100 ml.
- Be aware that vitamin D is necessary for the absorption of calcium compounds.
- Monitor the patient for hypophosphatemia (e.g., anorexia, muscle weakness, malaise). Aluminum agents can accumulate in the lungs, bones, and nerve tissue, thus they should be used only as a last resort.
- Monitor the patient for bone disease and dementia, which indicates aluminum toxicity.

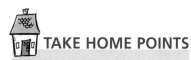

Older patients may be predisposed to constipation and fecal impaction.

TAKE HOME POINTS

Constipation resulting from vitamin D intake can be managed with a stool softener or laxative.

Aluminum hydroxide is to be avoided as a phosphate-binding agent whenever possible because aluminum accumulates in body tissues, causing aluminum toxicity.

Do You UNDERSTAND?

DIRECTIONS: **Provide the appropriate responses to the following questions from the italicized choices.**

1. The preferred phosphate-binding agent is what product?
   _____ (*aluminum, calcium*)

2. How long should the patient wait after ingesting phosphate-binding agents before taking other oral drugs?
   _____ (*30 minutes, 2 hours*)

What IS a Cation-Exchange Resin?

Cation-Exchange Resin	Trade Name	Use
sodium polystyrene sulfonate [pol-ee-STYE-reen]	Kayexalate	Treatment of hyperkalemia

Action

A cation-exchange resin releases sodium in exchange for other cations. Following oral administration, sodium is released from the cation-exchange resin in exchange for hydrogen ions in the acidic stomach environment. When this drug reaches the intestines, hydrogen cations are exchanged for potassium cations. Following rectal administration, sodium ions are released in exchange for other cations that are present (e.g., potassium, calcium, magnesium, iron, organic cations, lipids, steroids, proteins).

Uses

Cation-exchange resins are used in the treatment of hyperkalemia or excess potassium.

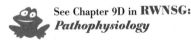 See Chapter 9D in **RWNSG:** *Pathophysiology*

What You NEED TO KNOW

Contraindications/Precautions

Sodium polystyrene sulfonate should be used with caution for patients with severe hypertension, CHF, marked edema, or those who are unable to tolerate an increase in sodium.

 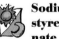 **Sodium polystyrene sulfonate should be used cautiously in women during pregnancy and in older adults.**

Sodium polystyrene sulfonate should also be used with caution in patients who are taking digitalis.

Drug Interactions

When sodium polystyrene sulfonate is given concurrently with cation-donating antacids and laxatives (e.g., magnesium hydroxide, calcium carbonate), a drug interaction may cause metabolic alkalosis in patients with renal impairment.

Adverse Effects

Adverse effects include anorexia, nausea, vomiting, diarrhea, constipation, hypokalemia, hypocalcemia, hypomagnesemia, and sodium retention. Intestinal necrosis has occurred with rectal administration.

What You DO

Nursing Responsibilities

Sodium polystyrene sulfonate, when administered orally, is diluted in 20 to 100 ml of fluid. When using rectal administration, sodium polystyrene sulfonate should be preceded by a cleansing enema, which should be retained for 30 to 60 minutes and longer, when possible. Following elimination of the sodium polystyrene sulfonate enema, the colon should be irrigated with 1 to 2 quarts of a nonsodium solution. A fresh solution should be prepared for each dose of cation-exchange resin.

When giving cation exchange resins, the nurse should:

- Monitor serum electrolyte levels, particularly sodium, potassium, calcium, and magnesium levels, in patients who are taking sodium polystyrene sulfonate.
- Monitor bicarbonate levels at least once a week for early detection of metabolic alkalosis.
- Monitor digitalis levels when the patient is taking sodium polystyrene sulfonate and digitalis concurrently.
- Monitor the patient who is taking a cation-exchange resin for confusion, irregular pulse, severe GI distress, and constipation.

Do You UNDERSTAND?

DIRECTIONS: Provide appropriate responses to the following questions.

1. Which two administration routes are appropriate for sodium polystyrene sulfonate?

   _____

   _____

2. The nurse should monitor which electrolytes?

   _____

   _____

   _____

   _____

Answers: 1. oral, rectal enema; 2. sodium, potassium, calcium, magnesium.

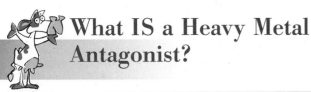

What IS a Heavy Metal Antagonist?

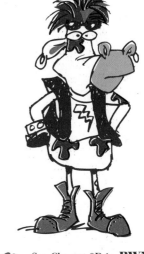

Heavy Metal Antagonist	Trade Name	Use
deferoxamine [de-fer-OX-a-meen]	Desferal	Treatment of aluminum toxicity in renal failure

Action

The heavy metal antagonist, deferoxamine mesylate, chelates iron or aluminum by enclosing the metal and rendering it nonactive and nontoxic. One gram of deferoxamine mesylate is capable of sequestering 85 mg of iron. This action is pH dependent and is more rapid in acid pH compared to alkaline pH.

Uses

Deferoxamine is used to treat iron or aluminum toxicity.

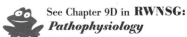

See Chapter 9D in **RWNSG:** *Pathophysiology*

What You NEED TO KNOW

Contraindications/Precautions

Deferoxamine is contraindicated for patients with severe renal disease.

Deferoxamine is contraindicated for women during pregnancy and for children under 3 years of age.

Drug Interactions

No drug interactions have been noted for deferoxamine.

Adverse Effects

Adverse effects of deferoxamine include anaphylactoid reactions, visual disturbances, tinnitus, hearing impairment, fever, abdominal discomfort, nausea, vomiting, diarrhea, leg cramps, and myasthenia gravis. Pain at injection site, skin irritation, and swelling may occur. Deferoxamine may cause tachycardia and hypotension. Adverse effects usually occur with rapid IV infusions.

Deferoxamine should be given cautiously to patients with a history of pyelonephritis.

What You DO

Nursing Responsibilities

Adding 2 ml of sterile water to a 500 mg vial for injection reconstitutes deferoxamine mesylate. The drug should be completely dissolved before withdrawal from the vial. For IV use, the drug may be added to 0.9% sodium chloride, D_5W,

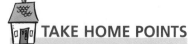

TAKE HOME POINTS

A laxative should be given in conjunction with the cation-exchange resin to facilitate passage of potassium from the body and to prevent constipation. Hypokalemia predisposes a patient to digitalis toxicity when digitalis is taken concurrently with sodium polystyrene sulfonate.

or lactated Ringer's solution. When administering heavy metal antagonists, the nurse should:

* Monitor the patient's vital signs throughout administration.
* Avoid storing solutions that are reconstituted with sterile water at room temperature for longer than 1 week.
* Teach the patient who is taking deferoxamine to have ophthalmic and otic examinations every 3 months. When ophthalmic or otic toxicities have developed, the dose should be temporarily reduced or discontinued.
* Warn patients who are taking deferoxamine that their urine will turn a characteristic reddish color.

Do You UNDERSTAND?

DIRECTIONS: Fill in the blanks with the appropriate response.

1. What two types of examinations should a patient have when taking deferoxamine?

2. What warning should the nurse give the patient about urine when taking deferoxamine?

What IS a Systemic Antacid?

Systemic Antacids	Trade Names	Uses
sodium bicarbonate [bye-CAR-bon-ayt]	Citrocarbonate	Correct metabolic acidosis
sodium citrate [SIH-trate]	Bicitra	Correct metabolic acidosis

Action

Systemic antacids buffer excess hydrogen ions and elevate blood pH, which reverses acidosis. As renal failure progresses, acid retention increases, resulting in metabolic acidosis, which requires alkali replacement to neutralize or counteract the acidosis.

Uses

Systemic antacids are used as alkalizing agents to prevent and treat metabolic acidosis resulting from renal failure.

See Chapter 9D in **RWNSG:** *Pathophysiology*

Answers: 1. ophthalmic, otic; 2. the urine will turn reddish color.

What You NEED TO KNOW

Contraindications/Precautions

Sodium bicarbonate is contraindicated for patients with hypertension, heart disease, peptic ulcer, and those who are losing chlorides because of vomiting, diuresing, or via GI suction.

Drug Interactions

Drug interactions with sodium bicarbonate include increased effects of anorexiants and sympathomimetics. Increased duration of effects occurs when sodium bicarbonate is given concurrently with amphetamines and ephedrine. Drugs that have decreased effects when given in combination with sodium bicarbonate include lithium, salicylates, tetracyclines, and sulfonylureas.

  Sodium bicarbonate is contraindicated during pregnancy. Sodium bicarbonate is to be used cautiously in older adults.

Adverse Effects

Adverse effects of systemic antacids include flatulence, gastric distention, electrolyte imbalance, metabolic alkalosis, sodium and fluid retention, dehydration, renal calculi, and milk-alkali syndrome. Because an increase in serum pH causes a translocation of potassium from extracellular fluids, hypokalemia may result. Severe tissue damage may follow infiltration of IV site. Rapid IV administration in neonates may cause hypernatremia, decreased cerebral spinal fluid pressure, and intracranial hemorrhage. Overtreatment causes alkalosis, the evidence of which includes decreased consciousness from hypernatremia, tetany from hypocalcemia, dysrhythmias from hypokalemia, and seizures from alkalosis.

 Sodium bicarbonate is to be used cautiously in patients with edema and sodium-retaining disorders.

What You DO

Nursing Responsibilities

Sodium bicarbonate and sodium citrate are equally effective in treating chronic acidosis and are given orally. Because citrate enhances absorption of toxic elements, including aluminum and sodium bicarbonate, it is the preferred drug. When administering systemic antacids, the nurse should:

- Monitor serum carbon dioxide and arterial pH values to determine the effectiveness of systemic antacid therapy.
- Monitor electrolytes and vital signs in patients who are taking systemic antacids.
- Monitor cardiac rhythm carefully when the patient is receiving IV administration of systemic antacids.

 TAKE HOME POINTS

When sodium bicarbonate is given IV, the rate of administration should not exceed 50 mEq/hr.

> ⚠ **Discontinue an infiltrated sodium bicarbonate IV immediately to prevent severe tissue damage.**

 Instruct the patient who is taking long-term sodium bicarbonate that milk-alkali syndrome is likely to occur, the symptoms of which include headache, mental confusion, anorexia, nausea, vomiting, soft-tissue calcification, hypercalcemia, hypophosphatemia, renal and ureteral calculi, and metabolic alkalosis.

Do You UNDERSTAND?

DIRECTIONS: **Indicate in the space provided whether the statement is *true* or *false*.**

_____ 1. The action of lithium and tetracyclines is increased when given concurrently with sodium bicarbonate.

_____ 2. Administration of IV sodium bicarbonate should not exceed 50 mEq/hr.

10 Drugs Affecting the Reproductive System

SECTION A
MALE AND FEMALE HORMONES

Estrogen, progesterone, and androgens can be replaced with synthetic substitutions, alone or in combination. The goal of replacement hormones is to perform the function of naturally produced hormones and to treat certain medical conditions.

What IS Estrogen?

Noncontraceptive Estrogens	Trade Names	Uses
conjugated estrogens [ESS-troh-jenz]	Premarin	Decreases menopausal symptoms; prevents osteoporosis
estradiol [ess-trah-DYE-ohl]	Estraderm	Decreases menopausal symptoms; prevents osteoporosis

Action

Estrogen is a hormone that produces several physiologic actions. These actions involve developmental changes, suppression of androgen production, and alteration in mineral, carbohydrate, protein, and lipid metabolism. Estrogens, similar to other hormones, are thought to act primarily through gene expression. The hormones pass through the cellular membrane and bind to a receptor in the nucleus. Estrogen receptors are present in the female reproductive system, breast, pituitary, hypothalamus, bone, and liver, as well as numerous tissues in males. Estrogen also promotes the development of the uterine lining.

Estrogen blocks bone-resorption and promotes the accumulation of minerals in bones. Estrogen decreases the low-density lipoprotein (LDL) and increases the high-density lipoprotein (HDL) cholesterol levels, thereby altering lipid

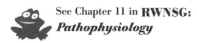 Estrogen assists in retaining bone mass in postmenopausal women.

See Chapter 11 in **RWNSG:** *Pathophysiology*

 Estrogen is contraindicated for women during pregnancy, unsuccessful abortions, and lactation, as well as for adolescents with incomplete epiphyseal closure.

 Estrogen should be used with caution in multiparous women with irregular menses.

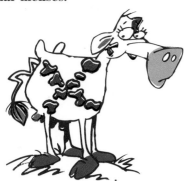

Cautious use of estrogen is necessary in patients with depression, renal disease, hypertension, migraines, seizures, asthma, diabetes mellitus, obesity, gallbladder disease, systemic lupus erythematosus (SLE), and those who are heavy smokers (more than 15 cigarettes per day).

metabolism. This factor is protective in nature because elevated LDL and decreased HDL levels predispose the individual to coronary artery disease (CAD) and resultant myocardial infarction (MI).

Uses

Estrogens are most commonly used as hormone replacement therapy (HRT) in postmenopausal women to decrease menopausal symptoms. HRT is usually life-long for suppressing vasomotor symptoms (e.g., hot flashes, sweating) and for preventing urogenital atrophy (e.g., vaginal dryness), osteoporosis, and CAD. However, HRT is also used to treat primary ovarian failure, hypermenorrhea, endometriosis, developmental delay or hypogonadism, and acne in adults. Because the growth of prostate cancer depends on the androgen hormone, the use of estrogen to suppress androgen provides a useful treatment for prostate cancer.

What You NEED TO KNOW

Contraindications/Precautions

Estrogen is contraindicated for patients with a history of thrombophlebitis, peripheral vascular disorders, thromboembolic disorders, breast or endometrial cancer, undiagnosed genital bleeding, cystic mastitis, cerebral vascular accident (CVA), CAD, MI, and hepatic dysfunction.

Drug Interactions

Carbamazepine, barbiturates, or rifampin decrease estrogen effectiveness when taken concurrently. Estrogen can increase the effects of corticosteroids and hepatotoxic medications (e.g., dantrolene). Cyclosporine has an increased risk of toxicity when administered with estrogen. Concurrent estrogen therapy and anticoagulants may cause a decrease in anticoagulation. Estrogen may interfere with the action of tamoxifen. Estrogen may increase caffeine levels when taken together. Estrogen may also increase cardiovascular adverse effects in smokers.

Adverse Effects

Common adverse effects of estrogen therapy involving gastrointestinal (GI) distress (e.g. nausea,, vomiting, abdominal cramps) usually decrease with continued use within 2 to 3 months. When estrogen therapy is initiated in low doses, GI distress may be eliminated. Adverse central nervous system (CNS) and cardiovascular effects include headache, dizziness, muscular twitching (chorea), depression, thrombophlebitis, hypertension, fluid retention, and weight gain. Worsening of myopia or astigmatism and intolerance of contact lenses are adverse effects related to eyesight. Amenorrhea, cervical erosion, enlargement of uterine fibromas, vaginal candidiasis, abnormal breast secretions, and libido changes have occurred. Other adverse effects include anorexia, increased appetite, jaundice, hyperglycemia, reduced carbohydrate tolerance, leg cramps, hair loss, urticaria, red nodules on the legs (erythema nodosum), dermatitis, colitis, acute pancreatitis, excessive thirst, and hypercalcemia. Gynecomastia, testicular atrophy, and reversible impotence may occur in men.

When deprived of estrogen, the endometrium will bleed within 48 to 72 hours. Hypomenorrhea, mid-cycle breakthrough bleeding, and increased spotting are adverse effects of estrogen deficiency. The adverse effects of excess estrogen include nausea, vomiting, bloating, diarrhea, dysmenorrhea, brown skin discoloration (**melasma**), polyps, hypertension, migraines, breast fullness, breast tenderness, and edema.

What You DO

Nursing Responsibilities

The patient should have a thorough physical examination before estrogen therapy is initiated. Estrogen therapy may be administered orally, intramuscularly (IM), intravenously (IV), intravaginally, and via a transdermal method. HRT may be given in a continuous-dose regimen with the same dose every day or a cyclic schedule. In the cyclic schedule, estrogen is taken for 21 days and stopped for 7 days. The discontinuation of estrogen will lead to menstrual bleeding.

When administering estrogens, the nurse should:
- Instruct the patient to rotate transdermal application sites and allow 1 week before reapplication to the previous site to avoid skin irritation. The patient should remain in a recumbent position for 30 minutes to prevent dislodging the medication.
- Monitor the patient's weight and blood pressure for early detection of fluid retention, weight gain, and hypertension.
- Counsel the patient who is experiencing nausea to take estrogen with or immediately following solid food.
- Keep estrogen tablets in a dry container that is protected from light damage.
- Instruct the patient to apply a transdermal application to a clean, dry area on the body trunk. Instruct the patient that when the transdermal patch falls off, reapply it and return to the original treatment schedule.
- Encourage the patient to avoid caffeine intake and smoking to prevent thromboembolism or an MI.
- Instruct the patient to direct the vaginal applicator of intravaginal estrogen back toward the sacrum when it is inserted.
- Advise the patient to urinate before the application to avoid having to ambulate after the medication is inserted.
- Instruct the patient to wash the hands before and after administration and report signs of irritation, such as redness, swelling, or excoriated skin in the perineal area.
- Teach the patient the self-breast examination technique for early detection of breast cancer.
- Monitor blood glucose levels regularly in patients with diabetes who are taking estrogen because hyperglycemia may occur.

 Life-threatening adverse effects of estrogen therapy include seizures, hepatic adenoma, breast cancer, thromboembolism, CVA, pulmonary embolism, and MI.

 Prolonged estrogen therapy in postmenopausal women may lead to an increased risk of uterine cancer. Excessive uterine development from estrogen may lead to uterine hyperplasia (excessive tissue growth) with prolonged exposure to estrogen alone.

TAKE HOME POINTS
Avoid transdermal application on irritated areas or those with excessive oil production, such as the breast and waistline.

- Monitor hepatic function and serum lipid levels for early detection of dysfunction.
- Teach patients the importance of ambulation and exercise to reduce vascular complications.
- Inform the patient that estrogen therapy should be stopped 4 weeks before procedures that are associated with prolonged immobilization.
- Advise the patient to report immediately a suspected pregnancy, intermittent vaginal bleeding or discharge, unexplained or sudden abdominal pain, numbness, stiffness in legs, shortness of breath, chest pain or pressure, visual changes, flashing lights, severe headaches, vaginal bleeding or discharge, breast changes, swelling of extremities, yellow skin or sclera, dark urine, and light-colored stools.
- Reassure male patients who are taking estrogen therapy that impotence and estrogen-induced female characteristics will disappear after treatment is discontinued.

Do You UNDERSTAND?

DIRECTIONS: **Complete the following statements with the appropriate terms from the list provided.**

1. Estrogen therapy is _____ for patients with a negative pregnancy test.
2. Estrogen therapy is _____ for patients with a history of thrombophlebitis.
3. Estrogen therapy with anticoagulants may cause a decrease in

_____.

| unknown | indicated | contraindicated |
| anticoagulation | coagulation | |

What IS Progestin?

Progestins	Trade Names	Uses
Hormone replacement therapy progesterone [proh-JESS-ter-one]	Progestasert	Treatment of amenorrhea or dysfunctional uterine bleeding
norethindrone [nor-eth-IN-drone]	Norlutin	Treatment of amenorrhea or dysfunctional uterine bleeding
medroxyprogesterone acetate [meh-DROX-ee-proh-JESS-ter-one]	Provera	Treatment of amenorrhea or dysfunctional uterine bleeding
Oral contraceptive minipill norethindrone [nor-eth-IN-drone]	Micronor	Birth control; treatment of amenorrhea and endometriosis
norgestrel [nor-JESS-trell]	Ovrette	Birth control

Answers: 1. indicated; 2. contraindicated; 3. anticoagulation.

Action

Progesterone is a steroid hormone that is synthesized and released in the testes, ovary, adrenal cortex and placenta. This hormone maintains uterine development in the second half of the menstrual cycle, preparing it for implantation. Progestin is a synthetic drug that has a progesterone-like effect on the uterus. Similar to estrogen, progestin produces developmental changes and alterations in mineral, carbohydrate, protein, and lipid metabolism. Progestin also opposes estrogen-mediated uterine proliferation and reverses hyperplasia.

Progestins suppress the secretion of luteinizing hormone (LH), thereby controlling ovulation. With the suppression of LH, ovulation cannot occur, even with full development of the follicle. Progestin also initiates endometrial changes that prevent an egg from implanting in the uterus and promotes the production of thick endometrial secretions. The thickened mucus of the cervix causes increased difficulty for the sperm to migrate and a less favorable uterine environment for egg implantation. Ultimately, these changes block ovulation and follicular maturation.

Uses

Progestin is used in the treatment of amenorrhea, dysfunctional uterine bleeding, cancer, endometriosis, and premenstrual syndrome. This agent is used as a progestin-only type of oral contraceptive, known as the "minipill." Progestin is also used to treat infertile women who have progestin deficiency.

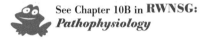 See Chapter 10B in **RWNSG:** *Pathophysiology*

 # What You NEED TO KNOW

Contraindications/Precautions

Progestin is contraindicated for patients with hypersensitivity, thrombophlebitis, vascular disorders, thromboembolism, CVA, and liver disease. Progestins are contraindicated for patients with peanut allergies because the drug contains peanut oil. Progestin is contraindicated for patients with undiagnosed vaginal bleeding, breast or genital malignancy, and unsuccessful abortion.

Progestin is contraindicated during pregnancy and lactation.

 When progestins are given within the first 4 months of pregnancy, birth defects (teratogenic effects) may occur.

Drug Interactions

No drug interactions have been clinically reported.

Adverse Effects

Common adverse effects include dizziness, nausea, vomiting, abdominal cramps, breakthrough bleeding, and edema. Other adverse effects include migraines, somnolence, insomnia, hepatic disease, cholestatic jaundice, and hyperglycemia. Decreased libido, transient increase in sodium and chloride excretion, fever, itching, allergic rashes, urticaria, photosensitivity, hirsutism, alopecia, and pain at injection site have also been reported. Gynecological adverse effects include gynecomastia, galactorrhea, vaginal candidiasis, brown skin discolorations, vaginal dryness, cervical erosion, dysmenorrhea, and amenorrhea.

Progestins should be used with caution for women who have had an abnormal Papanicolaou (pap) smear, as well as those with genital bleeding of unknown origin, previous ectopic pregnancy, sexually transmitted diseases, and previous pelvic surgery. Progestins should be used cautiously in patients with anemia, diabetes mellitus, depression, suspected acute porphyria, salpingitis, and liver disease, as well as conditions in which fluid retention is a factor.

Life-threatening adverse effects include thrombolytic disorders and pulmonary embolism.

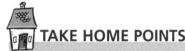

TAKE HOME POINTS

Inform the patient to expect withdrawal bleeding 48 to 72 hours after the last injection and that bleeding ordinarily stops by the sixth day.

Downward displacement of the eye, diplopia, papilledema, and retinal vascular lesions have occurred from progestin therapy.

Late menstrual cycle bleeding and amenorrhea are adverse effects of progestin deficiency. Hypomenorrhea, breast regression, vaginal candidiasis, depression, fatigue, weight gain, increased appetite, acne, oily scalp, hair loss are adverse effects of excess progestin.

What You DO

Nursing Responsibilities

Progestin may be administered orally, IM, intravaginally, and via a transdermal method. Progestin crystals may require dissolving in a vial under warm water before they are drawn into a syringe for IM injection. When administering progestins, the nurse should:

- Inform the patient to use an alternative form of birth control during the first 3 months to prevent contraception.
- Instruct the patient to have a thorough physical examination before progestin therapy is initiated.
- Monitor the patient's blood pressure, weight, and intake and output ratio for early detection of adverse effects.
- Monitor blood sugar levels regularly of the patient with diabetes.
- Monitor hepatic function studies. Because progestins affect the results of hepatic tests, the results should not be considered definitive until the patient has stopped the therapy and waited at least 60 days.
- Inject IM progestin deeply to avoid skin irritation. The site of administration of the drug should be rotated.
- Inform the patient that progestin is usually given for 6 to 8 days to treat amenorrhea and that progestin is usually given for 10 days for dysfunctional uterine bleeding.
- Advise the patient who is undergoing progestin therapy to avoid missing annually scheduled physical examinations.
- Advise the patient who is using the intrauterine progesterone contraceptive system (Progestasert) to expect spotting, cramping, and discomfort during the first 3 months.
- Encourage the patient to return to the health care provider to assess the efficacy and placement of the Progestasert device within 3 months of initial placement.
- Warn the patient to expect a slightly heavier menstruation while the Progestasert device is in place.
- Instruct the patient to inspect the Progestasert threads on a regular basis to ensure placement, and warn the patient that pulling on the threads for any reason will harm the uterus.
- Warn the patient to avoid exposure to ultraviolet light, which may cause a severe photosensitive reaction or exaggerated sunburn.

- Advise the patient to use sunscreen as necessary.
- Instruct the patient who is taking progestins to report fever, acute pelvic pain, and unusual bleeding to the health care provider immediately for early detection of infection.
- Instruct the patient to obtain an annual pelvic examination with a pap smear, breast examination, and assessment of hematocrit level.
- Advise the patient who is undergoing progestin therapy to report suspected pregnancy immediately.

Do You UNDERSTAND?

DIRECTIONS: Indicate in the space provided whether the statement is true or false.

_____ 1. Progestin is used for secondary amenorrhea, dysfunctional uterine bleeding, endometriosis, premenstrual syndrome, menopausal use, and to treat infertile women with progestin deficiency.

_____ 2. Progesterone is a steroid hormone synthesized and released in the testes, ovary, adrenal cortex, and placenta.

_____ 3. Progestin is an intrauterine agent that also provides fertility control.

_____ 4. Progestin is a hormone that increases LH secretion.

What IS Combination Estrogen and Progestin?

Estrogen and Progestin Combinations	Trade Names	Uses
Hormone replacement therapy conjugated estrogens/ medroxyprogesterone acetate	Prempro	Treat menopausal symptoms
estradiol/norgestimate	Ortho-Prefest	Treat menopausal symptoms
Oral contraceptives ethinyl estradiol/levonorgestrel (monophasic)	Alesse	Prevention of pregnancy
ethinyl estradiol/norethindrone (biphasic 10/11)	Ortho-Novum	Prevention of pregnancy
ethinyl estradiol/norethindrone (triphasic 7/7/7)	Ortho-Novum	Prevention of pregnancy

Action

In addition to the aforementioned actions of estrogen and progestins, these drugs have further actions when taken in combination. Estrogen and progestins control ovulation, the cyclical preparation of fertilization, and implantation.

Answers: 1. true; 2. true; 3. true; 4. false.

Estrogen reduces the release of the follicle-stimulating hormone (FSH) from the pituitary gland, thereby blocking follicle development. Consequently, this action prevents transport of the ovum through the fallopian tube, inhibiting ovulation. Estrogen also inhibits contraception through a negative feedback system with the hypothalamus and pituitary gland.

Progestin with estrogen promotes mammary gland development without causing lactation and increased body temperature during ovulation. A sudden decrease in progestin and estrogen levels causes bleeding.

Uses

Estrogen and progesterone are widely prescribed drugs, alone or in combination. This drug combination is most commonly prescribed for contraception measures and HRT in postmenopausal women to reduce menopausal symptoms. Estrogen and progesterone are also used to treat developmental delay or hypogonadism, primary ovarian failure, postcoital contraception, and acne in adults. Estrogen and progesterone receptor antagonists may also be used to decrease the amount of estrogen that the body produces, which may be beneficial in treating estrogen-dependent neoplasm, cancer chemotherapeutic strategies, and infertility. The progestin portion of this drug combination is present to protect the patient against estrogen-induced uterine cancer.

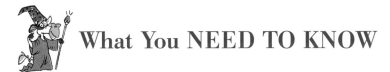 # What You NEED TO KNOW

Contraindications/Precautions

The contraindications and precautions are the same as those that are listed for estrogen and progestin in the previous discussion.

Drug Interactions

The drug interactions are the same as those that are listed for the estrogen and progestin. When used for contraception, estrogen will also interact with aminocaproic acid, barbiturates, anticonvulsants, antibiotics, and antifungals, causing an increase incidence of breakthrough bleeding and risk of pregnancy.

Adverse Effects

Estrogen therapy alone may lead to uterine cancer. When progestin is given in combination with estrogen, little or no risk of uterine cancer is present. However, the risk of breast cancer increases as a result of the addition of progestin. Women who are without a uterus may take estrogen alone with a 1% risk for breast cancer. Women with a uterus who are taking progestin and estrogen combination increase the risk of breast cancer to 8%. Other adverse effects are the same as those that are listed for estrogen and progestin.

What You DO

Nursing Responsibilities

Estrogen and progestin are combined in three combinations for oral contraceptive regimens. *Monophasic* is a set dose of estrogen and progestin, which remains constant throughout the menstrual cycle. *Biphasic* includes a constant amount of estrogen throughout the month, but the progestin increases as the cycle progresses. *Triphasic* is a varied amount of estrogen in two phases and varied amounts of progestin in three phases. Estrogen doses should be gradually reduced after the patient has been on high doses or after an extended period.

HRT is scheduled in two regimens. Continuous dosing indicates that a continuous dose of estrogen and progestin is administered every day of the month. Cyclic scheduling means that estrogen is given for 21 days and stopped for 7 days, and progestin is given the last 10 days of the cycle. In addition to the nursing responsibilities that have been mentioned for estrogen and progestins, the nurse should:

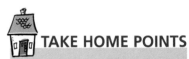

TAKE HOME POINTS

The possibility of ovulation, spotting, or bleeding increases with each dose that is missed.

- Instruct the patient to use an alternative form of birth control during the first 3 months to prevent contraception.
- Instruct the patient to wait 24 hours between doses when using contraceptive therapy.
- Advise the patient to take a missed dose as soon as possible or take two tablets the next day. When two doses are missed, take two tablets for the next 2 days; when three tablets are missed, the patient should start a new monthly cycle of tablets starting 7 days after the last tablet was taken.
- Instruct the patient that additional forms of birth control are recommended for a week after two missed doses or 14 days after three missed doses.
- Inform the patient that when she does not experience ovulation within two cycles, pregnancy should be ruled out before continuing therapy.
- Instruct the patient to discontinue estrogen and start a new cycle after 5 days when the patient experiences intracyclic bleeding that resembles menstruation, and notify the health care provider when the problem persists for the early detection of endometrial cancer.
- Explain to the patient who is undergoing cyclic therapy that withdrawal bleeding may occur during the time the patient is not taking the drug, and pregnancy cannot occur when fertility is not restored.
- Inform the patient that when two consecutive menstrual periods are missed, a pregnancy evaluation is required.
- Warn the patient that after discontinuation of oral contraceptives, 1 to 3 months may pass before normal menstruation resumes.
- When nursing, the patient should be advised to use an alternative form of birth control. When the mother is not nursing, oral contraception may be started immediately following the birth of the child.

 Inform the patient that she may experience spotting, cramping, and discomfort during the first 3 months of intrauterine progesterone contraception.

 Instruct the patient to consult the health care provider when pregnancy is suspected or menstruation is delayed or missed.

Do You UNDERSTAND?

DIRECTIONS: **Provide appropriate responses for the following statements and questions.**

1. When progestin is given with estrogen, what cancer risk is reduced?

   _____

   What cancer risk is increased?

   _____

2. List three combinations of oral contraceptive regimens.

   _____

   _____

   _____

3. List two regimens for HRT.

   _____

   _____

What IS an Androgen?

Androgens	Trade Names	Uses
danazol [DAN-ah-zole]	Cyclomen	Treatment of endometriosis and fibrocystic breast disease
nandrolone [NAN-droh-lone]	Durabolin	Treatment of metastatic breast cancer
testosterone [tess-TOSS-ter-one]	Testoderm	Treatment of delayed puberty and male hypogonadism

Action

An androgen is a steroid hormone that suppresses the pituitary output of FSH and LH, causing anovulation and amenorrhea. Testosterone, the male sex hormone, is the principle testicular androgen. In women, the ovary and adrenal gland produce minimal amounts of testosterone. The testes convert testosterone to dihydrotestosterone in the tissues. Testosterone esters can cause an increase in plasma concentrations of estrogens, thus feminizing effects are observed. Androgens cause atrophy and interruption of normal and ectopic endometrial tissue, thereby stopping endometriosis.

Answers: 1. uterine, breast; 2. monophasic, biphasic, triphasic; 3. continuous dosing, cyclic scheduling.

Uses

Androgen therapy is most commonly used for male hypogonadism because the replacement of the androgen or testosterone will encourage all testosterone functions, except for spermatogenesis. Other uses include refractory anemia, angioedema, mild and moderate endometriosis, fibrocystic breast disease, delayed puberty, palliation of breast cancer in women, breast cancer in postmenopausal women, cryptorchidism, and postpartum breast pain and engorgement. In the belief that these drugs will improve performance, athletes have also used androgens. However, this belief is proven to be false.

What You NEED TO KNOW

Contraindications/Precautions

Androgens are contraindicated for patients with a hypersensitivity to anabolic steroids, undiagnosed genital bleeding, porphyria, breast or prostate cancer, renal impairment, cardiac disorders, and hepatic dysfunction.

Drug Interactions

Danazol combined with carbamazepine may increase carbamazepine levels. Androgens increase the risk of nephrotoxicity. Combined with warfarin, androgens may cause a prolonged prothrombin time. Androgens may also affect the patient's insulin level.

Adverse Effects

An adverse effect of androgens is the presence of masculine secondary sex changes in adult women. Masculine sex changes include acne, facial hair growth, coarse voice, and menstrual irregularities. When androgen therapy is stopped immediately after symptoms are noticed, they will normally subside. Continued treatment may produce male baldness, body hair, and hypertrophy of the clitoris.

Androgen replacement in men may cause excessive erections when first initiated. Feminizing effects and toxic effects in adolescent and adult men depend on the dose and the length of exposure.

Additional adverse reactions of androgens include dizziness, headache, sleep disorders, fatigue, tremor, irritability, excitation, lethargy, sleep apnea, emotional lability, depression, paresthesia, elevated blood pressure, edema, and visual disturbances. GI and genitourinary adverse effects include nausea, vomiting, diarrhea, constipation, appetite changes, hematuria, vaginal bleeding, and testicular atrophy. Hepatic effects include irreversible jaundice, polycythemia, hepatitis, liver cell tumors, and hepatic dysfunction. Finally, muscle cramps, hypersensitive skin manifestations, hypercalcemia, chills, and allergic reactions have been noted.

See Chapters 10A and 10B in
RWNSG: *Pathophysiology*

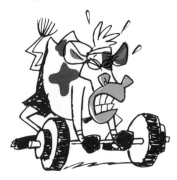

Androgens are contraindicated for pregnant women and nursing mothers because they can cause development of male characteristics in the female infant. Androgens should be used with great care in children because profound masculinization may occur.

Androgens should be used cautiously in patients with seizure disorders or migraine headaches.

Feminizing adverse effects include gynecomastia, which is significantly increased in children and adult males with liver disease.

Patients who have received androgens for prolonged periods may develop hepatic carcinoma. Androgens increase the concentration of thyroid-binding globulin and affect thyroid function test results, plasma proteins, lipids, lipoproteins, urine tests, glucose tolerance test, cholesterol readings, and hepatic function test results.

What You DO

TAKE HOME POINTS

Rotate IM injection sites to prevent atrophy. The transdermal patch should not be applied directly to the scrotum.

Nursing Responsibilities

When administering androgens, the nurse should:

- Instruct the patient to consume a high-calorie diet when using oral androgen therapy.
- Advise the patient to take the drug with food or meals when gastric upset occurs during androgen therapy.
- Inject the drug deeply into the upper outer quadrant of the gluteal muscle when the androgen is administered IM.
- Teach the patient the proper way to apply the transdermal system, when appropriate.
- Avoid bony prominences and rotate transdermal sites for at least 1 week before returning to the same site.
- Inform the patient that the transdermal patch does not have to be removed during sexual intercourse.
- Encourage the patient to follow up with regular laboratory work and semen evaluation.
- Remind the patient who is taking androgen that the buccal form can be stronger than other androgen forms.
- Instruct the patient who is taking androgens for fibrocystic disease to perform breast self-examinations regularly for early detection of masses.
- Advise the patient to use nonhormonal contraceptive methods while undergoing androgen therapy.
- Suggest that the patient wear cotton undergarments and wash the genital area immediately after intercourse, thereby decreasing the risk of vaginitis.
- Instruct the female patient to report masculinization adverse effects, such as acne, facial hair growth, coarse voice, sudden weight gain, and menstrual irregularities.

Inform parents that children may require regular bone assessment to determine maturation while undergoing therapy.

Do You UNDERSTAND?

DIRECTIONS: Provide the appropriate responses to the following questions from the italicized choices.

1. A negative feedback system influences testosterone. _____ testosterone suppresses the release of FSH and LH.
   (*increased, decreased*)
2. Athletes have also used androgens in the belief that they will improve performance, although this is _____.
   (*indicated, contraindicated*)
3. In women, the ovary and adrenal gland produce testosterone in _____ amounts.
   (*moderate, minimal*)

Answers: 1. increased; 2. contraindicated; 3. minimal.

SECTION B
AGENTS AFFECTING UTERINE MOTILITY

Natural conditions of the reproductive system require medications that promote and maintain pregnancy, induce or inhibit labor, promote or inhibit lactation, and terminate pregnancy. The drugs that are discussed in this section include tocolytics, oxytocics, prostaglandins, and ergot alkaloids.

What IS a Tocolytic?

Tocolytics	Trade Names	Uses
ritodrine [RYE-toe-dreen]	Yutopar	Stops premature labor
terbutaline [ter-BYOO-tah-leen]	Brethine	Stops premature labor
magnesium sulfate	MgSO4	Treatment of seizures in preeclampsia and eclampsia

Action

Tocolytics (uterine relaxants) are β-adrenergic agonists that mimic the sympathetic nervous system effects at β_2 sites. Tocolytics relax smooth muscle and stop or slow uterine contractions.

Uses

Tocolytics are used to stop preterm labor and to help maintain a pregnancy for days or weeks. Uterine contractions before 36 weeks are considered preterm or premature labor. Ritodrine and terbutaline decrease the intensity and frequency of uterine contractions, thereby suppressing premature labor and delivery and lengthening the gestation period. Magnesium sulfate can suppress preterm labor but is used most frequently as an anticonvulsant to prevent or treat the complication of seizures in eclampsia and severe preeclampsia.

What You NEED TO KNOW

Contraindications/Precautions

Tocolytics are contraindicated for patients with hemorrhage, diabetes mellitus, hypovolemia, hypertension, dysrhythmias, heart disease, and chorioamnionitis.

 Tocolytics are not used before 20 weeks of gestation because no adequate studies have been conducted that indicate safety before that time. Terbutaline is widely used to delay preterm labor, although the Food and Drug Administration (FDA) has not approved terbutaline for this use.

 See Chapter 2D in **RWNSG:** *Pathophysiology*

 Tocolytics are contraindicated for patients with the cervix that is dilated 4 cm or more, gestation of less than 20 weeks or greater than 36 weeks, severe preeclampsia, eclampsia, and intrauterine infection.

Tocolytics are used with caution in patients with hyperthyroidism.

When corticosteroids are combined with tocolytics, the risk of potentially fatal postpartal pulmonary edema is increased.

Fetal adverse effects include hypotension, tachycardia, hyperglycemia, and paralytic ileus.

Drug Interactions

When tocolytics are given with sympathomimetic drugs, the sympathetic effects are increased. Conversely, when tocolytics are combined with β-adrenergic blockers, the sympathetic effects are decreased.

Adverse Effects

Adverse effects are usually associated with IV administration of tocolytics but are rare following oral administration. Maternal adverse effects of tocolytics include allergy, headache, tremor, anxiety, nervousness, restlessness, malaise, temporary hyperglycemia, rash, nausea, vomiting, palpitations, tachycardia, hypotension, hypertension, and widening pulse pressure. More serious adverse effects include chest pain, dysrhythmias, increased cardiac output, and pulmonary edema.

Magnesium intoxication effects include flushing, sweating, hypotension, hypothermia, cardiac and CNS depression, circulatory collapse, flaccid paralysis, depressed reflexes, and hypocalcemia with tetany.

What You DO

Nursing Responsibilities

Generally, tocolytics are initiated IV and maintained for approximately 12 hours to quickly stop labor. These agents are then continued orally to maintain suppression of labor. Oral therapy usually begins 30 minutes before termination of IV administration. When uterine contractions reoccur, tocolytics are restarted IV. When administering tocolytics, the nurse should:

- Position the patient who is receiving tocolytics in the left lateral recumbent position throughout the infusion period to reduce the risk of hypotension.
- Use a micro-drip and infusion pump for tocolytic IV administration to prevent circulatory overload.
- Monitor the patient who is undergoing tocolytic therapy for pulmonary edema, particularly when the patient is taking corticosteroids. Continuously monitor maternal and fetal heart rate and maternal blood pressure during tocolytic infusions for early detection of adverse effects.
- Administer oral tocolytics with food when GI distress is present.
- Monitor the blood glucose levels of the patient with diabetes for early detection of hyperglycemia.

Do You UNDERSTAND?

DIRECTIONS: Fill in the blanks with the appropriate responses.

1. Tocolytics act to _____ the uterus and _____ delivery.
2. The route for tocolytic administration that is usually used first is _____ then given _____.

1. relax, delay; 2. IV, orally.

What IS an Oxytocic?

Oxytocic	Trade Name	Uses
oxytocin [ox-eh-TOE-sin]	Pitocin	Initiates uterine contractions and stimulates letdown reflex in nursing mothers

Action

An oxytocic is a drug that functions similarly to the hormone oxytocin, which is produced in the hypothalamus and is stored in the posterior pituitary gland. Oxytocin promotes an increase in the force, frequency, and duration of uterine contractions. The uterus becomes progressively sensitive to oxytocin during the gestational period, peaking before delivery. Oxytocin produces vasodilation of vascular smooth muscles to increase cerebral, coronary, and renal blood flow. Oxytocin also promotes the release of breast milk through the process of contracting cells that surround the alveoli of the breast, forcing milk from the alveoli into the larger ducts and facilitating milk ejection in nursing mothers.

Uses

Oxytocin is used at term to stimulate or improve uterine contractions during labor, delivery, and the immediate postpartum period. Oxytocin is the drug of choice in the antepartum period to induce near-term labor after the cervix is dilated and presentation of the fetus has occurred. Oxytocin is also useful in managing inevitable, incomplete, or missed abortions. The stimulation of uterine contractions can also prevent or control postpartal hemorrhage and promote postpartal uterine involution (decrease in uterine size) to control bleeding. Oxytocin is also used to stimulate the milk letdown reflex in nursing mothers and as a diagnostic agent in the oxytocin challenge test to detect abnormal fetal heart rates.

What You NEED TO KNOW

Contraindications/Precautions

Oxytocin is contraindicated for patients with hypersensitivity and invasive cervical carcinoma. Oxytocin is contraindicated for patients with borderline cephalopelvic disproportion, partial placenta previa, hydramnios, previous major surgery of cervix or uterus, uterine overdistension, grand multiparity, history of uterine sepsis or traumatic delivery, and severe toxemia.

Oxytocin is contraindicated during prematurity and fetal distress.

Drug Interactions

When oxytocin is given with vasoconstrictors, severe hypertension may develop. A drug interaction with cyclopropane anesthesia leads to hypotension, dysrhythmias, and maternal bradycardia.

Oxytocin should not be used to induce labor when a vaginal delivery is contraindicated.

With excessive doses or in sensitive patients, maternal adverse effects include amniotic fluid embolism, hyperstimulation of the uterus, prolonged tetanic uterine contractions, uterine rupture, cervical and vaginal lacerations, postpartum hemorrhage, and abruptio placentae. Fetal adverse effects include intracranial hemorrhage, deceleration of heart rate, hypoxia, hypercapnia, CNS impairment, and perinatal hepatic necrosis.

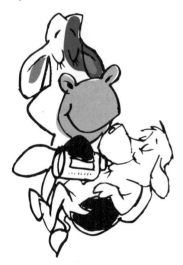

TAKE HOME POINTS

When inducing labor antepartally, administer the oxytocin IV rather than IM because IM administration is unpredictable to control. Never administer oxytocin via more than one route at a time.

Adverse Effects

Adverse effects of oxytocin include hypotension, severe hypertension, headache, subarachnoid hemorrhage, uterine cramping, tachycardia, dysrhythmias, impaired renal flow, anaphylaxis, seizures, coma, and death. Severe water intoxication usually occurs with an excessive volume of IV solution without electrolytes, an IV rate that is too rapid, or prolonged IV administration.

 # What You DO

Nursing Responsibilities

Oxytocin is administered IV when stimulating uterine contractions, whenever possible. When delivery is rapidly eminent without time to initiate an IV, oxytocin is usually given IM after delivery. When given for milk letdown in lactation, oxytocin may be administered intranasally. When administering an oxytocin, the nurse should:

- Always administer oxytocin intravenous piggyback (IVPB) in the smallest amount of fluid allowed in the antepartum period and never in the main IV to prevent overdosing and water intoxication.
- Monitor patients who are receiving IV oxytocin properly.
- Always dilute IV oxytocin with a physiologic electrolyte solution of 0.9% sodium chloride, lactated Ringer's solution, or 5% dextrose.
- Use a micro-drip and infusion pump for oxytocin IV administration to prevent water intoxication. Monitor uterine contractions, fetal and maternal heart rate, maternal blood pressure, and intrauterine pressure during oxytocin administration for early detection of adverse effects. Discontinue oxytocin immediately when uterine hyperactivity occurs to prevent adverse effects (e.g., uterine rupture) and fetal hypoxia.
- 🍎 Instruct patients to report a sudden, severe headache immediately, which may indicate a hypertensive episode.

Do You UNDERSTAND?

DIRECTIONS: **Indicate in the space provided whether the statement is** *true* **or** *false*. **If false, then correct the statement to make it true using the margin space at right.**

_____ 1. Oxytocin is given to promote milk letdown in nursing mothers.

_____ 2. In the gestation period, the uterus becomes progressively sensitive to oxytocin, peaking at delivery.

_____ 3. Initially, oxytocin is given IV in the antepartum period, then orally postpartum.

Answers: 1. true; 2. true; 3. false; IV initially then nasally as oxytocin is destroyed in the GI tract.

What IS a Prostaglandin?

Prostaglandins	Trade Names	Uses
dinoprostone [dye-nah-PROS-tone]	Cervidil, Prepidil	Induction of labor, evacuation of uterus, and control of postpartal hemorrhage
carboprost tromethamine [CAR-bo-prost]	Hemabate	Induction of labor, evacuation of uterus, and control of postpartal hemorrhage

Action

Prostaglandins are hormones that are synthesized in all body tissues. The mechanism of action has yet to be determined. These agents are thought to stimulate the myometrium (i.e., the smooth muscle layer of the uterus). These contractions of the pregnant uterus (**gravid**) are comparable to labor contractions in the full-term uterus and are usually adequate to evacuate the uterus. In the postpartal period, prostaglandins contract the myometrium to provide hemostasis (inhibit bleeding) at the placental attachment site.

Uses

Clinically, the use of prostaglandins is limited. In obstetrics, these agents are used to induce abortion and cervical ripening, as well as to control postpartal hemorrhage. Dinoprostone and carboprost are used to induce abortion during the second trimester of pregnancy. Prostaglandins are usually given in conjunction with oxytocin to shorten the induction-to-abortion time and reduce adverse effects. These agents are also used to evacuate the uterus in a missed abortion, the benign hydatidiform mole, or intrauterine fetal death up to 28 weeks of gestation.

What You NEED TO KNOW

Contraindications/Precautions

Prostaglandins are contraindicated for patients with acute pelvic inflammatory disease, uterine fibroids, cervical stenosis, and cardiac, pulmonary, renal, or hepatic disease.

Drug Interactions

Prostaglandins increase the action of oxytocic drugs. Recommendations are that these drugs should not be used concurrently.

Adverse Effects

Adverse effects of prostaglandins include headache, dizziness, fainting, flushing, hypertension, acute hypotension, chest pain, and dysrhythmias from the stimulation of vascular smooth muscle. Nausea, vomiting, and diarrhea may occur because of the stimulation of GI smooth muscles. Other adverse effects include

Prostaglandins should be used with caution in patients with hypotension, hyper--tension, diabetes mellitus, asthma, epilepsy, chorioam-nionitis, or uterine scarring.

fever, chills, shivering, bronchospasm, wheezing, and dyspnea. Sustained uterine contractility may cause cervical laceration and uterine rupture.

What You DO

Nursing Responsibilities

Prostaglandins are administered intravaginally. For cervical ripening, prostaglandin gel may be placed into the cervical canal immediately below the level of the internal mouth or opening of vagina (**internal os**) via a prefilled syringe. When administering prostaglandins, the nurse should:

- Allow prostaglandin intravaginal suppositories to warm to room temperature before removing the foil wrapper.
- Insert the prostaglandin suppository high into the posterior vagina, and have the patient remain supine for 10 minutes.
- Be aware that a dilute IV oxytocin solution may be started 1 hour after the first dose of dinoprostone.
- Carefully monitor uterine activity and fetal status throughout administration of prostaglandins for early detection of hypertonic uterine contractility and fetal distress.

Do You UNDERSTAND?

DIRECTIONS: **Place a check next to the potential adverse effects of prostaglandin.**

_____ 1. Seizures

_____ 2. Dyspnea

_____ 3. Dysrhythmias

_____ 4. Coma

What IS an Ergot Alkaloid?

Ergot Alkaloids	Trade Names	Uses
ergonovine maleate [er-go-NOH-veen]	Ergotrate Maleate	Treatment of postpartal hemorrhage
methylergonovine maleate [meth-ill-er-go-NOH-veen]	Methergine	Treatment of postpartal hemorrhage

Action

Ergot alkaloids stimulate adrenergic, dopaminergic, and serotonergic receptors, which stimulate uterine contractions and constrict arterioles and veins, thereby affecting uterine and vascular smooth muscle. In small doses following delivery, the uterine contractions are of moderate strength, with alternating uterine relaxation of a normal degree and duration. However, in large doses, uterine contractions are greatly increased in force and frequency, with reduced uterine relaxation. Sustained contractions are common with large doses and, when given during labor, can lead to maternal and fetal trauma. Sustained contractions result in a reduction of placental blood flow, leading to cervical laceration, uterine rupture, and fetal hypoxia.

Uses

The therapeutic use of ergot alkaloids in the postabortion and postpartal period is to increase uterine tone and decrease bleeding. The resulting sustained uterine contractions are desirable in this period. Because of the prolonged contractions, ergot alkaloids are not used to induce labor.

 # What You NEED TO KNOW

Contraindications/Precautions

Ergot alkaloids are contraindicated for patients with hypersensitivity and hypertension.

Drug Interactions

Drug interactions of ergot alkaloids involve parenteral sympathomimetics and other ergot alkaloids. When these agents are administered together, vasomotor action is increased, leading to hypertension.

Adverse Effects

The adverse effects of ergot alkaloids usually occur with IV administration. The most common adverse effects include severe hypertension, bradycardia, nausea, vomiting, allergic reaction, and shock. Other adverse effects include headache, dizziness, hallucinations, tinnitus, nasal congestion, dyspnea, foul taste, diaphoresis, palpitations, transient chest pain, thrombophlebitis, leg cramps, diarrhea, hematuria, and water intoxication. When IV methylergonovine is given undiluted, too rapidly, or in conjunction with regional anesthesia or vasoconstrictors, serious adverse effects may occur (e.g., particularly, severe hypertension, severe dysrhythmias, generalized headaches, CVA).

Ergot alkaloids are contraindicated for patients before delivery of the placenta, as well as those with threatened spontaneous abortion, uterine sepsis, and toxemia.

Ergot alkaloids should be used with caution in patients with a history of cardiovascular, renal, or hepatic dysfunction.

 Severe overdose effects include seizures and gangrene.

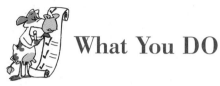

What You DO

Nursing Responsibilities

Because most adverse effects follow IV administration, IV use of ergot alkaloids is usually reserved for severe uterine bleeding or other life-threatening emergencies. When the situation necessitates the IV route, the drug should be diluted in at least 5 ml of 0.9% normal saline and administered at a slow rate over a period of not less than 1 minute to avoid serious adverse effects. When administering ergot alkaloids, the nurse should:

- Discard ampuls of methylergonovine that contain discolored solution or visible particles.
- Protect these agents from light when in storage.
- Monitor the vital signs and uterine response during and after parenteral administration of methylergonovine until the patient is stabilized, which is approximately 1 to 2 hours.
- Notify the health care provider in cases of sudden blood pressure increases or frequent periods of uterine relaxation.

Do You UNDERSTAND?

DIRECTIONS: Fill in the blanks with the appropriate responses.

1. _____ use of ergot alkaloids is usually reserved for severe uterine bleeding or other life-threatening situations.
2. IV solutions should be diluted in a least 5 ml of 0.9% _____ _____ and given at a slow rate over a period of not less than _____ to avoid serious adverse effects.

11 Drugs Affecting the Musculoskeletal System

SECTION A
ANTIINFLAMMATORY AGENTS

This section reviews the nurse's use of pharmacologic drugs that affect inflammatory conditions of the musculoskeletal system. Because antiinflammatory agents are the most widely used drugs of prescription and over-the-counter (OTC) use, the nurse must have a thorough understanding of these drugs to evaluate patient responses, identify adverse effects, and teach patients appropriately. This section discusses nonsteroidal antiinflammatory drugs, which included salicylates, propionic acid derivatives, acetic acid derivatives, pyrazolones, anthranilic acids, oxicams, and COX-$_2$ inhibitors, as well as acetaminophen, antiarthritics, and antigout agents.

What IS a Nonsteroidal Antiinflammatory?

Nonsteroidal Antiinflammatory Agents	Trade Names	Uses
Salicylate acetylsalicylic acid [ah-SEE-till-sal-ih-SILL-ick]	Aspirin Ecotrin	Treatment of arthritis, gout, and SLE
Propionic acid derivatives **ibuprofen** [eye-byoo-PROH-fen]	Motrin Advil	Treatment of arthritis
naproxen [nah-PROX-en]	Naprosyn Aleve	Treatment of arthritis, gout, and ankylosing spondylitis
Acetic acid derivative indomethacin [in-doe-METH-ah-sin]	Indocin	Treatment of arthritis, gout, and ankylosing spondylitis
Pyrazolone phenylbutazone [fen-ill-BYOO-tah-zone]	Butazolidin	Treatment of arthritis and ankylosing spondylitis

343

Continued

Nonsteroidal Antiinflammatory Agents—cont'd	Trade Names	Uses
Fenamate meclofenamate [me-kloh-fen-AM-ate]	Meclofen	Treatment of arthritis
Oxicam piroxicam [peer-OX-ih-cam]	Feldene	Treatment of arthritis
COX-$_2$ inhibitors nabumetone [nah-BU-meh-tone]	Relafen	Treatment of arthritis
celecoxib [CELL-ah-COX-ib]	Celebrex	Treatment of arthritis
rofecoxib [ROW-feh-COX-ib]	Vioxx	Treatment of arthritis

Action

Nonsteroidal antiinflammatory drugs (NSAIDs) suppress inflammation, relieve pain, and reduce fever. These responses are reached through the inhibition of cyclooxygenase, which is the enzyme that is responsible for the synthesis of prostaglandins. Prostaglandins are chemical mediators that are released at inflammatory sites, causing vasodilation, redness, warmth, increased capillary permeability, swelling, and sensitization of nerve cells to pain.

NSAIDs inhibit the formation and release of prostaglandin, which is one of the chemical mediators that is responsible for vasodilation, edema, and pain that is associated with inflammation. NSAIDs inhibit the two forms of cyclooxygenase: COX-$_1$ and COX-$_2$. Inhibiting COX-$_1$ decreases the protection of the stomach lining and platelet aggregation. Inhibiting COX-$_2$ decreases inflammation and pain.

Uses

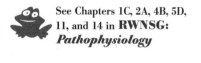

See Chapters 1C, 2A, 4B, 5D, 11, and 14 in **RWNSG:** *Pathophysiology*

NSAIDs are used for their analgesic effects in mild-to-moderate pain and inflammation in the treatment of arthritis, bursitis, tendonitis, ankylosing spondylitis, and systemic lupus erythematosus (SLE). Aspirin is the drug of choice in patients with arthritis. NSAIDs are also used for pain in headache and dysmenorrhea. Aspirin is also used in coronary artery disease (CAD), deep venous thrombosis (DVT), and transient ischemic attacks (TIAs) for their suppression of platelet aggregation. NSAIDs are safer than are opioids in older adults for short-term use.

What You NEED TO KNOW

Contraindications/Precautions

All NSAIDs are contraindicated for patients with hypersensitivity. Salicylates are contraindicated for patients with viral illnesses, such as influenza or chickenpox, because this combination is associated with Reye's syndrome. Indomethacin is contraindicated for patients who are taking triamterene because the combination may increase the risk of nephrotoxicity.

Drug Interactions

NSAIDs may exacerbate bleeding effects when given concurrently with warfarin. Prolonged use of NSAIDs and acetaminophen increases the risk of renal impairment. NSAIDs may induce lithium toxicity when these drugs are taken together. When phenytoin and NSAIDs are taken concurrently, drug levels may be altered, resulting in phenytoin toxicity. Acetylsalicylic acid (ASA) inhibits valproic acid metabolism, thereby causing valproic acid levels to rise. Hypoglycemia may occur when oral hypoglycemics are used with NSAIDs. NSAIDs reduce the antihypertensive effect of beta blockers and angiotensin-converting enzyme (ACE) inhibitors. NSAIDs reduce the effects of loop and thiazide diuretics, which may lead to induced congestive heart failure (CHF). When NSAIDs and potassium-sparing diuretics are given together, hyperkalemia may occur.

Adverse Effects

The most common adverse effects of NSAIDs include gastrointestinal (GI) effects of dyspepsia, anorexia, nausea, vomiting, diarrhea, and peptic ulcer formation. Other common adverse effects include headache, dizziness, and sodium and water retention. Renal adverse effects include reversible impairment of glomerular filtration, leading to chronic renal failure. Administering 1 to 2 g of salicylates per day decreases uric acid excretion. NSAIDs affect platelet aggregation and prolong bleeding time. Large doses of NSAIDs cause auditory and visual disturbances. Tinnitus is usually the first sign of toxicity. High doses of salicylate stimulate the respiratory center, resulting in hyperventilation and respiratory alkalosis. Toxic doses depress the respiratory center and cause metabolic acidosis.

 # What You DO

Nursing Responsibilities

NSAIDs are nearly always administered orally. When administering NSAIDs, the nurse should:
- Instruct the patient to take NSAIDs with food or milk to decrease GI distress.
- Instruct the patient to avoid the use of smoking products, alcohol, and other drugs that cause gastric irritation when taking NSAIDs.
- Advise the patient who is taking NSAIDs to avoid high-sodium foods because fluid retention may occur.
- Explain to the patient that some NSAIDs may take several weeks to produce maximal therapeutic effects.

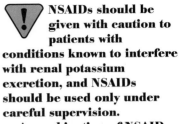 **NSAIDs should be given with caution to patients with conditions known to interfere with renal potassium excretion, and NSAIDs should be used only under careful supervision.**

A combination of NSAIDs, anticoagulants, and alcohol can be lethal.

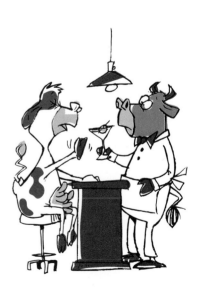

TAKE HOME POINTS

Instruct the patient to avoid crushing enteric coated or extended-release tablets.

Aspirin should be discontinued 1 week before elective surgery or childbirth because of the decrease in platelet aggregation and the risk of hemorrhage.

- Instruct the patient who is taking anticoagulant drugs concurrently with NSAIDs to observe for bleeding tendencies (e.g., black or tarry stools, bruising, nosebleeds).
- Monitor renal and hepatic function test for patients who are undergoing long-term therapy for early detection of dysfunction.
- Inform the patient who is taking NSAIDs to notify the health care provider when pain or fever persists for 3 days or when tinnitus occurs.
- Counsel the patient who is taking NSAIDs to consult with the health care provider before taking OTC drugs.

Do You UNDERSTAND?

DIRECTIONS: **Match the descriptions in Column A with the appropriate responses in Column B.**

Column A

_____ 1. The most common adverse effects after ingesting NSAIDs.

_____ 2. Primary reason for taking NSAIDs.

_____ 3. Nursing implications with concurrent NSAID and oral anticoagulant.

Column B

a. To decrease inflammation

b. GI disturbances

c. Monitor bleeding and petechiae

What IS Acetaminophen?

Acetaminophen	Trade Name	Use
acetaminophen [ah-SEAT-ah-MIN-ah-fen]	Tylenol	Relief of pain

Action

Acetaminophen, a nonprostaglandin derivative, has an unknown analgesic action. Acetaminophen acts on the hypothalamic heat-regulating-center to dissipate heat through the process of vasodilation and sweating, thereby reducing fever. Acetaminophen has weak antiinflammatory activity because of the minimal inhibition of peripheral prostaglandins. Acetaminophen neither decreases platelet aggregation nor alters prothrombin activity.

Uses

Acetaminophen is used in the treatment of pain and fever that is associated with a variety of conditions, including influenza and the relief of arthritic musculoskeletal pain. Acetaminophen is also used for patients who are receiving immunizations or those with viral illnesses because salicylates may cause Reye's syndrome.

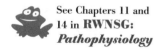

See Chapters 11 and 14 in RWNSG: *Pathophysiology*

Answers: 1. b; 2. a; 3. c.

What You NEED TO KNOW

Contraindications/Precautions

Acetaminophen is contraindicated for patients with renal dysfunction, hypersensitivity, and anemia.

Drug Interactions

Alcohol exacerbates the effects of acetaminophen, increasing the risk of hepatotoxicity when taken together. Long-term concurrent administration of barbiturates, carbamazepine, rifampin, or phenytoin with acetaminophen can increase the risk of hepatotoxicity. Cholestyramine decreases the absorption of acetaminophen.

Adverse Effects

Adverse effects of acetaminophen include headache, fever, skin rash, hemolytic anemia, and renal dysfunction.

What You DO

Nursing Responsibilities

Acetaminophen may be administered either with food or on an empty stomach. When administering acetaminophen, the nurse should:

- Advise the patient to avoid alcohol when taking more than one to two doses of acetaminophen per day.
- Instruct the patient who is taking acetaminophen and oral anticoagulants to report any increased bleeding, bruising, and nosebleeds.
- Counsel patients who are taking acetaminophen to consult their health care provider when fever lasts longer than 3 days or is over 103° F.
- Inform the patient that acetaminophen is available as chewable tablets, granules, extended-release tablets, solutions, liquids, elixirs, and suppositories.
- Instruct the patient to avoid acetaminophen use for more than 10 days for adults and 5 days for children without consulting the health care provider because abuse potential is high.
- Be aware that emptying the patient's stomach contents and immediately administrating acetylcysteine (Mucomyst), can minimize liver damage from toxic acetaminophen overdose.

 This agent should be used cautiously in patients with hepatic dysfunction or chronic alcoholism.

 Acetaminophen should be used cautiously during pregnancy and lactation.

Hepatotoxicity is a potentially fatal adverse effect that is associated with prolonged chronic use or overdose. Acute hepatic necrosis occurs when doses of 10 to 15 grams are administered. Doses greater than 25 g are fatal. Acetaminophen toxicity is defined as a plasma concentration of 200 μg/ml.

 TAKE HOME POINTS

Warn patients that psychologic dependence can occur with acetaminophen.

Do You UNDERSTAND?

DIRECTIONS: Provide appropriate responses to the following questions.

1. Acetaminophen toxicity is defined as a plasma concentration of what?

   _____

2. What symptoms should the patient who is taking acetaminophen report?

   _____

   _____

   _____

3. What organ is damaged from an acetaminophen overdose?

   _____

What IS an Antiarthritic?

Antiarthritics	Trade Names	Uses
Gold preparation gold sodium thiomalate [thigh-oh-MAH-late]	Myochrysine	Treatment of rheumatoid arthritis
Antimalarial medication hydroxychloroquine [hye-drox-ee-KLOR-oh-kwin]	Plaquenil	Treatment of rheumatoid arthritis and SLE
Immunosuppressive methotrexate [meth-oh-TREX-ate]	Mexate	Treatment of rheumatoid arthritis
Immunomodulator etanercept [eh-TAN-er-sept]	Enbrel	Treatment of rheumatoid arthritis
Glucocorticoid **prednisone** [PRED-nih-sone]	Deltasone	Treatment of rheumatoid arthritis
Miscellaneous medications penicillamine [pen-ih-SILL-ah-meen]	Cuprimine	Treatment of rheumatoid arthritis
sulfasalazine [sul-fa-SAL-ah-zeen]	Azulfidine	Treatment of rheumatoid arthritis
hyaluronic acid [HYE-al-your-ON-ic]	Hyalgan	Treatment of arthritis

Action

Antiarthritic drugs, also known as disease-modifying antirheumatic drugs (DMARDs), relieve symptoms of rheumatoid arthritis. DMARDs retard disease progression through the actions of decreasing the erythrocyte sedimentation rate (ESR); reducing inflammation, stiffness, and joint tenderness and pain; decreasing duration of early morning stiffness; improving grip strength; maintaining joint function; and preventing deformity.

Answers: 1. 200 µg/ml; 2. fever that lasts longer than 3 days or over 103° F, bleeding, bruising, and nosebleeds when also taking oral anticoagulants; 3. liver.

Gold compounds (**chrysotherapy** or **heavy metal therapy**) interrupt the progression of rheumatoid arthritis in the early synovitis stage and prevent deformities. Gold drugs suppress prostaglandin activity and are thought to inhibit destructive lysosomal enzyme activity in the joints. Gold therapy cannot reverse existing structural joint damage. The mechanism of action by which antimalarial drugs suppress the progression of disease is unclear at present.

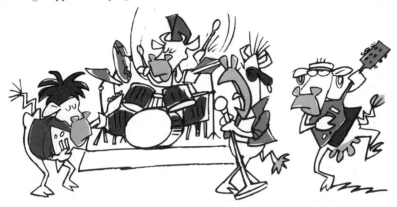

Because low-dose immunosuppressive agents suppress cancer growth and proliferation, they are useful in suppressing the inflammatory process of rheumatoid arthritis. Methotrexate treats rheumatoid arthritis through immunosuppressive or antiinflammatory effects or both. Etanercept is an immunomodulator, known as a tumor necrosis factor (TNF)–receptor antagonist, that binds to the TNF and blocks it from attaching to cell surface TNF receptors, thereby mediating the inflammatory response. Glucocorticoids act as antiinflammatory and immunosuppressant agents.

Penicillamine literally encloses a toxic substance to render it nonactive or nontoxic. Through suppression of T-cell activity, penicillamine has an immunosuppressive action. Sulfasalazine is metabolized into a salicylate and acts as an NSAID. Hyaluronic acid derivatives have elastic and viscous properties, which tend to cushion and lubricate the joint, thereby relieving pain.

Uses

Aspirin, other salicylates, and NSAIDs were used in the past as first-line drugs in the early stages of rheumatoid arthritis. Because only the synovial membranes are inflamed with painful swelling in the early stages, NSAIDs controlled the symptoms adequately. DMARDs were reserved for severe cases of rheumatoid arthritis or cases in which NSAIDs were ineffective.

Currently, some rheumatologists believe that aggressive therapy with DMARDs, initiated early in the disease, can interrupt joint degeneration. Recently, a combination of two or more DMARDs has been used for greater effectiveness in the treatment of rheumatoid arthritis.

Glucocorticoids have a role on a short-term basis at any point throughout the course of rheumatoid arthritis in treating severe exacerbations. Although the effect of gold compounds on the immune mechanism is limited, they are prescribed to relieve inflammation and pain. Antimalarial drugs are typically used

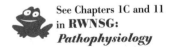

See Chapters 1C and 11 in **RWNSG:** *Pathophysiology*

Sulfasalazine is contra-indicated for children under 2 years of age. Gold agents, methotrexate, and sulfasalazine are contraindicated during pregnancy. Patients should take contraceptive precautions to prevent pregnancy for at least 12 weeks following methotrexate therapy. Etanercept is contraindicated for women during lactation and for children under 4 years of age.

Etanercept should be used cautiously during pregnancy. Hydroxychloroquine should be given cautiously during pregnancy and lactation. Methotrexate should be used with caution in older adults.

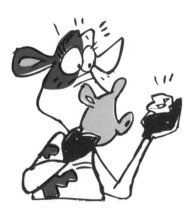

Gold agents are used with caution in patients with diabetes mellitus and CHF. Methotrexate is given cautiously to patients with peptic ulcers, ulcerative colitis, infections, poor nutritional status, and bone marrow dysfunction.

in combination with NSAIDs in the treatment of rheumatoid arthritis. Hydroxychloroquine is an antimalarial drug that can produce remission of rheumatoid arthritis. Low-dose immunosuppressives and miscellaneous DMARDs have been useful in treating rheumatoid arthritis. Hyaluronic acid may produce remission for 6 to 12 months in patients with rheumatoid arthritis and degenerative joint disease.

What You NEED TO KNOW

Contraindications/Precautions

Gold agents are contraindicated for patients with urticaria, colitis, hemorrhagic conditions, eczema, SLE, blood dyscrasias, and severe hepatic or renal disease. Etanercept is contraindicated for patients with sepsis. Penicillamine is contraindicated for patients who are hypersensitive to penicillin.

Drug Interactions

Folic acid preparations may decrease the effectiveness of methotrexate therapy. When penicillamine is combined with phenylbutazone, serious hematologic and renal toxicities may develop. Sulfasalazine can exacerbate anticoagulant and oral antidiabetic agents. Iron and antacids decrease penicillamine levels when taken concurrently.

Adverse Effects

The most common adverse effects of gold agents include rash, itching, and oral ulcers (**stomatitis**). Other adverse effects include photosensitivity, redness, anorexia, gastritis, abdominal cramps, colitis, diarrhea, hepatitis, and hair loss (**alopecia**). Unique adverse effects of gold therapy include a metallic taste, nitritoid reaction, and ocular gold deposits. Nitritoid reactions include dizziness, flushing, fainting, sweating, nausea, vomiting, headache, and weakness. Other serious adverse effects include hematuria, bradycardia, severe blood dyscrasias, interstitial pneumonitis, nephrotoxicity, and anaphylactic shock.

Prolonged high-dose hydroxychloroquine therapy (which is frequently necessary for rheumatoid arthritis) may result in serious and, occasionally, irreversible toxicities, such as hematologic and hepatic toxicity, retinopathy, and cardiomyopathy. Adverse effects of methotrexate include GI ulceration (particularly of the oral mucosa), gingivitis, glossitis, stomatitis, anorexia, nausea, vomiting, diarrhea, headache, hypotension, drowsiness, blurred vision, rash, itching, chills, fever, and muscle pain. More serious adverse effects include pericarditis, pericardial effusion, thromboembolism, Stevens-Johnson syndrome, bone marrow depression, pulmonary toxicity, hepatotoxicity, and sudden death.

Adverse effects from sulfasalazine include rash, itching, fever, anorexia, nausea, abdominal pain, vomiting, diarrhea, bone marrow depression, and hepatitis. Male infertility has been observed but is reversible following discontinuance of the drug.

What You DO

Nursing Responsibilities

Sulfasalazine is administered orally at least every 8 hours and should be given with food, in divided doses, or with enteric-coating to prevent gastric distress. When gastric distress occurs and persists, sulfasalazine should be discontinued for 5 to 7 days. Fluid intake should be increased to prevent crystalluria when the condition allows.

Methotrexate and penicillamine should be given 1 hour before or 2 hours after meals. Hydroxychloroquine is administered orally and should be given with food. Gold agents are injected intramuscularly (IM), and etanercept is injected subcutaneously (SC). When administering antiarthritic agents, the nurse should:

- Instruct the patient to take antacids or laxatives at least 4 hours before or after hydroxychloroquine.
- Monitor complete blood count (CBC) and platelet count throughout sulfasalazine, gold, methotrexate, and hydroxychloroquine therapy for early detection of bone marrow depression.
- Monitor patients who are receiving gold, methotrexate, and hydroxychloroquine for hepatic, renal, and pulmonary toxicities.
- Advise patients to decrease exposure to sunlight and ultraviolet light when taking gold to prevent gray-blue skin pigmentation from gold deposits (chrysiasis).
- Instruct patients who are taking gold or hydroxychloroquine to have eye examinations performed at least every 3 months.
- Instruct patients who are taking gold to perform careful oral hygiene to decrease discomfort from stomatitis.
- Instruct patients who are taking methotrexate to inspect their mouth daily and report any discomfort, patchy necrotic areas, bleeding, or overgrowth of black furry tongue to the health care provider.
- Monitor blood glucose periodically because methotrexate can precipitate diabetes mellitus.
- Warn patients who are taking methotrexate that exposure to ultraviolet light or sunlight may increase the risk of dermatologic reactions.
- Counsel the patient who is taking methotrexate to avoid alcohol to prevent hepatotoxicity.
- Instruct the patient to avoid taking OTC drugs without consulting the health care provider because many of these medications contain folic acid, which alters methotrexate response.
- Inform patients to report any sore mouth, weakness, unusual bleeding, bruising, skin eruptions, and visual or hearing impairment.
- Inject gold agents into the gluteus muscle.
- Inject etanercept SC into thigh, abdomen, or upper arm, with a rotation of sites.
- Carefully monitor the patient who is taking etanercept for signs of infection and immediately report these to the health care provider.

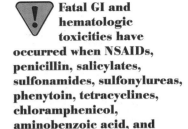

Fatal GI and hematologic toxicities have occurred when NSAIDs, penicillin, salicylates, sulfonamides, sulfonylureas, phenytoin, tetracyclines, chloramphenicol, aminobenzoic acid, and phenylbutazone are given with methotrexate.

TAKE HOME POINTS

Exposure to sunlight may aggravate chrysiasis. The patient who is receiving gold injections should remain in a recumbent position at least 30 minutes to avoid a nitritoid reaction. Never inject etanercept into an old injection site or into an area that is tender, bruised, red, or hard.

Never administer vaccinations, particularly live vaccines, to patients who are taking etanercept.

Do You UNDERSTAND?

DIRECTIONS: List six types of DMARDs, with an example of each that may be used for arthritis.

Types of DMARD　　　　　Examples

1. _____　　_____
2. _____　　_____
3. _____　　_____
4. _____　　_____
5. _____　　_____
6. _____　　_____

SECTION B

ANTIGOUT AGENTS

Antigout medications treat painful gouty attacks and prevent further attacks from occurring. A supersaturation of serum uric acid and crystal deposits that form in joints and surrounding tissue are characteristics of gout, thus antigout medications are focused on altering uric acid. Drugs are available that reduce uric acid production, increase renal uric acid excretion, and prevent recurrent attacks (e.g., antimitotics, NSAIDs, analgesics, corticosteroids, xanthine oxidase inhibitors, uricosurics).

In the first stage of gout (**asymptomatic hyperuricemia**), drugs are rarely required. In the second stage (**acute gouty arthritis**), antimitotics are the drugs of choice for the first attack. NSAIDs (particularly indomethacin) are preferred for subsequent attacks. Glucocorticoids may be used for patients who fail to respond to other drugs. The third stage (**asymptomatic intercritical period**) is treated with antimitotics, xanthine oxidase inhibitors, or uricosurics. The final stage of gout (**chronic tophaceous**) is treated primarily with xanthine oxidase inhibitors. This section reviews xanthine oxidase inhibitors, uricosurics, and antimitotics.

What IS an Antimitotic?

Antimitotic	Trade Name	Use
colchicine [KOHL-chi-seen]	Colchicine	Treatment of gout

Action

Antimitotics (the oldest gout medication) are antiinflammatory drugs, the effects of which are specific for gout. Colchicine inhibits the phagocytic response to

Answers: 1. *gold prepara-tions*—gold sodium thiomalate (Myochrysine); 2. *antimalari-als*—hydroxychloroquine (Plaquenil); 3. *immunosuppres-sives*—methotrexate (Mexate); 4. *immunomodulators*—etanercept (Enbrel); 5. *glucocorticoids*—prednisone (Deltasone); 6. *miscellaneous*—sulfasalazine (Azulfidine), peni-cillamine (Cuprimine), hyaluronic acid (Hyalgan).

urate crystals, thereby decreasing the inflammatory response. Colchicine causes neutrophils to block the release of the chemical mediators that are required in the inflammatory response, reduces mobility and adhesion of polymorphonuclear leukocytes, and inhibits production of leukotriene. Colchicine inhibits the inflammatory response, thereby generally eliminating pain within 48 hours of the onset of an acute gout attack and decreasing gouty signs and symptoms both rapidly and dramatically.

Uses

Colchicine has three uses: treating acute gouty attacks, aborting an impending attack, and reducing the incidence of chronic gout attacks. Colchicine is the drug of choice to relieve acute gouty attacks.

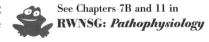

See Chapters 7B and 11 in
RWNSG: *Pathophysiology*

What You NEED TO KNOW

Contraindications/Precautions

Colchicine is contraindicated for patients with severe GI, cardiac, hepatic, or renal disorders.

Drug Interactions

When cimetidine and erythromycin are given concurrently with colchicine, the risk of colchicine toxicity is increased. Colchicine may decrease absorption of vitamin B_{12}.

  Antimitotics should be used with caution in women during pregnancy and lactation and in older or debilitated patients.

Adverse Effects

The common adverse effects of colchicines include nausea, abdominal cramping, vomiting, and diarrhea. Intravenous (IV) administration may lead to tissue necrosis from extravasation. Early signs of colchicine toxicity include nausea, anorexia, abdominal pain, vomiting, diarrhea, and paralytic ileus. Diarrhea may be severe and bloody. Other signs of colchicine toxicity include stomatitis, fever, malaise, rash, joint pain, hypocalcemia, dehydration, and oliguria.

 Life-threatening adverse effects include bone marrow suppression, renal failure, and disseminated intravascular coagulation.

What You DO

Nursing Responsibilities

Usually joint pain and swelling decrease within 8 to 12 hours and disappear within 24 to 72 hours after oral colchicine therapy and 6 to 12 hours after IV therapy. Colchicine should be discontinued when an acute gouty attack is

TAKE HOME POINTS

Take care to prevent IV extravasation of colchicine because severe tissue irritation and nerve damage may result. The patient with gout should have colchicine on hand.

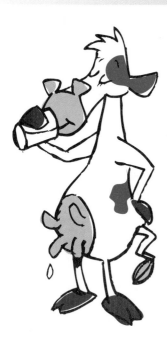

relieved. To avoid colchicine toxicity, therapy is not usually repeated within 3 days. When administering antimitotics, the nurse should:

- Inform the patient that colchicine may be given with food or milk to decrease the risk of GI distress.
- Counsel the patient to avoid beer, ale, and wine because these substances may cause sudden, unexpected gouty attacks.
- Instruct the patient that colchicine is effective only when taken at the first warning sign of an acute gout attack, not several days later.
- Instruct the patient to discontinue colchicine and immediately report any nausea, vomiting, and severe diarrhea to the health care provider because these are the first signs of toxicity. IV administration of colchicine eliminates most GI adverse effects.
- Advise the patient to report fever, fatigue, bleeding gums, sore mouth or throat, or any unusual bleeding or bruising to the health care provider for early detection of bone marrow suppression.

Do You UNDERSTAND?

DIRECTIONS: Circle the beverages that should be encouraged when undergoing colchicine therapy. Place a square around the beverages that should be avoided.

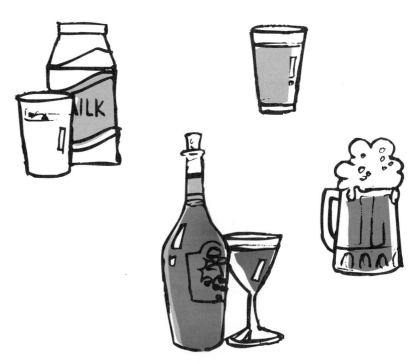

Answers: *encouraged beverages:* milk, water; *avoided beverages:* beer, wine.

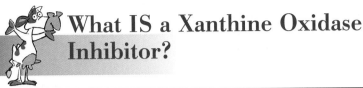

What IS a Xanthine Oxidase Inhibitor?

Xanthine Oxidase Inhibitor	Trade Name	Use
allopurinol [al-oh-PURE-ih-nohl]	Zyloprim	Treatment of hyperuricemia in gout

Action

Xanthine oxidase inhibitors inhibit the xanthine oxidase enzyme, thereby decreasing the serum uric acid level. Because the xanthine oxidase enzyme is responsible for converting hypoxanthine into xanthine and xanthine into uric acid, the inhibition of the xanthine oxidase enzyme blocks the production of uric acid.

Uses

Allopurinol is the drug of choice in the treatment of chronic tophaceous gout. Allopurinol reduces uric acid production and serum levels, which prevents tophus formation and promotes regression of preformed tophi.

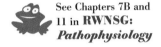 See Chapters 7B and 11 in **RWNSG:** *Pathophysiology*

 # What You NEED TO KNOW

Contraindications/Precautions

Xanthine oxidase inhibitors are contraindicated for patients with hypersensitivity. These drugs should be used with caution in patients with a history of peptic ulcer disease, bone marrow depression, and hepatic or renal dysfunction.

Drug Interactions

An increased effect of ACE inhibitors, theophylline, warfarin, phenytoin, and oncology drugs occurs when allopurinol is given concurrently. The risk of allopurinol toxicity is increased when given with thiazide diuretics, particularly in patients with renal dysfunction. Antacids decrease the absorption and action of allopurinol.

Adverse Effects

The adverse effects of allopurinol include drowsiness, headache, dizziness, metallic taste, rash, nausea, vomiting, abdominal discomfort, diarrhea, bone marrow depression, and hepatotoxicity. Cataracts and retinopathy may occur from prolonged allopurinol therapy.

Fatal hypersensitivity syndrome is the most serious (although rare) toxicity of xanthine oxidase inhibitors. Fever, rash, eosinophilia, and hepatic or renal dysfunction are characteristics of fatal hypersensitivity syndrome.

What You DO

Nursing Responsibilities

Allopurinol should be taken with food to eliminate GI distress. Tablets may be crushed and mixed with food or taken with fluids. When administering xanthine oxidase inhibitors, the nurse should:

- Monitor serum uric acid levels at least every 1 to 2 weeks to verify dose adequacy and maintain uric acid levels at 6 mg/dl.
- Monitor baseline CBC before beginning therapy and monthly for early detection of toxicity.
- Monitor baseline renal and hepatic function tests before therapy and monthly for early detection of toxicity.
- Instruct the patient who is taking allopurinol to report the first sign of a rash immediately to the health care provider.
- Inform the patient that a therapeutic response to allopurinol is usually expected in 1 to 3 weeks.
- When allopurinol is to be taken concurrently with an antineoplastic, the allopurinol should be initiated 1 to 2 days before administrating an antineoplastic.
- Inform the patient that periodic ophthalmic examinations are required when undergoing long-term allopurinol therapy.

Do You UNDERSTAND?

DIRECTIONS: Provide appropriate responses to the following questions.

1. When undergoing allopurinol therapy, which laboratory tests require periodic monitoring?

2. When undergoing allopurinol therapy, what adverse effect should be reported immediately?

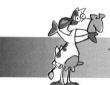

What IS a Uricosuric?

TAKE HOME POINTS

Because acute gouty attacks are likely to occur during the first 6 weeks of therapy, antimitotics may be given in combination therapy for the first 3 to 6 months of allopurinol treatment. Allopurinol should be immediately discontinued at the first sign of a rash because of a potentially fatal hypersensitivity reaction. Therapeutic responses to allopurinol include normal uric acid levels, gradual decrease in tophi, joint pain relief, and increased joint mobility.

Uricosurics	Trade Names	Uses
probenecid [pro-BEN-ih-sid]	Benemid	Treatment of hyperuricemia in gout
sulfinpyrazone [sul-fin-PEER-ah-zone]	Anturane	Treatment of hyperuricemia in gout

Answers: 1. CBC, hepatic, and renal function tests. 2. rash.

Action

Uricosurics block renal tubular reabsorption, which promotes excretion of uric acid.

Uses

Uricosurics are used in the treatment of hyperuricemia in gout to reduce the urate concentration in serum.

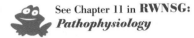 See Chapter 11 in **RWNSG:** *Pathophysiology*

 # What You NEED TO KNOW

Contraindications/Precautions

Uricosurics are contraindicated for patients with hypersensitivity, blood dyscrasias, uric acid kidney stones, and those who are taking β-lactam antibiotics or low-dose salicylates.

Drug Interactions

Probenecid increases the therapeutic effects of indomethacin and other NSAIDs. Salicylates counteract the action of uricosuric. Uricosurics inhibit the metabolism of tolbutamide, leading to hypoglycemia, and they inhibit the metabolism of warfarin, causing a bleeding tendency. Uricosurics also increase the concentrations of penicillins, cephalosporins, and other β-lactam antibiotics. Alcohol increases serum urate levels when taken together with uricosurics.

Adverse Effects

Uricosurics are usually well tolerated and have a low incidence of adverse effects. Common adverse effects of uricosurics include headache, dizziness, flushed skin, rash, sore gums, anorexia, nausea, vomiting, alopecia, peptic ulcer aggravation, urinary frequency, renal calculi, and blood dyscrasias. Hypersensitivity (e.g., itching, fever, sweating, hypotension, anaphylactic reaction) may also occur.

> **Uricosurics should be used cautiously in patients with a history of peptic ulcer disease and renal dysfunction.**

 # What You DO

Nursing Responsibilities

The goal is to reduce the uric acid level to 5 to 6 mg/dl, which depletes urate body storage, prevents the formation of tophi, and prevents renal damage. When gouty attacks have been absent for at least 6 months and serum urate levels are controlled, daily doses of uricosurics may be reduced to the lowest effective dose that maintains gout control. When administering uricosurics, the nurse should:

🍎 Instruct patients who are taking uricosurics to increase their fluid intake to at least 3000 ml/day to promote uric acid excretion and prevent renal calculi.

TAKE HOME POINTS

When gastric distress continues, a dose reduction may be required. An irregular dose schedule, such as skipped doses, may drastically increase serum urate levels and lead to gout attacks. Salicylates decrease uric acid excretion, which counteracts the uricosuric action.

- Instruct the patient to take uricosurics in divided doses with meals, milk, or antacids to prevent gastric distress.
- Advise the patient who is taking uricosurics to avoid alcohol to prevent GI distress and increased serum urate levels.
- Inform the patient who is taking uricosurics that the frequency of acute gouty attacks may increase during the first 6 to 12 months of uricosuric treatment, thus the health care provider may prescribe another concurrent prophylactic drug.
- Monitor blood glucose for patients who are taking uricosurics and concurrent sulfonylureas because these patients may require a dose adjustment to prevent hypoglycemia.
- Instruct the patient to take uricosurics as ordered and to avoid discontinuing the medication without consulting the health care provider.
- Instruct the patient who is taking uricosurics to avoid taking aspirin or OTC drugs without consulting the health care provider.

Do You UNDERSTAND?

DIRECTIONS: Fill in the blanks with the appropriate response.

1. Identify the drug that counteracts the uricosuric action when given concurrently.

   _____

2. Identify four of the most common adverse effects of uricosurics.

   _____
   _____
   _____
   _____

Answers: 1. salicylates; 2. headache, loss of appetite, nausea, vomiting.

12 Drugs for Nutritional Imbalances

Vitamins and minerals are essential to the body's metabolic activities and necessary in maintaining dynamic equilibrium that is required for good health. These substances are generally obtained from the diet. However, when the intake of vitamins or minerals is inadequate, deficiencies may occur and the health of the individual is affected. Factors that affect the dietary requirement and function of minerals and vitamins are environmental, genetic predisposition, hormone balance, growth, drugs, and disease processes. Vitamins and minerals that are used for nutritional imbalances are discussed in this chapter.

What IS a Vitamin?

Two types of vitamins have been classified: fat-soluble and water-soluble.

Fat-Soluble Vitamins

Fat-Soluble Vitamins	Trade Names
vitamin A	Aquasol A
vitamin D (calcitriol)	Rocaltrol
vitamin E	Aquasol E
vitamin K (phytonadione)	Aqua-Mephyton

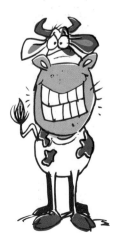

Action

The fat-soluble vitamins (A, D, E, and K) are found in the oil or fats of foods. Fat-soluble vitamins bind with specific plasma proteins and are then stored in the fat areas of the body. An excess accumulation in storage may cause toxicity. For the body to absorb fat-soluble vitamins, fat or bile salts are required.

Uses

Vitamin A is used in the growth and development of bones, teeth, retina, and epithelial and embryonic tis-

359

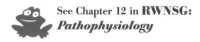

See Chapter 12 in **RWNSG:**
Pathophysiology

Water-Soluble Vitamins	Trade Names
vitamin C (ascorbic acid) [ah-SKOR-bic]	Ascorbicap
vitamin B_1 (thiamine) [THIGH-ah-min]	Betalin
vitamin B_2 (riboflavin) [RYE-bow-fly-vin]	None listed
vitamin B_3 (niacin) [NYE-ah-sin]	Nicobid
vitamin B_6 (pyridoxine) [peer-ih-DOX-een]	Hexa Betalin
vitamin B_9 (folic acid) [FOE-lick]	Folvite
vitamin B_{12} (cyanocobalamin) [sye-ANN-oh-koh-BAL-ah-min]	Cyanabin

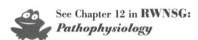

See Chapter 12 in **RWNSG:**
Pathophysiology

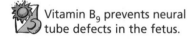

Vitamin B_9 prevents neural tube defects in the fetus.

Vitamin A should be used with caution in patients with renal dysfunction, women who are taking contraceptives, and with prolonged administration. Vitamin D should be used with caution in patients with coronary disease, renal dysfunction, dialysis, arteriosclerosis, asthma, and hypoparathyroidism. Vitamin K should be used with caution in those with hepatic impairment.

sue. Vitamin A is also used in the synthesis of hydrocortisone. Vitamin D prevents and treats rickets; promotes calcium, magnesium, and phosphorus absorption and metabolism; and controls parathyroid hormone levels. Vitamin E is an antioxidant that prevents formation of free radicals that damage cell membranes. Vitamin E also promotes the growth and development of muscles, increases fat metabolism, aids the body's use of vitamin A, and prevents the formation of blood clots. Vitamin K affects the synthesis of blood coagulation factors II (**prothrombin**), VII, IX, and X in the liver. Vitamin K is also the antidote for oral anticoagulant overdose.

Water-Soluble Vitamins

Action

Vitamin C and the B-complex vitamins are water-soluble and are found in the watery portion of foods. The B-complex vitamins include vitamins B_1, B_2, B_3 (niacin), B_6, B_9 (**folic acid**), and B_{12}. These vitamins are readily excreted, and small amounts of these vitamins are stored in the body. Therefore water-soluble vitamins rarely cause toxicity, and regular daily intake is required.

Uses

Vitamin C is an antioxidant that promotes collagen formation, tissue repair, wound healing, gastrointestinal (GI) absorption of iron, and the synthesis of peptide and epinephrine. Vitamin C also prevents and treats scurvy. Vitamin B_1 promotes carbohydrate and aerobic metabolism, transmission of nerve impulses, maintenance of normal growth and development, and synthesis of acetylcholine. Vitamin B_2 acts as a catalyst in oxidation-reduction reactions of glucose, amino acid, and the metabolism of fatty acids. Vitamin B_3 acts as a catalyst in oxidation-reduction reactions of cholesterol and fatty acids. Vitamin B_3 also causes vasodilation and prevents and treats pellagra. Vitamin B_6 promotes protein, fat, and carbohydrate metabolism; facilitates release of glucose from liver and muscles; promotes formation of neurotransmitters; and treats neuropathy. Vitamin B_9 helps in protein synthesis and erythropoiesis and stimulates production of red blood cells, white blood cells, and platelets. Vitamin B_{12} is essential for growth, cell reproduction, hematopoiesis; synthesis of nucleic acid and myelin; and treatment of vitamin B_{12} deficiency and pernicious anemia.

What You NEED TO KNOW

Contraindications/Precautions for Fat-Soluble Vitamins

Vitamin E has no contraindications. Vitamin K is contraindicated for patients with hypersensitivity.

Drug Interactions

Mineral oil decreases the absorption of vitamin A. Oral contraceptives increase levels of vitamin A. Mineral oil decreases absorption of vitamin D. Use of vitamin D in patients on chronic renal dialysis may lead to hypomagnesemia. Concurrent use of digitalis or verapamil with vitamin D may precipitate dysrhythmias. Concurrent administration of phenobarbital and phenytoin may decrease vitamin D levels. Corticosteroids counteract vitamin D effects. Mineral oil and sucralfate decrease the absorption of vitamin E. Vitamin E may also enhance the action of oral anticoagulants. Mineral oil and sucralfate decrease the absorption of vitamin K. Vitamin K antagonizes the effect of warfarin.

 Vitamin A should be used with caution during pregnancy and lactation. Vitamin D should be used with caution in older adults. Vitamin K should be used with caution in women during pregnancy and lactation and in children.

Adverse Effects

Vitamin A may cause inflammation of the skin, conjunctiva, and lips; dry mucus membranes; baldness; and peeling of the palms of hands and soles of feet. Overdosing of vitamin A causes malaise, anorexia, abdominal discomfort, lethargy, and vomiting (**hypervitaminosis syndrome**). Overdosing of vitamin A also causes headache, dizziness, irritability, increased intracranial pressure (ICP), dry cracked skin, edema, jaundice, hypomenorrhea, blurred vision, and irreversible bone demineralization.

Early adverse effects of vitamin D include headache, dizziness, weakness, nausea, vomiting, dry mouth, constipation, diarrhea, metallic taste, and muscle and bone pain. Late adverse effects of vitamin D include anorexia, irritability, polyuria, polydipsia, photophobia, itching, and decreased libido.

Vitamin E is nontoxic. Prolonged use of excessive doses of vitamin E causes skeletal muscle weakness, headache, blurred vision, nausea, diarrhea, abdominal cramps, and fatigue. Adverse effects of vitamin K include transient flushing and alteration in taste.

 Following intravenous (IV) use of vitamin A, anaphylactic shock and death has been reported.

Contraindications/Precautions for Water-Soluble Vitamins

Vitamin B$_3$ is contraindicated for patients with liver impairment, severe hypotension, active peptic ulcer or bleeding, and hypersensitivity. Vitamin B$_9$ is contraindicated for the treatment of pernicious anemia and other megaloblastic anemias when vitamin B$_{12}$ is deficient. Vitamin B$_{12}$ is contraindicated for patients with hypersensitivity.

 Vitamin B$_3$ is contraindicated during pregnancy and lactation.

Drug Interactions

Vitamins B$_1$, B$_2$, and B$_{12}$ have no known drug interactions. Large doses of vitamin C may decrease the response to oral anticoagulants and disulfiram. Vitamin C requirements may be increased with concurrent use of salicylates, oral contraceptives, and smoking. The absorption of iron is increased when vitamin C is taken with iron-rich foods. Vitamin B$_3$ enhances antihypertensive agents, causing hypotensive effects. Concurrent use of isoniazid, hydralazine, penicillamine, or oral contraceptives decreases therapeutic effects of vitamin B$_6$. Vitamin B$_6$ may reverse or antagonize the effects of levodopa. Concurrent use of sulfasalazine, methotrexate, trimethoprim, oral contraceptives, and aminosalicylic acid decreases vitamin B$_9$ folic acid levels. Folic acid (vitamin B$_9$) decreases hydantoin concentrations.

 Vitamin C should be used with caution in patients with diabetes and those who are prone to renal calculi, on a sodium restricted diet, or those who are taking anticoagulants. Vitamin B$_1$ should be used with caution in patients with hypersensitivity. Vitamin B$_3$ should be used with caution in patients with a history of gallbladder disease, liver disease, glaucoma, angina, gout, diabetes, and coronary artery disease.

 Vitamins C, B$_1$, B$_2$, and B$_6$ should be used cautiously during pregnancy and lactation.

Adverse Effects

Vitamin C is usually nontoxic, except when excessive doses are taken. Transient soreness at intramuscular (IM) and subcutaneous (SC) injection sites, temporary dizziness, and faintness following rapid IV administration. Overdosing of vitamin C causes nausea, vomiting, diarrhea, gout attacks, and renal stones. Adverse effects of vitamin B_1 include a warm feeling, itching, weakness, sweating, restlessness, nausea, angioedema, pulmonary edema, hypersensitivity, anaphylactic shock, and death. Vitamin B_2 is nontoxic but may cause yellow discoloration of urine when taken in large doses. Adverse effects of vitamin B_3 include transient headache, generalized flushing, feeling of warmth, nausea, vomiting, flatulence, bloating, dry skin, itching, tingling of extremities, jaundice, and elevated hepatic function tests. Adverse effects of vitamin B_6 include a slight flushing and warm feeling. Although rare, vitamin B_6 causes paresthesia and seizures, usually with large parenteral doses. Adverse effects of vitamin B_9 include hypersensitivity reactions, decreased vitamin B_{12} serum levels, altered sleep patterns, difficulty concentrating, irritability, excitement, overactivity, mental depression, confusion, anorexia, impaired judgment, bitter taste, and flatulence. Adverse effects of vitamin B_{12} include allergic reactions and hypersensitivity.

What You DO

Nursing Responsibilities for Fat-Soluble Vitamins

Fat-soluble vitamins are generally given orally. Vitamin K may also be given SC or IM. When administering fat-soluble vitamins, the nurse should:

- 🍎 Advise the patient to avoid concurrent use of mineral oil with fat-soluble vitamins because it decreases absorption of the vitamins.
- 🍎 Instruct the patient to take vitamins A and E on an empty stomach. When the patient has GI distress, vitamins A and E may be taken with food or milk. Vitamins D and K may be taken without regard to food.
- 🍎 Advise the patient to swallow oral vitamin D whole and avoid chewing or crushing the vitamin.
- 🍎 Counsel the patient to avoid magnesium antacids when taking vitamin D.
- 🍎 Instruct the patient to obtain sufficient exposure to sunlight to help satisfy vitamin D requirements.
- • Protect vitamin K medication from the light.
- 🍎 Instruct the patient who is taking vitamin K to avoid alcohol, ibuprofen, and aspirin and to report any bleeding.
- 🍎 Inform the patient that food sources of vitamin A include liver, butter, cheese, whole milk, egg yolk, meat, fish, dark-green leafy vegetables, carrots, squash, sweet potatoes, and cantaloupes. Food sources of vitamin D include fish, liver, and oils. Food sources of vitamin E include wheat germ, vegetable oils, green leafy vegetables, dairy products, nuts, meat, liver, eggs, and cereals. Food sources of vitamin K include cauliflower, spinach, fish, liver, eggs, meats, cereal grain products, dairy products, and fruits.

TAKE HOME POINTS

- • Monitor calcium and phosphorus levels at least twice weekly, then once weekly for 12 weeks until the patient with chronic renal failure (CRF) who is taking vitamin D stabilizes; monitor monthly thereafter.
- • Heparin is the antidote for vitamin K overdose.

🍎 Warn the patient to report hypervitaminosis (e.g., malaise, anorexia, nausea, vomiting, diarrhea, headache, dizziness, irritability, dried and cracked skin, edema, jaundice, hypomenorrhea, blurred vision).

Nursing Responsibilities for Water-Soluble Vitamins

Most water-soluble vitamins are given orally. Vitamin B_1 may also be given IM or IV. When GI absorption is severely impaired, vitamin B_9 may be given SC, IM, or IV. Parenteral vitamin B_{12} should be given IM or deep SC. When administering water-soluble vitamins, the nurse should:

🍎 Instruct the patient to take oral vitamins C, B_1, B_3, and B_{12} with food. Large doses of vitamins C and B_3 should be given in small, divided doses because the body will excrete excessive amounts beyond the current requirement. Vitamin B_6 may be given without regard to food.

🍎 Instruct patients that the need for vitamin B_1 and B_6 is increased when the diet is high in carbohydrates.

🍎 Instruct the patient to taper vitamin C doses when discontinuing. Abrupt discontinuation of large doses may lead to bleeding gums, gingivitis, and loosened teeth (**rebound scurvy**).

• Rotate IM injection sites of vitamin B_1 and apply cold compresses to relieve pain at injection site.

🍎 Inform the patient that food sources of vitamin C include citrus fruits, such as oranges, limes, lemons and strawberries, tomatoes, leafy vegetables, melons, and cabbage. Food sources of vitamin B_1 include brewer's yeast, beef, pork, milk, liver, nuts, legumes, whole grains, enriched flour, and cereal. Food sources of vitamin B_2 include meat, fish, poultry, dairy products, broccoli, asparagus, spinach, mushrooms, grains, cereal, and bakery products. Food sources of vitamin B_3 include organ and lean meats, brewer's yeast, poultry, fish, and peanuts. Food sources of vitamin B_6 include yeast, whole-grain cereals, liver, legumes, green vegetables, and bananas. Food sources of vitamin B_9 include liver, oranges, asparagus, broccoli, Brussels sprouts, spinach, beets, whole-wheat products, peas, dried beans, and lentils. Food sources of vitamin B_{12} include liver, fish, dairy products, clams, oysters, and crabs.

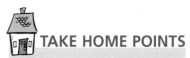

TAKE HOME POINTS

Warn the patient to take the oral **vitamin B_{12}** dose promptly when it is mixed with juice because ascorbic acid affects the stability of vitamin B_{12}.

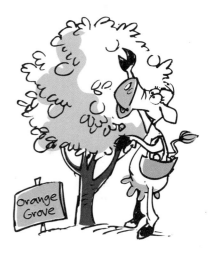

Orange Grove

Do You UNDERSTAND?

DIRECTIONS: Match the correct vitamin in Column A with the appropriate word from the scrambled letters in Column B.

Column A

_____ 1. Vitamin B_3
_____ 2. Vitamin K
_____ 3. Vitamin D
_____ 4. Vitamin B_{12}

Column B

a. incain
b. trillaccoi
c. diyhpnatooen
d. manboaycilocan

Answers: 1. niacin; 2. phytonadione; 3. calcitriol; 4. cyanocobalamin.

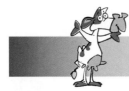

What IS a Mineral?

Minerals	Trade Names
sodium (sodium bicarbonate)	None listed
potassium (potassium chloride)	K-Dur Micro-K
calcium (calcium citrate)	Citra Cal
phosphorus	K-Phos Neutro-Phos
magnesium (magnesium oxide)	Mag-Ox 400
iron (ferrous gluconate)	Fergon
zinc	None listed

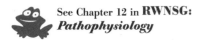

See Chapter 12 in **RWNSG:**
Pathophysiology

Action

Minerals function as structural components, forming bones, teeth, and nails and acting as components of enzymes. Minerals are essential for the body's regulation of water metabolism, blood volume, cell membrane permeability, tissue excitability, and the maintenance of acid-base balance. The body excretes minerals, thus they must be replaced through the intake of food or supplements.

Uses

Sodium regulates fluids, tissues, water, and acid-base balance and conducts electrical impulses of muscles and nerves. Sodium also prevents or treats extracellular volume depletion and dehydration or sodium depletion. Sodium prevents heat prostration.

Potassium is the principle intracellular cation of most body tissues. Potassium maintains intracellular tonicity, cell metabolism, transmission of impulses, acid-base balance, and renal function. Potassium also maintains contraction of cardiac, skeletal, and smooth muscles, as well as prevents and treats hypokalemia.

Calcium maintains the integrity of nervous and muscular systems, normal cardiac function, cell permeability, and blood coagulation. Calcium promotes bone growth and the activity of endocrine and exocrine glands. Calcium also treats calcium deficiency, end-stage renal failure (calcium acetate), hypoparathyroidism, osteoporosis, rickets, and osteomalacia.

Phosphorus functions at the intracellular level for energy transport and energy production (adenosine diphosphate [ADP] and adenosine triphosphate [ATP]). Phosphorus aids calcium transport, acts as phospholipids in cell membranes, is a component of deoxyribonucleic acid (DNA) and ribonucleic acid (RNA) molecules, lowers urinary calcium levels, and increases urinary phosphate levels.

Magnesium aids in sodium and potassium transport, phosphate transfer, muscular contraction, nerve conduction, enzyme systems, energy release with conversion of ATP to ADP, and treats hypomagnesemia, preeclampsia, and cardiac dysrhythmias.

Iron, a component of hemoglobin, myoglobin, and enzymes, maintains heat production, aids in muscle and catecholamine metabolism, and prevents and treats iron deficiency. Iron supplements are needed in CRF to correct the iron deficiency anemia, which is a major abnormality in renal failure.

Zinc promotes the growth and repair of tissue, is an integral part of enzymes that are required for protein and carbohydrate metabolism, and controls copper absorption in the long-term treatment of Wilson's disease.

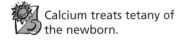
Calcium treats tetany of the newborn.

What You NEED TO KNOW

Contraindications/Precautions

Potassium is contraindicated for patients with severe renal impairment, crush syndrome, Addison's disease, hyperkalemia, severe hemolytic reactions, acute dehydration, anuria, heat cramps, and in those who are receiving potassium-sparing diuretics or angiotensin-converting enzyme (ACE) inhibitors. Calcium is contraindicated for patients with hypercalcemia, hypophosphatemia, and renal calculi. Phosphorus is contraindicated for patients with hyperkalemia, Addison's disease, severe renal impairment, hyperphosphatemia, and hypercalcemia. Magnesium is contraindicated for patients who are experiencing abdominal pain, nausea, vomiting, diarrhea, fecal impaction, intestinal obstruction, and heart block following delivery. Iron is contraindicated for patients with hemolytic anemia, hemosiderosis, cirrhosis of the liver, peptic ulcer, hemochromatosis, and ulcerative colitis.

Drug Interactions

Sodium has no known drug interactions. Concurrent use of potassium with potassium-sparing diuretics or ACE inhibitors may cause hyperkalemia.

Calcium may enhance inotropic and toxic effects of digoxin. Calcium decreases absorption and the effects of verapamil, tetracycline, quinolones, iron, and atenolol. Concurrent use of calcium with thiazide diuretics may result in hypercalcemia. Calcium supplements reduce zinc absorption. When hypocalcemic agents are taken concurrently with antacids that contain magnesium, hypermagnesemia may occur. Reduced absorption may occur when hypocalcemics are taken with cholestrylamine or mineral oil. Phosphates absorption and action are decreased when given concurrently with vitamin D and antacids with magnesium, aluminum, or calcium. When phosphates and potassium-containing agents are given together, hyperkalemia may occur. Magnesium salts decrease the absorption of quinolones, digoxin, nitrofurantoin, penicillamine, and tetracyclines. When given concurrently, antacids lower iron absorption. Ascorbic acid and chloramphenicol enhance the absorption of iron. Iron decreases the absorption of tetracyclines, ofloxacin, penicillamine, and ciprofloxacin, and may delay the effects of chloramphenicol. Drugs that may have a decreased absorption or effectiveness when given with iron include levodopa, levothyroxine, methyldopa, penicillamine, quinolones, and tetracyclines. When zinc is given concurrently, the absorption and effectiveness of fluoroquinolones and tetracyclines are decreased.

Adverse Effects

Sodium overdosing causes electrolyte imbalances, GI irritation, anorexia, nausea, vomiting, diarrhea, abdominal cramps, restlessness, confusion, weakness, irritability, convulsions, coma, hypertension, tachycardia, and pulmonary edema.

 Sodium and zinc are contraindicated during pregnancy and lactation.

 Potassium and calcium should be used cautiously during pregnancy. Phosphorus should be used cautiously during pregnancy and lactation.

Sodium should be used cautiously in patients with kidney dysfunction, preeclampsia, and peripheral or pulmonary edema. Potassium should be used cautiously in patients with severe burns and cardiac or renal disease. Calcium should be used cautiously in patients with hypoparathyroidism who are also receiving high doses of vitamin D and in patients who have aspirin hypersensitivity (because some calcium products contain tartrazine that may cause allergic reactions, including bronchial asthma). Phosphorus should be used cautiously in patients who are on a sodium- or potassium-restricted diet or those with cardiac disease, acute dehydration, renal and hepatic dysfunction, edema, hypernatremia, hypertension, preeclampsia, acute pancreatitis, hypoparathyroidism, osteomalacia, and renal calculi. Magnesium should be used cautiously in patients with renal disease.

Potassium's adverse effects include nausea, vomiting, diarrhea, abdominal pain, and oliguria. Hyperkalemia (i.e., a potassium level greater than 5.5 mEq/L) can cause muscle weakness, paresthesias, nausea, diarrhea, hypotension, bradycardia, dysrhythmias, and cardiac arrest.

Calcium's adverse effects include mild hypercalcemia (i.e., a calcium level greater than 10.5 mg/dl), which can be asymptomatic or in the form of headache, anorexia, nausea, vomiting, abdominal pain, constipation, dry mouth, thirst, metallic taste, and polyuria. Severe hypercalcemia (i.e., a calcium level greater than 12.5 mg/dl) displays neuromuscular irritability, confusion, delirium, and coma. Hypercalcemia occurs more frequently with calcitrate and calcium carbonate compared with calcium acetate.

Adverse effects of phosphorus that include nausea, vomiting, abdominal pain, and diarrhea are common. Less frequently, phosphorus causes headache, dizziness, weakness, confusion, muscle cramps, numbness, tingling, pain, shortness of breath, swelling of lower extremities, weight gain, thirst, and bone and joint pain.

Overdosing of magnesium causes hypermagnesemia, weakness, hypotension, bradycardia, electrocardiogram changes, nausea, vomiting, urinary retention, and hyporeflexia.

Iron's adverse effects include nausea, vomiting, diarrhea, constipation, and dark-colored stools. Liquid iron preparations may stain teeth. Iron overdosing may also produce lethargy, abdominal pain, weak thready pulse, hypotension, fever, hyperglycemia, decreased tissue perfusion, leukocytosis, dyspnea, metabolic acidosis, coma, convulsions, shock, vascular congestion, pulmonary edema, anuria, and death.

Zinc's adverse effects include nausea and vomiting. Zinc overdosing causes nausea, severe vomiting, dehydration, and restlessness.

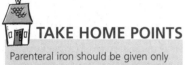

TAKE HOME POINTS

Parenteral iron should be given only in the muscle of the upper-outer buttock quadrants using the Z-track technique.

What You DO

Nursing Responsibilities

Mineral supplements are generally given orally, but may be administered IV in acute situations. When administering mineral supplements, the nurse should:

- Give sodium tablets with 8 ounces of water up to 10 times a day in the treatment of heat cramps and dehydration.
- Give potassium with an 8-ounce glass of water or fruit juice to ensure that the drug is swallowed and does not cause esophagitis by dissolving and irritating the mucous membranes.
- Administer calcium with meals to increase the absorption of fats and carbohydrates.
- Instruct the patient to avoid chewing any extended-release or long-acting potassium preparation.

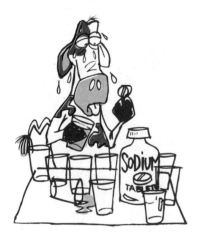

🍎 Instruct the patient to drink an 8-ounce glass of water with calcium and to report any anorexia, nausea, vomiting, constipation, abdominal pain, polyuria, thirst, or dry mouth (signs and symptoms of hypercalcemia) to the health care provider.

🍎 Inform the patient that foods high in fiber decrease calcium absorption time because of decreased transit time.

🍎 Advise the patient that swallowing phosphorus capsules whole should be avoided. Rather, the capsule should be opened and the powder inside dissolved in water.

🍎 Inform the patient that iron pills should not be crushed or the contents of the capsule emptied.

• Administer iron and calcium 2 hours apart from tetracyclines, fluoroquinolones, or any medication that affects the absorption of iron.

🍎 Instruct the patient that iron should be taken on an empty stomach. When GI distress occurs, the drug may be taken with meals. However, iron should not be taken within 1 hour of bedtime.

• Warn the patient that tarry black stools may result from iron therapy.

• Absorption of iron may be decreased when taken with milk, eggs, and caffeine-containing drinks.

• Administer zinc 1 hour before, or 2 to 3 hours after meals. When GI distress occurs, zinc may be taken with food.

🍎 Advise patients to avoid coffee because it reduces zinc absorption by 50%.

🍎 Instruct the patient to report signs and symptoms of potassium toxicity (e.g., muscle weakness, paresthesias, nausea, diarrhea, hypotension, bradycardia) because potassium toxicity can occur with therapeutic doses.

• Monitor serum calcium levels two times a week initially after beginning therapy and periodically thereafter.

• Report serum sodium level that is over 146 mEq/L.

• Monitor serum phosphorus, calcium, potassium, sodium (because phosphate products contain high amounts of potassium and sodium), and renal function tests.

• Monitor the pulse and blood pressure every 15 minutes or at more frequent intervals as indicated when giving IV magnesium sulfate.

• Check the patient's patellar reflex before each repeated dose of parenteral magnesium. Signs of early magnesium toxicity include depressed or absent reflexes.

• Monitor the respirations and urine output in patients with renal dysfunction.

• Monitor hemoglobin and reticulocyte values for drug effectiveness. Iron therapy is usually continued for 2 to 3 months after the hemoglobin level returns to normal. As a rule, iron therapy should not exceed 6 months.

🍎 Inform patients that excessive consumption of sodium chloride may lead to acidosis and hypokalemia.

🍎 Inform patients who are on sodium- and potassium-restricted diets that phosphate products contain high amounts of potassium and sodium.

TAKE HOME POINTS

• Give calcium preparations with caution to digitalized patients because of the increased risk of digitalis toxicity.

• Administer iron with citrus juice or fruits to enhance absorption.

• Administer liquid iron through a straw, adequately diluted, and then rinse the mouth with water immediately after taking the medication to prevent staining the teeth. Hypercalcemia may develop when given in therapeutic doses for a prolonged period.

• Parenteral iron should be given with the Z-track technique.

Inform the patient that good sources of potassium in foods are milk, bananas, raisins, prunes, dates, avocado, beef, lamb, chicken, turkey, veal, watermelon, cantaloupe, apricots, pears, broccoli, brussels sprouts, spinach, potatoes, and lentils. Sources of calcium include milk, milk products, and dark green vegetables. Food sources of magnesium include nuts, meats, legumes, fish, whole-grain cereals, milk, and green leafy vegetables. Food sources of iron include red meat, liver, dark-green leafy vegetables, carrots, raisins, prunes, and apricots.

Counsel the patient to avoid foods that are high in copper (e.g., liver, pork, tofu, shellfish, nuts, dried beans, mushrooms, broccoli, avocado, cocoa, chocolate), calcium, and phosphorus when taking zinc.

Do You UNDERSTAND?

DIRECTIONS: **Provide the appropriate responses to the following questions from the italicized choices.**

1. Vitamins A, D, E, and K are _____. (*fat-soluble, water-soluble*)

2. _____ is an antioxidant essential for collagen formation and tissue repair. (*folic acid, vitamin C*)

CHAPTER

13 Drugs Affecting the Sensory System

Section A
OPHTHALMICS AND OTICS

Visual disorders present a danger to patients, largely because vision is one of the most cherished senses. Although many eye disorders are correctable with eyeglasses or contact lenses, others require medications to control or treat. Hearing and balance disorders interfere with the patient's involvement in social activities, constructive use of leisure time, and ability to communicate, leading to social isolation. Removing earwax (**cerumen**) helps the patient avoid problems that are associated with impaired sound reception. This section reviews selected medications that are used in the treatment of eye and ear disorders, including ocular lubricants, decongestants, miotics, and osmotics; carbonic anhydrase inhibitors; mydriatic and cycloplegics; and ceruminolytic agents.

What IS an Ocular Lubricant?

Ocular Lubricants	Contents
artificial tears	White petrolatum, mineral oil, and anhydrous lanolin
tyloxapol (Enuclene)	Benzalkonium chloride

Action

Ocular lubricants include single-ingredient formulations, such as sodium chloride and polyvinyl alcohol. Combination formulations include petrolatum, mineral oil, and lanolin. Ocular lubricants keep the eyes moist with isotonic solutions and wetting agents. The most important properties of artificial tear formulations are that they stabilize the tear film while preventing tear evaporation.

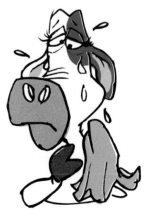

369

Uses

Ocular lubricants alleviate dry eyes and provide lubrication for patients with an artificial eye. These agents offer lubrication and protection for exposure-related inflammation of the cornea (keratitis), decreased corneal sensitivity, corneal erosions, dry cornea (during or following eye surgery), and removal of a foreign body. Lubricants with high thickness (viscosity) alone do not necessarily provide relief for all dry eye conditions.

 # What You NEED TO KNOW

Contraindications/Precautions

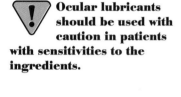 **Ocular lubricants should be used with caution in patients with sensitivities to the ingredients.**

Ocular lubricants should be used with caution in patients with sensitivities to the ingredients.

Drug Interactions

Ocular lubricants may alter the effects of other concurrently administered medications that are used in the eye.

Adverse Effects

Ocular lubricants generally cause no irritation or toxicity to eye tissues. Adverse effects of ocular lubricants include photophobia, lid edema, stinging, temporarily blurred vision, and eye discomfort.

 # What You DO

Nursing Responsibilities

Ocular lubricants are used for their local effects in the eye. Because nearly all ocular lubricants are available without a prescription, the health care provider and pharmacist frequently carry the primary responsibility of assisting and counseling the patient regarding their selection and proper use. When administering ocular lubricants, the nurse should:

- Advise the patient to consult with the health care provider regarding the concurrent use of ocular lubricants and contact lenses.
- Inform the patient that no single formulation of natural tears has been identified that universally improves the signs and symptoms of dry eyes while maintaining patient comfort and acceptance.

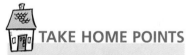 **TAKE HOME POINTS**

Some contact lenses may absorb the medications or their additives.

Do You UNDERSTAND?

DIRECTIONS: **Provide appropriate responses to the following questions and statements.**

1. List five ingredients that are common in ocular lubricants.

   _____

   _____

   _____

   _____

   _____

2. Ocular lubricants are indicated for patients with what?

   _____

3. High _____ alone does not provide relief for all dry eye problems.

What IS an Ocular Decongestant?

Ocular Decongestants	Trade Names
naphazoline [naf-AZ-oh-leen]	Allerest
oxymetazoline 0.025% [ox-ih-met-AZ-oh-leen]	OcuClear
tetrahydrozoline 0.05% [tet-ra-high-DROZ-ah-leen]	Visine Murine

Action

Ocular decongestants (ocular vasoconstricting medications) stimulate α-receptors on the vascular smooth muscle of the eye and nasal mucosa. The result is local vasoconstriction and a decrease in ocular congestion. Strong solutions of the ocular decongestant also dilate the pupil (mydriasis).

Uses

Ocular decongestants are typically used for the short-term local treatment of ocular congestion, itching, minor irritation, and red eyes (hyperemia).

What You NEED TO KNOW

Contraindications/Precautions

Ocular decongestants should be used cautiously in patients with hyperthyroidism, heart disease, hypertension, diabetes mellitus, eye disease, infection, and injury.

> **!** **Ocular decongestants should be used cautiously in patients with hyperthyroidism, heart disease, hypertension, diabetes mellitus, eye disease, infection, and injury. Naphazoline should be used cautiously in patients with diabetes mellitus and those who are prone to ketoacidosis.**

Answers: 1. sodium chloride, polyvinyl alcohol, petrolatum, mineral oil, lanolin; 2. dry eyes, artificial eyes; 3. viscosity.

Drug Interactions

When ocular decongestants are given concurrently with monoamine oxidase inhibitors (MAOIs) or inhalation anesthetics, a greater adrenergic response and hypertensive crisis may occur. When absorbed systemically, oxymetazoline can increase the effect of tricyclic antidepressants. Local ophthalmic anesthetics increase the absorption of oxymetazoline. Beta blockers (BBs) increase the systemic effects of oxymetazoline when given together.

Adverse Effects

Adverse effects of ocular decongestants include transient burning, stinging, dryness, blurred vision, pupillary dilation, and increased or decreased IOP. Rebound congestion and eye redness may occur when the medication is overused. The adverse effects from systemic absorption include headache, nervousness, dizziness, weakness, hypertension, chest pain, and dysrhythmias.

What You DO

TAKE HOME POINTS

Applying pressure to the inner canthus for 3 to 5 minutes is useful to prevent systemic absorption of all eye medications. Advise the patient to use the ocular decongestant sparingly to avoid rebound redness and congestion.

Nursing Responsibilities

When administering ocular decongestants, the nurse should:

- Teach the patient proper eye administration technique and that applying pressure to the inner canthus for 3 to 5 minutes after drug administration can minimize systemic absorption of ocular decongestants.
- Explain to the patient that systemic absorption from conjunctival membranes can occur.
- Advise the patient to remove contact lenses before applying an ocular decongestant.
- Instruct the patient to contact the health care provider before using an over-the-counter ocular decongestant.
- Instruct the patient to contact the health care provider when the ocular decongestant provides no relief after using the drug for 2 days.
- Warn the patient that the drug should be used only in the prescribed dose when needed and to avoid sharing the medication with family members or others.
- Instruct the patient to report any systemic reactions (e.g., dizziness, chest pain) to the health care provider. The medication may be discontinued.
- Warn patients that oxymetazoline may cause bradycardia, hypotension, dizziness, and weakness with excessive use.
- Store ocular decongestants away from heat, light, and humidity (not in the bathroom medicine cabinet) and out of children's reach.
- Instruct the patient to avoid using the medication when the solution is brown or contains a precipitate.

Do You UNDERSTAND?

DIRECTIONS: Provide appropriate responses to the following questions and statements.

1. Ocular decongestants should be used with caution in patients with what?

   _____

   _____

   _____

   _____

2. Name the brand name for the ocular decongestant tetrahydrozoline that is commonly used to clear red eyes.

   _____

3. In susceptible individuals, systemic absorption of an ocular decongestant may cause what?

   _____

   _____

What IS an Ocular Miotic?

Miotic Medications	Trade Names
Anticholinesterase Miotics	
demecarium [dem-ee-CARE-ee-um]	Humorsol
echothiophate [ek-oh-THIGH-oh-fate]	Phospholine Iodide
Cholinergic Miotics	
carbachol [CAR-ba-coal]	Isopto-carbachol
pilocarpine [pie-low-CAR-peen]	Pilocar
Beta-Blocker Miotics	
betaxolol [be-TAX-oh-lole]	Betoptic
timolol 0.25% [TIE-moe-lole]	Timoptic

Action

The classes of ocular miotics include cholinergic miotics, anticholinesterase miotics, and BBs. Each class of ocular miotics produces miosis through different mechanisms. Anticholinesterase miotics inhibit the breakdown of acetylcholine (ACh) (a parasympathetic nervous system transmitter) by the enzyme cholinesterase, allowing ACh to accumulate. The additional ACh acts on the ciliary muscles and the sphincters of the iris, causing ciliary muscles to contract and pupils to dilate.

Answers: 1. acute-angle glaucoma, diabetes mellitus, hypertension, cardiac disease, eye disease; 2. Visine; 3. chest pain, dizziness.

Cholinergic miotics enhance the action of ACh. Contraction of the sphincter of the iris, contraction of ciliary muscles, and deepening of the anterior chamber occur. The filtration angle is made larger, which increases outflow of aqueous humor and decreases IOP. The exact action of BBs is unknown, although all ocular formulations antagonize circulating catecholamines on β_2-receptors in the ciliary epithelium. Thus a fall in the production of aqueous humor and IOP takes place.

Uses

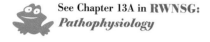

See Chapter 13A in **RWNSG**: *Pathophysiology*

Anticholinesterase miotics and cholinergic miotics are used to treat chronic, open-angle glaucoma. However, BBs are now preferred for initial therapy. Miotics may also be used to treat conditions that obstruct the outflow of aqueous humor.

What You NEED TO KNOW

Contraindications/Precautions

Cholinergic miotics should be used with caution in patients with peptic ulcer disease, Parkinson's disease, seizures, and hyperthyroidism.

Generally, ocular miotics are contraindicated for patients with hypersensitivity, severe bradycardia, greater than first-degree heart block, cardiogenic shock, uncontrolled heart failure, asthma, and chronic airflow limitation.

Drug Interactions

Epinephrine, cyclopentolate, belladonna alkaloids, and ocular anticholinesterase drugs decrease the effectiveness of ocular miotics. Echothiophate increases the effects of succinylcholine, organic insecticides, cholinesterase inhibitors, and systemic anticholinesterase drugs. When cholinergic agents are given together with physostigmine, additive toxicity is produced. Anticholinesterase miotics decrease the effects of cholinergic miotics. A greater reduction in IOP occurs when pilocarpine is given concurrently with epinephrine and timolol. When ocular BBs are given with systemic BBs or reserpine, systemic effects are increased. Pilocarpine, epinephrine, and carbonic anhydrase inhibitors enhance the lowering of IOP when given with ocular BBs. Systemic absorption may result in additive bradycardia and hypotension when ocular miotics are used concurrently with antihypertensives and antiarrhythmics.

Adverse Effects

Adverse effects of anticholinesterase miotics generally include decreased visual acuity, ocular burning, and rash. These agents produce accommodative myopia and can be problematic in young patients because pupillary constriction and eyelid twitching interferes with vision. Other adverse effects of anticholinesterase miotics include brow ache, headache, eye pain, ciliary and conjunctival congestion, and tearing. Long-term use of these agents can cause thickening of the conjunctiva and obstruction of the nasolacrimal canals.

Pilocarpine is tolerated better than are other miotics. The adverse effects of cholinergic miotics include irritation, conjunctivitis, and blepharitis. Allergic reactions and systemic effects are uncommon. With prolonged use, cholinergic miotics may cause tolerance, resistance, retinal detachment, obstruction of tear ducts, cysts on the iris, and cataracts.

Ocular BBs are usually well tolerated. The adverse effects are most noticeable during the first 2 weeks of therapy, including mild eye irritation, conjunctival redness, eye pain, headache, decreased corneal sensitivity, transient dry eye syndrome, and blurring of central vision. Refractive changes resulting from withdrawal of miotics may be responsible for some reports of blurred vision. Occasionally, ocular BBs can mask the symptoms and increase the frequency of hypoglycemic episodes in patients with type 1 diabetes mellitus. Systemic absorption of ocular miotics is minimal but may result in bradycardia and hypotension.

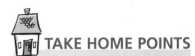 Systemic reactions, such as bronchospasm and delirium may occur in older patients who are taking an ocular miotic.

 # What You DO

Nursing Responsibilities

When administering ocular miotics, the nurse should:

- Obtain a current medication history because many systemically administered medications affect the eyes.
- Ask the patient specifically about chronic, systemic diseases that are associated with eye disorders (e.g., diabetes mellitus, arthritis, hypertension, thyroid disease).
- Determine when the patient's last eye examination was performed and when the eyeglass prescription was last changed.
- Inquire specifically about nearsightedness (myopia), farsightedness (hyperopia), glaucoma, and uncontrollable eye deviation (strabismus).
- Teach patients who are taking ocular miotics the importance of washing hands before drug administration.
- Instruct the patient that pressure on the inner canthus of the eye after ocular drug administration of BBs will help prevent systemic absorption.
- Assess for redness, swelling, or other irritation and systemic effects that were not present before treatment was started.
- Inform the patient that only ocular formulations are to be used in the eye.
- Advise the patient that eye drops that have changed color or become cloudy should be discarded.
- Warn patients to move about carefully until the full effect of the medication is known.

TAKE HOME POINTS

A miotic medication may cause blurred vision, thus taking the drug at bedtime is preferable to any other time of day.

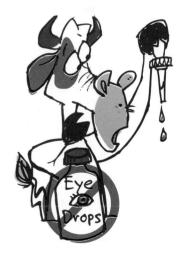

Do You UNDERSTAND?

DIRECTIONS: Match the drug actions in Column A with the medication classes in Column B.

Column A	Column B
_____ 1. Inhibits the breakdown of ACh by the enzyme cholinesterase, thereby allowing ACh to accumulate.	a. BBs b. Anticholinesterase medications
_____ 2. Enhances the effects of ACh, the parasympathetic nervous system neurotransmitter.	c. Cholinergic medications
_____ 3. Antagonizes circulating catecholamines on β_2-receptors in the ciliary epithelium.	

What IS an Ocular Osmotic?

Ocular Osmotics	Trade Names
glycerin (50%–75%) [GLI-sir-in]	Ophthalgan
isosorbide [eye-so-SORE-bide]	Isomotic
mannitol (20%) [MAN-ih-tole]	Osmitrol
urea (30%) [your-EE-ah]	Ureaphil

Action

The ocular osmotic medications are "diuretics for the eye." These agents reduce the fluid volume in the posterior portion of the eye, which aids in opening the angle. Ocular osmotics make the plasma more hypertonic than does intraocular fluid. The action of these agents causes the fluid to be drawn from the epithelium tissue of the cornea to the tear film for elimination from the eye. Ocular osmotics also decrease the production of aqueous humor by acting on hypothalamic osmoreceptors.

Uses

See Chapter 13A in **RWNSG:** *Pathophysiology*

Osmotics are used for short-term reduction of intraocular fluid and IOP in patients with glaucoma, corneal edema, and corneoscleral lacerations. Osmotics are used for preoperative and postoperative surgical repair of a detached retina, cataract extraction, and surgical repair of the cornea. Ocular osmotics are also used to interrupt an acute attack of glaucoma before laser or surgical intervention.

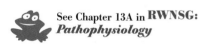

Answers: 1. b; 2. c; 3. a.

What You NEED TO KNOW

Contraindications/Precautions

Ocular osmotics are contraindicated for patients with hypersensitivity, anuria, and severe dehydration. Ocular isosorbide is contraindicated for patients with acute pulmonary edema and hemorrhagic glaucoma. Mannitol and urea are contraindicated for patients with severe heart failure, progressive renal or hepatic dysfunction, active intracranial bleeding, or sickle cell disease with central nervous system (CNS) involvement.

Drug Interactions

Glycerin produces additive effects with slight elevation of serum and urine glucose levels when given together with diuretics. Mannitol increases the risk of digitalis toxicity when given concurrently with cardiac glycosides. Mannitol increases the effects of diuretics, including carbonic anhydrase inhibitors. Urea and mannitol decreases lithium levels when given together.

Adverse Effects

The adverse effects of ocular osmotics include a pounding headache (because of a decrease in cerebrospinal fluid volume), nausea, vomiting, and occasional diarrhea. The shift in body fluids increases the workload on the heart and may precipitate heart failure. Glycerin may cause hyperglycemia and glycosuria.

What You DO

Nursing Responsibilities

Ocular osmotics, glycerin and isosorbide, are given orally, while mannitol and urea are given intravenously (IV). When administering ocular osmotics, the nurse should:
- Avoid administering a hypotonic IV solution following the administration of an osmotic medication because these fluids cancel the effect of the osmotic.
- Ensure that the IV line is patent before administering the medication to avoid extravasation of the medication and subsequent tissue necrosis.
- Administer oral glycerin with lemon, lime, or orange juice, or use the commercially prepared flavored solution to improve taste and minimize nausea and vomiting. The medication may also be mixed with unsweetened fruit juice. Pour over cracked ice and sip through a straw to increase palatability.
- Monitor the patient for 5 to 10 minutes after oral glycerin administration for evidence of persistent or increased eye pain and decreased visual acuity.
- Inform the patient that glycerin or ocular isosorbide may cause thirst.

 Osmotics should be used cautiously in patients with cardiac disease, renal or hepatic dysfunction, and diabetes mellitus. Ocular isosorbide should be used with caution in patients with diseases that are associated with sodium retention, such as heart failure.

  The oral form of glycerin is used cautiously in older or dehydrated patients. Osmotics should be used with caution during pregnancy and lactation.

 TAKE HOME POINTS

 Confusion and amnesia are adverse effects of ocular osmotics that may occur in older adults.

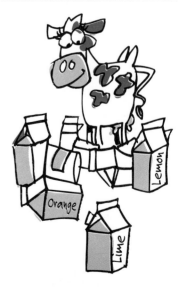

Monitor older adults who are taking glycerin for disorientation or seizure activity.

TAKE HOME POINTS

Lying down during and after administration of glycerin helps prevent or relieve the headache.

 Advise the patient to call the health care provider when a severe headache develops.
• Monitor patients with diabetes who are taking glycerin for alterations in serum glucose levels.

Do You UNDERSTAND?

DIRECTIONS: **Fill in the blanks with the appropriate response.**

1. Four ocular osmotic medications that are used in the treatment of increased IOP include _____, _____, _____, and _____.
2. Patients with an acute attack of glaucoma may receive an osmotic medication that acts to _____.
3. Necrosis may result when extravasation of urea occurs. Thus the most important nursing intervention is to be certain of a _____.

What IS a Carbonic Anhydrase Inhibitor?

Carbonic Anhydrase Inhibitors	Trade Names
acetazolamide [ah-set-ah-ZOLE-ah-mide]	Diamox
brinzolamide [brin-ZOL-ah-mide]	Azopt
dichlorphenamide [dye-klor-FEN-ah-mide]	Daranide
dorzolamide [dor-ZOL-ah-mide]	Trusopt
methazolamide [meth-ah-ZOL-ah-mide]	Neptazane

Action

Carbonic anhydrase is an enzyme that promotes the conversion of carbonic acid to carbon dioxide and water. Carbonic anhydrase inhibitors block enzyme activity in ciliary epithelium, thereby decreasing the production of aqueous humor and IOP. The reduction in pressure usually results in pupillary constriction (miosis) and opening of the anterior chamber of the eye.

Uses

See Chapter 13A in **RWNSG:** *Pathophysiology*

Carbonic anhydrase inhibitors are used for the long-term treatment of open-angle glaucoma and other glaucoma that is refractory to cholinergic miotics, BBs, and epinephrine. Emergency treatment of acute closed-angle glaucoma includes use of BBs and osmotics, in addition to carbonic anhydrase inhibitors. Carbonic anhydrase inhibitors are also used to decrease IOP for preoperative and postoperative eye surgery patients.

Answers: 1. glycerin, isosorbide, mannitol, urea; 2. decease IOP until laser or surgical intervention is possible; 3. patent IV line.

What You NEED TO KNOW

Contraindications/Precautions

Acetazolamide and methazolamide are contraindicated for patients with acute-angle glaucoma, decreased sodium or potassium levels, kidney or liver disease, adrenal gland dysfunction, or acid-base imbalance that is characterized by hyperchloremic acidosis.

Drug Interactions

Acetazolamide decreases the elimination of methenamine, procainamide, and quinidine when given together. Diflunisal increases the therapeutic and toxic effects of acetazolamide. Methazolamide decreases elimination of amphetamines, procainamide, quinidine, and flecainide. Conversely, methazolamide increases the elimination of salicylates and phenobarbital. Additionally, methazolamide augments the effects of thiazide diuretics when given concurrently and exacerbates hypokalemia when given together with glucocorticosteroids.

Adverse Effects

The adverse effects of carbonic anhydrase inhibitors include transient myopia, alteration in taste, anorexia, nausea, vomiting, diarrhea, malaise, fatigue, weakness, nervousness, and loss of libido. Lethargy and depression are common but are frequently unnoticed until the medication is discontinued.

> ⚠️ **Acetazolamide and methazolamide should be used cautiously in patients with respiratory acidosis, emphysema or pulmonary obstruction, or diabetes mellitus.**

What You DO

Nursing Responsibilities

When administering carbonic anhydrase inhibitors, the nurse should:
- Be aware that dorzolamide is a sulfonamide and is absorbed systemically, therefore the same adverse effects of sulfonamides may occur with topical administration of dorzolamide.
- Be certain to administer the correct medication.
- Discourage the patient from using an eye cup because of the risk of contamination and spreading disease.
- Crush oral formulations of acetazolamide tablets and mix with highly flavored syrup, such as raspberry, cherry, or chocolate. Tablets can also be softened in hot water and added to honey or syrup.
- Monitor older adults and debilitated patients for medication-induced diuresis because diuresis promotes rapid dehydration, hypovolemia, hypokalemia, hyponatremia, and may cause circulatory collapse. Reduced doses may be indicated for these patients.

> ⚠️ **Do not administer two or more carbonic anhydrase inhibitors concurrently. Two or more oral carbonic anhydrase inhibitors increase the risk of additive effects. Do not open or crush sustained release capsules.**

TAKE HOME POINTS

Medication containers of ophthalmic and otic medications are similar in appearance in many cases. Ear formulations should not be used in the eye. Similarly, eye medications should not be used in the ear.

 Warn the patient who is taking carbonic anhydrase inhibitors to use caution when driving or performing tasks that require alertness, coordination, or physical dexterity because the medication may cause drowsiness.

 Instruct the patient to discard medications that have changed color or become cloudy.

Do You UNDERSTAND?

DIRECTIONS: Provide the appropriate answer to the following questions.

1. Is the action of ocular carbonic anhydrase inhibiting medications that are used for reducing IOP different from that observed when the medication is used for other purposes (e.g., epilepsy, overdose)?

2. Why or why not?

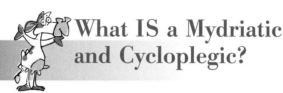

What IS a Mydriatic and Cycloplegic?

Mydriatic and Cycloplegic Agents	Trade Names
Ocular anticholinergics	
homatropine [hoe-MA-troe-peen]	AK-Homatropine
cyclopentolate [sye-kloe-PEN-toe-late]	Cyclogyl
Adrenergics	
dipivefrin [dye-PI-ve-frin]	Propine
phenylephrine [fen-ill-EH-frin]	AK-Dilate

Action

Mydriatics and cycloplegic agents dilate the pupil (mydriasis) to visualize the inner workings of the eye and diagnose eye problems. Either anticholinergic medications or adrenergic medications can be used to dilate the pupil.

The autonomic nervous system plays an important role in controlling the amount of light entering the eye and in focusing on images. The size of the iris controls the amount of light penetrating the eye, which contains two sets of muscles: the sphincter muscles and the dilator muscles. The pupil is constricted when the sphincter muscles contract, thus only a small amount of light passes

Answers: 1. No differences exist, except in the use of the medications 2. The action of the drug is the same.

through the pupil. The dilator muscles contain α-receptors that are innervated by the sympathetic nervous system. As the name implies, the pupil is dilated when these radial muscles contract after stimulation of the α-receptors. A mydriatic medication dilates the pupil without affecting accommodation.

Ocular anticholinergics block the action of the parasympathetic nervous system to stimulation. Paralysis of ciliary muscles and relaxation of the muscles of the iris occurs, resulting in dilation of the pupil and loss of accommodation (cycloplegia).

Adrenergic medications activate β_2-receptors in the canal of Schlemm, thereby increasing the outflow of aqueous humor. Epinephrine, when used alone, produces a 30% to 35% decrease in the rate of aqueous humor production. The duration of mydriasis and cycloplegia differs. Cycloplegia lasts a shorter period than does mydriasis, with recovery of accommodation taking several days. The outflow of aqueous humor is decreased with all of the ocular anticholinergics because of the miotic effect.

Uses

Ocular anticholinergic and adrenergic medications (mydriatics and cycloplegics) are used to dilate the pupil for refraction and other diagnostic purposes. These agents can be used in the treatment of anterior uveitis and keratitis, as well as secondary forms of glaucoma. These medications also facilitate pupillary dilation during eye surgery and help decrease postoperative complications.

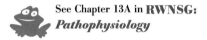 See Chapter 13A in **RWNSG:** *Pathophysiology*

 # What You NEED TO KNOW

Contraindications/Precautions

Ocular anticholinergics are contraindicated for patients with a shallow anterior chamber, closed-angle glaucoma, and hypersensitivity to the medication or to belladonna alkaloids. These agents are also contraindicated for patients with scar tissue between the iris and the lens. Topical epinephrine and its analogs are contraindicated before removal of a piece of the iris (iridectomy) in closed-angle glaucoma because they may precipitate an acute attack.

Anticholinergic medications should be used with caution in older adults.

Drug Interactions

Anticholinergics cause additive effects when given together with atropine. When anticholinergics are given concurrently with amantadine, the anticholinergic adverse effects are increased. CNS depression is intensified when anticholinergics are given with alcohol, antianxiety drugs, or sedative-hypnotics. The risk of tachycardia and hypertension is increased when anticholinergics are given together with ocular adrenergic drugs. Indomethacin inhibits the action of epinephrine when given concurrently. The effects of phenylephrine are enhanced when given with atropine and tricyclic antidepressants.

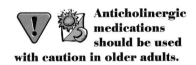 **Phenylephrine should be used with caution in patients with a history of cardiovascular disease or diabetes mellitus.**

Adverse Effects

The adverse effects of ocular anticholinergic and adrenergic medications include blurred vision, photophobia, and precipitation of closed-angle glaucoma. Chronic use of adrenergics causes rebound congestion of the conjunctiva. Absorption through the tear ducts and blood vessels of the eye causes systemic effects, including dry mouth, constipation, fever, tachycardia, and CNS effects.

What You DO

Nursing Responsibilities

When administering mydriatics and cycloplegics, the nurse should:

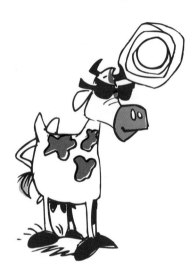

- Wash the hands before administering an eye medication.
- Double check the medication order.
- Gently retract the lower lid with your thumb or index finger against the cheekbone to expose the lower conjunctival sac with the patient looking upward. Rest your hand holding the dropper or tube of ointment on the patient's forehead. Without touching the dropper to the eye structures, instill the prescribed number of drops into the conjunctival sac.
- Apply an ointment evenly in a thin stream along the inside edge of the entire lower eyelid from the inner to the outer canthus. Instruct the patient to gently close the eyes. Using a clean tissue, gently wipe away excess medication, moving from the inner canthus to the outer canthus.
- Record medication administration, noting which eyes received the medication.
- Advise patients to wear sunglasses to reduce the discomfort of photophobia caused by mydriatic-cycloplegic medications.

Do You UNDERSTAND?

DIRECTIONS: **Provide appropriate answers to the following questions.**

1. What are the first two steps in administering mydriatic-cycloplegic medications?

2. What is the last step in administering a mydriatic-cycloplegic medication?

Answers: 1. wash your hands and check the medication order; 2. record medication administration, noting which eyes received the medication.

What IS a Ceruminolytic?

Ceruminolytic Agents	Trade Names
carbamide peroxide	Debrox Ear Drops
triethanolamine, polypeptide oleate, condensate	Cerumenex Ear Drops

Action

A ceruminolytic medication contains glycerin to soften cerumen and carbamide peroxide to loosen debris through the action of oxygen effervescence. These agents emulsify and disperse excess or impacted cerumen.

Uses

Removal of cerumen is frequently necessary for otoscopy examination, audiometry, tympanometry, and when the patient experiences discomfort or hearing loss from excessive or dry cerumen. Additionally, ceruminolytic medications provide antiseptic protection.

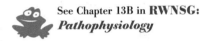

See Chapter 13B in **RWNSG:** *Pathophysiology*

What You NEED TO KNOW

Contraindications/Precautions

Ceruminolytics are contraindicated for patients with a perforated eardrum, swimmer's ear, and itching of the ear canal, as well as those with an allergy to preservatives (e.g., benzethonium chloride, sulfites, thimerosal) because many otic medications contain these products.

Ceruminolytics should not be administered to children under 12 years of age.

Drug Interactions

No known drug interactions have been noted with ceruminolytics.

Adverse Effects

Ceruminolytic medications are irritating to the ear and may cause an allergic reaction, particularly with prolonged exposure.

What You DO

Nursing Responsibilities

When administering ceruminolytics, the nurse should:
- Inform patients that ceruminolytics may be used over a 2- to 3-day period to soften the wax.

TAKE HOME POINTS

Instill drops on the side of the auditory canal, allowing them to flow in without falling directly on the eardrum (**tympanic membrane**). When drops are ordered for the other ear, wait 15 minutes and repeat this procedure with the other ear. Ceruminolytic medications may be used once a week to prevent recurrence of the problem.

 Gently pull the auricle (**pinna**) down and back for children under 3 years of age or up and back for children over 3 years of age and adults.

- Inform the patient that holding the medication in the hand before use will warm the otic solution.
- Teach the patient the correct way to use ceruminolytics.
- Fill the ear canal with the medication while the patient's head is tilted at a 45-degree angle.
- Place the ceruminolytic directly on the affected ear tissue without touching the dropper to the ear or ear canal.
- Straighten the ear canal using one hand. Rest your hand holding the medication dropper 1 cm ($^1/_2$ inch) above the ear canal.
- Apply gentle pressure on the tragus (cartilage projection anterior to the external ear opening) or gently massage the tragus with your finger.
- Instruct the patient to remain in a side-lying position for 2 to 3 minutes.
- Mechanically remove the cerumen using a soft rubber otic bulb syringe and warm water to gently irrigate the ear.
- Warn the patient to avoid using the otic preparation for more than 4 consecutive days and to avoid contact with the eyes. Accidental ocular exposure causes immediate pain and irritation; however, severe injury is rare.
- Inform the patient that some individuals have a continual problem with cerumen impaction.
- Advise the patient to contact the health care provider when inflammation or irritation persists after using a ceruminolytic medication.

Do You UNDERSTAND?

DIRECTIONS: **Indicate in the space provided whether the statement is** *true* **or** *false.*

_____ 1. Ceruminolytics are safe for children under 10 years of age.

_____ 2. Patients can experience hearing loss because of excessive earwax.

_____ 3. A patient with a perforated eardrum can safely receive ceruminolytic medications.

SECTION B
DERMATOLOGICS

This section reviews the use of pharmacologic methods to treat common skin diseases. Dermatologic complaints are frequently treated on an outpatient basis. The skin is the body's largest organ, the primary goal of which is to act as a barrier against the influences of the outside environment. The functions of the skin include protection, temperature regulation, immune responsiveness, biochemical synthesis, and improved appearance. Dermatologic medications correct dysfunction of the skin topically and systemically. Systemic medication is most commonly delivered through oral medication, and topical medication is

Answers: 1. false; 2. true; 3. false.

absorbed through the skin layers. This section provides information about agents that are used for the treatment of burns, poison ivy, and acne. Emulsions, lotions, creams, ointments, antipruritics, and keratolytics are also discussed.

What IS a Burn Treatment Agent?

Burn Treatment Agents	Trade Names
mafenide [meh-FEN-ide]	Sulfamylon
nitrofurazone [nye-troh-FYOOR-ah-zone]	Furacin
silver sulfadiazine [sul-fah-DYE-ah-zeen]	Silvadene

Action

Burn treatment agents prevent bacterial growth, thereby assisting with the healing of burned tissue. Mafenide interferes with bacterial cellular metabolism and reduces bacteria in burns, which allows for spontaneous healing of deep burns. Nitrofurazone and silver sulfadiazine are bactericidal agents that exert broad-spectrum antibacterial action on gram-positive and gram-negative microorganisms. Nitrofurazone inhibits the aerobic and anaerobic cycles of carbohydrate metabolism in bacteria. Silver sulfadiazine exerts a bactericidal action on the bacterial cell membrane and cell wall to reduce bacteria.

Uses

Burn treatment agents are useful in the treatment of burns, and they prevent bacterial infection in burns, skin grafts, and donor sites.

What You NEED TO KNOW

Contraindications/Precautions

Burn agents are contraindicated for patients with atrophy or hypersensitivity to the drug or sulfites. Silver sulfadiazine is contraindicated for patients with glucose-6-phosphate dehydrogenase (G6PD) deficiency. Sulfite sensitivity tends to be more prevalent in patients with asthma compared with the general population.

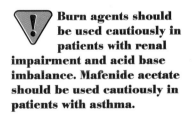

Burn agents should be used cautiously in patients with renal impairment and acid base imbalance. Mafenide acetate should be used cautiously in patients with asthma.

Burn agents are contra-indicated for women during pregnancy and lactation, as well as for premature infants, neonates, and children because these agents may increase the risk of bilirubin infiltration into the spinal cord and brain (**kernicterus**).

Drug Interactions

Silver sulfadiazine may cause inactivation of enzymes when interacted with topical proteolytic enzymes.

Adverse Effects

Topical burn medication interactions generally cause few life-threatening crises, except when the patient experiences an allergic reaction. Allergic reactions include skin irritation, rashes, pruritus, burning, hives, blisters, redness, skin discoloration, and swelling of the lips or face.

Mafenide may cause tachypnea, diarrhea, G6PD deficiency, bone marrow suppression, and disseminated intravascular coagulation. Mafenide also inhibits carbonic anhydrase, leading to metabolic acidosis, which is usually compensated through hyperventilation.

Nitrofurazone has a polyethylene glycol base, which may be absorbed through unprotected (**denuded**) skin. Impaired kidneys may not adequately eliminate nitrofurazone and may lead to metabolic acidosis and progressive renal impairment.

Photosensitivity and an increased risk of kernicterus may occur with silver sulfadiazine. When extensive systemic absorption occurs, silver sulfadiazine administration may result in decreased neutrophil count, indicating reversible leukopenia. Prolonged use of these agents may result in superinfections, including overgrowth of other microorganisms, such as Candida albicans.

What You DO

Nursing Responsibilities

To avoid allergic reactions, culture and sensitivity tests are recommended before applying medication. When administering burn agents, the nurse should:

- Teach the patient to use the medication only as prescribed, and avoid sharing the medication with others.
- Discard the agent when the color is incorrect, according to the package.
- Store medications in tight containers to avoid exposure to direct sunlight, prolonged heat, and alkaline materials.
- Adhere strictly to sterile technique and gloved hands to avoid wound contamination.
- Flush the dressing with sterile saline to facilitate dressing removal.
- Inspect patient's skin daily, and note any changes.
- Continuously monitor signs of rash, infection, and toxicity.
- Use burn agents only on affected areas, and keep the burn medicated at all times.
- Apply burn preparations to a clean, débrided wound to enhance absorption.
- Protect skin around the wound with zinc oxide when using a wet dressing.
- Document marked discomfort, acidosis, and fungal infections.

TAKE HOME POINTS

Sterile technique and gloved hands help avoid wound contamination. Dressings are not always necessary, but when used, they should be nonocclusive and light.

- Monitor renal function studies and acid-base balance for patients who are undergoing nitrofurazone therapy.
- Report metabolic acidosis to the health care provider because mafenide will usually be discontinued for 24 to 48 hours to allow restoration of acid-base balance.
- Monitor the complete blood count of patients who are undergoing silver sulfadiazine therapy for early detection of leukopenia.
- Instruct the patient to report rash, irritation, swelling, or other evidence of an allergic reaction to the health care provider.
- Caution the patient to report to the health care provider when no improvement occurs, the condition worsens, or systemic and adverse reactions occur.

Do You UNDERSTAND?

DIRECTIONS: Match the following descriptions in Column A to the medications in Column B.

Column A	Column B
_____ 1. Careful use with patients who are diagnosed with renal failure and asthma.	a. Silver sulfadiazine
_____ 2. Used cautiously when patient has renal insufficiency.	b. Mafenide acetate

What IS an Acne Treatment Agent?

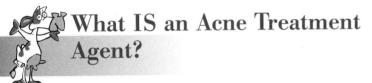

Acne Treatment Agents	Trade Names
isotretinoin [eye-so-TREAT-ih-noyn]	Accutane
azelaic acid [ah-zih-LAY-ick]	Azelex
tetracycline [te-trah-SIGH-clean]	Topicycline
erythromycin [eh-RIH-throw-MY-sin]	Akne-Mycin
clindamycin [klin-dah-MY-sin]	Cleocin

Action

Acne treatment agents decrease the sebaceous gland size and inhibit sebaceous gland differentiation, thereby causing a decrease in oil secretion. Acne treatments may also inhibit follicular keratinization. Antibiotics disrupt bacterial protein synthesis.

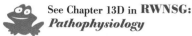

See Chapter 13D in **RWNSG:**
Pathophysiology

Uses

Broad-spectrum antibiotics are frequently used to treat acne vulgaris. Topical treatment is usually prescribed first, and when no clinical improvement takes place, systemic therapy is then introduced.

What You NEED TO KNOW

Contraindications/Precautions

Acne treatment agents are contraindicated for patients with hypersensitivity. Isotretinoin is also contraindicated for patients with allergies to isotretinoin, parabions, or combinations of these products, and tetracycline is contraindicated for patients with sensitivity to sodium bisulfate.

Adverse Effects

Adverse effects of acne medications include temporary stinging or burning on application, tingling, itching, yellow discoloration of skin, redness, irritation, swelling, and peeling. Tetracycline interacts with isotretinoin, causing dryness or oiliness and excessive skin irritation. Intolerance to contact lenses and photosensitive reactions may occur. Prolonged use may cause overgrowth of bacterial or fungal infections.

 These acne agents are contraindicated during pregnancy and lactation. Clindamycin is contraindicated for infants. Tetracycline is contraindicated for children under 11 years of age.

Azelaic acid should be used with caution in children under 12 years old.

Isotretinoin must be used cautiously in patients with diabetes mellitus, coronary artery disease, obesity, alcoholism, pancreatitis, hepatitis, renal or hepatic impairment, retinal disease, and rheumatology disorders. Tetracycline must be used cautiously in patients with myasthenia gravis and asthma. Azelaic acid should be used with caution in patients with dark complexions.

What You DO

Nursing Responsibilities

Acne medications are usually topical, but some may be taken orally when necessary. When administering acne agents, the nurse should:

- Inform the female patient that a pregnancy test is required with contraceptive use before treatment is prescribed.
- Apply lotions and creams with a gloved hand, and wash hands thoroughly before and after treatment.
- Instruct patients to wash their hands before applying a generous amount of medication to the affected area.
- Warn the patient that medicated soaps, cleansers, and other acne treatments contain peeling agents.
- Inform the patient that individual medications may have instructions regarding safe storage.
- Remind the patient that the application may cause stinging, local irritation, or dryness.
- Warn the patient to avoid exposure to direct sunlight to prevent photosensitivity.

 TAKE HOME POINTS

Adhere strictly to the use of gloves and thorough hand washing before and after treatment. Avoid application of acne medication in the mouth, nose, and eyes.

🍎 Caution the patient to avoid sharing the medication.

🍎 Inform the patient that topical medications may stain clothes.

🍎 Advise the patient to report to the health care provider when no improvement occurs, when the condition worsens, or when adverse effects occur.

🍎 Encourage patients with diabetes who are taking isotretinoin to monitor blood glucose levels regularly.

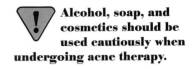

Alcohol, soap, and cosmetics should be used cautiously when undergoing acne therapy.

Do You UNDERSTAND?

DIRECTIONS: Provide appropriate responses to the following questions.

1. How does a broad-spectrum antibiotic assist in clinically improving acne?

2. What route is the first-line defense against acne?

What IS an Emollient?

Action

Topical emollients are agents that soften, lubricate, moisturize, and soothe skin surfaces. These agents promote hydration through topical absorption and remove excess keratin in dry skin.

Uses

Topical emollients, frequently offered in more than one formula, are used to provide temporary relief of discomfort resulting from skin irritation, itching, minor burns, sunburns, diaper rash, chapped or dry skin, and poison ivy.

Emollients
Lanolor Cream
Desitin Ointment
Lubriderm Cream
Zinc Oxide Ointment
Nivea Moisturizing Lotion
Vitamin E Lotion, Oil, and Cream
Neutrogena Body Lotion
Vitamin A and D Ointments
Alpha Keri Emollient
Retinol Cream

What You NEED TO KNOW

Contraindications/Precautions

Emollients are contraindicated for patients with an allergy to the medication.

Drug Interactions

Emollients have no known drug interactions.

Adverse Effects

Adverse effects of emollients include local irritation, stinging, burning, and redness.

Answers: 1. antibiotics disrupt bacterial protein synthesis; 2. topical treatment is usually prescribed first, and systemic therapy is then introduced when no clinical improvement occurs.

What You DO

Nursing Responsibilities

Emollients are available in the form of emulsions, lotions, creams, gels, oils, ointments, and bath preparations. These agents are applied topically for external use only. When administering emollients, the nurse should:

- Avoid contact of emollients with the patient's eyes and open wounds.
- Instruct the patient to report increased irritation, allergic reaction, or worsening of the condition.
- Document all irritation, stinging, burning, redness, and swelling.

Do You UNDERSTAND?

DIRECTIONS: Indicate in the space provided whether the statement is true or false.

_____ 1. Eye contact must be avoided.

_____ 2. Avoid open wounds.

_____ 3. Report increased irritation, allergic reaction, or worsening condition.

What IS an Antipruritic?

Antipruritics	Trade Names
benzocaine [BEN-zo-cane]	Americaine
crotamiton [kroh-TAM-ih-ton]	Eurax
dyclonine [DYE-kloh-neen]	Dyclone
pramoxine [prah-MOX-een]	Tronothane

Action

Antipruritics are surface anesthetics that stop discomfort and itching and inhibit the conduction of the nerve impulses from the sensory nerve endings.

Uses

Antipruritic agents are used for temporary relief of pain and discomfort of minor burns, sunburn, wounds, insect bites, toothache, sore throat pain, canker sores, hemorrhoids, rectal fissures, and itching of the anus or vulva. Some of these agents are used for catheter and endoscope insertion. Systemic antipruritic agents can relieve allergic conditions that are associated with allergic dermatoses.

What You NEED TO KNOW

Contraindications/Precautions

Antipruritics are contraindicated for patients with hypersensitive or allergic reaction to the medication or any components.

Drug Interactions

Antipruritics have no known drug interactions.

Adverse Effects

Adverse effects of antipruritics medications include allergic reactions, burning, rash, and redness. Skin irritation may occur, particularly with prolonged use. Adverse effects following systemic absorption of dyclonine include dizziness, drowsiness, blurred vision, nervousness, tremors, depression, seizures, hypotension, bradycardia, and cardiac or respiratory arrest.

What You DO

Nursing Responsibilities

Antipruritic preparations are available in gels, creams, sprays, and lotions. When administering antipruritics, the nurse should:

- Thoroughly clean and dry the affected area before application.
- Apply lotions and creams with a gloved hand, and wash hands thoroughly before and after treatment.
- Massage crotamiton gently into the skin. Application is usually effective for 6 to 10 hours.
- Instruct the patient to avoid contact of antipruritics with the eyes or nasal membranes.
- Teach the patient to hold the spray medication at arms length to avoid eye contamination.
- Advise the patient to avoid eating for 1 hour after the medication is sprayed into the mouth because the numbing affect may impede swallowing.
- Instruct the patient to contact the health care provider and stop treatment when the condition worsens, fails to improve, or when signs of sensitivity, irritation, or infection occur.

  Antipruritics are contra-indicated for women during pregnancy and for children under 2 years of age. Antipruritic use is discouraged for use in children under 6 years of age.

 Antipruritics should be used cautiously in older adults.

  Antipruritics should be used cautiously in patients with denuded skin, severely traumatized mucosa, or sepsis.

 Serious adverse effects of ben-zocaine include toxicity, anaphylaxis, and methemoglobinemia in infants.

TAKE HOME POINTS

When antipruritic accidentally comes in contact with the eyes, thoroughly flush the eyes with water for 15 minutes. Test the return of the gag reflex by gently touching the soft palate with a cotton tipped applicator while holding the tongue down with a depressor. If the patient does not swallow or gag, then wait another hour before allowing the patient to drink or eat to prevent aspiration.

Do You UNDERSTAND?

DIRECTIONS: Name four problems or complications that antipruritics agents treat or procedures during which antipruritics may be used.

1. _____
2. _____
3. _____
4. _____

What IS a Keratolytic?

Keratolytics	Trade Names
podophyllum resin [pode-oh-FILL-um]	Pod-Ben-25
podofilox [poh-DAHF-ih-lox]	Condylox
masoprocol [mah-SOH-proh-kol]	Actinex

Action

Keratolytic agents directly affect epithelial cell metabolism, causing degeneration and a pause in mitosis, a slow disruption of cell movement, and an erosion of tissue. This action is caustic, affecting embryonic and tumor cells selectively before they develop into adult cells. The caustic action promotes shedding of the horny layer of skin, ranging from skin peeling to an extensive shedding of the epidermal layer of the skin.

Uses

Keratolytic agents are used to treat benign growths including warts (genital and perianal), papillomas, and fibroids. Keratolytic agents are also clinically used to treat hyperkeratotic skin disorders, verrucae, xerosis, ichthyosis, and photo aging. Irritated, friable, and bleeding skin fails to respond to treatment.

What You NEED TO KNOW

Contraindications/Precautions

Keratolytic agents are contraindicated for patients with birthmarks; moles; warts with hair growth; oral, cervical, or urethral warts; normal skin and mucous

Answers: 1. otic preparation are available for otitis itching; 2. gels, creams, and lotion preparations are available for toothaches, sore throat pain, and canker sores; 3. preparations are available for hemorrhoids, rectal fissures, itching of the ani or vulva, and as genital desensitizers; 4. aesthetic lubricants for catheter insertion and endoscopes.

membranes that surround affected areas. These agents are contraindicated for patients with hypersensitivity to the drug or an allergy to sulfites, diabetes mellitus, and impaired circulation.

Drug Interactions

Keratolytics have no known drug interactions.

Adverse Effects

The adverse effects of keratolytics include skin irritation, burning, itching, tingling, blistering, wrinkling, flaking, dryness, and peeling. Other adverse effects include bleeding, crusting edema, leatherlike skin, and painful intercourse. Systemic adverse effects include vomiting, diarrhea, insomnia, peripheral neuropathy, coma, seizures, respiratory and renal failure, and bone marrow depression.

What You DO

Nursing Responsibilities

Because of the potency of podophyllum resin, the health care provider is usually responsible for application. When administering keratolytics, the nurse should:

- Teach the patient the proper technique of drug self-administration.
- Instruct the patient to remove the last drug application thoroughly from the affected area with soap and water before the next application.
- Caution the patient that medication application over a large area is discouraged.
- Instruct the patient to apply the drug to the lesion, allow the area to dry, apply a loose bandage to cover the site, cover with tape, and remove as per the prescribed frequency instructions.
- Warn the patient that when contact with the eyes occurs, flush with warm water for 15 minutes, remove film that is precipitated by flush, and report the incident to the health care provider.
- Caution the patient to avoid applying the drug to normal body tissue, and when it occurs, wipe the area with alcohol to remove.
- Avoid applying the medication when the wart is inflamed or irritated.
- Inform the patient that when application causes extreme pain, pruritus, or swelling, remove the application with alcohol and notify the health care provider.
- Podophyllum resin should be stored in an airtight, light-resistant container, and avoid exposure to heat.
- Warn the patient that keratolytics may cause itching, burning, discomfort, and tenderness of the affected site and surrounding area for 2 to 6 days.
- Inform the patient that the wart will become blanched, then necrotic within 24 to 48 hours. Sloughing begins at 72 hours, with no scarring. A mild antiinfective can be applied until fully healed.
- Advise the patient that the sexual partner should be referred for examination when the keratolytic treatment is intended for sexually transmitted warts.

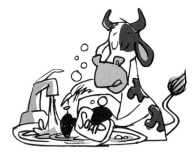

Keratolytics are contraindicated for women during pregnancy and lactation and for children.

TAKE HOME POINTS

Proper disposal of all used applicators is important to prevent contamination of the growth. Protect the surrounding skin or tissue with petrolatum. When keratolytics are spilled on the skin, wipe off with alcohol, acetone, or tape remover.

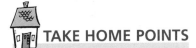

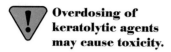

Overdosing of keratolytic agents may cause toxicity.

- Use the minimal amount of medication to avoid excess systemic absorption.
- Counsel the patient to call the health care provider immediately when symptoms of toxicity occur (e.g., seizures, peripheral neuropathy, respiratory depression).
- Emphasize adverse effects of keratolytic agents to the patient because the danger of misuse and systemic toxicity is high.
- Warn the patient who is using masoprocol to protect clothing and linen because the medication may cause staining.
- Instruct the patient to avoid exposure to sunlight and cosmetics while using keratolytic agents.

Do You UNDERSTAND?

DIRECTIONS: **Fill in the blanks in the following statements.**

1. Keratolytic agents directly affect _____
   metabolism, causing degeneration and a pause in

   _____.

2. When applying keratolytics, protect the surrounding skin or tissue with

   _____.

3. Avoid keratolytic application when the wart is _____
   or _____.

Agents Used for Pain Relief

SECTION A
OPIOID AGENTS

This chapter reviews pharmacologic control of pain. Harmful effects of unrelieved pain include confusion, prolonged stress response, depressed immune response, tumor growth, and increased hypercoagulation. Because nurses are the primary pain managers, nurses must have a thorough understanding of analgesics to provide adequate pain relief for patients.

Many types of receptor sites are present in body cells. Analgesics bind to certain receptors in the cells that influence the perception of pain. Opiate (**narcotic**) analgesics are classified as agonists and agonist-antagonists. Agonists are drugs that mimic the regulatory function of the body and have an affinity for their respective receptor sites. Antagonists may either block interaction at certain receptor sites or compete for those receptor sites. Agonists-antagonists have some characteristics of both agonists and antagonists. This section discusses opioid agonists, agonists-antagonists, and antagonists, as well as antimigraine agents, which includes ergot derivatives and triptans.

What IS an Opiate Agonist?

Opiate Agonists	Trade Names
morphine sulfate [MOR-feen]	Duramorph MS Contin
fentanyl [FEN-tah-nil]	Sublimaze Duragesic
meperidine [meh-PER-ih-deen]	Demerol
oxycodone [OX-ee-KOH-doan]	Percodan
codeine sulfate [KOH-deen]	Paveral

395

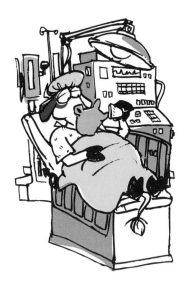

See Chapter 14 in **RWNSG:**
Pathophysiology

Action

Opiate agonists relieve pain without loss of consciousness. These drugs interact at specific receptor-binding sites (e.g., limbic system, thalamus, hypothalamus, mid-brain, spinal cord). Agonist activity at the receptor site can result in analgesia, euphoria, depression, hallucinations, miosis, sedation, decreased body temperature, decreased gastrointestinal (GI) motility, cardiac stimulation, and respiratory depression. Opiate agonists alter pain at the spinal cord and higher levels in the central nervous system (CNS), as well as the patient's emotional response.

Uses

Opiate agonists are used to relieve mild to severe pain or as a preoperative medication. These drugs are usually given when nonnarcotic analgesics are unsuccessful. Low-dose opioids are generally safer than are nonsteroidal antiinflammatory drugs (NSAIDs) for long-term use in older adults. The first choice of severe pain control via the patient-controlled analgesia (PCA) pump is morphine. MS Contin is a recommended choice for oral controlled-release pain medication. Meperidine has been used for the pain of myocardial infarction (MI) but is not as effective as is morphine. Some sources state that meperidine is not recommended for use other than the GI laboratory and for the treatment of shivering. Fentanyl transdermal relieves severe chronic pain. Oxycodone relieves moderate-to-severe pain. Codeine sulfate relieves mild-to-moderate pain.

What You NEED TO KNOW

Contraindications/Precautions

Opiate agonists are contraindicated for patients with hypersensitivity, increased intracranial pressure, suspected head injuries, seizures, asthma, severe respiratory depression, hepatic and renal dysfunction, acute alcoholism, biliary tract surgery, and acute ulcerative colitis. Meperidine is contraindicated for patients with renal insufficiency because dysfunctional kidneys cannot eliminate the toxic metabolite (normeperidine) that this drug produces.

Drug Interactions

CNS effects are increased when opiate agonists are given concurrently with sedatives, barbiturates, benzodiazepines, tricyclic antidepressants, and alcohol. When opiate agonists are given with monoamine oxidase inhibitors (MAOIs), seizures, hypertensive crisis, hyperpyrexia, and respiratory depression may occur. Phenothiazines may antagonize analgesic effects when given together with opiate agonists.

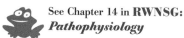 **Caution should be used in patients who are very young, older, debilitated, pregnant, or in labor.**

Caution should be used in patients with dysrhythmias and emphysema.

Adverse Effects

Opiate agonists have adverse effects that include rash, itching, anaphylaxis, euphoria, dizziness, fainting, sweating, confusion, seizures, visual disturbances, drowsiness, palpitations, bradycardia, flushing of neck and face, orthostatic hypotension, and decreased respirations. Other adverse effects affecting the GI system include anorexia, dry mouth, nausea, vomiting, constipation, urinary retention, and decreased libido. Overdose effects include bronchoconstriction, severe respiratory depression or arrest, skeletal muscle flaccidity, coma, and cardiac arrest. Meperidine produces a toxic metabolite (normeperidine) that may remain in the body for 8 to 21 hours. In patients with renal dysfunction, normeperidine may accumulate more than 30 hours in the body, leading to an increased risk of neurotoxicity.

What You DO

Nursing Responsibilities

Opiates (**narcotics**) are among the "scheduled" drugs, which are strictly regulated because of their potential for abuse. Opiates require strict documentation because they are considered as controlled substances. Documentation is required on the institution's narcotic sheet and on the nurses' notes. Additionally, two nurses at set intervals count the narcotics to validate the narcotic sheet. Any waste of narcotics must be witnessed and documented.

Multiple routes of administration are available: oral, transdermal, subcutaneous (SC), intramuscular (IM), IV, and rectal. Anesthetists may also use spinal, epidural, inhalation, and transmucosal routes. When administering opioids, the nurse should:

- Assess the nature of the patient's pain, status, and vital signs before and after drug administration. Opioid naives (patients who are receiving the first opioid dose) are more likely to develop respiratory depression than are patients who are receiving daily doses.
- Document the intensity of the patient's pain, medication administered, route, dose, and response.
- Instruct the patient to avoid crushing or chewing controlled-release tablets.
- Inform the patient that immediate-release capsules may be swallowed intact or that the contents may be sprinkled on food or mixed in juice to decrease the bitter taste.
- Aspirate before IM injections to avoid inadvertent IV administration.
- Advise the patient who is taking opiate agonists to breath deeply, cough, and turn from side to side frequently to decrease the risk of atelectasis.
- Provide safety for the patient because opiate agonists may cause dizziness and drowsiness.
- When the opiate agonist is ineffective, notify the health care provider to increase the dose or change drugs until the pain is relieved.

 TAKE HOME POINTS

- The nurse must sign out each narcotic before administration.
- Pain is typically undertreated.
- Agonist-antagonists should not be administered when the patient has a respiratory rate less than 12 respirations per minute, shallow respirations, constricted or dilated pupils, or CNS hyperactivity.
- Closely monitor patients who are taking opioid agonists for respiratory depression.
- Check doses carefully, particularly in children, and follow agency protocols for documentation.
- Describe the nature of pain before giving the drug and the degree of relief after the drug's onset of action.
- Intravenous (IV) injection of undiluted opiate agonists may lead to tachycardia and fainting.
- Provide side rails and assistance with ambulation after administering opiate agonists.
- Abrupt discontinuation of morphine and meperidine may lead to withdrawal effects (e.g., nausea, vomiting, diarrhea, dilated pupils, muscle twitching, nervousness, restlessness).

- Instruct the patient to avoid alcohol and other CNS depressants when taking opiate agonists.
- Be aware that emergency treatment for overdosing includes bag and mask ventilation, naloxone, and several hours of observation.
- Inform patients that opiate agonists should be tapered during discontinuation.

Do You UNDERSTAND?

DIRECTIONS: Indicate in the space provided whether the statement is true or false.

_____ 1. Monitor patients who are taking opioid agonists for respiratory depression.
_____ 2. Meperidine is contraindicated for patients with renal dysfunction.
_____ 3. Controlled-release tablets are to be crushed or chewed for better pain control.

What IS an Agonist-Antagonist?

Action

Agonist-antagonists act as an opioid agonist on one type of receptor and as a competitive antagonist on other receptors. Theories suggest that these agents produce analgesia at a subcortical level in the limbic system.

Uses

Agonist-antagonists are used for moderate to severe pain or as a preoperative medication. These drugs are useful to treat pain for patients with renal colic, burns, and cancer.

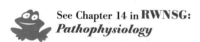

Agonist-Antagonists	Trade Names
pentazocine [pen-TAZ-oh-seen]	Talwin
butorphanol [byoo-TOR-fah-nole]	Stadol

See Chapter 14 in **RWNSG:** *Pathophysiology*

What You NEED TO KNOW

Contraindications/Precautions

Agonist-antagonists should be used with caution in patients with a head injury, increased intracranial pressure, acute MI, coronary insufficiency, hypertension, biliary tract surgery, hepatic or renal dysfunction, respiratory depression, chronic obstructive pulmonary disease (COPD), and those who have a history of drug dependency.

Answers: 1. true; 2. true; 3. false.

Drug Interactions

When agonist-antagonists are given together with other CNS depressants or alcohol, both CNS and respiratory depression are increased.

Adverse Effects

Adverse effects of agonist-antagonists are similar to those of opioid agonists, including rash, itching, headache, drowsiness, dizziness, fainting, sweating, euphoria, confusion, palpitations, bradycardia, nausea, flushing, difficulty urinating, and respiratory depression. Because these agents have agonist and antagonist actions, acute withdrawal effects can develop in opiate-dependent individuals. Opioid withdrawal effects peak 48 hours after drug discontinuation. Withdrawal effects include nausea, vomiting, anorexia, abdominal cramps, restlessness, fainting, and increased blood pressure. These agents have habit-forming potential.

What You DO

Nursing Responsibilities

Agonist-antagonists may be administered orally, SC, IM, and IV. For frequent long-term injections, IM is the preferred route over SC. When administering agonist-antagonists, the nurse should:

- Closely monitor patients who are taking agonist-antagonists for respiratory depression.
- Instruct patients to avoid combining agonist-antagonists with alcohol or other CNS depressants.
- Instruct patients to avoid activities that require alertness (e.g., driving) when taking opioid agonist-antagonists.
- Advise patients that abrupt discontinuation may cause withdrawal effects, including nausea, vomiting, anorexia, abdominal cramps, restlessness, chills, fainting, and increased blood pressure. Be aware that opioid withdrawal effects peak 48 hours after drug discontinuation.

Do You UNDERSTAND?

DIRECTIONS: **Indicate in the space provided whether the statement is *true* or *false*. If false, then correct the statement to make it true using the margin space to the right.**

_____ 1. Agonist-antagonists should not be administered when the patient's respiratory rate is less than 10 respirations per minute.

_____ 2. Opioid withdrawal effects peak 48 hours after drug discontinuation.

 Agonist-antagonists should be used with caution in patients with head injury, increased intracranial pressure, acute MI, coronary insufficiency, hypertension, biliary tract surgery, hepatic or renal dysfunction, respiratory depression, COPD, and those who have a history of drug dependency.

Safe use in pregnant women before labor and during lactation and in children under 18 years of age has not been established.

TAKE HOME POINTS

Do not administer opioid agonist-antagonists when the patient's respiratory rate is less than 12 respirations per minute. Agonist-antagonists may cause dizziness and drowsiness.

Answers: 1. false; respirations should be 12 or greater before giving agonist-antagonists; 2. true.

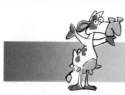

What IS an Opiate Antagonist?

Opiate Antagonists	Trade Names
naloxone [nal-OX-ohn]	Narcan
nalmefene [NAL-meh-feen]	Revex
naltrexone [nal-TREX-ohn]	Revia

Action

Opiate antagonists block (or antagonize) receptor sites. These agents are antidotes to opiate agonists and agonist-antagonists.

Uses

Opiate antagonists are used to reverse the opiate effects of narcotic overdose. These agents are also used to reverse respiratory depression.

What You NEED TO KNOW

 Safe use of opiate antagonists during pregnancy and lactation has not been established.

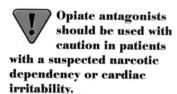 **Opiate antagonists should be used with caution in neonates and children.**

Opiate antagonists should be used with caution in patients with a suspected narcotic dependency or cardiac irritability.

Contraindications/Precautions

Opiate antagonists are contraindicated for patients with respiratory depression resulting from nonopioid agents.

Drug Interactions

When flumazenil is given together with nalmefene, seizures may result.

Adverse Effects

The adverse effects of opiate antagonists include slight drowsiness, hypertension, hyperventilation, tremors, and reversal of analgesia. When reversal is too rapid, the patient may develop sweating, nausea, vomiting, elevated partial thromboplastin time (PTT), and tachycardia.

What You DO

Nursing Responsibilities

Opiate antagonists are given IV because of the urgency of the situation of overdose and respiratory depression. When administering opiate antagonists, the nurse should:

- Continue to monitor the patient who is taking opiate antagonists because the duration of the narcotic analgesics may be longer than that of the opiate antagonist, and respiratory depression may reoccur. Administer repeated doses of opiate antagonists as required.
- Be aware that when reversal of opiate antagonists is too rapid, the patient may develop sweating, nausea, vomiting, and tachycardia.
- Monitor the patient for bleeding, particularly in surgical and obstetrical patients because opiate antagonists may alter coagulation.

 TAKE HOME POINTS

Monitor vital signs, particularly respirations, after administering opiate antagonists.

Do You UNDERSTAND?

DIRECTIONS: Provide the appropriate responses to the following statements from the italicized choices.

1. Duration of opiate antagonist is usually _____ compared with narcotic analgesics. (*longer, shorter*)

2. Evidence of an excessive opiate antagonist administration is _____. (*bradycardia, tachycardia*)

SECTION B
ANTIMIGRAINE AGENTS

Antimigraine agents are drugs that control the severe periodic headaches that usually have throbbing or stabbing pain as characteristics. Because migraines are a result of a dysfunction in the neurotransmitter serotonin and low serotonin levels, pharmacologic migraine control focuses on altering the serotonin concentration. Antimigraine agents are used to terminate an acute attack and prevent further attacks from occurring. Agents that are used to treat an acute migraine attack include aspirinlike analgesics, opioid analgesics, ergot derivatives, and triptans. Agents that are used to prevent migraine attacks include β-adrenergic blockers, calcium channel blockers, amitriptyline, methysergide, and valproic acid. An explanation of many of these drug categories is covered in other chapters of this text. This section contains information regarding ergot derivatives and triptans.

What IS an Ergot Derivative?

Ergot Derivatives	Trade Names
ergotamine tartrate *[er-GOT-ah-meen]*	Ergostat
ergotamine tartrate with caffeine	Cafergot
dihydroergotamine *[dye-high-droh-er-GOT-ah-meen]*	Migranal DHE 45
methysergide maleate *[meth-ih-SIR-jide]*	Sansert

Action

Ergot derivatives block or alter α-adrenergic, dopaminergic, and serotonin receptor sites in the brain and depress the vasomotor center, causing constriction of cranial blood vessels, decrease in the pulsation of cranial arteries, and decrease in basil artery perfusion. Because serotonin is a vasoconstrictor, ergot derivatives reduce the hyperperfusion of the dilated basilar artery and vascular bed. Methysergide is a semisynthetic ergot derivative that inhibits serotonin at postsynaptic receptors. Methysergide acts as a competitive antagonist of serotonin peripherally and may act as a serotonin agonist in the CNS. The antiserotonin effects of methysergide are greater compared with other ergot derivatives and result in inhibiting the peripheral vasoconstrictor effects of serotonin and serotonin-induced inflammation.

Uses

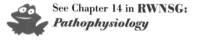

See Chapter 14 in **RWNSG:** *Pathophysiology*

Ergot derivatives are used to prevent or treat acute migraine or vascular headache. Ergot derivatives are the drugs of choice in the treatment of an acute migraine attack. Dihydroergotamine is the drug of choice for rapid treatment of severe, refractory migraine, and cluster headaches. Combinations with ergot derivatives include an anticholinergic (e.g., belladonna), a sedative (e.g., pentobarbital), or an antihistamine (e.g., diphenhydramine) to prevent nausea and vomiting, which usually accompany migraines.

What You NEED TO KNOW

Ergot derivatives are contraindicated during pregnancy and lactation because these agents are potent uterine stimulants and decrease uterine blood flow. Methysergide is also contraindicated for children and older adults.

Contraindications/Precautions

Ergot derivatives are contraindicated for patients with angina, coronary artery disease, peripheral vascular disease, hypertension, hypersensitivity, malnutrition, sepsis, and hepatic or renal dysfunction. Methysergide is also contraindicated for patients with peptic ulcers, collagen diseases, debilitation, or severe infection.

Drug Interactions

When ergot derivatives are given in combination with beta blockers and other vasoconstrictors, the risk of peripheral ischemia and gangrene is increased. Examples of vasoconstrictors include cocaine, epinephrine, norepinephrine, metaraminol, methoxamine, phenylephrine, and tobacco. Therefore smoking increases the risk of vasoconstriction when it is concurrent with an ergot derivative. Antibiotics, troleandomycin, and erythromycin may lead to ergot toxicity when given together with ergotamine. When ergotamine is combined with caffeine (Cafergot), GI absorption is enhanced.

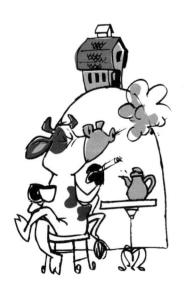

Adverse Effects

The most common adverse effects of ergot derivatives are nausea and peripheral ischemia. Transient cold fingers and toes accompanied by tingling and numbness is indicative of peripheral ischemia from vasoconstriction. Other adverse effects include vomiting, tachycardia, bradycardia, diminished or absent pulses, dysrhythmias, edema, itching, leg weakness, muscle pain, paresthesia, and chest pain. Other adverse effects from methysergide include visual changes, drowsiness, insomnia, restlessness, depression, euphoria, and peripheral edema. A rare adverse effect after prolonged therapy is fibrosis in cardiac, pulmonary, retroperitoneal, or penile tissue. When methysergide is discontinued abruptly, rebound headaches may occur. Because methysergide is chemically related to the hallucinogen lysergic acid diethylamide (LSD), overdose symptoms include visual changes, excitement, thought impairment, unsteadiness, dissociation, nightmares, hallucinations, convulsions, and impaired respirations.

Serious toxicity from an excessive amount of ergot agents is called ergotism and may lead to peripheral ischemia (e.g., cold, pale, numb extremities, gangrene). Because continuous excessive doses of ergot agents can cause physical dependence, rebound headache, increased frequency of headaches, dilated pupils, mental depression, restlessness, thirst, nausea, vomiting, diarrhea, and convulsions are among the withdrawal symptoms. Dihydroergotamine causes little nausea and vomiting and no physical dependence, but diarrhea is a common adverse effect.

 # What You DO

Nursing Responsibilities

Ergot derivatives may be given orally, IV, sublingually, rectally, or via inhalation. When administering ergot derivatives, the nurse should:

- Instruct the patient that ergot derivatives should be taken at the first symptoms of a headache. Then, the patient should lie down and relax in a quiet, darkened room for 2 to 3 hours for the medication to be most effective.
- Advise the patient to take methysergide with food to decrease GI distress. Inform the patient that intranasal and IV routes usually relieve migraines in less than 5 minutes.
- Counsel the patient to avoid chewing or swallowing sublingual tablets, but rather, they should be allowed to dissolve completely.
- Advise the patient that methysergide should be taken for no longer than 6 months. After 6 months of methysergide therapy, allow 3 to 4 weeks to pass without the drug.
- Instruct the patient that when no response to methysergide therapy appears within 3 weeks, treatment should be discontinued, and the health care provider should be notified.
- Be aware that the normal peak of methysergide is 60 ng/ml and that the normal trough level is 17 ng/ml.
- Inform patients that although migraine relief is achieved from dihydroergotamine, the headache usually returns in approximately 18% of patients within 24 hours.
- Instruct the patient to avoid increasing the dose without consulting the health care provider because overdosing is the leading cause of ergotamine adverse effects.

 TAKE HOME POINTS

- Teach the patient that ergot derivatives should be taken at the first warning or aura of a migraine.
- Instruct the patient that intranasal and rectal routes of antimigraines are usually preferred over oral therapy when nausea or vomiting is present.
- Gradually discontinue methysergide over a 2- to 3-week period, never abruptly.
- Warn the patient that prolonged use or excessive doses may lead to ergotism and gangrene.

Instruct the patient who is taking ergot derivatives to report shortness of breath, persistent paresthesia, leg muscle pain or weakness, cold or numb fingers or toes, pain in the chest, edema, abdomen, or muscles, and irregular heartbeat to the health care provider immediately.

Do You UNDERSTAND?

DIRECTIONS: Provide appropriate responses to the following questions.

1. What are two routes of administration that relieve migraine headaches?

_____

2. What is added to ergotamine to facilitate GI absorption?

_____

3. What type of tablets should not be chewed or swallowed but allowed to dissolve completely?

_____

What IS a Triptan?

Triptans	Trade Names
sumatriptan [soo-mah-TRIP-tan]	Imitrex
naratriptan [nar-ah-TRIP-tan]	Amerge
rizatriptan [rye-za-TRIP-tan]	Maxalt
zolmitriptan [zole-mih-TRIP-tan]	Zomig

Action

Triptans, the newest migraine agents on the market, are also known as serotonin 5-HT_1 receptor agonists. These agents bind to serotonin receptors $5\text{-HT}_1\text{B}$ or $5\text{-HT}_1\text{D}$ or both to cause vasoconstriction of cerebral blood vessels and inhibit the release of pain-producing inflammatory neuropeptides.

Uses

Triptans are used to relieve acute migraine attacks. Sumatriptan is usually more effective than is ergotamine for treating acute cluster attacks.

What You NEED TO KNOW

Contraindications/Precautions

Triptans should be used with caution in patients with coronary artery disease.

Drug Interactions

The major drug interaction of triptans involves severe vasoconstriction when they are given with ergot derivatives within 24 hours of each other. MAOIs

Triptans should be used with caution in patients with coronary artery disease.

decrease absorption of sumatriptan when they are given together or within 2 weeks of each other. Weakness, incoordination, and hyperreflexia have been reported when triptans are taken with selected serotonin reuptake inhibitors (SSRIs).

Adverse Effects

Most of the adverse effects of triptans are mild and transient, usually occurring within 1 hour after oral or SC administration and subside within 1 hour after onset from an oral dose and 10 to 30 minutes after an SC dose. The adverse effects include hypersensitivity, weakness, fatigue, nausea, hearing deficit, ocular irritation, visual disturbance, dizziness, drowsiness, edema, polyuria, urgency, tachycardia, palpitations, hypertension, and dysrhythmias. Angina has occurred in rare instances after sumatriptan administration. An overdose can lead to a reduced respiratory rate, tremors, seizures, cyanosis, reddened extremities, muscular incoordination, and pupil dilation.

  Triptans are contraindicated for women during lactation and pregnancy and in those who may become pregnant.

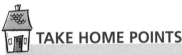 **Triptans should be used with caution in children and older adults.**

What You DO

Nursing Responsibilities

Triptans may be administered orally, intranasally, and SC. Although food does not appear to affect absorption, it delays peak concentration by approximately 30 minutes. When administering triptans, the nurse should:

- Administer the first dose of sumatriptan SC and under medical supervision.
- Inform the patient that when the first dose of oral naratriptan is ineffective, the dose may be repeated in 4 hours. When required, a second dose of rizatriptan may be repeated in 2 hours. With zolmitriptan administration, repeated doses may be taken every 2 hours for 24 hours. However, when no response to naratriptan, rizatriptan, or zolmitriptan is forthcoming, the health care provider should be consulted before taking another tablet.
- Instruct patients to report tingling, flushing, or dizziness to the health care provider.
- Inform the patient that although migraine relief is achieved from sumatriptan in all stages of an acute attack, the headache usually returns in approximately 40% of patients within 24 hours.
- Advise patients that while taking triptans, they should immediately report wheezing, facial swelling, rash, hives, chest pain, or tightness in the throat or chest to the health care provider.
- Warn patients that sumatriptan should be taken as soon as possible after migraine onset.
- Instruct the patient to use safety precautions when taking triptans when visual alterations and unsteadiness occur (e.g., when driving).

TAKE HOME POINTS

Monitor for unexpected cardiovascular responses following the first dose of sumatriptan.

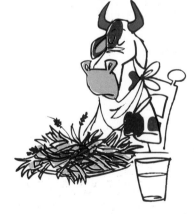

Do You UNDERSTAND?

DIRECTIONS: Indicate in the space provided whether the statement is *true* or *false*. If false, then correct the statement to make it true using the margin space at left.

_____ 1. A major drug interaction of triptans when given with ergot is severe vasoconstriction.

_____ 2. Migraines usually diminish within 30 minutes after administering oral triptans.

References

Chapter 1

Abramowicz M: Gatifloxacin and Moxifloxacin: two new fluoroquinolones, *Med Let Drugs Ther* 42(1072):315, 2000.

Abrams AC: *Clinical drug therapy: rationales for nursing practice*, ed 6, Philadelphia, 2001, Lippincott.

Burke MB, Wilkes GM, Ingwersen K: *Cancer chemotherapy: a nursing process approach*, Sudbury, MA, 1996, Jones and Bartlett Publishers.

Clayton BD, Stock YN: *Basic pharmacology for nurses*, ed 11, St Louis, 1997, Mosby.

Cleveland L et al: *Nursing management in drug therapy*, Philadelphia, 1999, Lippincott.

Eisenhauer LA et al: *Clinical pharmacology and nursing management*, ed 5, Philadelphia, 1998, Lippincott.

Fishman M, Mrozek-Orlowski M: *Cancer chemotherapy guidelines and recommendations for practice*, Pittsburgh, 1999, Oncology Nursing Press.

Freeman Clark JB, Queener SF, Karb VB: *Pharmacologic basis of nursing practice*, ed 6, St Louis, 2000, Mosby.

Gutierrez K: *Pharmacotherapeutics: clinical decision-making in nursing*, Philadelphia, 1999, WB Saunders.

Hardman JG, Limbird LE: *Goodman & Gilman's: the pharmacological basis of therapeutics*, ed 9, New York, 1996, McGraw-Hill.

Ignatavicius DD, Workman ML, Mishler MA: *Medical-surgical nursing across the health care continuum*, ed 3, Philadelphia, 1999, WB Saunders.

Karch AM: *Focus on nursing pharmacology*, Philadelphia, 2000, Lippincott.

Kee JL, Hayes ER: *Pharmacology: a nursing process approach*, ed 3, Philadelphia, 2000, WB Saunders.

Kuhn M: *Pharmacotherapeutics: a nursing process approach*, ed 4, Philadelphia, 1998, FA Davis.

Lehne RA et al: *Pharmacology for nursing care*, ed 4, Philadelphia, 2001, WB Saunders.

Peterson PG, Burns M: Antineoplastic drugs. In Gutierrez K: *Pharmacotherapeutics: clinical decision-making in nursing*, Philadelphia, 1999, WB Saunders.

Rang HP, Dale MM, Ritter JM: *Pharmacology*, ed 4, London, 1999, Churchill Livingstone.

Smeltzer SC, Bare BG: *Brunner and Suddarth's textbook of medical-surgical nursing*, ed 9, Philadelphia, 2000, Lippincott.

Wilkes GM, Ingwersen K, Burke MB: *1997-1998 Oncology nursing drug handbook*, Sudbury, Mass, 1997, Jones and Bartlett Publishers.

Williams BR, Baer CL: *Essentials of clinical pharmacology in nursing*, ed 3, Springhouse, Pa, 1998, Springhouse.

Wilson BA, Shannon MT, Stang CL: *Nurses drug guide*, Stamford, Conn, 2001, Appleton & Lange.

Chapter 2

Abrams AC: *Clinical drug therapy: rationales for nursing practice*, ed 6, Philadelphia, 2001, Lippincott.

Arky R, consultant: *Physician's desk reference 2001*, ed 55, Montvale, NJ, 2001, Medical Economic.

Clark JBF, Queener SF, Karb VB: *Pharmacologic basis of nursing practice*, St Louis, 2000, Mosby.

Clayton BD, Stock YN: *Basic pharmacology for nurses*, ed 11, St Louis, 1997, Mosby.

Cleveland L et al: *Nursing management in drug therapy*, Philadelphia, 1999, Lippincott.

Deglin JH, Vallerand AH: *Davis's drug guide for nurses*, ed 6, Philadelphia, 1999, FA Davis.

Dipiro J et al: *Pharmacology, a pathophysiologic approach*, ed 3, Stamford Conn, 1997, Appleton & Lang.

Eisenhauer L, Murphy M: *Pharmacotherapeutics and advanced nursing practice*, New York, 1998, McGraw-Hill.

Eisenhauer LA et al: *Clinical pharmacology and nursing management*, ed 5, Philadelphia, 1998, Lippincott.

Freeman Clark JB, Queener SF, Karb VB: *Pharmacologic basis of nursing practice*, ed 6, St Louis, 2000, Mosby.

Gutierrez K: *Pharmacotherapeutics: clinical decision-making in nursing*, Philadelphia, 1999, WB Saunders.

Hardman JG, Limbird LE: *Goodman & Gilman's: the pharmacological basis of therapeutics*, ed 9, New York, 1996, McGraw-Hill.

Hodgson B, Kizior R: *Saunders nursing drug handbook 2002*, ed 10, Philadelphia, 2001, WB Saunders.

Ignatavicius DD, Workman ML, Mishler MA: *Medical-surgical nursing across the health care continuum*, ed 3, Philadelphia, 1999, WB Saunders.

Julian R: Central nervous system depressants: traditional sedative-hypnotic drugs and antiepileptic drugs. In *A primer of drug action*, ed 8, New York, 1998, WH Freeman.

Karch AM: *Focus on nursing pharmacology*, Philadelphia, 2000, Lippincott.

Kee JL, Hayes ER: *Pharmacology: a nursing process approach*, ed 3, Philadelphia, 2000, WB Saunders.

Kuhn M: *Pharmacotherapeutics: a nursing process approach*, ed 4, Philadelphia, 1998, FA Davis.

Lehne RA et al: *Pharmacology for nursing care*, ed 4, Philadelphia, 2001, WB Saunders.

Porter R, Meldrum B: Antiepileptic drugs. In Katzung B, editor: *Basic and clinical pharmacology*, ed 7, New York, 1998, Lang Medical Books–McGraw-Hill.

Schull P: Pharmacologic classes. In *Physician's drug handbook*, ed 8, Springhouse, Pa, 1999, Springhouse.

Schwinghammer T: *Pharmacotherapy: a patient-focused approach*, Stamford, Conn, 1997, Appleton & Lang.

Smeltzer SC, Bare BG: *Brunner and Suddarth's textbook of medical-surgical nursing*, ed 9, Philadelphia, 2000, Lippincott.

Spratto G, Woods A: *PDR nurse's drug handbook*, Montvale, NJ, 2001, Delmar Publishers and Medical Economics.

Whitehouse S: Seizure disorders. In Beers M, Berkow R, editors: *The Merk manual of diagnosis and therapy*, ed 17, Montvale, NJ, 1999, Medical Economics.

Williams BR, Baer CL: *Essentials of clinical pharmacology in nursing*, ed 3, Springhouse, Pa, 1998, Springhouse.

Wilson BA, Shannon MT, Stang CL: *Nurses drug guide*, Stamford, Conn, 2001, Appleton & Lange.

Chapter 3

Brieger DB et al: Heparin-induced thrombocytopenia: a review, *J Am Coll Cardiol* 31:1449, 1998.

Cleveland L et al: *Nursing management in drug therapy*, Philadelphia, 1999, Lippincott.

Eisenhauer LA et al: *Clinical pharmacology and nursing management*, ed 5, Philadelphia, 1998, Lippincott.

Gutierrez K: *Pharmacotherapeutics: clinical decision-making in nursing*, Philadelphia, 1999, WB Saunders.

Hansen M: *Pathophysiology: foundations of disease & clinical interventions*, Philadelphia, 1998, WB Saunders.

Kee JL, Hayes ER: *Pharmacology: a nursing process approach*, ed 2, Philadelphia, 1997, WB Saunders.

Kuhn M: *Pharmacotherapeutics: a nursing process approach*, ed 4, Philadelphia, FA Davis.

Lehne RA et al: *Pharmacology for nursing care*, ed 4, Philadelphia, 2001, WB Saunders.

Ortel TL, Chong BH: New treatment options for heparin-induced thrombocytopenia, *Sem Hematol* 35(suppl 5):26, 1998.

Williams BR, Baer CL: *Essentials of clinical pharmacology in nursing*, ed 3, Springhouse, Pa, 1998, Springhouse.

Wilson BA, Shannon MT, Stang CL: *Nurses drug guide*, Stamford, Conn, 2001, Appleton & Lange.

Chapter 4

Abrams AC: *Clinical drug therapy: rationales for nursing practice*, ed 6, Philadelphia, 2001, Lippincott.

Clark JBF, Queener SF, Karb VB: *Pharmacologic basis of nursing practice*, St Louis, 2000, Mosby.

Clayton BD, Stock YN: *Basic pharmacology for nurses*, ed 11, St Louis 1997, Mosby.

Cleveland L et al: *Nursing management in drug therapy*, Philadelphia, 1999, Lippincott.

Drug facts and comparisons, 2001 edition, St Louis, 2001, Wolters-Kluwer.

Eisenhauer LA: *Clinical pharmacology and nursing management*, ed 5, Philadelphia, 1998, Lippincott.

Freeman Clark JB, Queener SF, Karb VB: *Pharmacologic basis of nursing practice*, ed 6, St Louis, 2000, Mosby.

Gutierrez K: *Pharmacotherapeutics: clinical decision-making in nursing*, Philadelphia, 1999, WB Saunders.

Hardman JG, Limbird LE: *Goodman & Gilman's: the pharmacological basis of therapeutics*, ed 9, New York, 1996, McGraw-Hill.

Ignatavicius DD, Workman ML, Mishler MA: *Medical-surgical nursing across the health care continuum*, ed 3, Philadelphia, 1999, WB Saunders.

Karch AM: *Focus on nursing pharmacology*, Philadelphia, 2000, Lippincott.

Karch AM: *Lippincott's nursing drug guide 2001*, Philadelphia, 2001, Lippincott–Williams & Wilkins.

Kee JL, Hayes ER: *Pharmacology: a nursing process approach*, ed 3, Philadelphia, 2000, WB Saunders.

Kuhn M: *Pharmacotherapeutics: a nursing process approach*, ed 4, Philadelphia, 1998, FA Davis.

Lehne RA et al: *Pharmacology for nursing care*, ed 4, Philadelphia, 2001, WB Saunders.

McEvoy G: *American Hospital Formulary Service (AHFS) drug information 2001*, Bethesda, MD, 2001, American Society of Health-System Pharmacists.

Smeltzer SC, Bare BG: *Brunner and Suddarth's textbook of medical-surgical nursing*, ed 9, Philadelphia, 2000, Lippincott.

Spratto G, Woods A: *PDR nurse's drug handbook*, Montvale, NJ, 2001, Delmar Publishers and Medical Economics.

Williams BR, Baer CL: *Essentials of clinical pharmacology in nursing*, ed 3, Springhouse, Pa, 1998, Springhouse.

Wilson BA, Shannon MT, Stang CL: *Nurses drug guide*, Stamford, Conn, 2001, Appleton & Lange.

Chapter 5

Abrams AC: *Clinical drug therapy: rationales for nursing practice*, ed 6, Philadelphia, 2001, Lippincott.

Braunwald E, Zipes DP, Libby P: *Heart disease: a textbook of cardiovascular medicine*, ed 6, Philadelphia, 2001, WB Saunders.

Clayton BD, Stock YN: *Basic pharmacology for nurses*, ed 11, St Louis, 1997, Mosby.

Cleveland L et al: *Nursing management in drug therapy*, Philadelphia, 1999, Lippincott.

Deglin JH, Vallerand AH: *Davis's drug guide for nurses*, ed 6, Philadelphia, 1999, FA Davis.

Eisenhauer LA et al: *Clinical pharmacology and nursing management*, ed 5, Philadelphia, 1998, Lippincott.

Freeman Clark JB, Queener SF, Karb VB: *Pharmacologic basis of nursing practice*, ed 6, St Louis, 2000, Mosby.

Gutierrez K: *Pharmacotherapeutics: clinical decision-making in nursing*, Philadelphia, 1999, WB Saunders.

Hardman JG, Limbird LE: *Goodman & Gilman's: the pharmacological basis of therapeutics*, ed 9, New York, 1996, McGraw-Hill.

Ignatavicius DD, Workman ML, Mishler MA: *Medical-surgical nursing across the health care continuum*, ed 3, Philadelphia, 1999, WB Saunders.

Karch AM: *Focus on nursing pharmacology*, Philadelphia, 2000, Lippincott.

Kee JL, Hayes ER: *Pharmacology: a nursing process approach*, ed 3, Philadelphia, 2000, WB Saunders.

Kuhn M: *Pharmacotherapeutics: a nursing process approach*, ed 4, Philadelphia, 1998, FA Davis.

Lehne RA et al: *Pharmacology for nursing care*, ed 4, Philadelphia, 2001, WB Saunders.

Opie LH, Gersh BJ: *Drugs for the heart*, ed 5, Philadelphia, 2001, WB Saunders.

Physician's desk reference, ed 55, Montage, NJ, 2001, Oradell: Medical Economics Data.

Smeltzer SC, Bare BG: *Brunner and Suddarth's textbook of medical-surgical nursing*, ed 9, Philadelphia, 2000, Lippincott.

Williams BR, Baer CL: *Essentials of clinical pharmacology in nursing*, ed 3, Springhouse, Pa, 1998, Springhouse.

Wilson BA, Shannon MT, Stang CL: *Nurses drug guide*, Stamford, Conn, 2001, Appleton & Lange.

Chapter 6

Abrams AC: *Clinical drug therapy: rationales for nursing practice*, ed 6, Philadelphia, 2001, Lippincott.

Drug facts and comparisons, 2001 edition, St Louis, 2001, Wolters-Kluwer.

Gutierrez K: *Pharmacotherapeutics: clinical decision making in nursing*, Philadelphia, 1999, WB Saunders.

Hansen M: *Pathophysiology: foundations of disease and clinical intervention*, Philadelphia, 1998, WB Saunders.

Lehne RA et al: *Pharmacology for nursing care*, ed 4, Philadelphia, 2001, WB Saunders.

McEvoy G: *American Hospital Formulary Service (AHFS) drug information 2001*, Bethesda, MD, 2001, American Society of Health-System Pharmacists.

Monahan FD, Neighbors M: *Medical-surgical nursing: foundations for clinical practice*, ed 2, Philadelphia, 1998, WB Saunders.

Schrefer J: *Mosby's GenRx: a comprehensive reference for generic and brand drugs*, St Louis, 2000, Mosby.

Spratto G, Woods A: *PDR nurse's drug handbook*, Montvale, NJ, 2001, Delmar Publishers and Medical Economics.

Wilson BA, Shannon MT, Stang CL: *Nurses drug guide*, Stamford, Conn, 2001, Appleton & Lange.

Chapter 7

Abramowicz M: Somatrem and somatropin, *Med Let Drugs Ther* 41:2. 1999.

Abrams AC: *Clinical drug therapy: rationales for nursing practice*, ed 6, Philadelphia, 2001, Lippincott.

Abrams AC: *2001 Lippincott's nursing drug guide*, Philadelphia, 2001, Lippincott–Williams & Wilkins.

Drug facts and comparisons, 2001 edition, St Louis, 2001, Wolters-Kluwer.

Gelman CR, Rumack BH: *DrugDex information system*, Denver, 1999, Micromedex.

Gutierrez K: *Pharmacotherapeutics: clinical decision-making in nursing*, Philadelphia, 1999, WB Saunders.

Hudak CM, Gallo BM, Morton PG: Common endocrine disorders. In *Critical care nursing: a holistic approach*, ed 7, Philadelphia, 1998, Lippincott.

Johnson PH, editor: *Nurse practitioner's drug handbook*, ed 2, Springhouse, Pa, 1998, Springhouse.

Karch AM: Drugs that act on the endocrine system. In *Focus on nursing pharmacology*, Philadelphia, 2000, Lippincott.

Lehne RA et al: *Pharmacology for nursing care*, ed 4, Philadelphia, 2001, WB Saunders.

McEvoy G: *American Hospital Formulary Service (AHFS) drug information 2001*, Bethesda, MD, 2001, American Society of Health-System Pharmacists.

Monahan FD, Neighbors M: Nursing care of patients with other endocrine disorders. In *Medical-surgical nursing foundations for clinical practice*, ed 2, Philadelphia, 1998, WB Saunders.

Schrefer J: *Mosby's GenRx: a comprehensive reference for generic and brand drugs*, St Louis, 2000, Mosby.

Smeltzer S, Bare B: *Brunner and Suddarth's textbook of medical-surgical nursing*, ed 9, Philadelphia, 2000, Lippincott.

Spratto G, Woods A: *PDR nurse's drug handbook*, Montvale, NJ, 2001, Delmar Publishers and Medical Economics.

Wilson BA, Shannon MT, Stang CL: *Nurses drug guide*, Stamford, Conn, 2001, Appleton & Lange.

Chapter 8

Abrams AC: *Clinical drug therapy: rationales for nursing practice*, ed 6, Philadelphia, 2001, Lippincott.

Arky R, consultant: *Physician's desk reference 2001*, ed 55, Montvale, NJ, 2001, Medical Economic.

Clayton BD, Stock YN: *Basic pharmacology for nurses*, ed 11, St Louis, 1997, Mosby.

Cleveland L et al: *Nursing management in drug therapy*, Philadelphia, 1999, Lippincott.

Eisenhauer LA et al: *Clinical pharmacology and nursing management*, ed 5, Philadelphia, 1998, Lippincott.

Fauci AS et al: *Harrison's principles of internal medicine*, ed 14, New York, 1998, McGraw-Hill.

Freeman Clark JB, Queener SF, Karb VB: *Pharmacologic basis of nursing practice*, ed 6, St Louis, 2000, Mosby.

Gutierrez K: *Pharmacotherapeutics: clinical decision-making in nursing*, Philadelphia, 1999, WB Saunders.

Hansen M: *Pathophysiology: foundations of disease & clinical interventions*, Philadelphia, 1998, WB Saunders.

Hardman JG, Limbird LE: *Goodman & Gilman's: the pharmacological basis of therapeutics*, ed 9, New York, 1996, McGraw-Hill.

Ignatavicius DD, Workman ML, Mishler MA: *Medical-surgical nursing across the health care continuum*, ed 3, Philadelphia, 1999, WB Saunders.

Karch AM: *Focus on nursing pharmacology*, Philadelphia, 2000, Lippincott.

Kee JL, Hayes ER: *Pharmacology: a nursing process approach*, ed 3, Philadelphia, 2000, WB Saunders.

Kuhn M: *Pharmacotherapeutics: a nursing process approach*, ed 4, Philadelphia, 1998, FA Davis.

Lehne RA et al: *Pharmacology for nursing care*, ed 4, Philadelphia, 2001, WB Saunders.

Skidmore-Roth L: *Nursing drug reference*, St Louis, 1999, Mosby.

Smeltzer SC, Bare BG: *Brunner and Suddarth's textbook of medical-surgical nursing*, ed 9, Philadelphia, 2000, Lippincott.

Williams BR, Baer CL: *Essentials of clinical pharmacology in nursing*, ed 3, Springhouse, Pa, 1998, Springhouse.

Wilson BA, Shannon MT, Stang CL: *Nurses drug guide*, Stamford, Conn, 2001, Appleton & Lange.

Chapter 9

Beers MH, Berkow R: *The Merck manual of diagnosis and therapy, centennial edition*, Montvale, NJ, 1999, Merck.

Cleveland L et al: *Nursing management in drug therapy*, Philadelphia, 1999, Lippincott.

Eisenhauer LA et al: *Clinical pharmacology and nursing management*, ed 5, Philadelphia, 1998, Lippincott.

Gutierrez K: *Pharmacotherapeutics: clinical decision-making in nursing*, Philadelphia, 1999, WB Saunders.

Hansen M: *Pathophysiology: foundations of disease & clinical interventions*, Philadelphia, 1998, WB Saunders.

Ignatavicius DD, Workman ML, Mishler MA: *Medical-surgical nursing across the health care continuum*, ed 3, Philadelphia, 1999, WB Saunders.

Johnson PH, editor: *Nurse practitioner's drug handbook*, ed 3, Springhouse, Pa, 2000, Springhouse.

Karch AM: *Lippincott's nursing drug guide 2001*, Philadelphia, 2001, Lippincott–Williams, & Wilkins.

Kuhn M: *Pharmacotherapeutics: a nursing process approach*, ed 4, Philadelphia, 1998, FA Davis.

Lehne RA et al: *Pharmacology for nursing care*, ed 4, Philadelphia, 2001, WB Saunders.

McEvoy G: *American Hospital Formulary Service (AHFS) drug information 2001*, Bethesda, MD, 2001, American Society of Health-System Pharmacists.

Williams BR, Baer CL: *Essentials of clinical pharmacology in nursing*, ed 3, Springhouse, Pa, 1998, Springhouse.

Wilson BA, Shannon MT, Stang CL: *Nurses drug guide*, Stamford, Conn, 2001, Appleton & Lange.

Chapter 10

Abrams AC: *Clinical drug therapy: rationales for nursing practice*, ed 6, Philadelphia, 2001, Lippincott.

Karch A: *2001 Lippincott's nursing drug guide*, Philadelphia, 2001, Lippincott.

Karch AM: *Focus on nursing pharmacology*, Philadelphia, 2000, Lippincott.

Lehne RA et al: *Pharmacology for nursing care*, ed 4, Philadelphia, 2001, WB Saunders.

McEvoy G: *American Hospital Formulary Service (AHFS) drug information 2001*, Bethesda, MD, 2001, American Society of Health-System Pharmacists.

Wilson B, Shannon M, Stang C: *Nurses drug guide 2001*, Stamford, Conn, 2001, Appleton & Lange.

Chapter 11

Abrams AC: *Clinical drug therapy: rationales for nursing practice*, ed 6, Philadelphia, 2001, Lippincott.

Clark JF, Queener SF, Karb VB: *Pharmacologic basis of nursing practice*, ed 6, St Louis, 2000, Mosby.

Clayton BD, Stock YN: *Basic pharmacology for nurses*, ed 11, St Louis, 1997, Mosby.

Cleveland L et al: *Nursing management in drug therapy*, Philadelphia, 1999, Lippincott.

Eisenhauer LA et al: *Clinical pharmacology and nursing management*, ed 5, Philadelphia, 1998, Lippincott.

Freeman Clark JB, Queener SF, Karb VB: *Pharmacologic basis of nursing practice*, ed 6, St Louis, 2000, Mosby.

Gutierrez K: *Pharmacotherapeutics: clinical decision-making in nursing*, Philadelphia, 1999, WB Saunders.

Hardman JG, Limbird LE: *Goodman & Gilman's: the pharmacological basis of therapeutics*, ed, 9 New York, 1996, McGraw-Hill.

Ignatavicius DD, Workman ML, Mishler MA: *Medical-surgical nursing across the health care continuum*, ed 3, Philadelphia, 1999, WB Saunders.

Karch AM: *Focus on nursing pharmacology*, Philadelphia, 2000, Lippincott.

Kee JL, Hayes ER: *Pharmacology: a nursing process approach*, ed 3, Philadelphia, 2000, WB Saunders.

Kuhn M: *Pharmacotherapeutics: a nursing process approach*, ed 4, Philadelphia, 1998, FA Davis.

Lehne RA et al: *Pharmacology for nursing care*, ed 4, Philadelphia, 2001, WB Saunders.

McEvoy G: *American Hospital Formulary Service (AHFS) drug information 2001*, Bethesda, MD, 2001, American Society of Health-System Pharmacists.

Smeltzer SC, Bare BG: *Brunner and Suddarth's textbook of medical-surgical nursing*, ed 9, Philadelphia, 2000, Lippincott.

Williams BR, Baer CL: *Essentials of clinical pharmacology in nursing*, ed 3, Springhouse, Pa, 1998, Springhouse.

Wilson BA, Shannon MT, Stang CL: *Nurses drug guide*, Stamford, Conn, 2001, Appleton & Lange.

Chapter 12

Drug facts and comparisons, 2001 edition, St Louis, 2001, Wolters-Kluwer.

Gelman CR, Rumack BH: *DrugDex information system*, Denver, 1999, Micromedex.

Gutierrez K: *Pharmacotherapeutics: clinical decision making in nursing*, Philadelphia, 1999, WB Saunders.

Lehne RA et al: *Pharmacology for nursing care*, ed 4, Philadelphia, 2001, WB Saunders.

Spratto G, Woods A: *PDR nurse's drug handbook*, Montvale, NJ, 2001, Delmar Publishers and Medical Economics.

Thomas CL, editor: *Taber's cyclopedic medical dictionary*, ed 18, Philadelphia, 1997, FA Davis.

Wilson BA, Shannon MT, Stang CL: *Nurses drug guide*, Stamford, Conn, 2001, Appleton & Lange.

Chapter 13

Deglin J, Vallerand A: *Davis's medication guide for nurses*, ed 6, Philadelphia, 1999, FA Davis.

Gutierrez K: *Pharmacotherapeutics: clinical decision-making in nursing*, Philadelphia, 1999, WB Saunders.

Johnson PH, editor: *Nurse practitioner's medication handbook*, ed 2, Springhouse, Pa, 1999, Springhouse.

Chapter 14

Baker B: Avoid triptans for migraine in pregnant patients, *Ob Gyn News* 35(17):9, 2000.

Bateman N: Triptans and migraine, *Lancet* 355(9207):860, 2000.

Clark JF, Queener SF, Karb VB: *Pharmacologic basis of nursing practice*, ed 6, St Louis, 2000, Mosby.

Gutierrez K: *Pharmacotherapeutics: clinical decision-making in nursing*, Philadelphia, 1999, WB Saunders.

Karch AM: *Focus on nursing pharmacology*, Philadelphia, 2000, Lippincott.

Kee JL, Hayes ER: *Pharmacology: a nursing process approach*, ed 3, Philadelphia, 2000, WB Saunders.

Lehne RA et al: *Pharmacology for nursing care*, ed 4, Philadelphia, 2001, WB Saunders.

McCaffery M, Pasero C: *Pain clinical manual*, ed 2, St Louis, 1999, Mosby.

McEvoy G: *American Hospital Formulary Service (AHFS) drug information 2001*, Bethesda, MD, 2001, American Society of Health-System Pharmacists.

Wilson BA, Shannon MT, Stang CL: *Nurses drug guide*, Stamford, Conn, 2001, Appleton & Lange.

Illustration Credit Listing

Page 141: Redrawn from Kee J, Hayes E, editor: *Pharmacology: a nursing process approach*, ed 3, Philadelphia, 2000, WB Saunders.

NCLEX Section

CHAPTER *1*

Section A

1. Which of the following statements about natural penicillins is true?
   1 The spectrum of action is wider than that of any other penicillin.
   2 Natural penicillins have a structure that was developed to resist splitting of the beta-lactam ring.
   3 Bacteria may develop a protective mechanism and become resistant to natural penicillins.
   4 Natural penicillins have an amino group attached to the nucleus that increases the action against gram-negative bacteria.

2. Bacteriocidal means that the antibacterial drug has which of the following characteristics?
   1 A narrow spectrum of action against bacteria
   2 A wide spectrum of action against bacteria
   3 Inhibits the formation and growth of new bacteria
   4 Inhibits enzymes that are necessary for bacterial cell wall maintenance and life

3. When administering sulfonamides, an important nursing responsibility is to instruct the patient to do which of the following?
   1 Limit fluid intake.
   2 Drink 2 liters of fluid per day.
   3 Take the drug with orange juice.
   4 Lie down for 30 minutes after the initial dose of the drug.

4. The nurse should monitor the patient who is taking aminoglycosides for which of the following adverse effects?
   1 Seizures
   2 Ototoxicity
   3 Photosensitivity
   4 Teeth discoloration

5. Many antibiotics should be used with caution in pregnant individuals. Which of the following are contraindicated for women during pregnancy?
   1 Penicillins
   2 Macrolides
   3 Aminoglycosides
   4 Fluoroquinolones

Section B

6. Which of the following statements about AZT is incorrect?
   1 AZT must be converted to the nucleotide form to express antiviral activity.
   2 AZT is incorporated into growing viral but not mammalian nuclear DNA.
   3 AZT is currently used to treat severe herpesvirus and respiratory syncytial viral infections, as well as AIDS.
   4 AZT is toxic to bone marrow and causes adverse hematologic effects.

7. Retroviruses contain which of the following substances?
   1 Fungi
   2 DNA only
   3 RNA only
   4 Reverse transcriptase

8. Protease inhibitors should be taken with which food or drink?
   1 Wine
   2 Meals
   3 Acidic juice
   4 Chocolate milk

9. Identify one of the principles of retroviral therapy.
   1 Use monotherapy regime.
   2 Initiate treatment before immunodeficiency becomes evident.
   3 Discontinue one drug when plasma viral loads decrease.
   4 Antiviral agents do not affect the viral replication cycle.

10. Which antifungal medication is considered as a first-line drug for systemic use?
   1 Nystatin
   2 Clotrimazole
   3 Oxiconazole
   4 Amphotericin B

Section C

11. Interleukin-11 is an example of a drug that is designed to perform which action?
   1 Stimulates platelet production
   2 Stimulates red blood cell production
   3 Increases the body's ability to produce antibodies
   4 Regulates the production of neutrophils

12. Interleukin therapy should continue until the postnadir platelet count is greater than what values?
   1 0.005 to 0.015 μmol/ml
   2 15 to 35 μmol/ml
   3 50,000 cells/μl
   4 500,000 cells/mm

13. Which of the following drugs exert antitumor activity?
   1 Cyclosporine
   2 Interleukin-11
   3 Interferon alfa-2a
   4 Sargramostim

14. Which one of the following drug actions prevent rejection of organ transplantation?
   1 Erythropoietin
   2 Interferon alfa-2a
   3 Cyclosporine or Imuran
   4 Interleukin-1 or interleukin-2

15. By what method should cyclosporine be administered?
   1 IM
   2 In a plastic container
   3 Mixed with grapefruit juice
   4 Mixed with chocolate milk or orange juice

Section D

16. Doses for chemotherapy are based on which of the following factors?
   1 The patient's ideal body weight
   2 Milligrams per kilogram
   3 Body surface area
   4 The patient's actual weight

17. When preparing chemotherapy drugs, special precautions must be taken because the drugs have which of the following characteristics?
   1 Irritating to the GI tract
   2 Liable to cause vomiting
   3 Acidic
   4 Biohazardous substances

18. Cytotoxic agents tend to exert their effect on which type of cells?
   1 Rapidly growing cells
   2 Cells that are poorly supplied with oxygen
   3 Cells with a long doubling time
   4 Cells with a poor blood supply

19. Patients with a low white blood cell count may experience which of the following problems?
   1 Acidosis
   2 Delayed wound healing
   3 Hyperviscosity of the blood
   4 Prolonged bleeding times

20. Which of the following drugs is not a vesicant?
   1 Vincristine
   2 Methotrexate
   3 Vinblastine
   4 Melphalan

CHAPTER 2

Section A

1. A patient who is diagnosed with emphysema is receiving albuterol treatments via a nebulizer. The most important responsibility is for the nurse to assess the _____ and _____ during and after each treatment.
   1 Pupils, breath sounds
   2 Capillary refill, heart sounds
   3 Pulse rate, blood pressure
   4 Bowel sounds, skin color

2. α-Adrenergic antagonists may cause which of the following conditions?
   1 Mydriasis and decreased gastric motility
   2 Miosis and increased gastric motility
   3 Hypertension
   4 Hemorrhage

3. Administering a β-adrenergic antagonist to a patient who is receiving a calcium channel blocker may result in which of the following conditions?
   1 Hypertension and bradycardia
   2 Hypotension and bradycardia
   3 Tachycardia and hypertension
   4 Tachycardia and hypotension

4. The nurse is ready to administer a β-adrenergic antagonist to a patient. Before administering the drug, the patient complains of shortness of breath, and the nurse auscultates crackles throughout the lung fields. Which of the following is the appropriate nursing intervention for this patient?
   1 Administer the drug as ordered and notify the health care provider.
   2 Hold the drug and notify the health care provider.
   3 Wait 1 hour and then administer the drug.
   4 Hold the drug and administer the next dose.

5. A β-adrenergic antagonist should not be administered when which of the following is assessed in the patient?
   1 Bilateral wheezing
   2 A heart rate of 80 beats per minute
   3 A blood pressure of 120/72
   4 A blood pressure of 170/100

Section B

6. Which of the following is the antidote for an overdose of a direct-acting cholinergic agonist?
   1 Procainamide
   2 Lidocaine
   3 Artane
   4 Atropine

7. A patient who takes pyridostigmine for myasthenia gravis is given an edrophonium (Tensilon) test. The patient's skeletal muscle weakness improves. How would the dose of pyridostigmine be classified?
   1 Not enough
   2 Too much
   3 Therapeutic
   4 Overdose level

8. Which drug or drugs may precipitate a hypertensive crisis when taken with a dopaminergic?
   1 Methyldopa
   2 Tricyclic antidepressants
   3 Alcohol
   4 MAOIs

9. Opioids may cause possible life-threatening reactions when taken with which of the following drugs?
   1 Selegiline
   2 Bromocriptine
   3 Amantadine
   4 Ropinirole

10. Which of the following agents is used as maintenance therapy for myasthenia gravis?
    1 Ambenonium and pyridostigmine
    2 Edrophonium and neostigmine
    3 Donepezil and rivastigmine
    4 Neostigmine and pyridostigmine

Section C

11. For which reason is the psychomotor stimulant methylphenidate (Ritalin) used in children?
    1 To overcome obesity
    2 As a sleeping aid at bedtime
    3 Found to be safe for long-term use
    4 Primarily for ADHD therapy

12. When are anorexiants best administered?
    1 Before breakfast
    2 Midmorning
    3 With the evening meal
    4 At bedtime

13. Which substance does not contain caffeine?
    1 Cola
    2 Ritalin
    3 Excedrin
    4 Chocolate

14. Baclofen is used primarily to treat which of the following disorders?
    1 Leg cramps
    2 Hyperactivity
    3 Narcolepsy
    4 Muscle spasms

15. Which laboratory values are important to monitor when administering peripheral-acting muscle relaxants?
    1 Sodium level
    2 Phenytoin levels
    3 Potassium level
    4 Liver function studies

Section D

16. Which anticonvulsant causes slurred speech, enlargement of facial features, nystagmus, or gingival hyperplasia as possible adverse effects?
    1 Phenytoin
    2 Phenobarbital
    3 Lorazepam
    4 Carbamazepine

17. When taking barbiturates, elderly patients usually develop which of the following adverse effects?
    1 Lethargy, drowsiness, and faintness
    2 Excitement, confusion, or depression
    3 Hypertension and diuresis
    4 Bleeding or gingival hyperplasia

18. What can be assumed about patients who are taking benzodiazepines?
    1 Patients should take benzodiazepines with antacids.
    2 Patients develop an increased tolerance for alcohol.
    3 Patients may develop toxicity of short-term memory.
    4 Patients are generally affected by CNS-stimulating properties of benzodiazepines.

19. SLE and Stevens-Johnson syndrome may develop as adverse effects of which of the following substances?
    1 Ethosuximide
    2 Lorazepam
    3 Phenytoin
    4 Valproic Acid

20. Which is the drug of choice in treating status epilepticus?
    1 Phenytoin
    2 Diazepam
    3 Phenobarbital
    4 Valproic acid

21. In which of the following would procaine be contraindicated?
    1 Heart block
    2 Spinal block
    3 Older adult
    4 Peripheral nerve block

Section E

22. Which anesthetic agent would be least likely to cause laryngospasm?
    1 Regional
    2 Inhalation
    3 IV barbiturate
    4 IV nonbarbiturate

23. Which of the following might indicate a local anesthetic overdose?
    1 Hypertension
    2 Bradycardia
    3 Tachycardia
    4 Alkalosis

24. Which anesthetic agent would require cautious use or be contraindicated in patients with acute alcohol intoxication?
    1 Fentanyl
    2 Enflurane
    3 Midazolam
    4 Thiopental sodium

25. Which of the following agents is known as the dissociative anesthetic?
    1 Propofol
    2 Droperidol
    3 Fentanyl
    4 Ketamine

Section F

26. Which of the following is the drug of choice for mild-to-moderate depression?
    1 Lithium
    2 An MAOI
    3 A cyclic depressant
    4 An SSRI

27. Short-acting benzodiazepines are preferred for elderly patients because of which of the following characteristics?
    1 Benzodiazepines improve visual ability.
    2 Benzodiazepines are less apt to accumulate in the body.
    3 Benzodiazepines promote more wakeful hours of the day.
    4 Benzodiazepines cause less GI disturbances.

28. Which of the following represents the maximal therapeutic level for lithium?
    1 0.6 mEq/L
    2 1.2 mEq/L
    3 1.5 mEq/L
    4 2.0 mEq/L

29. Buspirone should not be given concurrently with MAOIs because of which of the following possible complications?
    1 Insomnia
    2 Hypotension
    3 Hypertension
    4 Suicidal tendencies

30. Buspirone should be tapered gradually on discontinuation of therapy to avoid which of the following complications?
    1 Seizures
    2 Laryngospasms
    3 Agranulocytosis
    4 Excessive bleeding

CHAPTER 3

1. Which of the following is an adverse effect of heparin?
    1 Central nervous system depression
    2 Increased seizure activity
    3 Thrombocytopenia
    4 Lens opacity

2. Which of the following is an adverse effect of thrombolytics?
    1 Central nervous system depression
    2 Increased seizure activity
    3 Leukocytopenia
    4 Bleeding

3. Alteplase recombinant is approved as a thrombolytic for which of the following conditions?
    1 Viral gastroenteritis
    2 TIAs
    3 Thrombotic stroke
    4 Angina

4. Which of the following is a symptom of salicylate overdose?
    1 Tinnitus
    2 Bruising
    3 Nausea
    4 Bradycardia

5. Which of the following is a therapeutic PTT value during heparin therapy?
    1 Half of normal
    2 Equal to normal
    3 $1^{1}/_{2}$ to 2 times of normal
    4 3 to $3^{1}/_{2}$ times of normal

CHAPTER 4

Section A

1. The nurse should monitor the patient for adverse effects of ACE inhibitors, including which of the following?
    1 Seizures
    2 Hemorrhage
    3 Dysrhythmias
    4 First-dose phenomenon

2. When initiating angiotensin II inhibitor therapy, maximal BP reduction can usually be expected within which of the following time frames?
    1 24 hours
    2 3 to 4 days
    3 3 to 6 weeks
    4 2 months

3. α_1-Adrenergic blockers are associated most with which of the following characteristics?
    1 Reduction of diastolic pressure
    2 Reduction of systolic pressure
    3 Adverse effect of seizures
    4 Adverse effect of constipation

4. BBs are most associated with which of the following adverse effects?
    1 Tachycardia
    2 Bronchospasm
    3 Hyperglycemia
    4 Constipation

5. Which of the following adrenergic responses to CCBs is considered as normal?
    1 Reflex vasoconstriction
    2 Reflex vasodilation
    3 Risk of hyperactivity
    4 Increased bone density

Section B

6. Initial detection of which of the following adverse effects indicates rhabdomyolysis?
   1 Tinnitus
   2 Muscle pain
   3 Palpitations
   4 Photosensitivity

7. When rhabdomyolysis is suspected, what further laboratory test should be evaluated?
   1 Red blood cell count
   2 CK level
   3 White blood cell count
   4 PT time assessment

8. Antilipidemics are contraindicated or used with caution in patients with which of the following disorders?
   1 Seizures
   2 Depression
   3 Hypertension
   4 Renal and liver dysfunction

9. Which of the following assumption can be made when giving HMG-CoA reductase inhibitors and bile acid sequestrants combination therapy?
   1 They may be given at the same time.
   2 They must both be given early in the morning.
   3 Bile acid sequestrants should be taken without fluids.
   4 The HMG-CoA reductase inhibitor should be given at least 2 hours after the bile acid sequestrant.

10. Which of the following agents is unlikely to increase the risk of bleeding?
    1 Niacin
    2 Bile acid sequestrants
    3 HMG-CoA reductase inhibitor
    4 Fibric acid derivative

CHAPTER 5

Section A

1. Which of the following drugs would be most beneficial for immediate relief of an acute anginal attack?
   1 Verapamil
   2 Propranolol
   3 Sublingual nitroglycerin
   4 Sustained-released isosorbide mononitrate

2. Which of the following antianginal adverse effects is most closely related to vasodilation?
   1 Dizziness
   2 Depression
   3 Bradycardia
   4 Hypoglycemia

3. Which of the following is the normal therapeutic range of digoxin?
   1 0.8 to 2.0 ng/ml
   2 0.6 to 3.5 ng/ml
   3 3.5 to 5.0 ng/ml
   4 3.0 to 8.0 ng/ml

4. Phosphodiesterase inhibitors cause which of the following events?
   1 Decreased contractility
   2 Increased PVR
   3 Increased PCWP
   4 Increased CO

5. When teaching the patient the proper way to take sublingual nitroglycerin tablets in an acute anginal attack, the nurse instructs the patient to place one tablet under the tongue. If the pain in unrelieved, then this procedure may be repeated. The patient should notify the health care provider when the chest pain continues after how many tablets?
   1 One
   2 Two
   3 Three
   4 Four

Section B

6. A class IA antiarrhythmic may cause torsades de pointes under which of the following circumstances?
   1 When it is taken with food
   2 When it is taken with verapamil
   3 When its serum level becomes toxic
   4 When its serum level is below therapeutic level

7. Which of the following drugs, when taken with flecainide, causes an increased risk of dysrhythmias?
   1 Digoxin
   2 Lidocaine
   3 Warfarin
   4 CCBs

8. Which agent may cause hypotension in a patient who is taking a class II antiarrhythmic?
   1 Dopamine
   2 Alcohol
   3 Dobutamine
   4 Norepinephrine

9. Which of the following adverse effect may occur during or after administering adenosine?
   1 Torsades de pointes
   2 Atrial tachycardia
   3 Chest pain
   4 Ventricular tachycardia

10. The nurse should discontinue isoproterenol and notify the health care provider immediately when the patient develops which of the following complications?
    1 Bradycardia
    2 Chest pain
    3 A heart rate of 90 beats per minute
    4 A systolic BP of 130 mm Hg

CHAPTER 6

Section A

1. Which of the following drugs is an example of an opioid antitussive?
   1 Pseudoephedrine (Sudafed)
   2 Naphazoline (Allerest)
   3 Hydrocodone (Vicodin)
   4 Benzonatate (Tessalon)

2. OTC combination preparations commonly contain which of the following substances?
   1 Acetylcysteine (Mucomyst)
   2 Guaifenesin (Robitussin)
   3 Codeine
   4 Hydrocodone (Vicodin)

3. Dextromethorphan, when given concurrently with MAOIs, may cause which of the following adverse effects?
   1 Drowsiness and lethargy
   2 Excitation and hyperpyrexia
   3 Hypertension and nausea
   4 An anesthetic effect and choking

4. Which of the following drugs is the antidote for an opioid overdose?
   1 Acetylcysteine (Mucomyst)
   2 Diphenhydramine (Benadryl)
   3 Naloxone (Narcan)
   4 Acetaminophen (Tylenol)

5. Rebound congestion may result from nasal decongestants that are used longer than which of the following time frames?
   1 That which is less than prescribed
   2 24 hours
   3 1 to 2 days
   4 3 to 5 days

Section B

6. Which of the following classifications of antihistamines is referred to as nonsedating?
   1 Alkylamines
   2 Ethylenediamines
   3 Phenothiazines
   4 Piperazines

7. Before skin test procedures for allergy, antihistamines should be discontinued at least how many days before administration to avoid false results?
   1 1
   2 2
   3 4
   4 10

8. Concurrent use of MAOIs with H_1-receptor antagonists (ethanolamines) may prolong or increase which of the following type of effects of antihistamines?
   1 Emetic
   2 Anticholinergic
   3 Antiemetic
   4 Hypnotic

9. Because of the life-threatening adverse effects present with overdose, recommendations are that children should not be given which of the following medications?
   1 Sustained-release tripelennamine (PBZ-SR)
   2 Oral brompheniramine (Dimetane)
   3 Oral diphenhydramine (Benadryl)
   4 Rectal promethazine (Phenergan)

10. Most H_1-receptor antagonists are contraindicated in patients with which of the following conditions?
    1 Anxiety disorders
    2 Narrow-angle glaucoma
    3 Skin infections
    4 Elevated temperature

Section C

11. Which of the following actions decreases the edema and mucus production of the airways as part of the action of inhaled corticosteroids?
    1 Inhibiting protein synthesis
    2 Blocking α-adrenergic receptors
    3 Inhibiting the inflammatory response
    4 Blocking the opiate receptors

12. Excessive use of corticosteroids may cause which of the following results?
    1 Adrenal insufficiency
    2 Status asthmaticus
    3 Sudden death
    4 Vaginal bleeding

13. Montelukast is classified as which of the following?
    1 β-Agonist
    2 Corticosteroid
    3 Leukotriene antagonist
    4 Xanthine derivative

14. Which of the following drugs is a long-acting β-agonist?
    1 Bitolterol
    2 Metaproterenol
    3 Salmeterol
    4 Terbutaline

15. Which of the following is considered as the therapeutic level of theophylline?
    1 0 to 5 µg/ml
    2 5 to 10 µg/ml
    3 10 to 20 µg/ml
    4 25 to 30 µg/ml

CHAPTER 7

Section A

1. A health care provider would evaluate that desmopressin therapy has been effective when which of the following findings is noted during reassessment?
    1 Increased pulse rate
    2 Increased blood glucose
    3 Decreased urinary output
    4 Decreased blood pressure

2. A health care provider who is preparing to administer corticotropin would obtain which of the following pieces of equipment?
    1 Syringe
    2 Glass measuring device
    3 Plastic medicine cup
    4 Medicine dropper

3. A patient is receiving glucocorticosteroid replacement therapy. How should the health care provider administer the total daily dose?
    1 The entire dose is given in the morning.
    2 The entire dose is given in the late afternoon.
    3 One third of the dose is given in the early morning and two thirds is given in the late afternoon.
    4 Two thirds of the dose is given in the early morning and one third is given in the late afternoon.

4. The objective of drug therapy for patients with adrenal insufficiency has been met when mineralocorticoids accomplish which of the following results?
    1 Decreased cardiac output
    2 Decreased adrenal steroids
    3 Maintained fluid and electrolyte balance
    4 Counteracted destructive activities of the immune system

5. A patient who is taking an adrenal inhibiting drug should have which of the following monitored to determine drug efficacy?
    1 CBC
    2 Blood chemistries
    3 24-hour urine samples
    4 Routine urinalysis tests

Section B

6. Which of the following actions are representative of antithyroid drugs?
   1 Decreases production or release of thyroid hormone
   2 Increases release of parathyroid hormone
   3 Increases production and release of thyroid hormone
   4 Decreases the release of parathyroid hormone

7. Iodine solutions may cause which of the following effects?
   1 Yellow eyes
   2 Staining of teeth
   3 Loss of teeth
   4 Gray hair

8. When should propylthiouracil be given?
   1 Only at bedtime
   2 Only as a single dose
   3 Every 2 hours
   4 In divided doses around the clock

9. Which of the following are possible actions of thyroid hormones?
   1 Decreases the potency of oral anticoagulants
   2 Increases the effectiveness of digitalis
   3 Increases the potency of oral anticoagulants
   4 Acts as antiinflammatories

10. Hypercalcemic agents will reduce calcium levels for patients with all but which of the following conditions?
    1 Hyperparathyroidism
    2 Malignancies
    3 Adrenal disorders
    4 GI disorders

Section C

11. When the patient is scheduled for radiologic studies during which iodinated dye is administered, for what length of time should metformin be held (not given)?
    1 24 hours before and after the test
    2 36 hours before and after the test
    3 48 hours before and after the test
    4 2 weeks after the test

12. Which of the following is an action of thiazolidinediones?
    1 Increases the effects of circulating insulin
    2 Stimulates the production of insulin
    3 Increases the production of glucose by the liver
    4 Decreases the uptake of insulin by the skeletal muscles

13. When does the onset of ultra rapid-acting insulin (Lispro) occur?
    1 Less than 15 minutes
    2 30 to 60 minutes
    3 1 to 2 hours
    4 4 to 8 hours

14. When a patient with diabetes is being treated with a sulfonylurea and uses alcohol, the nurse knows to monitor for which of the following reactions?
    1 Bradycardic episode
    2 Hyperglycemic reaction
    3 Disulfiramlike reaction
    4 Edema

15. α-Glucosidases (acarbose and miglitol) are contraindicated in patients with diabetes who have which of the following complications?
    1 Hypothyroidism
    2 Colon ulcers
    3 Severe acne
    4 Freckles

CHAPTER *8*

Section A

1. Misoprostol (Cytotec) is used in patients with gastric ulcers. Indications for use are ulcers caused by which of the following?
   1 Stress
   2 Excessive gastric acid production
   3 NSAIDs
   4 Helicobacter pylori

2. One of the undesirable drug actions of Misoprostol (Cytotec) causes which of the following conditions?
   1 Uterine contractions
   2 Blurred vision
   3 Dry mouth
   4 Tardive dyskinesia

3. The nurse assesses a patient who is taking metoclopramide (Reglan) after the nurse's aide notices "something different" about the patient. The nurse notices that the patient is grimacing and her tongue keeps protruding in a rhythmic, repetitive motion. The nurse recognizes this as a sign of which of the following?
   1 Parkinson's disease
   2 The prodrome phase of a seizure
   3 Pain
   4 Tardive dyskinesia

4. The drugs that are ordered for the new 79-year-old male patient include digoxin 0.25 mg po qid, norfloxacin 400 mg po bid, Dilantin 150 mg po bid, Maalox 2 tsps po qid, and Carafate 1 g po ac and hs. Assume that routine hospital medication administration times for qid are 9:00 AM, 1:00 PM, 5:00 PM, 9:00 PM, that antibiotics should be given to maintain a steady blood level, and meals are delivered at 7:00 AM, 12:00 PM, 5:00 PM. What times should you schedule the Carafate?
   1 6:00 AM, 11:00 AM, 4:00 PM, and 9:00 PM
   2 7:00 AM, 12:00 PM, 5:00 PM, and 9:00 PM
   3 9:00 AM, 1:00 PM, 5:00 PM, and 9:00 PM
   4 6:00 AM, 12:00 PM, 6:00 PM, and 12:00 AM

5. How should proton pump inhibitors be administered?
   1 Chewed
   2 Given before meals
   3 Given after meals
   4 Followed by two glasses of water

Section B

6. Extrapyramidal reactions are more common with metoclopramide when taken concurrently with which of the following drugs?
   1 Phenothiazines
   2 Antacids
   3 Antidysrhythmics
   4 Anticoagulants

7. Phenothiazines act as antiemetics in which of the following ways?
   1 Blocking dopamine receptors in the CTZ
   2 Increasing GI motility
   3 Inhibit vomiting center directly
   4 Blocking muscarinic receptors from the cholea

8. The serotonin antagonists, granisetron and ondansetron, are administered by which of the following routes?
   1 Per rectum
   2 Intrathecal
   3 Intravenous
   4 Subcutaneous

9. Granisetron is approved as an antiemetic for which of the following conditions?
   1 Viral gastroenteritis
   2 Radiologic enteral intubation
   3 Cancer chemotherapy nausea
   4 Preoperative and postoperative nausea

10. Absorption or overdose of ipecac syrup can produce which of the following effects?
    1 Cardiotoxicity
    2 Vertigo
    3 Tinnitus
    4 Dermatitis

Section C

11. Mr. M., a 56-year-old man, has a recent history of peptic ulcer and Helicobacter pylori. Which of the following medications might he be taking in combination with other drugs to treat his disease?
    1 Docusate (Surfak)
    2 Mineral oil
    3 Diphenoxylate with atropine
    4 Bismuth subsalicylate

12. Mrs. B., an 84-year-old woman, is admitted to your unit and is under your care. She has a history of six to eight watery stools per day for the last 3 days. What nursing assessment is most important for Mrs. B.?
    1 Her pain level
    2 Intake and output
    3 CBC and blood glucose
    4 Heart rate and rhythm

13. Mrs. B.'s health care provider orders diphenoxylate hydrochloride with atropine sulfate (Lomotil) to treat her diarrhea. While reviewing her current medication history, you notice that she is taking the MAOI tranylcypromine (Parnate). What drug interaction effect is possible with an MAOI and her antidiarrheal?
    1 It may exacerbate the effects of the MAOI.
    2 It may cause a hypertensive crisis.
    3 It may decrease the absorption of the MAOI.
    4 It may increase the risk of bleeding.

14. Mr. T., a 57-year-old man, has severe diarrhea and oral ulcers as a result of antibiotic use. What drug would most likely be ordered to treat his diarrhea?
    1 Lactobacillus acidophilus
    2 Polycarbophil (FiberCon)
    3 Deodorized opium tincture
    4 Loperamide (Imodium)

15. Which laxative is prone to decrease absorption of food and fat-soluble vitamins?
    1 Bisacodyl
    2 Mineral oil
    3 Psyllium
    4 Bismuth subsalicylate

CHAPTER 9

Section A

1. Adverse effects that can occur following nitrofurantoin (Macrodantin) administration include which of the following?
    1 Hemolytic anemia
    2 EPS
    3 Stevens-Johnson syndrome
    4 Pseudomembranous enterocolitis

2. Which of the following is a life-threatening adverse effect of ofloxacin (Floxin)?
    1 Urticaria
    2 Agranulocytosis
    3 Seizures
    4 Dystonia

3. Which of the following is an adverse effect of phenazopyridine (Pyridium)?
    1 CNS depression
    2 Increased seizure activity
    3 Orange-red urine
    4 Lens opacity

4. Oxybutynin (Ditropan) is contraindicated for which of the following conditions?
    1 Hypertension
    2 Dysphonia
    3 Paraplegia
    4 Bowel obstruction

5. Which of the following is an adverse effect of loop diuretics?
    1 Black stools
    2 Increased seizure activity
    3 Leukopenia
    4 Lens opacity

Section B

6. When the hematocrit level rises 5 points in 2 weeks for a patient who is taking epoetin alfa, which of the following is the nurse's best course of action?
    1 Continue to monitor hematocrit levels daily.
    2 Call the health care provider and expect a dose reduction.
    3 Change the frequency of monitoring the hematocrit to every month.
    4 Take no action because a rise in hematocrit is the expected action of this drug.

7. Which of the following is true about iron supplements?
    1 Iron tablets may be crushed.
    2 Antacids increase iron absorption.
    3 Liquid forms should be given undiluted for greater efficacy.
    4 Liquid forms may stain teeth when not taken with a straw.

8. Which of the following is a major adverse effect of calcitriol?
    1 Hypocalcemia
    2 Hypercalcemia
    3 Anemia
    4 Hypotension

9. Cation-exchange resins are used in which of the following conditions?
    1 Hypocalcemia
    2 Hypercalcemia
    3 Hypokalemia
    4 Hyperkalemia

10. Which of the following characteristics is true for systemic antacids?
    1 Systemic antacids are not absorbed well in the GI tract.
    2 Systemic antacids are considered as treatment for metabolic alkalosis.
    3 Systemic antacids are commonly found to decrease anorexiant effects when given concurrently.
    4 Systemic antacids are apt to lead to milk-alkali syndrome when given long-term.

CHAPTER *10*

Section A

1. A woman who is receiving estrogen therapy should be advised to see her health care provider immediately when she experiences which of the following conditions?
   1 Osteoporosis
   2 Water retention
   3 Shortness of breath
   4 Diarrhea

2. Which of the following is not a contraindication of estrogen replacement therapy?
   1 Pregnancy
   2 Breast cancer
   3 Vascular disease
   4 Osteoporosis

3. Which of the following does not release the steroid hormone progestin?
   1 Testes
   2 Ovary
   3 Adrenal cortex
   4 Bone

4. Which of the following medications reduces the effectiveness of oral contraceptives with estrogen and progestin?
   1 Rifampin
   2 Theophylline
   3 Digoxin
   4 Cyclosporin

5. Your patient wants to know how oral contraceptives with estrogen and progestin prevent pregnancy. Which of the following is the principal goal of this therapy?
   1 Blocks the passage of sperm
   2 Decreases progesterone levels
   3 Inhibits ovulation and implementation of the egg
   4 Decreases estrogen levels

Section B

6. The tocolytic magnesium sulfate is used to prevent which of the following complications of severe preeclampsia?
   1 Hypotension
   2 Seizures
   3 Depressed reflexes
   4 GI distress

7. How do tocolytic agents act on the reproductive system?
   1 Induce ovulation
   2 Maintain pregnancy
   3 Facilitate milk letdown
   4 Induce abortion

8. During oxytocic treatment, which of following is a serious adverse effect?
   1 Water intoxication
   2 Ovarian hyperstimulation
   3 Cephalopelvic disproportion
   4 Invasive cervical carcinoma

9. Which of the following statements about dinoprostone treatment is incorrect?
   1 They are administered intravaginally.
   2 They may cause bronchospasm and chest pain.
   3 They are contraindicated in patients with pelvic inflammatory disease.
   4 The nurse should remove the foil wrapper of the intravaginal suppository when it is chilled.

10. Which of the following statements about ergot alkaloid use during labor is correct?
    1 Large doses can lead to maternal and fetal trauma.
    2 Hypotension is a common adverse effect of ergot alkaloids.
    3 IV administration is the most common.
    4 Ergot alkaloids are the drugs of choice in patients with renal disease.

CHAPTER *11*

1. Which of the following is a type of NSAID?
   1 Oxicam
   2 Uricosuric
   3 Immunosuppressive
   4 Gold agent

2. Which of the following represents the action of an NSAID?
   1 Reduces serum urate levels
   2 Inhibits formation of prostaglandins
   3 Inhibits destructive lysosomal enzyme activity in joints
   4 Reduces xanthine oxidase enzyme production

3. The COX-2 form of cyclooxygenase is associated with the reduction of which of the following symptoms?
   1 Pain
   2 Fever
   3 Stomach distress
   4 Platelet aggregation

4. Which DMARD requires periodic eye examinations?
   1 Gold agents
   2 Methotrexate
   3 Etanercept
   4 Hyaluronic acid

5. The goal of antigout therapy is to maintain which of the following serum uric acid levels?
   1 2 mg/dl or below
   2 4 mg/dl or below
   3 6 mg/dl or below
   4 10 mg/dl or below

CHAPTER 12

1. Which of the following vitamins is essential for the synthesis of blood coagulation factors in the liver?
   1 Vitamin B
   2 Vitamin C
   3 Vitamin D
   4 Vitamin K

2. Vitamin C is used for the treatment or prevention of which of the following conditions?
   1 Thiamine deficiency
   2 Scurvy
   3 An overdose of anticoagulants
   4 Chapped or dry skin

3. Sodium is used in the treatment and prevention of which of the following conditions?
   1 Beriberi
   2 Scurvy
   3 Heat prostration
   4 Anemia

4. To evaluate the effectiveness of iron therapy, the nurse should monitor which of the following tests?
   1 Renal function studies
   2 Hepatic function studies
   3 Sodium and potassium levels
   4 Hemoglobin and reticulocyte levels

5. Which of the following is the best food source of vitamin B_9 (folic acid)?
   1 Fish
   2 Milk
   3 Asparagus
   4 Strawberries

CHAPTER 13

Section A

1. The health care provider would recommend which of the following products to a patient who complains of dry eyes?
   1 Naphazoline
   2 Polyvinyl alcohol
   3 Timolol
   4 Demecarium

2. The use of carbachol for a patient with glaucoma would have which of the following effects?
   1 Dilation of the iridic sphincter
   2 Increased outflow of aqueous humor
   3 Mydriasis
   4 Vasoconstriction of collecting channels

3. Which of the following adverse effects is most commonly associated with pilocarpine?
   1 Iridic cysts
   2 Eye irritation
   3 Lacrimal system obstruction
   4 Retinal detachment

4. The health care provider is teaching a parent the proper way to administer an ear medication to a child. Which of the following points is important to include in the teaching?
   1 Pull the pinna down and back.
   2 Pull the pinna up and back.
   3 Pull the pinna down and forward.
   4 Pull the pinna up and forward.

5. A patient who is learning to take an otic medication should be taught to do which of the following?
   1 Keep the cap to the solution loosely closed.
   2 Hold the medication in the hands to warm it.
   3 Administer an otic medication at cold temperatures.
   4 Warm the medication in a microwave oven before use.

Section B

6. Which of the following is an agent that prevents bacterial growth, thereby helping to heal burned tissue?
   1. Silver sulfadiazine
   2. Antipruritic
   3. Tetracycline
   4. Keratolytic

7. Which of the following is not a primary function of the skin?
   1. Protection
   2. Support colonization of bacteria
   3. Immune responsiveness
   4. Thermoregulation

8. Which of the following is inappropriate when applying silver sulfadiazine to a burned area of skin?
   1. Cover the burned area with airtight dressing.
   2. Keep the burned area covered with medication at all times.
   3. Apply the medication in a thin layer over the burned area.
   4. Use a sterile technique when applying the medication.

9. Which of the following about crotamiton, an antipruritic dermatologic medication, is correct?
   1. It should be administered using a sterile technique.
   2. It should be gently massaged into the affected area.
   3. When an antipruritic comes into contact with the eyes, immediately close eyes and bandage for 2 hours.
   4. When given for endoscope insertion, the patient may eat immediately after the procedure.

10. Silver sulfadiazine is associated with which of the following adverse effects?
    1. Discoloration of skin
    2. Peeling of skin layers
    3. Elevated blood glucose
    4. Requires previous pregnancy test

CHAPTER *14*

1. Which of the following migraine preparations has increased GI absorption?
   1. Dihydroergotamine
   2. Ergotamine tartrate
   3. Ergotamine tartrate with caffeine
   4. Methysergide maleate

2. Which of the following adverse effects are the most common for ergot derivatives?
   1. Vomiting and diarrhea
   2. Tachycardia or bradycardia
   3. Itching and rebound headache
   4. Nausea and cold fingers and toes

3. The onset of action for intranasal dihydroergotamine occurs within which of the following time frames?
   1. 5 minutes
   2. 30 minutes
   3. 2 hours
   4. 4 hours

4. Which opiate is responsible for producing toxic metabolites?
   1. Codeine sulfate
   2. Fentanyl
   3. Meperidine
   4. Oxycodone

5. Which adverse effect of opiates is the most serious?
   1. Dilated pupils
   2. Seizures
   3. Orthostatic hypotension
   4. Respiratory depression

NCLEX CHAPTER *1* ANSWERS

Section A

1. 3 Bacteria may develop a protective mechanism and become resistant to natural penicillins. The spectrum of action is wider with extended-spectrum penicillins compared with any other penicillin. Penicillinase-resistant penicillins have a structure that was developed to resist splitting of the beta-lactam ring. Aminopenicillins have an amino group that is attached to the penicillin nucleus, which increases the action against gram-negative bacteria.

2. 4 Bacteriocidal indicates that the antibiotic inhibits enzymes that are required for bacterial cell wall maintenance, thus they kill bacteria. Narrow- or wide-spectrum action refers to the antibiotic's effectiveness against a variety of microorganisms. Bacteriostatic means that these antibiotics inhibit the formation and growth of new bacteria thus keeping bacteria in check but not killing them.

3.2 When taking sulfonamides, the patient should drink 2 L of fluid per day to prevent crystalluria and resultant renal damage. Therefore limiting fluid intake is incorrect. Taking the drug with orange juice is incorrect because sulfonamides should preferably be taken on an empty stomach. The patient need not lie down after the initial dose.

4.2 Aminoglycosides are known to cause ototoxicity as an adverse effect; the nurse should monitor for this effect. Penicillins, sulfonamides, aztreonam, and imipenem-cilastatin may lead to seizures but not aminoglycosides. Sulfonamides, tetracyclines, and fluoroquinolones may lead to photosensitivity but not aminoglycosides. Tetracyclines may lead to teeth discoloration but not aminoglycosides.

5.4 Fluoroquinolones are contraindicated in women during pregnancy, as are tetracyclines, sulfonamides, aztreonam, clindamycin, vancomycin, and imipenem-cilastatin. Penicillins, macrolides, and aminoglycosides should be used cautiously during pregnancy.

Section B

6.3 AZT is currently used only in the treatment of HIV infections. AZT must be converted to the nucleotide form to express antiviral activity, is incorporated into growing viral but not mammalian nuclear DNA, and is toxic to bone marrow and causes adverse hematologic effects.

7.4 Retroviruses contain reverse transcriptase and tumor viruses, which induce tumors (e.g., sarcomas, leukemias, lymphomas). Reverse transcriptase is essential for the production of a DNA molecule from RNA. Retroviruses do not contain fungi, but rather, DNA only or RNA only.

8.4 Protease inhibitors should be taken with water, milk, or chocolate milk. Protease inhibitors should not be mixed with acidic juices or wine or taken with meals.

9.2 A principle of retroviral therapy is to initiate treatment before immunodeficiency is evident. NRTIs have greater effectiveness in HIV and AIDS treatment when used in combination with at least three drugs. A drug should not be discontinued when plasma viral loads decrease. Antivirals inhibit single steps in the viral replication cycle.

10.4 The first-line antifungal drug for systemic use is amphotericin B. Nystatin has little systemic effect. Clotrimazole is used topically for skin and Candida albicans infections. Oxiconazole is used for cutaneous candidiasis.

Section C

11.1 Oprelvekin is a thrombopoietic growth factor that stimulates platelet production. Erythropoietin stimulates red blood cell production. An immunosuppressant suppresses the body's natural response to an antigen. Filgrastim (Neupogen) is a colony-stimulating factor that regulates the production of neutrophils.

12.3 Interleukin therapy should continue until the postnadir platelet count is greater than 50,000 cells/μl. The desirable dATP trough level is 0.005 to 0.015 μmol/ml. The desirable ADA trough level is 15 to 35 μmol/ml. Interleukin therapy should not continue if the postnadir count is at 500,000 cells/mm.

13.3 Interferon alfa-2a is an immunomodulator that exerts antitumor activity. Cyclosporine is an immunosuppressant that prevents rejection of transplanted organs. Interleukin-11 is a thrombopoietic growth factor that stimulates platelet production. Sargramostim is a colony-stimulating factor that restores red bone marrow after transplantation.

14.3 Immunosuppressants, cyclosporine, and Imuran prevent rejection of organ transplantation. Erythropoietin is a colony-stimulating factor that stimulates red blood count production. Interferon alfa-2a is an immunomodulator that treats leukemia and Kaposi's sarcoma. Interleukin-1 or interleukin-2 treats melanoma or renal cell cancer.

15.4 Cyclosporine should be mixed with milk, chocolate milk, and apple or orange juice for oral administration. Cyclosporine is given orally or, when not tolerated, IV but never IM. Cyclosporine must be given in a glass container. Cyclosporine may adhere to a plastic container, which reduces the dose. Styrofoam is also porous and may absorb the drug. Grapefruit juice affects cyclosporine metabolism.

Section D

16.3 Chemotherapy doses are based on body surface area, which is calculated based on height and weight. Chemotherapy doses should not be based on ideal body weight, mg/kg of body weight, or actual weight.

17.4 Special precautions must be taken when preparing chemotherapy drugs because these agents are irritating to the skin, are liable to cause hypersensitivity reactions, and are biohazardous. Chemotherapy drugs may cause GI tract irritability and vomiting, but this reaction is not the reason for which these agents are administered with special precautions. Chemotherapy drugs are not acidic.

18. 1   Cytotoxic drugs tend to exert their effect on rapidly growing cells. These drugs do not exert their effect on cells that have poor oxygen or blood supply or on cells with a long doubling time.

19. 2   Patients with a low white blood cell count experience delayed wound healing because white blood cells (leukocytes) are involved in the inflammatory response to injury and aid in tissue repair. Acidosis is associated with a low red blood cell count. Viscosity of blood is related more to a high red blood cell count. Bleeding times are associated more with platelets, which affect blood coagulation and hemostasis.

20. 2   Methotrexate is not a vesicant. Vincristine, vinblastine, and melphalan are vesicants.

NCLEX CHAPTER *2* ANSWERS

Section A

1. 3   Albuterol, an adrenergic that stimulates β-receptors (primarily β_2-receptors), has adverse effects of tachycardia and hypertension. α-Agonists, not β-agonists, cause pupil dilation. Capillary refill, heart sounds, bowel sounds, and skin color are unrelated to β_2-adrenergic agonists.

2. 2 α-Adrenergic antagonists cause pupil constriction (miosis) and increased GI motility. Mydriasis and decrease gastric motility are opposite effects. α-Adrenergic antagonists cause vasodilation and decreased blood pressure. Hemorrhage is unrelated to α-adrenergic antagonists.

3. 2   When β-adrenergic antagonists are given concurrently with drugs that have similar effects, such as calcium channel blockers, adverse effects of decreased pulse and blood pressure are increased. Hypertension and tachycardia are opposite of β-adrenergic antagonist effects.

4. 2   Because β-adrenergic antagonists cause bronchoconstriction and possible bronchospasms, these agents are contraindicated until the patient is ruled out of any diagnosis of asthma or emphysema. The nurse should therefore hold the drug and notify the health care provider. Administering the drug now, an hour later, or at the next dose time is contraindicated.

5. 1   A β-adrenergic antagonist should not be administered to a patient with bilateral wheezing because these agents could exacerbate the problem that results from bronchoconstriction and bronchospasm. These agents also decrease pulse and blood pressure.

Section B

6. 4   A cholinergic (which stimulates muscarinic glandular secretions; stimulates receptors in the heart, CNS, and smooth muscles of organs; and excites nicotinic responses) requires a drug that produces the opposite for an antidote. Atropine is the antidote for cholinergic overdose because it blocks muscarinic responses with an antisecretory action and blocks vagal impulses to the heart. Procainamide and lidocaine are incorrect because these drugs are antiarrhythmics. Artane is used as a treatment of Parkinson's disease and extrapyramidal disorders. Procainamide, lidocaine, and Artane do not block muscarinic responses.

7. 1   When the edrophonium (Tensilon) test is performed and the patient's skeletal muscle weakness improves, the patient is experiencing a myasthenic crisis from underdosing of a cholinesterase inhibitor. When the patient's condition worsens, the patient is experiencing a cholinergic crisis from overdosing or receiving excessive pyridostigmine.

8. 3   MAOIs may precipitate a hypertensive crisis when taken with a dopaminergic. When a dopaminergic is given with methyldopa, the risk of toxic effects in the CNS is increased. When combined with tricyclic antidepressants, postural hypotension may occur. Alcohol exacerbates CNS depression, not a hypertensive crisis, when given with a dopaminergic.

9. 1   Opioids may cause life-threatening reactions when taken with selegiline. Bromocriptine, amantadine, and ropinirole have no drug interaction with opioids.

10. 1   Ambenonium and pyridostigmine are used as maintenance therapy for myasthenia gravis. Edrophonium and neostigmine are used for diagnosing myasthenia gravis and for differentiating between myasthenic and cholinergic crisis. Donepezil and rivastigmine are used to improve memory in patients with Alzheimer's disease.

Section C

11. 4   Ritalin is primarily used in children for ADHD therapy. Anorexiants are used to treat obesity. Ritalin should be given early in the day, no later than 6 hours before bedtime, not at bedtime. The long-term effects of Ritalin are unknown.

12. 2   Anorexiants should be administered midmorning or midafternoon, depending on the patient's eating habits. Anorexiants should be given on an empty stomach, approximately 30 to 60 minutes before meals and no later than 6 hours before bedtime.

13. 2   Ritalin contains no caffeine. Caffeine is found in many beverages, such as coffee, tea, cola, and chocolate. Caffeine is also an ingredient in many OTC headache medications (e.g., Anacin, Excedrin).

14.4 Baclofen is a centrally acting muscle relaxant that is used primarily to treat muscle spasms. Leg cramps are treated by quinine, a peripherally acting muscle relaxant. Ritalin is used to treat hyperactivity. A psychomotor stimulant treats narcolepsy.

15.4 Liver function studies should be monitored when administering peripherally acting muscle relaxants for early detection of hepatotoxicity. Peripherally acting muscle relaxants do not affect sodium, phenytoin, and potassium levels.

Section D

16.1 Hydantoins are associated with the peculiar adverse effects of nystagmus and gingival hyperplasia. Phenobarbital and lorazepam do not cause these adverse effects. Carbamazepine may cause nystagmus but not slurred speech, enlargement of facial features, or gingival hyperplasia.

17.2 Older patients commonly develop the adverse effects of depression, confusion, and the paradoxic effect of excitement when taking barbiturates. Barbiturates lead to hypotension but not hypertension and excitement but not lethargy. Although barbiturates can cause thrombocytopenia, gingival hyperplasia is not an adverse effect.

18.3 Benzodiazepines are associated with toxicity, ranging from short-term memory, confusion, and vertigo to bradycardia, ataxia, severe weakness, shortness of breath, and depression. Antacids delay absorption of benzodiazepines. A reduced, not increased, tolerance for alcohol occurs when taking benzodiazepines. Benzodiazepines lead to CNS-depressing effects.

19.1 Ethosuximide is associated with causing the adverse effect of SLE. Lorazepam, phenytoin, and valproic acid are not associated with these adverse effects.

20.2 Diazepam is the drug of choice in treating status epilepticus. Phenytoin and valproic acid are not used for the treatment of status epilepticus. Phenobarbital may be used to control status epilepticus, but it is not the drug of choice.

Section E

21.1 Procaine is contraindicated for the patient who has heart block. Common uses of procaine include infiltration anesthesia in spinal and peripheral nerve block. Procaine may be given to older adults when caution is taken.

22.1 Regional anesthetic agents are least likely to cause laryngospasm. Inhalation, IV barbiturate, and IV nonbarbiturate anesthetics are all likely to cause laryngospasm as an adverse effect.

23.2 Bradycardia is an indication of local anesthetic overdose, not tachycardia. Other indications of local anesthetic overdose include hypotension, not hypertension, and acidosis, not alkalosis.

24.3 Midazolam is contraindicated in patients with acute alcohol intoxication. Fentanyl, enflurane, and thiopental sodium do not require cautious use nor are they contraindicated in patients with acute alcohol intoxication.

25.4 Ketamine is known as the dissociative anesthetic by blocking consciousness of body sensation. Propofol, droperidol, and fentanyl are not known as dissociative anesthetics.

Section F

26.1 Lithium is the drug of choice for mild-to-moderate depression. MAOIs, cyclic depressants, and SSRIs are not the drugs of choice.

27.2 Short-acting benzodiazepines are preferred for elderly patients because these agents are less likely to accumulate in the body. Benzodiazepines do not improve visual ability. Benzodiazepines lead to insomnia, not wakeful hours. Benzodiazepines do not cause fewer GI disturbances.

28.4 The maximal therapeutic level for lithium is 2.0 mEq/L. Levels of 0.6 mEq/L, 1.2 mEq/L, and 1.5 mEq/L are too low.

29.3 Buspirone should not be given within 14 days of MAOIs to avoid a lethal elevation in blood pressure or hypertensive crisis. Combining buspirone and MAOIs does not lead to insomnia, hypotension, or suicidal tendencies.

30.1 Buspirone should be tapered gradually on discontinuation of therapy to avoid seizures. Laryngospasms, agranulocytosis, and excessive bleeding are not reasons to taper buspirone gradually.

NCLEX CHAPTER 3 ANSWERS

1.3 Heparin may cause an adverse effect of thrombocytopenia. Central nervous system depression, seizures, and lens opacity are not adverse effects of heparin.

2.4 Thrombolytics may cause bleeding as an adverse effect. Central nervous system depression, seizures, and leukocytopenia are not adverse effects of thrombolytics.

3.3 tPA is approved for use in thrombotic stroke because it breaks down an existing thrombus. No thrombus exists in viral gastroenteritis, TIAs, or angina.

4.1 Tinnitus is the most common symptom of salicylate overdose. Bruising and nausea are adverse effects of aspirin but not of aspirin overdose. Bradycardia is not an adverse effect of aspirin.

5.3 The therapeutic PTT value for the patient on heparin therapy is $1^{1}/2$ to 2 times the normal PTT. Half of or equal to the normal PTT value is too low to be therapeutic, and 3 to $3^{1}/2$ times the normal PTT value is too high to be therapeutic.

NCLEX CHAPTER *4* ANSWERS

Section A

1.4 After initiation of ACE therapy or a rapid increase in doses, the first-dose phenomenon with severe hypotension and fainting is common. Seizures, hemorrhage, and dysrhythmias are not adverse effects of ACE inhibitors.

2.3 Maximal BP reduction following angiotensin II inhibitors occurs in 3 to 6 weeks. The time frames of 24 hours and 3 to 4 days are insufficient to gauge BP reduction. Two months is well past the optimal time to record maximal BP reduction.

3.1 α_1-Adrenergic blockers are more effective in reducing diastolic BP, not systolic BP. Seizures and constipation are not adverse effects of α_1-adrenergic blockers. Diarrhea is an adverse effect.

4.2 BBs are associated most with bronchospasm. Tachycardia is incorrect because BBs usually cause bradycardia. Hyperglycemia is incorrect because BBs may lead to hypoglycemia. BBs usually lead to diarrhea but not constipation.

5.1 The normal adrenergic response to CCBs is reflex vasoconstriction. In the older adult patient with diminished reflexes, this protective vasoconstriction is decreased and occasionally leads to excessive hypotension. Reflex vasodilation is incorrect because the effect is directly opposite. Hyperactivity is incorrect because CCBs usually cause weakness. CCBs do not increase bone density.

Section B

6.2 Rhabdomyolysis is a fatal disease that causes acute destruction of skeletal muscle. Initial evidence includes muscle pain. Tinnitus, palpitations, and photosensitivity are adverse effects but are not evidence of rhabdomyolysis.

7.2 Rhabdomyolysis may be accompanied by renal damage and is associated with elevated CK levels. Rhabdomyolysis are not associated with elevated red or white blood cell counts or elevated PT time.

8.4 Antilipidemics are contraindicated or used with caution in patients with renal and liver dysfunction. Antilipidemics are not contraindicated or to be used cautiously for patients with seizures, depression, or hypertension.

9.4 When HMG-CoA reductase inhibitors and bile acid sequestrants are given together, HMG-CoA reductase inhibitors should be given at least 2 hours after the bile acid sequestrant, thus they may not be given at the same time. HMG-CoA reductase inhibitors should not be given early in the morning because they are more effective when taken in the evening because cholesterol is synthesized mostly at night. Bile acid sequestrants may be taken without regard to meals.

10.4 Fibric acid derivatives do not increase the chance of bleeding. An increased risk of bleeding occurs when giving fibric acid derivatives, bile acid sequestrants, and HMG-CoA reductase inhibitors. Niacin may lead to hypoprothrombinemia, bile acid sequestrants may increase prothrombin time and GI bleeding, and HMG-CoA reductase inhibitors may cause nosebleeds and thrombocytopenia.

NCLEX CHAPTER *5* ANSWERS

Section A

1.3 Sublingual nitroglycerin is the drug of choice in an acute anginal attack because of the rapid onset of action. Verapamil is incorrect because CCBs are not used in the immediate relief of angina attacks nor to prevent expected attacks. Propranolol, a BB, is used in long-term prevention of angina, not for immediate relief of acute angina. Sustained-release isosorbide mononitrate is a drug that provides coverage in a time-released manner, not immediately.

2.1 The adverse effect that is most closely related to vasodilation is dizziness. When vessels dilate, flushing, headache, dizziness, fainting, weakness, tachycardia, and orthostatic hypotension are expected. Depression, bradycardia, and hypoglycemia are not expected.

3.1 The normal therapeutic range of digoxin is 0.8 to 2.0 ng/ml. All of the remaining options (0.6 to 3.5 ng/ml, 3.5 to 5.0 ng/ml, and 3.0 to 8.0 ng/ml) are excessive therapeutic ranges for digoxin.

4.4 Phosphodiesterase inhibitors exert an inotropic effect on the heart, which causes increased myocardial contractility and CO. Decreased contractility is incorrect. Increased PVR is incorrect because phosphodiesterase inhibitors dilate arteries and veins, thereby decreasing PVR. PCWP is decreased, not increased, by phosphodiesterase inhibitors.

5.3 The nurse should teach the patient the proper way to relieve an acute anginal attack by taking sublingual or buccal nitroglycerin tablets according to established protocol. The dose may be repeated twice at 5-minute intervals if chest pain is unrelieved. When pain persists after three nitrates, the health care provider should be notified.

Section B

6.4 Class IA antiarrhythmics may cause torsades de pointes when its serum level is subtherapeutic, not at a toxic level. Class IA antiarrhythmics are poorly absorbed with food and should be taken on an empty stomach. Class IAs should not be given with verapamil. Giving class IAs and verapamil together may cause excess prolonging of conduction time and decreased CO.

7.4 An increased risk of dysrhythmias occurs when flecainide is taken together with a CCB. Digoxin levels are increased by flecainide when taken with a class IC antiarrhythmic. Lidocaine and warfarin have no drug interaction with flecainide.

8.2 Alcohol, nitrates, and antihypertensives may cause hypotension when taken together with a class II antiarrhythmic. Dopamine, dobutamine, and norepinephrine increase BP.

9.3 An adverse effect of adenosine that may occur during or after administration is 3 to 6 seconds of asystole, which leads to ischemia and chest pain. Torsades de pointes may occur when a class IA antiarrhythmic level is subtherapeutic. Tachycardia does not occur with class IA antiarrhythmics.

10.2 When the patient develops chest pain while receiving isoproterenol, the nurse should discontinue the drug and notify the health care provider immediately. Isoproterenol can trigger ventricular dysrhythmias, hypotension, and tachycardia. Therefore bradycardia, a pulse of 90 beats per minute, and a systolic BP of 130 mm Hg are incorrect.

NCLEX CHAPTER *6* ANSWERS

Section A

1.3 Hydrocodone is an opioid antitussive. Pseudoephedrine and naphazoline are decongestants. Benzonatate is a nonopioid antitussive.

2.2 Guaifenesin is commonly found in OTC cold preparations. Acetylcysteine requires a prescription. Codeine and hydrocodone are controlled substances that also require a prescription.

3.2 Excitation and hyperpyrexia may occur when dextromethorphan is given concurrently with an MAOI. Drowsiness, lethargy, hypertension, and nausea are not adverse effects of dextromethorphan. An anesthetic effect and choking are adverse effects of benzonatate.

4.3 Naloxone is the antidote for an opioid overdose. Acetylcysteine is the antidote for acetaminophen, not opioid overdose. Diphenhydramine and acetaminophen are not antidotes.

5.4 Rebound congestion may result from nasal decongestants that are used longer than 3 to 5 days. Rebound congestion occurs with the overuse or abuse of nasal decongestants, not with the short-term use. Therefore taking less than prescribed, taking the medication for 24 hours, or taking for 1 to 2 days do cause rebound congestion.

Section B

6.4 The second-generation antihistamines produce low to no CNS adverse effects of sedation, do not cross the blood-brain barrier, and are called nonsedating. Piperazines are second-generation antihistamines. The most common adverse effect of alkylamines is drowsiness. Ethylenediamines and phenothiazines are first-generation antihistamines.

7.3 Antihistamines should be discontinued at least 4 days before skin testing to avoid false results. Discontinuing antihistamines 1 day, 2 days, or 10 days before skin testing is inappropriate.

8.2 Use of MAOIs together with H_1-receptor antagonists may prolong or intensify anticholinergic effects because MAOIs interfere with the detoxification of antihistamines and phenothiazines. Taking MAOIs with H_1-receptor antagonists does not cause emetic, antiemetic, or hypnotic effects.

9.1 The sustained-release form of tripelennamine is not recommended for use in children because overdose may cause hallucinations, convulsions, coma, and cardiovascular collapse. Brompheniramine and diphenhydramine are incorrect because they are not contraindicated in children. Promethazine is contraindicated only in acutely ill, dehydrated children.

10.2 Most ethanolamines (H_1-receptor antagonists) are contraindicated in patients with narrow-angle glaucoma. Antihistamines, particularly ethanolamines, are contraindicated in patients with anxiety disorders, skin infections, or an elevated temperature.

Section C

11.3 Inhaled corticosteroids inhibit the inflammatory process, thereby decreasing edema and mucus production of the airways. Inhaled corticosteroids do not inhibit protein synthesis, block α-adrenergic receptors, nor block opiate receptors.

12.1 Excessive use of corticosteroids may result in adrenal insufficiency. Excessive use of corticosteroids does not cause status asthmaticus, sudden death, or vaginal bleeding.

13.3 Montelukast is classified as a leukotriene antagonist, not as a β-agonist, corticosteroid, or a xanthine derivative.

14.3 Salmeterol is the only long-acting β-agonist that is available. Bitolterol, metaproterenol, and terbutaline are short-acting β-agonists.

15.3 The therapeutic level of theophylline is 10 to 20 μg/ml. Levels of 0 to 5 μg/ml and 5 to 10 μg/ml are subtherapeutic. A level of 25 to 30 μg/ml is a toxic range.

NCLEX CHAPTER 7 ANSWERS

Section A

1.3 Desmopressin acts in the renal distal tubules and collecting ducts to increase water reabsorption and decrease urinary output in the treatment of diabetes insipidus, which is characterized by large amounts of dilute urine. No evidence exists that desmopressin causes an increased pulse rate and blood glucose level. Desmopressin usually causes a slightly elevated, not decreased, blood pressure.

2.1 Because replacement hormones are made of protein, they are digested in the GI tract and must therefore be administered parenterally with a syringe. A glass measuring device, plastic medicine cup, and a medicine dropper all indicate oral administration.

3.4 Two thirds of the dose that is given in the early morning and one third that is given in the late afternoon mimics the body's normal glucocorticoid secretion cycle. The entire dose given in the morning, the entire dose given in the late afternoon, and one third of the dose given in the early morning and two thirds given in the late afternoon do not mimic the body's normal glucocorticoid secretion cycle.

4.3 Mineralocorticoids exert an effect on sodium, chloride, and potassium and maintain extracellular and intracellular fluid volume, thus they maintain fluid and electrolyte balance. Mineralocorticoids do not decrease cardiac output or adrenal steroid production. Mineralocorticoids counteract destructive activities of the immune system.

5.3 The nurse should monitor 24-hour urine samples of 17-hydroxyglucocorticosteroids and 17-ketogenic steroids, which reveal increased elimination of glucocorticosteroids byproducts to validate drug efficacy. A CBC, blood chemistries, and routine urinalysis are not indicative of adrenal inhibitor drug therapy.

Section B

6.1 Antithyroid drugs decrease production or the release of thyroid hormone in the treatment of hyperthyroidism. The action of antithyroid drugs does not increase the release of the parathyroid hormone, increase the production and release of the thyroid hormone, and decrease the release of the parathyroid hormone.

7.2 Iodine solutions may cause staining of the teeth. Iodine solutions do not cause yellow eyes, loss of teeth, or gray hair.

8.4 Propylthiouracil should be given in divided doses around the clock. Giving propylthiouracil only at bedtime, only as a single dose, or every 2 hours is inappropriate.

9.3 Thyroid hormones may increase the potency of oral anticoagulants but do not decrease the potency of oral anticoagulants, increase the effectiveness of digitalis, or act as antiinflammatories.

10.4 Hypercalcemic agents will not reduce calcium levels in patients with GI disorders. Hypercalcemic agents may be given to reduce the calcium levels for patients with hyperparathyroidism, adrenal disorders, and hypercalcemia that are associated with malignancies.

Section C

11.3 Metformin should be withheld for 48 hours before and after radiologic studies during which iodinated dye is administered. Withholding metformin 24 or 36 hours before and after the test or for 2 weeks after the test are inappropriate.

12.1 The action of thiazolidinediones increases the effects of circulating insulin. Thiazolidinediones do not stimulate the production of insulin, increase the production of glucose by the liver, or decrease the uptake of insulin by skeletal muscles.

13.1 The onset of ultra rapid-acting insulin (Lispro) is less than 15 minutes. The remaining options (30 to 60 minutes, 1 to 2 hours, and 4 to 8 hours) do not represent the time at which the onset of rapid-acting insulin occurs.

14.3 A disulfiramlike reaction may occur when the patient takes sulfonylureas and alcohol together. Sulfonylurea with alcohol does not cause bradycardia, hyperglycemia, or edema. Sulfonylureas may cause hypoglycemia.

15.2 α-Glucosidases are contraindicated in patients with diabetes who have colon ulcers. α-Glucosidases are not contraindicated in patients with hypothyroidism, severe acne, or freckles.

NCLEX CHAPTER *8* ANSWERS

Section A

1.3 Misoprostol is indicated for the prevention and treatment of ulcers caused by NSAIDs, including aspirin. NSAIDs decrease prostaglandin production, which decreases bicarbonate and mucus production in the stomach. Misoprostol increases bicarbonate and mucus, which helps protect the gastric lining. Misoprostol is not indicated for ulcers resulting from stress, excessive gastric acid production, or Helicobacter pylori.

2.1 Cytotec is a synthetic prostaglandin E1. Prostaglandins are found in the female reproductive system, as well as other systems in the body (e.g., prostaglandins are abundant in the uterus). When prostaglandins are given to either pregnant or non-pregnant women in sufficient amounts, uterine contractions occur and the cervix softens. Misoprostol does not cause blurred vision, dry mouth, or tardive dyskinesia.

3.4 Tardive dyskinesia is a potentially serious adverse effect of metoclopramide. Dyskinesia involves repetitive, rhythmic, uncontrollable movements, usually of the face, mouth, jaw, and tongue. Protrusion of the tongue, jaw movements, facial grimace, or pursing or smacking of the lips may occur. Tardive dyskinesia can become permanent, thus early detection and withdrawal of the medication is necessary. Rhythmic, repetitive tongue movement, and grimacing are not indicative of Parkinson's disease, prodrome phase of a seizure, or pain.

4.1 Give Carafate at 6:00 AM, 11:00 AM, 4:00 PM, 9:00 PM. Considerations include the following: Carafate should be given 1 hour before meals and at bedtime; oral medications should be given 2 hours before giving Carafate; antacids must be given 30 minutes before or after Carafate; and Carafate may decrease absorption of digoxin, Dilantin, and the quinolone antibiotic when they are administered too close together.

5.2 Proton pump inhibitors should be given before, not after, meals. Proton pump inhibitors should not be chewed or followed by two glasses of water.

Section B

6.1 EPS reactions are more common with metoclopramide when taken concurrently with phenothiazines. Extrapyramidal reactions are not common when metoclopramides are given with antacids, antidysrhythmics, and anticoagulants.

7.1 Phenothiazines act as antiemetics by blocking dopamine receptors in the CTZ, which is responsible for activating the vomiting reflex. The action of phenothiazines does not increase GI motility, directly inhibit the vomiting center, or block muscarinic receptors from the cholea.

8.3 The serotonin antagonists are administered orally or IV, not rectally, intrathecal, or SC.

9.3 Granisetron is approved and used as an antiemetic for emetogenic chemotherapy. Granisetron is not approved for use for viral gastroenteritis, radiologic enteral intubation, or preoperative and postoperative nausea.

10.1 **An** overdose or absorption of ipecac can produce cardiotoxic effects, such as dysrhythmias, chest pain, bradycardia, and tachycardia. Overdosing of ipecac does not cause vertigo, tinnitus, and dermatitis.

Section C

11.4 Bismuth subsalicylate has an antiinflammatory and antimicrobial effect and is frequently used in combination with antibiotics to treat *Helicobacter pylori* infection. Docusate is a stool softener. Mineral oil is a lubricant laxative. Diphenoxylate with atropine is an opioid antidiarrheal. Laxatives, stool softeners, or opioid antidiarrheals are not used to treat *Helicobacter pylori*.

12.2 Assess her intake and output to determine fluid volume deficit and dehydration, primarily because of her age, which makes her more susceptible to dehydration. A complete assessment is always necessary for your patients and should be performed. However, you should be aware that dehydration is the greatest concern in this case. Electrolytes would also be an important assessment but was not one of the choices. Pain level assessment, CBC and blood glucose assessment, and heart rate and rhythm assessment are incorrect because they are not related to dehydration as closely as is intake and output assessment.

13.2 The combination of MAOI and opioid antidiarrheal may cause hypertensive crisis. MAOIs that contain diphenoxylate hydrochloride with atropine sulfate do not enhance the MAOI, decease MAOI absorption, or increase bleeding.

14.1 Lactobacillus acidophilus is used to prevent and treat superinfections following antibiotic therapy. Polycarbophil, deodorized opium tincture, and loperamide are not used to treat superinfections.

15.2 Mineral oil is the laxative that is likely to decrease absorption of food and fat-soluble vitamins. Bisacodyl, psyllium, and bismuth subsalicylate do not decrease the absorption of food and fat-soluble vitamins.

NCLEX CHAPTER 9 ANSWERS

Section A

1.1 Hemolytic anemia is an adverse effect of nitrofurantoin. EPS, Stevens-Johnson syndrome, and pseudomembranous enterocolitis are not adverse effects of nitrofurantoin.

2.2 Agranulocytosis is a life-threatening adverse effect of ofloxacin. Urticaria, seizures, and dystonia are neither life threatening nor adverse effects of ofloxacin.

3.3 Orange-red urine is a distinctive adverse effect of phenazopyridine. Phenazopyridine does not cause CNS depression, an increase in seizures, or lens opacity.

4.4 Oxybutynin is contraindicated in patients with bowel obstruction. Oxybutynin is not contraindicated in patients with hypertension, dysphonia, or paraplegia.

5.3 Leukopenia is an adverse effect of loop diuretics. Loop diuretics do not cause black stools, increased seizure activity, or lens opacity.

Section B

6.2 When the hematocrit rises more than 5 points in 2 weeks, the best nursing action is to notify the health care provider and expect a dose reduction of epoetin alfa. When the hematocrit has not risen 5 points in 2 weeks and remains below the target range, the nurse should notify the health care provider and expect a dose increase. Monitoring hematocrit levels daily and every month are incorrect because frequent monitoring is considered to be twice weekly. Doing nothing because a rise in hematocrit is expected is incorrect because a rapid elevation of hematocrit may lead to seizures.

7.4 Liquid iron preparations may stain the teeth when not taken with a straw. Iron tablets should not be crushed. Antacids decrease iron absorption. The liquid form should be adequately diluted.

8.2 The primary adverse effect of calcitriol is hypercalcemia. Evidence includes headache, irritability, dizziness, tinnitus, metallic taste, GI distress, and weakness. Calcitriol is a vitamin D supplement that promotes absorption of calcium. Hypocalcemia is incorrect because the most common major adverse effect is hypercalcemia. Anemia is incorrect because it is a subsequent effect of hypercalcemia. Hypotension is incorrect because calcitriol does not appear to affect blood pressure.

9.4 Cation-exchange resins acts by releasing sodium in exchange for hydrogen ions in the acidic stomach environment. Hydrogen cations are exchanged for potassium cations, which are aided by a laxative to be eliminated in feces. Cation-exchange resins are therefore used in hyperkalemia to reduce high potassium levels, thus hypocalcemia, hypercalcemia, and hypokalemia are incorrect.

10.4 Systemic antacids may lead to milk-alkali syndrome. Systemic antacids are thoroughly absorbed. Antacids are considered as treatment for metabolic acidosis. Antacids increase the duration of anorexiant effects when given concurrently.

NCLEX CHAPTER 10 ANSWERS

Section A

1.3 Life-threatening adverse effects of estrogen therapy include seizures, thromboembolism, CVA, pulmonary embolism, MI, hepatic adenoma, and an increased risk of endometrial and breast cancer. Shortness of breath may indicate pulmonary embolism and should be reported immediately. Estrogen decreases the risk of osteoporosis, and patients may be unaware that they are experiencing it anyway. Water retention and diarrhea are effects that need not be reported immediately.

2.4 Estrogen replacement therapy is intended to prevent osteoporosis. Estrogen is contraindicated in women during pregnancy and in patients with breast cancer and vascular disease.

3.4 Estrogen, not progesterone, is found in the bone. Progesterone is a steroid hormone that is synthesized and released by the testes, ovary, adrenal cortex, and the placenta.

4.1 When carbamazepine, phenobarbital, and rifampin are taken with estrogen, estrogen effectiveness is decreased. Theophylline and digoxin have no drug interaction with estrogen and progestin. Cyclosporine increases the risk of toxicity when administered with estrogen, not reduced effectiveness.

5.3 When estrogen suppresses secretion of follicle-stimulating hormone, which blocks follicle development, the action consequently inhibits ovulation. With a depression of luteinizing hormone, ovulation cannot occur, even with full development of the follicle. Progestin also causes endometrium changes that may prevent an egg from being implanted in the uterus.

Section B

6.2 Magnesium sulfate can suppress preterm labor but is used primarily as an anticonvulsant to prevent or treat the complication of seizures in severe pre-eclampsia or eclampsia. Magnesium sulfate is not used to prevent hypotension, depressed reflexes, and GI distress.

7.2 Tocolytic agents act on the reproductive system to maintain a pregnancy. Tocolytics (uterine relaxants) are β-adrenergic agonists that mimic the sympathetic nervous system effects at β_2 sites, relax smooth muscle, and stop or slow uterine contractions. The action of tocolytics does not induce ovulation, facilitate milk letdown, or induce abortion.

8.1 The nurse should monitor the patient for water intoxication during oxytocic administration. Ovarian hyperstimulation and invasive cervical carcinoma are not adverse effects of oxytocics. Oxytocin is contraindicated in patients with cephalopelvic disproportion.

9.4 Dinoprostone should be allowed to warm to room temperature before removing the foil wrapper. Dinoprostone is administered by intravaginal suppository, is contraindicated in patients with pelvic inflammatory disease, and may cause bronchospasm and chest pain.

10.1 Large doses of ergot alkaloid during labor may cause maternal and fetal trauma. Hypertension, not hypotension, is a common adverse effect. IV ergot alkaloids are reserved for severe uterine bleeding or other life-threatening emergencies because most adverse effects follow IV administration. Ergot alkaloids are not the drugs of choice in patients with renal disease but should be used with caution in these individuals.

NCLEX CHAPTER *11* ANSWERS

1.1 An oxicam is a type of NSAID, as well as salicylates, propionic acid derivatives, acetic acid derivatives, pyrazolones, anthranilic acids, and COX-2 inhibitors. Uricosurics are antigout drugs. Immunosuppressives and gold agents are DMARDs.

2.2 The action of NSAIDs inhibits the formation of prostaglandins but does not reduce serum urate levels (action of antigout drugs), inhibit destructive lysosomal enzyme activity in joints (action of gold compounds), or reduce xanthine oxidase enzyme production (action of allopurinol, a xanthine oxidase inhibitor).

3.1 COX-2 decreases pain and inflammation. COX-2 is not associated with the reduction of fever, stomach distress, and platelet aggregation. COX-1 decreases the protection of the stomach lining and platelet aggregation.

4.1 Gold agents may cause corneal gold deposits and retinopathy. Methotrexate, etanercept, and hyaluronic acid do not cause adverse effects that require periodic eye examinations.

5.3 The goal of antigout therapy is to maintain serum uric acid levels between 5 and 6 mg/dl. The remaining options (2 mg/dl or below, 4 mg/dl or below, and 10 mg/dl or below) are incorrect serum uric acid levels in gout prevention.

NCLEX CHAPTER *12* ANSWERS

1.4 Vitamin K is essential for the synthesis of blood coagulation factors. Vitamins B, C, and D are not associated with blood coagulation.

2.2 Vitamin C is used for the prevention and treatment of scurvy. Vitamin C is not used for the treatment and prevention of thiamine deficiency, overdose of anticoagulants, or chapped or dry skin.

3.3 Sodium is used in the prevention and treatment of heat prostration. Sodium is not used in the treatment and prevention of beriberi, scurvy, or anemia.

4.4 The nurse should monitor hemoglobin and reticulocyte levels to evaluate the effectiveness of iron therapy. Iron therapy is usually continued for 2 to 3 months after the hemoglobin level returns to normal. Renal and hepatic function studies or sodium and potassium levels do not indicate the effectiveness of iron therapy.

5.3 The best food source that is listed of vitamin B_9 is asparagus. Fish, milk, and strawberries are not the best food sources of vitamin B_9.

NCLEX CHAPTER *13* ANSWERS

Section A

1.2 Drugs are ocular lubricants that relieve dry eyes and are composed of sodium chloride, polyvinyl, petrolatum, mineral oil, and lanolin. Naphazoline is an ocular decongestant. Timolol is an ocular BB. Demecarium is an anticholinesterase miotic that is used for the treatment of glaucoma.

2.2 Carbachol is a cholinergic miotic that contracts the sphincter of the iris and ciliary muscles. By deepening the anterior eye chamber, the larger filtration angle causes an increased outflow of aqueous humor and decreased IOP. Carbachol contracts, not dilates, the iridic sphincter. Carbachol causes miosis (pupil constriction), not mydriasis (pupil dilation). Carbachol does not cause vasoconstriction of the collecting channels.

3.2 Pilocarpine is an ocular cholinergic that commonly causes ocular burning and tearing adverse effects. Pilocarpine does not cause iridic cysts, obstruction of the lacrimal system, or retinal detachment.

4.1 When administering otic medication to a child, the nurse should instruct the mother to pull the pinna down and back for a child who is under 3 years of age. Pulling the pinna up and back should be performed for children over age 3 and for adults. Pulling the pinna forward is an inappropriate action.

5.2 When teaching an adult about eye medication administration, the patient should be taught to hold the container in the hand, thereby warming the otic solution. The patient should be taught to keep the solution cap tightly, not loosely, closed. Otic medication should be administered at a warm, not cold, temperature. The microwave oven would warm the medication excessively, possibly cause a burn.

Section B

6.1 Silver sulfadiazine is a burn treatment agent that is designed to prevent bacterial growth of burned tissue. An antipruritic is used to relieve itching. Tetracycline is used as an acne treatment. A keratolytic is a caustic agent that promotes shedding of the horny layer of skin.

7.2 Supporting colonization of bacteria is not a primary function of the skin. Primary functions of the skin include protection, immune responsiveness, and thermoregulation.

8.1 Burned areas should not be covered with occlusive dressings because healing would be impeded. Therefore covering the area with airtight dressing is an inappropriate intervention. Keeping the burn area covered with medication at all times, applying medication in a thin layer over the burned area, and using sterile technique are appropriate interventions.

9.2 Crotamiton should be gently massaged into the affect area. A clean technique is acceptable; it need not be sterile. When an antipruritic comes into contact with the eyes, the eyes should be thoroughly and immediately flushed with water for 15 minutes, not closed and bandaged. The patient should avoid eating for 1 hour after an antipruritic spray of the throat. The nurse must check for the return of the gag reflex before allowing the consumption of food or fluid.

10.1 Discoloration of skin is an adverse effect that is associated with silver sulfadiazine. Silver sulfadiazine is not associated with peeling of skin layers (action of keratolytic), elevated blood glucose (adverse effect of isotretinoin), or required pregnancy test before treatment (as is true for tetracycline).

NCLEX CHAPTER *14* ANSWERS

1.3 When caffeine is combined with ergotamine tartrate (Cafergot), GI absorption is increased. Dihydro-ergotamine, ergotamine tartrate alone, and methysergide maleate do not increase GI absorption.

2.4 The most common adverse effects of ergot derivatives are nausea and peripheral ischemia, which is evidenced by cold fingers or toes. Vomiting and diarrhea, tachycardia or bradycardia, and itching or rebound headache are not common adverse effects of ergot derivatives.

3.1 The onset of action for intranasal and IV ergot derivatives is rapid, less than 5 minutes. The remaining options (30 minutes, 2 hours, and 4 hours) are incorrect onsets of action for intranasal and IV ergot derivatives.

4.3 Meperidine is responsible for producing the toxic metabolite normeperidine, which may lead to neurotoxicity. Codeine, fentanyl, and oxycodone produce no toxic metabolites.

5.4 The most serious adverse effect of opiates is respiratory depression. Breathing oxygen is more essential to life than are dilated pupils, seizures, and orthostatic hypotension.

Index

A

AAPC. *See* Antibiotic-associated pseudomembranous colitis
Abciximab, 138
Acarbose (Precose), 249t, 250
Accolate. *See* Zafirlukast
Accupril. *See* Quinapril
Accutane. *See* Isotretinoin
ACE inhibitors. *See* Angiotensin-converting enzyme (ACE) inhibitors
Acetaminophen (Tylenol), 28, 193, 346-348
Acetazolamide (Diamox), 302, 378t, 379
Acetic acid derivatives, 343t
Acetohexamide (Dymelor), 247t
Acetylcholine (ACh), 70, 127, 272, 373
Acetylcholinesterase (AChE), 72
Acetylcysteine (Mucomyst), 199t
N-acetylprocainamide (NAPA), 181
Acetylsalicylic acid (ASA; Aspirin), 132t, 343t, 345
ACh. *See* Acetylcholine
AChE. *See* Acetylcholinesterase
Achlorhydria, 36
Achromycin. *See* Tetracycline
Acidifier-digestive enzymes, 281-283
Acidifiers, urinary, 197
Acidophilus Lactobacillus. *See* Lactobacillus acidophilus
Acidosis, lactic, 252
Acne treatment agents, 387-389
Acquired immune deficiency syndrome (AIDS), 27, 223
ACTH. *See* Corticotropin
Actinex. *See* Masoprocol
Actinomycin-D. *See* Dactinomycin
Activated partial thromboplastin time (APTT), 137
Actos. *See* Pioglitazone
Acute coronary syndrome, 135
Acycloguanosine. *See* Acyclovir
Acyclovir (Acycloguanosine), 31t
Adams-Stokes syndrome, 92
ADD. *See* Attention-deficit disorder
Adderall. *See* Amphetamine sulfate
Addison's disease, 365
Adenocard. *See* Adenosine
Adenosine (Adenocard), 190t, 191

Adenosine diphosphate (ADP), 131, 364
Adenosine triphosphate (ATP), 364
ADH. *See* Antidiuretic hormone; Vasopressin
ADHD. *See* Attention-deficit/hyperactivity disorder
ADP. *See* Adenosine diphosphate
Adrenal hormone inhibiting agents, 231-233
α₁-Adrenergic blockers, 145-147, 145t
β-Adrenergic blockers, 147-149, 147t, 261
Adrenocorticosteroids, 221
Adrenocorticotropic hormone (ACTH) deficiency, 223
Adriamycin. *See* Doxorubicin
Advanced Cardiac Life Support (ACLS), 182
Aerobes, 2
Agonist-antagonists, 398-399, 398t
Agonists
  adrenergic, (stimulators), 62, 63-66
  β-agonist, 211-213, 211t
  direct-acting cholinergic, 69-71
Agranulocytosis, 92, 94, 98, 133, 204, 273
AIDS. *See* Acquired immunodeficiency syndrome
AK-Dilate. *See* Phenylephrine
AK-Homatropine. *See* Homatropine
Akathisia, 54, 106, 273
Akinesia, 80
Akne-Mycin. *See* Erythromycin
Alanine aminotransferase (ALT), 7, 137
Albuminuria, 98
Albuterol (Proventil; Ventolin), 63t, 64t, 211
Alcohol, 9, 182, 211, 227, 232, 244, 248, 261, 309
Alcoholism, chronic, 36
Aldactone. *See* Spironolactone
Aldesleukin. *See* Interleukin-2
Aldomet. *See* Methyldopa
Aldosterone, 221
Aldosterone-like drugs, 233
Alesse. *See* Ethinyl estradiol/levonorgestrel
Aleve. *See* Naproxen

Alfentanil, 17, 37
Alkalinizers, urinary, 197
Alkylamines, 201, 201t
Alkylating agents, 55-57
Allegra. *See* Fexofenadine
Allerest. *See* Naphazoline
Allergy, drug, 3
Allopurinol (Zyloprim), 216, 355
Alopecia, 56, 60, 350
Alpha Keri Emollient, 389t
Alprazolam (Xanax), 30, 109
ALT. *See* Alanine aminotransferase
Altace. *See* Ramipril
Alteplase, 139
Aluminum carbonate (Basaljel), 315t
Aluminum hydroxide (Amphojel), 257t, 315t, 316-317
Aluminum, 264
Alupent. *See* Metaproterenol, 211t
Alzheimer's disease, 67, 72
Amantadine hydrochloride (Symmetrel), 76, 78, 78t, 311
Amaryl. *See* Glimepiride
Ambenonium chloride (Mytelase), 71t
Ambenonium hydrochloride, 72
Ambien. *See* Zolpidem
Amerge. *See* Naratriptan
Americaine. *See* Benzocaine
American Academy of Pediatrics, 311
American Heart Association (AHA), 182
Amikacin sulfate (Amikin), 11t, 12
Amikin. *See* Amikacin sulfate
Amiloride (Midamor), 311t
Amiloride, 312
Amino acids, 100
Aminocaproic acid, 138
Aminoglutethimide (Cytadren), 231, 231t, 232, 234
Aminoglycosides, 6, 11-13, 22, 34, 241, 307
Aminoketones, 123
Aminopenicillins, 2
Aminophylline, 42
Amiodarone (Cordarone), 20, 39, 174, 179, 182, 185, 187t, 188, 191
Amitriptyline (Elavil), 116t

Ammonium chloride, 133
Amnesia, anterograde, 110
Amoxicillin (Amoxil), 1t
Amoxil. *See* Amoxicillin
Amphetamine sulfate (Adderall), 81t
Amphetamines, 379
Amphojel. *See* Aluminum hydroxide
Amphotec. *See* Amphotericin B
Amphotericin B (Amphotec), 22, 33t, 34, 174, 191, 229, 241, 307, 309
Ampicillin, 263
Amrinone lactate (Inocor), 176t
Amrinone, 188
Anacin, 86
Anaerobes, 2
Analeptics, 81, 85-87
Anaphylaxis, 3
ANAs. *See* Antinuclear antibodies
Ancef. *See* Cefazolin
Androgens, 332-334
Anemia, 34, 42, 79, 98, 101, 112, 131, 133
Anesthesia, 103
Anesthetic agents, 103-107, 105t
Angina, 90, 147, 405
Angina pectoris, 155
Angioedema, 144
Angiotensin converting enzyme (ACE) inhibitors, 39, 313
Angiotensin II antagonists, 144
Angiotensin II inhibitors, 143-145
Angiotensin receptor blockers (ARBs), 144
Angiotensin-converting enzyme (ACE) inhibitors, 39, 140-143, 311, 313, 345, 355
Anistreplase, 138
Anorexia, 88, 101
Anorexiants, 81, 83-85, 321
Antacids, 174, 191, 302, 350
  nonsystemic, 257-259
  systemic, 320-322
Antagonists
  adrenergic, 62, 66-68
  β-adrenergic, 68, 147
Anterior pituitary hormone replacement agents, 222-225
Anthrax, 2
Antianemic agents, 314

Page numbers followed by *f* indicate figure; *t*, table; *b*, box.

435

Antiarrhythmics, 178-192
  class IA, 178-181
  class IB, 181-184
  class IC, 184-186
  class II, 186
  class III, 187-189
  class IV, 190
  miscellaneous, 190-192t
Antiarthritics, 348-352
Antiasthmatics and bronchodilators
  β-agonists, 211-213
  anticholinergics, 218-220
  corticosteroids, inhaled, 208-211
  leukotriene antagonists, 213-215
  xanthine derivatives, 215-218
Antibiotics, 1-24. See also Specific
    antibiotics
  aminoglycosides, 11-13
  fluoroquinolones, 19-21
  β-lactam, 1-8, 357
  macrolide, 16-18, 216
  miscellaneous, 21-24. See also
    Specific antibiotic
  oral, 294
  sulfonamides, 8-10
  tetracyclines, 14-16
Anticholinergic effects, 202
Anticholinergics, 74-78
  ocular, 380t
Anticoagulants, 135-137, 315
  oral, 229, 248, 361
Anticonvulsants, 91-102,
  barbiturates, 93-95
  benzodiazepines, 95-97
  hydantoin, 91-93
  miscellaneous, 99-102
  succinimide, 97-99
Antidepressant agents, 115-127
  tricyclic, 116-118
  lithium, 125-127
  miscellaneous, 123-124
  monoamine oxidase inhibitors,
    120-122
  selective serotonin reuptake
    inhibitors (SSRIs), 118-120
  tricyclic (TCAs), 20, 37, 76,
    114, 116-118, 123, 116t,
    148, 155, 157, 179, 206,
    261, 277
Antidiabetic agents, 229. See also
    Antidiabetics
Antidiabetics, 242-256
  biguanides, 251-253
  α-glucosidase inhibitors, 249-251
  insulin, 243-246
  meglitinides, 255-256
  sulfonylureas, 247-249
  thiazolidinediones, 253-255
Antidiarrheals, 293-299
  absorbent, 293-295
  intestinal flora modifiers, 297-299
  opioid and opioid-derivative,
    295-297
Antidiuretic hormone (ADH), 221

Antiemetics, 271-279
  miscellaneous, 277-279
  phenothiazines, 272-274
  serotonin antagonists, 275-276
Antiflatulents, 267-269, 267
Antifungals, 33-38
  azole, 36-38
  polyene, 33-35
Antigout agents, 352-358
  antimitotic, 352-354
  uricosuric, 356-358
  xanthine oxidase inhibitors,
    355-356
Antihistamines, 64, 76, 201-208
  first-generation sedating, 201-205
  second-generation nonsedating,
    206-208
Antihyperlipidemics, 160-168
  bile acid sequestrants, 163-165
  fibric acid derivatives, 165-166
  HMG-CoA reductase inhibitors,
    161-163
  miscellaneous, 167-168
Antihypertensives, 140-160
  ACE inhibitors, 140-143
  α$_1$-adrenergic blockers, 145-147
  β-adrenergic blockers, 147-149
  angiotensin II inhibitors, 143-145
  α-beta blocker, 149-151
  calcium channel blockers, 152-154
  central α-adrenergic agonist,
    154-156
  direct vasodilators, 158-160
  peripheral adrenergic neuron
    antagonist, 156-158
Antiinflammatory agents, 343-352
  acetaminophen, 346-348
  nonsteroidal antiinflammatory,
    343-346. See also Nonsteroidal
    antiinflammatory agents
Antimigraine agents, 401-406
Antimitotics, 352-354
Antimuscarinics, 315
Antineoplastic agents, 49-61. See
    also Specific drugs
  alkylating agents, 55-57
  antimetabolites, 50-52
  antitumor antibiotics, 57-59
  inhibitors, mitotic, 52-55
  miscellaneous, 59-61
Antinuclear antibodies (ANAs), 159
Antiparkinsonism agents. See
    Parasympathetic nervous
    system agents and
    antiparkinsonism agents
Antiplatelets, 131-134
Antipruritics, 390-392
Antipsychotic agents, 127-130
Antisecretory agents. See Proton
    pump inhibitors
Antiseptics, for urinary tract, 301t
Antithrombin III, 135
Antithyroid agents, 235-237
Antitumor antibiotics, 57-59

Antitussives, 193-195
Antivirals, 24-38. See also Specific
    antivirals
  nucleoside reverse transcriptase
    inhibitor antiretroviral, 27-29
  protease inhibitor retroviral, 25-26
Anturane. See Sulfinpyrazone
Anxiolytic agents, 108-113
  benzodiazepine anxiolytic agents,
    109-111
  nonbenzodiazepine, 111-113
Apresoline. See Hydralazine
APTT. See Activated partial throm-
    boplastin time
Aqua-Mephyton. See Vitamin K
Aquasol A. See Vitamin A
Aquasol E. See Vitamin E
ARA-C. See Cytarabine
ARBs. See Angiotensin receptor
    blockers
Aricept. See Donepezil hydrochloride
Aristospan. See Triamcinolone
Arthralgia, 34
Arthritis, agents used in, 348-352
  acute gouty, 352t
ASA. See acetylsalicylic acid
Ascorbic acid, 365. See also
    Vitamin C
Ascorbicap. See Vitamin C (ascorbic
    acid)
Asparaginase (L-Asparaginase), 59t,
    60
Aspartate aminotransferase (AST),
    7, 137
Aspartate proteinase, 25
Aspergillosis, disseminated, 33
Aspergillus, 34
Aspergillus fumigatus, 33
Aspergillus niger, 210
Aspirin, 132, 132t, 133, 138. See also
    Acetylsalicylic acid
Aspirin hypersensitivity, 133
AST. See Aspartate aminotransferase
Astemizole, 17, 20
Asthenia, 214
Asthma, 133, 208, 216
  exercise-induced, 212
Atacand. See Candesartan cilexetil
Ataxia, 10, 92, 96, 101
Atenolol, 365
Atherosclerosis, coronary, 160
Athlete's foot, 36
Ativan. See Lorazepam
Atorvastatin (Lipitor), 161t
Atracurium, 73
Atrioventricular (AV) conduction,
    150
Atrioventricular node, 190
Atromid-S. See Clofibrate
Atrophy, gonadal, 56
Atropine, 64, 73, 76, 148
Atropine sulfate (Isopto Atropine),
    74t, 297
Atrovent. See Ipratropium bromide

Attention-deficit disorder (ADD),
    81
Attention-deficit/hyperactivity
    disorder (ADHD), 81
Automaticity, 173
AV. See Atrioventricular conduction
Avandia. See Rosiglitazone
Avapro. See Irbesartan
Axid. See Nizatidine
Azactam. See Aztreonam
Azatadine, 206
Azatadine maleate (Optimine), 206t
Azathioprine (Imuran), 38t, 39
Azelaic acid (Azelex), 387t
Azelex. See Azelaic acid
Azithromycin (Zithromax), 16t
Azmacort. See Triamcinolone
Azole antifungal, 36-38
Azopt. See Brinzolamide
AZT. See Zidovudine
Aztreonam (Azactam), 21t, 22
Aztreonam, 22
Azulfidine. See Sulfasalazine

B

Bacilli, 2
Baclofen (Lioresal), 87t, 88
Bactrim. See Trimethoprim-
    sulfamethoxazole
Barbiturates, 9, 58, 174, 223, 296,
    324, 347
Basaljel. See Aluminum carbonate
Beclomethasone (Beclovent;
    Vanceril), 208t, 209
Beclovent. See Beclomethasone
Bedwetting. See Enuresis
Belladonna, 402
Belladonna alkaloids, 374
Benadryl. See Diphenhydramine
Benazepril (Lotensin), 140
Benemid. See Probenecid
Benzalkonium chloride, 369t
Benzocaine (Americaine), 4, 390t
Benzodiazepines (BZDs), 37, 79,
    95-97, 109-110, 182, 261
Benzonatate (Tessalon Perles), 193t
Benzphetamine (Didrex), 83t
Benztropine, 76
Benztropine mesylate, 271
Bepridil, 20
Berger's disease, 67, 155
α-Beta antagonists. See α-Beta
    blockers
Beta blockers, 147, 172, 216, 244
  ocular, 375
α-Beta blockers, 149-151. 149t
Betalin. See Vitamin B$_1$ (thiamine)
Betapace. See Sotalol
Betaxolol (Betoptic), 373t
Bethanechol, 70
Bethanechol chloride (Urecholine),
    69t
Betoptic. See Betaxolol
Biaxin. See Clarithromycin

Bicitra. *See* Sodium citrate
Biguanides, 251-253, 251t
Bile acid sequestering resins. *See* Bile acid sequestrants
Bile acid sequestrants, 163-165
Bile acid-binding resins. *See* Bile acid sequestrants
Biperiden, 76
Biphosphonates-alendronate (Fosamax), 240t
Biphosphonates-etidronate (Didronel), 240
Bipolar disorder, 125
Birth defects, alkylating drugs and, 56
Bisacodyl (Dulcolax), 283t
Bismuth subsalicylate (Pepto-Bismol), 293t
Bitolterol, 211
Bladder paralysis, 117
Bleomycin, 58
α_1-Blockers. *See* α_1-Adrenergic blockers
Blood dyscrasias, 90, 94
Blood pressure (BP), 140
Blood pressure and flow, drugs affecting, 140-168
    antihyperlipidemics, 160-168
    antihypertensives, 140-160
Blood urea nitrogen (BUN), 7, 149
Bone marrow depression, 101
BP. *See* Blood pressure
Bradycardia, 96
Bradykinesia, 78
Brethine. *See* Terbutaline
Bretylium (Bretylol), 187t, 188
Bretylol. *See* Bretylium
Brinzolamide (Azopt), 378t
Bromocriptine mesylate (Parlodel), 17, 78, 79
Brompheniramine (Dimetane), 201t
Bromsulphalein (BSP), 137
Bronchoconstriction, 69
Bronchodilation, 216
Bronchodilators, antiasthmatics and, 208-220
Bronchospasms, 218
BSP. *See* Bromsulphalein
Bumetanide (Bumex), 306t
Bumex. *See* Bumetanide
BUN. *See* Blood urea nitrogen
Bupivacaine (Marcaine), 103t
Bupropion (Wellbutrin; Zyban), 123, 124
Burns, treatment agents for, 385-387
BuSpar. *See* Buspirone
Buspirone (BuSpar), 37, 111t
Busulfan (Myleran), 55t, 56
Butabarbital (Butisol), 113t, 114
Butazolidin. *See* Phenylbutazone
Butisol. *See* Butabarbital
Butorphanol (Stadol), 398t
Butyrophenones, 79
BZDs. *See* Benzodiazepines

C

CAAs. *See* Central α-adrenergic antagonists
CAD. *See* Coronary artery disease
Cafergot. *See* Ergotamine tartrate with caffeine
Caffedrine. *See* Caffeine
Caffeine (Caffedrine; Vivarin), 19, 85t, 191, 216,
CAL disorders. *See* Chronic airway limitation disorders
Calan. *See* Verapamil
Calcimar. *See* Calcitonin-salmon
Calcitonin-human (Cibacalcin), 240t
Calcitonin-salmon (Calcimar), 240t
Calcium (Citra Cal), 364
Calcium acetate (Phos-Ex; PhosLo), 315t
Calcium antagonists. *See* Calcium channel blockers
Calcium carbonate (Caltrate; Os-Cal; Tums), 257t, 315t
Calcium channel blockers (CCBs), 152-154, 172
Caltrate. *See* Calcium carbonate
cAMP. *See* Cyclic adenosine monophosphate phospho-diesterase
Camptothecins (Topoisomerase I inhibitors), 53
Cancer
    antineoplastic agents for, 49
    mitotic inhibitors for, 53
Candesartan cilexetil (Atacand), 143t
Candida albicans, 34, 36, 210, 386
Capecitabine (Xeloda), 50t
Capillary leak syndrome (CLS), 45
Capoten. *See* Captopril
Capreomycin, 34
Captopril (Capoten), 140, 252
Carafate. *See* Sucralfate
Carbachol, 373t
Carbamazepine (Tegretol), 17, 37, 73, 99t, 100, 101, 125, 234, 261, 324, 347
Carbamide peroxide (Debrox Ear Drops), 383t
Carbidopa-levodopa (Sinemet; Sinemet-CR; Lodosyn), 78
Carbohydrate (CHO), 281
Carbonic anhydrase inhibitors, 90, 133, 374, 377, 378-380
Carboplatin, 34
Carboprost tromethamine (Hemabate), 339t
Carcinoma, hepatic, 333
Cardiac output (CO), 140, 169
Cardiac output, agents affecting, 169-192
    glycosides, cardiac, 172-175
    nitrates, 169-172, 169t
    phosphodiesterase inhibitors, 176

Cardiac system, drugs affecting
    agents affecting cardiac output, 169-177
    antiarrhythmics, 178-192
Cardizem. *See* Diltiazem
Cardura. *See* Doxazosin mesylate
Carisoprodol (Soma), 87
Carmustine, 56
Carvedilol, 149, 150
Cascara sagrada (Cascara), 283t
Cascara. *See* Cascara sagrada
Castor oil (Neolid), 283t
Catapres. *See* Clonidine
CBC. *See* Complete blood count
CCBs. *See* Calcium channel blockers
Cefamandole (Mandol), 5t, 6
Cefazolin (Ancef; Kefzol), 5t, 8
Cefepime (Maxipime), 5t
Cefoperazone, 6
Cefotaxime (Claforan), 5t
Cefotetan, 6
Ceftriaxone (Rocephin), 8
Celebrex. *See* Celecoxib
Celecoxib (Celebrex), 344t
Cell, bacterial, 2f
Cell cycle, 49
Celontin. *See* Methsuximide
Central α-adrenergic antagonists (CAAs), 154-156
Central agonists. *See* Central α-adrenergic antagonists
Central nervous system (CNS), 19
Central nervous system depressants, 206
Centrally acting muscle relaxants, 87-89
Cephalosporins, 5-8
Cephulac. *See* Lactulose
Cerebrovascular accident (CVA), 86, 132
Cerebrovascular disease, 155
Cerumen, 369, 383-384
Cerumenex Ear Drops. *See* Triethanolamine, poly-peptide oleate, condensate
Ceruminolytics, 383-384
Cervidil. *See* Dinoprostone
Cetirizine (Zyrtec), 206t
Chamber, anterior of eye, 374
Charcoal, 100, 250
Charcoal, inactivated, 280
Charcoal attapulgite, activated (Kaopectate), 293t
Chemoreceptor trigger zone (CTZ), 106, 269, 275
CHF. *See* Congestive heart failure
Chickenpox, 31, 39
Chlamydia, 17
Chlor Trimeton. *See* Chlorpheniramine
Chloramphenicol, 22, 182, 248, 365
Chloroquine, 261
Chlorothiazide (Esidrix), 308t
Chlorzoxazone (Parafon Forte), 87t

Chlorpheniramine (Chlor Trimeton), 193, 201t
Chlorpheniramine, 193
Chlorpromazine (Thorazine), 125, 127t, 128, 193
Chlorpropamide (Diabinese), 247t
CHO. *See* Carbohydrate
Choledyl (Oxtriphylline)
Cholesterol, 161
Cholestyramine (Questran), 100, 163t, 164, 167, 174, 191, 347
Cholinesterase inhibitors, 71-74, 71t-72t
Chronic airway limitation (CAL) disorders, 229
Chronic obstructive pulmonary disease (COPD), 86, 148, 204, 208
Chronic renal failure (CRF), 46, 141
Chronic renal failure, 46
Chrysotherapy, 349. *See also* Gold therapy
Cibacalcin. *See* Calcitonin-human
Cimetidine (Tagamet), 19, 37, 51, 86, 117, 148, 150, 179, 182, 216, 252, 260, 260t, 309, 311, 353
Cipro. *See* Ciprofloxacin
Ciprofloxacin, 19t, 20, 86, 300t, 302, 365
Cisapride, 20
Cisplatin, 34, 56, 307
Citra Cal. *See* Calcium
Citrocarbonate. *See* Sodium bicarbonate
Claforan. *See* Cefotaxime
Clarithromycin, 16t, 25, 30
Claritin. *See* Loratadine
Clemastine fumarate (Tavist), 201t
Cleocin. *See* Clindamycin
Clindamycin (Cleocin), 21t, 387t
Clindamycin, 22, 23
Clofibrate (Atromid-S), 165, 165t, 166, 244, 248
Clonazepam (Klonopin), 95t, 96
Clonidine (Catapres), 154t, 155
Clopidogrel (Plavix), 132, 133
Clorazepate (Tranxene), 95t, 96, 109
Clotrimazole (Lotrimin), 36t
CLS. *See* Capillary leak syndrome
CNS stimulants and muscle relaxants
    analeptics, 85-87, 85t
    anorexiants, 83-85, 83t
    centrally acting muscle relaxants, 87-89, 87t
    peripherally acting muscle relaxants, 89-91, 89t
    psychomotor stimulants, 81-83, 81f, 81t
CNS. *See* Central nervous system
CO. *See* Cardiac output
Coagulation, disseminated intravascular (DIC), 135

Coagulation disorders, 131. See also Hematologic system, drugs affecting
Cocaine, 402
Codeine, 193t
Codeine sulfate (Paveral), 395t
Colace. See Docusate sodium
Colchicine, 39, 352t
Colchicine toxicity, 353
Colestid. See Colestipol
Colestipol (Colestid), 163t, 167
Colistin, 22
Colitis, antibiotic-associated pseudomembranous (AAPC), 22, 23
Colony-stimulating factor, 46-48, 46t
Complete blood count, 10, 143
Compazine. See Prochlorperazine
Condylomata acuminata, 42
Condylox. See Podofilox
Confusion, 92
Congestion, pulmonary, 173
Congestive heart failure (CHF), 45, 101, 133, 179, 182
Constipation. See Laxatives
Contraceptives, oral, 37, 86, 117, 248, 309, 361
  effects of penicillin on, 3
Contractility, myocardial, 172
Controlled Substances Act of 1970
COPD. See Chronic obstructive pulmonary disease
Corbamazine, 191
Cordarone. See Amiodarone
Coreg. See Carvedilol
Coronary artery disease (CAD), 324
Coronary insufficiency, 155
Corticosteroids, 37, 244, 309
  inhaled, 208-211
Corticosterone, 221
Corticotropin (ACTH), 222t
Corticotropin-releasing hormone (CRH), 228
Cortisol, 221
Cortisone (Cortone), 221, 228
Cortone. See Cortisone
Cortrosyn. See Cosyntropin
Corvert. See Ibutilide
Cosyntropin (Cortrosyn), 222t
Coumadin. See Warfarin
COX₂ inhibitors, 344t
Cozaar. See Losartan
CPK. See Creatine phosphokinase
Cramps, menstrual, 75
Creatine phosphokinase (CPK), 162
CRF. See Chronic renal failure
CRH. See Corticotropin-releasing hormone
Crisis, cholinergic, 77
Crohn's disease, 284
Crotamiton (Eurax), 390t
Cryptococcus, 34
Cryptococcus neoformans, 33
Crystalluria, 9, 10

CTZ. See Chemoreceptor trigger zone
Cuprimine. See Penicillamine
Cushing's disease, 202
Cushing's syndrome, 210, 230
CVA. See Cerebrovascular accident
Cyanabin. See Vitamin B₁₂ (cyanocobalamin)
Cyanocobalamin. See Vitamin B₁₂
Cyclic adenosine monophosphate phosphodiesterase (cAMP), 176
Cyclobenzaprine (Flexeril), 87t
Cyclogyl. See Cyclopentolate
Cyclomen. See Danazol
Cyclooxygenase, 131, 132, 344. See also COX₁; COX₂
Cyclopentolate (Cyclogyl), 374, 380t
Cyclophosphamide (Cytoxan), 55t, 56
Cycloplegia, 381
Cyclopropane, 86
Cyclosporin, 229
Cyclosporine (Sandimmune), 9, 17, 38, 38t, 39, 162, 167, 191, 324
Cyproheptadine (Periactin), 201t
Cystitis, hemorrhagic, 56
Cytadren. See Aminoglutethimide
Cytarabine (ARA-C), 50
Cytomel. See Liothyronine
Cytoprotective agents. See Mucosal protectants
Cytotec. See Misoprostol
Cytoxan. See Cyclophosphamide

D

D₅W, 180
Dactinomycin (Actinomycin-D), 57t
Danazol (Cyclomen), 332t, 333
Dantrium. See Dantrolene
Dantrolene (Dantrium), 89t, 90, 324
Dapsone, 28, 30
Daranide. See Dichlorphenamide
Daunorubicin, 58
DDAVP. See Desmopressin acetate
Debris, cellular, 51
Debrox Ear Drops. See Carbamide peroxide
Decadron. See Dexamethasone
Decamethonium, 73
Decaspray. See Dexamethasone
Declomycin. See Demeclocycline
Decongestants, 196-198, 196t
  ocular, 371-373, 271t
Deep vein thrombosis (DVT), 135
Deferoxamine (Desferal), 319t
Delavirdine (Rescriptor), 29t, 30
Deltasone. See Prednisone
Demecarium (Humorsol), 373t
Demeclocycline (Declomycin), 14t
Demerol. See Meperidine
Deoxyribonucleic acid (DNA), 8, 138

Deoxyribonucleic acid gyrase, 301
Depakote. See Valproic acid
Depressants, 309
Depression, 96, 101, 155
Dermatitis, exfoliative, 94, 98
Dermatologics, 384-394
  acne treatment agents, 387-389, 387t
  antipruritics, 390-392, 390t
  burn treatment agents, 385-387, 385t
  emollients, 389-390, 389t
  keratolytics, 392-394, 392t
Dermatophytes, 33
Desferal. See Deferoxamine
Desitin Ointment, 389t
Desmopressin acetate (DDAVP), 226t
Desoxycorticosterone (DOCA), 221, 233
Dexamethasone (Decadron; Decaspray), 73, 208t, 228t
Dexedrine. See Dextroamphetamine sulfate
Dexpanthenol (Ilopan), 69t, 70
Dextroamphetamine sulfate (Dexedrine), 81
Dextromethorphan (Robitussin DM), 193t
Dextrothyroxine, 244
DHE 45. See Dihydroergotamine
DiaBeta. See Glyburide
Diabetes insipidus, 221
Diabetes, symptomatic, 269. See also Antidiabetics
Diabetes mellitus (DM), 82, 141
  type 1, 375
  type 2, 251
Diabinese. See Chlorpropamide
Dialose. See Docusate potassium
Diamox. See Acetazolamide
Diaphoresis, 3, 224
Diapid. See Lypressin
Diarrhea, 294b. See also Antidiarrheals
Diastole, 169-170
Diazepam (Valium), 95t, 96, 109, 159, 248, 263, 315
DIC. See Coagulation, disseminated intravascular
Dichlorphenamide (Daranide), 378t
Diclofenac, 191
Didanosine (Videx), 27
Didanosine, 28
Didrex. See Benzphetamine
Didronel. See Biphosphonates-etidronate
Diethylpropion (Tepanil), 83t
Diflucan. See Fluconazole
Diflunisal, 379
Digibind. See Digoxin immune Fab
Digitalis toxicity, 309
Digitalis, 172, 173, 238, 361

Digoxin (Lanoxin), 17, 39, 51, 64, 90, 109, 114, 172, 185, 188, 190, 190t, 191, 229, 232, 250, 263, 264, 294, 307, 265
Digoxin immune Fab (Digibind), 174
Digoxin toxicity, 141
Dihydroergotamine (Migranal; DHE 45), 340t, 401t, 402
Dihydrotestosterone, 332
Dihydroxyphenylalanine (DOPA), 79
Dilantin. See Phenytoin
Dilor. See Dyphylline
Diltiazem (Cardizem), 152t, 153, 191, 244
Dimenhydrinate (Dramamine), 11, 277t
Dimetane. See Brompheniramine
Dinoprostone (Cervidil; Prepidil), 339t
Diovan. See Valsartan
Diphenhydramine (Benadryl), 193, 194, 204, 271, 277t
Diphenoxylate with atropine (Lomotil), 295t
Diphtheria, 2, 17
Dipivefrin (Propine), 380t
Diprivan. See Propofol
Dipyridamole (Persantine), 132, 133, 138, 191
Direct vasodilators, 158-160, 158t
Direct-acting cholinergic agonists, 69-71, 69t
Dirithromycin (Dynabac), 16t
Disease-modifying antirheumatic drugs (DMARDs), 348. See also Antiarthritics
Disopyramide (Norpace), 73, 76, 176, 178, 179
Disulfiram, 86, 182, 361
Disulfiram reaction, 6, 7
Ditropan. See Oxybutynin
Diuretic agents, 140
Diuril. See Hydrochlorothiazide
DKA. See Ketoacidosis, diabetic
DM. See Diabetes mellitus
DMARDs. See Disease-modifying antirheumatic drugs
DNA. See Deoxyribonucleic acid
Dobutamine (Dobutrex), 63t, 244
DOCA. See Desoxycorticosterone
Docetaxel, 53
Docusate calcium (Surfak), 291t
Docusate potassium (Dialose), 291t
Docusate sodium (Colace), 291t
Donepezil hydrochloride (Aricept), 37, 72t
DOPA decarboxylase, 79
DOPA. See Dihydroxyphenylalanine
Dopamine (Intropin), 63t, 64t, 65, 272
Dopaminergics, 78-80, 78t
Dopram. See Doxapram

Dorzolamide (Trusopt), 378t, 379
Doxapram (Dopram), 85t
Doxazosin mesylate (Cardura), 66t, 67, 145t
Doxepin (Sinequan), 116t
Doxorubicin (Adriamycin), 56, 57t, 58
Doxycycline (Vibramycin), 14t, 114
Dramamine. *See* Dimenhydrinate
Drixoral. *See* Pseudoephedrine
Drooling, 80
Droperidol (Inapsine), 105t, 277t
Drug allergy, 3
Drugs
    affecting blood pressure and blood flow, 140-168
        antihyperlipidemics, 160-168
        antihypertensives, 140-160
    affecting cardiac system, 169-192
        agents affecting cardiac output, 169-177
        antiarrhythmics, 178-192
    affecting endocrine system, 221-256
    affecting gastrointestinal system, 257-299
        agents affecting hyperacidity, gastric mucosa, motility, and flatulence, 257-271
        laxative and antidiarrheal agents, 283-299
    affecting genitourinary tract and renal disorders, 300-322
    affecting hematologic system, 131-139
        anticoagulants, 135-137
        antiplatelets, 131-134
        thrombolytics, 135-137
    affecting the immune system, 1-61
        See also Specific drugs
    affecting musculoskeletal system, 343-358
        antigout agents, 352-358
        antiinflammatory agents, 343-358
    affecting the nervous system, 62-130
        anesthetics, 103-107
        anticonvulsants, 91-102
        CNS stimulants and skeletal muscle relaxants, 81-91
        parasympathetic nervous system agents and antiparkinsonism agents, 69-80
        psychotherapeutic agents, 107-130
        sympathetic nervous system agents, 62-68
    affecting reproductive system, 323-342
        agents affecting uterine motility and infertility, 335-342
    affecting the respiratory system, 193-220

Drugs—cont'd
    affecting the respiratory system—cont'd
        antihistamines, 201-208
        upper respiratory disorders, agents affecting, 193-201
    affecting the sensory system, 369-394
    affecting upper respiratory system, antiasthmatics and bronchodilators, 208-220
    for nutritional imbalances, 359-368
Dulcolax. *See* Bisacodyl
Durabolin. *See* Nandrolone
Duragesic. *See* Fentanyl transdermal
Duramorph. *See* Morphine sulfate
DVT. *See* Deep vein thrombosis
Dyclone. *See* Dyclonine
Dyclonine (Dyclone), 390t
Dymelor. *See* Acetohexamide
Dynabac. *See* Dirithromycin
Dyphylline (Dilor), 215, 216
Dyrenium. *See* Triamterene
Dyscrasias, blood, 92
Dysfunction
    hepatic, 104, 182
    renal, 104
Dyskinesia, tardive, 129, 157, 273
Dyslipidemia, 161
Dysphasia, 3
Dysrhythmias, 104
    cardiac, 42
Dystonia, 106, 273
    acute, 70
Dysuria, 88

E

E-Mycin. *See* Erythromycin
Earwax (cerumen), 369, 383-384
Ecchymoses, 134, 224
ECG. *See* Electrocardiogram
Echothiophate (Phospholine iodide), 373t, 374
Ecotrin (Ibuprofen), 343t
Edema, 306t
    peripheral, 170, 173
Edrophonium chloride (Tensilon; Ilopan), 71t, 72
EEG. *See* Electroencephalograms
Effexor. *See* Venlafaxine
Efflux, 91
Elavil. *See* Amitriptyline
Electrocardiogram (ECG), 230
Electroencephalograms (EEG), 97
Embolism, pulmonary (PE), 135
Emergencies, acute, from anesthetics, 104-105
Emetics, 279-281, 279t
Emollients, 389-390, 389t
Emphysema, 208
Enalapril (Vasotec), 140
Enbrel. *See* Etanercept
Encephalopathy, 125

Endocarditis, 2, 33
Endocrine system, drugs affecting, 221-256
    antidiabetics, 242-256
    pituitary and adrenal hormones, 221-235
    thyroid and parathyroid agents, 235-242
Endometriosis, 332
Enflurane, 86
Enoxacin, 86
Enoxaparin (Lovenox), 135
Enterobacter, 301
Enterococci, 2
Enterocolitis, pseudomembranous, 302
Enuclene. *See* Tyloxapol
Enuresis, 226
Enzymes, acidifier-digestive, 281-283, 281t
Enzymes, pancreatic, 281
Eosinophilia, 98, 305
Ephedrine (Ephedsol; Ectasule; Vantronol), 64t, 196t, 321
Ephedsol. *See* Ephedrine
Epinephrine, 62, 147, 244, 374, 402
    topical, 381
Epistaxis, 210, 226
Epithelium, ciliary, 374
Epogen. *See* Erythropoietin
EPS. *See* Extrapyramidal symptoms
Epstein-Barr virus, 31
Equanil. *See* Meprobamate
Erectile dysfunction, 90
Ergonovine maleate (Ergotrate Maleate), 340t
Ergostat. *See* Ergotamine tartrate
Ergot alkaloids, 17, 25, 30, 340-342, 340t
Ergot derivatives, 401-404, 401t
Ergotamine tartrate (Ergostat), 401t
Ergotamine tartrate with caffeine (Cafergot), 401t
Ergotrate Maleate. *See* Ergonovine maleate
Erythrocyte sedimentation rate (ESR), 348
Erythromycin (Akne-Mycin; E-Mycin), 16t, 20, 22, 162, 174, 214, 353, 387t, 402
Erythropoietin (Epogen), 46t
Escherichia coli, 296, 301
Esidrix. *See* Chlorothiazide
Esmolol, 147
Estazolam, 109
Estraderm. *See* Estradiol
Estradiol (Estraderm), 323t
Estradiol/norgestimate (Ortho-Prefest), 329t
Estrogen and progestin combination, 329-332, 329t
Estrogen, 100, 114, 323-326, 323t
Estrogens, 182, 244
    conjugated, 323t

Estrogens/medroxyprogesterone, conjugated, 329t
Etanercept (Enbrel), 348t
Ethacrynic acid, 244
Ethanolamines, 201, 201t
Ethinyl estradiol/levonorgestrel (Alesse), 329t
Ethinyl estradiol/norethindrone (Ortho-Novum), 329t
Ethmozine. *See* Moricizine
Ethosuximide (Zarontin), 97t, 98
Ethotoin, 92
Ethylenediamines, 201, 201t
Etoposide (Toposar), 52t
Eurax. *See* Crotamiton
Euthroid. *See* Liotrix
Excedrin, 86
Exelon. *See* Rivastigmine tartrate
Ex-Lax. *See* Phenolphthalein
Expectorants, 198-199, 198t
Expectorate, 198
Extrapyramidal symptoms (EPS), 203, 270
Eye. *See* Ophthalmics and otics, 369-384

F

Famciclovir (Famvir), 31t
Famotidine (Pepcid), 260t
Famvir. *See* Famciclovir
FDA. *See* Food and Drug Administration
Felbamate, 182
Feldene. *See* Piroxicam
Felodipine, 37
Fenamate, 344t
Fenofibrate, 167, 167t
Fentanyl (Sublimaze), 105t, 106
Fentanyl transdermal (Duragesic; Sublimaze), 395t
Fergon. *See* Iron
Fever, 194
Fexofenadine (Allegra), 206t, 207
FiberCon. *See* Polycarbophil
Fibric acid derivatives, 165-166
Fibrillation, ventricular
Fibrinolytics. *See* Thrombolytics
Filgrastim (Neupogen), 46t
First-dose syncope, 142
Fistula, arteriovenous, 47
Flatulence, agents affecting, 257-271
Flavoxate (Urispas), 304t
Flecainide (Tambocor), 184t, 185, 379
Flexeril. *See* Cyclobenzaprine
Flomax. *See* Tamsulosin hydrochloride
Flonase. *See* Fluticasone
Florinef. *See* Fludrocortisone
Flovent. *See* Fluticasone
Floxin. *See* Ofloxacin
Floxuridine (FUDR), 50t
Fluconazole (Diflucan), 36t, 37, 182
Flucytosine, 33

Fludrocortisone (Florinef), 233t
Fluoroquinolones, 19-21, 264, 290, 300t, 315, 365
Fluorouracil, 33
5-Fluorouracil (5-FU), 50t
Fluoxetine (Prozac), 118t, 125, 182
Flurazepam, 109
Fluticasone (Flonase; Flovent), 208t
Flux, ionic, 103
Folic acid. See Vitamin B$_9$
Folic acid preparations, 350
Follicle-stimulating hormone (FSH), 330
Folvite. See Vitamin B$_9$ (folic acid)
Food and Drug Administration (FDA), 335
Formaldehyde, 301
Fosamax. See Biphosphonates-alendronate
Foxglove, 172
FSH. See Follicle-stimulating hormone
5FU. See 5-fluorouracil
FUDR. See Floxuridine
Fungi, filamentous. See Molds
Furacin. See Nitrofurantoin
Furosemide (Lasix), 34, 244, 252, 306t

G

G-CSF. See Filgrastim
G6PD. See Glucose-6-phosphate dehydrogenase
GABA. See Gamma-aminobutyric acid
Gabapentin (Neurontin), 99t, 100
Gait, shuffling, 80
Gallium (Ganite), 240t
Gamma-aminobutyric acid (GABA), 100, 108
Ganite. See Gallium
Gantanol. See Sulfamethoxazole
Gantrisin. See Sulfisoxazole
Garamycin. See Gentamicin sulfate, 11t
Gastroesophageal reflux disease (GERD), 258, 260
Gastrointestinal agents, prokinetic, 269-271, 269t
Gastrointestinal system, drugs affecting, 257-299
  agents affecting hyperacidity, gastric mucosa, motility, and flatulence, 257-271
  antiemetics, emetics, and agents used for digestive problems, 271-283
  laxative and antidiarrheal agents, 283-299
Gated blood pool scan, 58
Gatifloxacin, 19
Gemfibrozil (Lopid), 162, 165
Gemonil. See Metharbital

Genitourinary (GU) tract, 75
Genitourinary tract and renal disorders, drugs affecting, 300-322
  agents used in renal failure, 313-322
  agents used in urinary tract disorders and to improve renal output, 300-313
Gentamicin sulfate (Garamycin), 11t, 12
GERD. See Gastroesophageal reflux disease
Gilles de la Tourette's syndrome, 82
Glaucoma, 378
  acute angle-closure, 109
  anterior chamber, closed-angle, 381
  open-angle, 374
Glimepiride (Amaryl), 247t
Glipizide (Glucotrol), 247t
Glucocorticoids, 191, 248
Glucocorticosteroids, 228-231
Gluconeogenesis, 228
Glucotrol. See Glipizide
Glucophage. See Metformin
Glucose-6-phosphate dehydrogenase (G6PD), 133
Glucose-6-phosphate dehydrogenase (G6PD) deficiency, 385
α-Glucosidase inhibitors, 249-251, 249t
Glutethimide, 150
Glyburide (DiaBeta; Micronase), 247t
Glycerin (Glycerol), 289
Glycerin (Ophthalgan), 376t
Glycerol. See Glycerin
Glycopyrrolate (Robinul), 74t
Glycosides, cardiac, 172-175, 377
Glyset. See Miglitol
GM-CSF. See Sargramostim
Gold sodium thiomalate (Myochrysine), 348t
Golytely. See Polyethylene glycol-electrolyte solution
Gonorrhea, 2
Gout, 133
  agents used in, 352-358. See also Antigout agents
  chronic tophaceous, 353, 355
Grand mal seizure, 100. See also Seizures, tonic-clonic
Granisetron (Kytril), 275, 275t
Gravid, 339
Griseofulvin, 114
GU tract. See Genitourinary tract
Guaifenesin (Robitussin), 193, 198t
Guanabenz, 155
Guanadrel (Hylorel), 156t, 157
Guanethidine (Ismelin), 84, 156t, 197, 244, 273
Gynecomastia, 333

H

Hallucinations, 94
Haloperidol, 125l, 128
Halothane, 86, 106, 150, 182, 216
HDLs. See High-density lipoproteins
Heart, drugs affecting. See Cardiac system, drugs affecting
Heart failure (HF), 173
Heart valve replacement therapy, 133
Heavy metal antagonist, 319-320, 319t
Heavy metal therapy, 349
Helicobacter pylori, 293
Hemabate. See Carboprost tromethamine
Hematologic system, drugs affecting, 131-139
  anticoagulants, 135-137
  antiplatelets, 131-134
  thrombolytics, 138-139
Hematuria, 98
Henle, loop of, 300, 306
Heparin, 135, 136, 138, 227
Heparin overdose, 137
Hepatic failure, 101
Hepatotoxicity, 92, 101
Herpes zoster, 39
Hexa Betalin. See Vitamin B$_6$
HF. See Heart failure
HHNK coma. See Hyperosmotic hyperglycemic nonketotic coma
5-HIAA. See Urine 5-hydroxy-indoleacetic acid
High-density lipoproteins (HDLs), 161, 222, 323
Hirsutism, 40
Histamine, 272
Histamine H$_2$ antagonists, 260-262, 260t
Histamine-1 (H$_1$) receptor antagonists, 201
Histamine-2 (H$_2$) receptor antagonists, 201
HIV protease inhibitors
HIV type I (HIV-1), 25
HIV type II (HIV-2), 25
HIV-1. See HIV type I
HIV-2. See HIV type II
HMG-CoA reductase inhibitors, 161-163, 161t
HMG-CoA reductase inhibitors, 161-163, 161t
Hodgkin's disease, 53, 55, 59t, 60, 133
Homatropine (AK-Homatropine), 380t
Hormone replacement therapy (HRT), 324
Hormones, 62
  male and female, 323-334
    androgens, 332-334, 332t
    combination estrogen and progestin, 329-332, 329t

Hormones—cont'd
  male and female—cont'd
    estrogen, 323-326, 323t
    progestin, 326-329, 326t
  pituitary and adrenal, 232-235
    adrenal hormone inhibiting agents, 231-233
    anterior pituitary hormone replacement agents, 222-225, 222t
    glucocorticosteroids, 228-231
    posterior pituitary hormone replacement agents, 226-228
    thyroid and parathyroid agents, 235-242
  thyroid, 237
HPA axis. See Hypothalamic-pituitary-adrenal axis
HRT. See Hormone replacement therapy
Humalog. See Insulin Lispro
Humatrope. See Somatropin
Humor, aqueous, 374
Humorsol. See Demecarium
Humulin L, 243t
Humulin N, 243t
Humulin R, 243t
Humulin U, 243t
Hyalgan. See Hyaluronic acid
Hyaluronic acid (Hyalgan), 348t
Hycamtin. See Topotecan
Hydantoins, 91-93
Hydralazine (Apresoline), 158t, 159, 361
Hydrea. See Hydroxyurea
Hydrochloric acid, 257
Hydrochlorothiazide (Diuril), 37, 308t
Hydrocodone bitartrate (Vicodin), 193t
Hydrocortisone (Hydrocortone), 228t
Hydrocortone. See Hydrocortisone
Hydrogen-potassium-ATPase gastric enzyme system, 262
Hydroxychloroquine (Plaquenil), 174, 348t
Hydroxychloroquine therapy, 350
17-Hydroxyglucocorticoids, 232
Hydroxyurea (Hydrea), 59, 60
Hydroxyzine (Vistaril), 277t
Hylorel. See Guanadrel
Hyoscine. See Scopolamine
Hyperacidity, 264
  agents affecting, 257-271
Hyperammonemia, 101
Hypercalcemia, 240. See also Hypercalcemic agents
Hypercalcemic agents, 240-242, 240t
Hypercholesterolemia, 133, 161
Hyperemia, 371
Hyperexcitability, 91
Hyperglycemia, 92, 223

Hyperkalemia, 136, 141, 144
Hyperkinetic syndrome, 81
Hypermagnesemia, 258
Hypernatremia, 224
Hyperosmotic hyperglycemic non-
ketotic (HHNK) coma, 242
Hyperparathyroidism, 240
Hyperplasia
adrenocortical, 224
congenital adrenal, 233
Hyperplasia, gingival, 92
Hyperpyrexia, 117, 194
Hypersalivation, 101
Hypertension, 64
Hyperthermia, 129
Malignant, 89
Hyperthyroidism, 133, 235, 236
Hyperuricemia, 159, 282
asymptomatic, 352t
Hyperuricosuria, 282
Hypervitaminosis syndrome, 361
Hypnotic agents. See Sedative-
hypnotic agents
Hypoaldosteronism, 136
Hypocalcemia, 224
Hypocalcemic agents, 239
Hypoglycemia, 133, 244
Hypoglycemics, oral, 89
Hypokalemia, 34, 224
Hypokalemia, 34
Hypomenorrhea, 325
Hypophosphatemia, 258
Hypotension, 94, 133, 159
orthostatic, 128, 129
Hypothalamic-pituitary-adrenal
(HPA) function, 210
Hypothalamic-pituitary-adrenal axis.
Hypothalamus, 221
Hypothermia, 90, 129
Hypothrombinemia, 302
Hypothyroidism, 224
Hypovolemia, 144
Hytrin. See Terazosin

I

Ibuprofen (Motrin; Ecotrin), 343t
Ibutilide (Corvert), 187t, 188
Idiopathic thrombocytopenic pur-
pura (ITP), 229
Ilene II, 243t
Iletin II, 243t
Ilopan. See Dexpanthenol
Imdur. See Isosorbide mononitrate
Imidazoles, 33
Imipenem, 21
Imipenem-cilastatin (Primaxin), 21t
Imipenem/cilastatin, 22, 23
Imipramine (Tofranil), 116t
Imitrex. See Sumatriptan
Immune reactions, cell-mediated, 39
Immune system, drugs affecting,
38-48
antibiotics, 1-24

Immune system, drugs affecting—
cont'd
antineoplastic agents, 49-61
antivirals and antifungals, 24-38
Immunoglobulins, 229
Immunomodulators, 41-43
Immunosuppressants, 38-41, 38t
Imodium. See Loperamide
Impetigo contagiosa, 17
Impulse conduction, 173
Imuran. See Azathioprine
Inapsine. See Droperidol
Inderal. See Propranolol
Indinavir, 25, 30
Indocin. See Indomethacin
Indomethacin (Indocin), 343t, 381
Indomethacin and potassium-sparing
diuretics, 311
Infection, soft-tissue, 2
Infections, urinary tract (UTIs), 2, 9
Infertility, agents affecting, 335-342
Inhibitor, mitotic, 52-55
Inocor. See Amrinone lactate
Inotrope, negative, 147
INR. See International normalized
ratio, 137
Insomnia, 109, 114
Insulard NPH, 243t
Insulin, 89, 243-246, 248
Insulin injection, 243t
Insulin Glargine, 243t
Insulin Lispro (Humalog), 243t
Insulin Zinc Suspension (Lente),
243t
Insulin Zinc Suspension Extended
(Ultralente), 243t
Insulin Zinc Suspension Prompt
(Semilente), 243t
α-Interferon, 51
Interferon α-2a (Roferon-A), 41t
Interferon α-2b (Intron A), 41t
Interleukin, 44-45, 44t
Interleukin-2 (Aldesleukin), 44t
Interleukin-11 (Oprelvekin), 44t, 45
Intermittent positive-pressure
breathing (IPPB), 65
International normalized ratio
(INR), 137
Intestinal flora modifiers, 297-299,
297t
Intraocular pressure (IOP), 372
Intravenous piggyback (IVPB), 338
Intron A. See Interferon α-2b
Intropin. See Dopamine
Invirase. See Saquinavir
Involution, uterine, 337
Iodine, protein-bound, 134
Iodine solution, strong (Lugol's
Solution), 235t
Iodism, 236
IOP. See Intraocular pressure
Ipecac, 279t, 280
Ipecac Syrup. See Ipecac

IPPB. See Intermittent positive
pressure breathing
Ipratropium (Atrovent), 196t, 218t
IPZ. See Insulin Protamine Zinc
Irbesartan (Avapro), 143
Iridectomy, 381
Irinotecan, 53, 54
Iris, 373
Iron (Fergon), 263, 315, 350, 364,
365
Iron supplements, 314
Ischemia, myocardial, 64
Ismelin. See Guanethidine
ISMO. See Isosorbide mononitrate
Isomotic. See Isosorbide
Isoniazid, 25, 98, 182, 225, 229, 315,
361
Isophane Insulin Suspension (NPH),
243t
Isopto Atropine. See Atropine sulfate
Isopto-carbachol. See Carbachol
Isordil. See Isosorbide dinitrate
Isosorbide (Isomotic), 376t
Isosorbide dinitrate (Isordil), 169t
Isosorbide mononitrate (ISMO;
Imdur), 169t, 170
Insulin Protamine Zinc (IPZ), 243t
Isuprel. See Isoproterenol
ITP. See Idiopathic thrombo-
cytopenic purpura
Itraconazole, 37, 174
IVPB. See Intravenous piggyback

J

Jock itch, 36

K

K-Dur. See Potassium
K-Phos. See Phosphorus
Kanamycin sulfate (Kantrex), 11t,
12
Kantrex. See Kanamycin sulfate
Kaolin, 174
Kaolin-pectin, 191
Kaopectate. See Charcoal
attapulgite, activated
Kaposi's sarcoma, 42
Kayexalate. See Sodium polystyrene
sulfonate
Kefzol. See Cefazolin
Keratitis, 370, 381
corneal, 32
Keratolytics, 392-294, 392t
Ketalar. See Ketamine
Ketamine (Ketalar), 105t, 106
Ketoacidosis, diabetic (DKA), 242
Ketoconazole (Nizoral), 25, 36t, 182,
229, 263
17-Ketogenic steroids, 232
Ketogenesis, 222
Klebsiella, 301

Klonopin. See Clonazepam
Kondremul Plain. See Mineral oil
Kytril. See Granisetron

L

Labetalol (Trandate), 149, 150
Lacrimation, 69
β-Lactam antibiotics, 1-8
Lactate dehydrogenase (LDH), 7
Lactinex. See Lactobacillus
acidophilus
Lactobacillus acidophilus
(Acidophilus Lactobacillus;
Lactinex), 297t, 298
Lactulose (Cephulac), 289, 289t
Lamotrigine, 100
Lanolin, 369
Lanolor Cream, 389t
Lanosterol x-demethylase, 33
Lanoxin. See Digoxin
Lansoprazole (Prevacid), 262t
Lantus R, 243t
Lasix. See Furosemide
Laxative and antidiarrheal agents,
283-299. See also Laxatives;
Antidiarrheal agents
Laxatives, 283-293
bulk, 285-287, 285t
hyperosmotic, 289-291, 289t
lubricant, 287-288, 287t
stimulant, 283-285, 283t
LDH. See Lactate dehydrogenase
LDLs. See Low-density lipoproteins
Legionnaires' disease, 17
Lente. See Insulin Zinc Suspension
Lente Iletin II, 243t
Lente Purified Pork Novolin L, 243t
Leukemia, 42
Leukine. See Sargramostim
Leukocytes, 229
Leukopenia, 79, 98, 101, 133
Leukotriene antagonists, 213-215,
213t
Leutrol. See Zileuton
Levaquin. See Levofloxacin
Levodopa, 123, 361
Levofloxacin (Levaquin), 19t
Levothyroxine (Synthroid), 237t, 365
Lidocaine (Xylocaine), 103, 179,
181t, 182, 183
Lincosamide, 21
Lioresal. See Baclofen
Liothyronine (Cytomel), 237t
Liotrix (Euthroid), 237t
Lipitor. See Atorvastatin
Lithium, 116, 125-127, 141, 216, 227,
273, 321
Lithium toxicity, 126, 141, 307, 309,
345
Lodosyn. See Carbidopa-levodopa
Lomefloxacin, 20
Lomotil. See Diphenoxylate with
atropine

Lomustine, 56
Loniten. *See* Minoxidil
Loop diuretics, 306-308, 306t
Loperamide (Imodium), 295t
Lopid. *See* Gemfibrozil
Loratadine (Claritin), 206t, 207
Lorazepam (Ativan), 95t, 109
   parenteral, 96
Losartan (Cozaar), 37, 143t
Lotensin. *See* Benazepril
Lotrimin. *See* Clotrimazole
Lovastatin (Mevacor), 39, 161t
Lovenox. *See* Enoxaparin
Low-density lipoproteins (LDLs), 39,
   160, 222, 323
Loxapine, 128
LSD. *See* Lysergic acid diethylamide
Lubricants, ocular, 369-371, 369t
Lubriderm Cream, 389t
Lugol's Solution. *See* Iodine solution,
   strong
Luminal. *See* Phenobarbital
Luteinizing hormone (LH), 327
Lypressin (Diapid), 226t
Lyse, 66
Lysergic acid diethylamide (LSD),
   403
Lysis, osmotic, 1
Lysodren (Mitotane), 231t

M

Macrodantin. *See* Nitrofurantoin
Macrolides, 16-18, 216
Mafenide (Sulfamylon), 385t, 386
Mag-Ox 400. *See* Magnesium
Magaldrate (Riopan), 257t
Magnesium (Mag-Ox 400), 364
Magnesium hydroxide (Milk of
   Magnesia), 289t
Magnesium sulfate (MgSO$_4$), 335t
Malaise, 34
Malaria, 14
Mandol. *See* Cefamandole
Mannitol (Osmitrol), 376t, 377
MAOIs. *See* Monoamine oxidase
   inhibitors
Marcaine. *See* Bupivacaine
Masoprocol (Actinex), 392t
Matulane. *See* Procarbazine
Maxalt. *See* Rizatriptan
Maxipime. *See* Cefepime
Mazindol (Sanorex), 83t
MDI. *See* Metered-dose inhaler
Mebaral. *See* Mephobarbital
Mecamylamine, 73
Meclofen. *See* Meclofenamate
Meclofenamate (Meclofen), 344t
Medroxyprogesterone acetate
   (Provera), 326t
Megacillin. *See* penicillin G
   potassium
Meglitinides, 255-256, 255t
Melanoma, malignant, 42

Melasma, 325
Mellaril. *See* Thioridazine
Meningitis, fungal, 36
Meperidine (Demerol), 395t
Mephenytoin (Mesantoin), 91t
Mephobarbital (Mebaral), 94t
Meprobamate (Equanil; Miltown),
   111t
Mesantoin. *See* Mephenytoin
Mesoridazine, 128
Metamucil. *See* Psyllium
Metaproterenol (Alupent), 211t
Metaraminol, 402
Metered-dose inhaler (MDI), 65
Metformin (Glucophage), 251t
Metharbital (Gemonil), 94t
Methazolamide (Neptazane), 378t,
   379
Methemoglobinemia, 170, 270
Methenamine (Urised), 301t
Methergine. *See* Methylergonovine
   maleate
Methimazole (Tapazole), 235t, 236,
   309
Methimazole, 236
Methocarbamol (Robaxin), 87t
Methotrexate (Mexate; MTX), 9,
   50t 348t
Methotrimeprazine, 76
Methoxamine, 402
Methsuximide (Celontin), 97t, 98
Methyldopa (Aldomet), 125, 154t,
   155, 197, 365
Methylergonovine maleate
   (Methergine), 340t
Methylphenidate (Ritalin), 81t, 182
Methysergide maleate (Sansert),
   340t, 401t
Metoclopramide (Reglan), 39, 69t,
   70, 79, 174, 182, 269-271
Metolazone (Zaroxolyn), 308t, 309
Metopirone. *See* Metyrapone
Metoprolol, 185
Metronidazole, 182
Metyrapone (Metopirone), 231t, 232
Mevacor. *See* Lovastatin
Mexate. *See* Methotrexate
Mexiletine (Mexitil), 181t, 182
Mexitil. *See* Mexiletine
Mezlocillin, 191, 223
MgSO$_4$. *See* Magnesium sulfate
MI. *See* Myocardial infarction
Miconazole, 182
Micro-K. *See* Potassium
Micronor. *See* Norethindrone
Midamor. *See* Amiloride
Midazolam (Versed), 25, 30, 105t,
   109
   oral, 37
Miglitol (Glyset) 249t, 250
Migraine. *See* Antimigraine agents
Migranal. *See* Dihydroergotamine
Milk letdown, 337

Milk of Magnesia. *See* Magnesium
   hydroxide
Milk-alkali syndrome, 258, 321
Milontin. *See* Phensuximide
Milrinone lactate (Primacor), 176t
Miltown. *See* Meprobamate
Mineral oil (Kondremul Plain), 287t,
   369
Mineralocorticoid agents, 233-235
Minerals, 364-368, 364t
Minipress. *See* Prazosin
Minoxidil (Loniten), 158t
Miosis, 69, 194
Miotics, ocular, 373-376, 373t
Misoprostol, 266t
Mitomycin-C, 58
Mitotane, 232
Mixtard, 243t
Molds, 33
Monamine oxidase inhibitors
   (MAOIs), 60, 64, 119,
   120-122, 120t, 206, 244,
   248, 277, 372
Mononucleosis, infectious, 31
Monotherapy, antibiotic, 1
Montelukast (Singulair), 213t, 214
Morbilliform rash, 232
Moricizine (Ethmozine), 178t
Morphine sulfate (Duramorph; MS
   Contin), 261, 395t
Motility, agents affecting, 257-271
Motrin. *See* Ibuprofen
Moxifloxacin, 19
MS Contin. *See* Morphine sulfate
MTX. *See* Methotrexate
Mucolytics, 199-201, 199t
Mucomyst (acetylcysteine), 199t,
   347
Mucosa, gastric, agents affecting,
   257-271
Mucosal protectants, 264-265, 264t
Murine. *See* Tetrahydrozoline
Muromonab-CD3 (Orthoclone
   OKT3), 38, 39, 40
Muscle relaxants, 81
   centrally acting, 87-89, 87t
   peripherally acting, 89-91, 89t
   skeletal, 81-91. *See* CNS
      stimulants and skeletal
      muscle relaxants,
Musculoskeletal system, drugs affect-
   ing, 343-358
   antigout agents, 352-358
   antiinflammatory agents,
      343-352
Myasthenia gravis, 75, 179
Mycostatin. *See* Nystatin
Mydriasis, 64, 75, 79, 196, 371, 380
Myleran. *See* Busulfan
Mylicon. *See* Simethicone
Myocardial infarction, 64, 141, 142,
   227, 284
Myocardium, 147

Myochrysine. *See* Gold sodium
   thiomalate
Myopathy, 162
Myopia, accommodative, 374
Mytelase. *See* Ambenonium chloride

N

Na-K-ATPase. *See* Sodium-
   potassium-ATPase
Nabumetone (Relafen), 344t
Nadir, 51
Nalidixic acid (NegGram), 301t
Nalmefene (Revex), 400t
Naloxone (Narcan), 400t
Naltrexone (Revia), 400t
Nandrolone (Durabolin), 332t
NAPA. *See* N-acetylprocainamide
Naphazoline (Allerest; VasoClear),
   196t, 371t
Naprosyn. *See* Naproxen
Naproxen (Naprosyn; Aleve), 343t
Naratriptan (Amerge), 404t
Narcan. *See* Naloxone
Narcolepsy, 82
Narcosis, 194
Narcotics, 395
Nardil. *See* Phenelzine
Nateglinide (Starlix), 255t
Nebcin. *See* Tobramycin sulfate
NegGram. *See* Nalidixic acid
Nelfinavir (Viracept), 25t
Neo-Synephrine. *See* Phenylephrine
   hydrochloride
Neolid. *See* Castor oil
Neomycin, 174
Neostigmine bromide (Prostigmin),
   71t, 72
Nephrotoxicity, 241
Neptazane. *See* Methazolamide
Nerve block, 103
Nervous system, drugs affecting,
   62-130
   anesthetics, 103-107
   anticonvulsants, 91-102
   CNS stimulants and skeletal mus-
      cle relaxants, 81-91
   parasympathetic nervous system
      agents and antiparkinsonism
      agents, 69-80
   psychotherapeutic agents, 107-130
   sympathetic nervous system
      agents, 62-68
Netilmicin, 12
Neupogen. *See* Filgrastim
Neuralgia, trigeminal, 100
Neuroleptic malignant syndrome,
   302
Neuron, 107
Neurontin. *See* Gabapentin
Neuropathies, peripheral, 92
Neurotransmitters, 107, 108f
Neutro-Phos. *See* Phosphorus
Neutrogena Body Lotion, 389t

Neutropenia, 133
Nevirapine (Viramune), 29t
Niacin (vitamin B₃) (Nicobid; Novo-Niacin), 167t
Nicotinic acid (Novo-Niacin), 167t, 248
Nifedipine (Procardia), 152t, 252, 261
Nisoldipine, 37
Nitrobid. See Nitroglycerin
Nitrofurantoin (Furacin; Macrodantin), 19, 294, 301t, 302, 385t
Nitroglycerin (Nitrobid), 169t
Nivea Moisturizing Lotion, 389t
Nizatidine (Axid), 260t, 261
Nizoral. See Ketoconazole
NNRTI. See Nonnucleoside reverse transcriptase inhibitor (NNRTI) antiretrovirals
Nonnucleoside reverse transcriptase inhibitor (NNRTI) anti-retrovirals, 29-31
Nonsteroidal antiinflammatory drugs (NSAIDs), 19-20,125, 133, 141, 266, 307
Norepinephrine, 62, 65, 115, 147, 157, 227, 272, 402
Norethindrone (Micronor; Norlutin), 326t
Norgestrel (Ovrette), 326t
Norlutin. See Norethindrone
Normeperidine, 397
Norpace. See Disopyramide
Nosebleeds, acute. See Epistaxis
Novo-Niacin. See Niacin; Nicotinic acid
Novocaine. See Procaine hydrochloride
Novolin 70/30, 243t
Novolin N, 243t
Novolin R, 243t
NPH. See Isophane Insulin Suspension
NRTIs. See Nucleoside reverse transcriptase inhibitors
NSAIDs. See Nonsteroidal antiinflammatory drugs
Nucleoside analog antiviral, 31-32
Nucleoside reverse transcriptase inhibitor antiretroviral, 27-29
Nucleoside reverse transcriptase inhibitors (NRTIs), 27
Nutritional imbalances, drugs for, 359-368
    minerals, 364-368
    vitamins, 359-363
Nystagmus, 88, 92, 101
Nystatin (Mycostatin), 33t, 34, 35

O

Oat cell carcinoma, 53
Obesity, exogenous, 82

OcuClear. See Oxymetazoline
Ocular vasoconstricting medications See Decongestants, ocular
Oculogyric crisis, 106
Ofloxacin (Floxin), 300t, 365
Omeprazole (Prilosec), 174, 182, 262t, 263
Oncology Nursing Society, 50
Oncovin. See Vincristine
Ondansetron (Zofran), 275, 275t
Ophthalgan. See Glycerin
Ophthalmics and otics
    carbonic anhydrase inhibitors, 378-380, 378t
    ceruminolytics, 383-384, 383t
    decongestants, ocular, 371-373, 371t
    miotics, ocular, 373-376, 373t
    mydriatic and cycloplegic agents, 380-382, 380t
    osmotics, ocular, 376-378, 376t
Opiate antagonists, 400-401, 400t
Opioid agonists, 395-398, 395t
Opioids, 193t
Oprelvekin. See Interleukin-11
Optimine. See Azatadine maleate
Organophosphate poisoning, 76, 77
Orinase. See Tolbutamide
Orphenadrine, 76, 88
Ortho-Novum. See Ethinyl Estradiol/norethindrone
Ortho-Prefest. See Estradiol/norgestimate
Orthoclone OKT3. See Muromonab-CD3
Os-Cal. See Calcium carbonate
Osmitrol. See Mannitol
Osmotics, ocular, 376-378, 376t
Osteoporosis, 136, 240
OTC. See Over-the-counter
Otitis media, 2
Ototoxicity, 34, 90
Over-the-counter (OTC), 65
Overdosage, 210
Ovrette. See Norgestrel
Oxacillin (Prostaphlin), 1t
Oxicam, 344t
Oxiconazole (Oxistat), 36t
Oxistat. See Oxiconazole
Oxtriphylline (Choledyl), 215
Oxybutynin (Ditropan), 74t, 304t
Oxycodone (Percodan), 395t
Oxymetazoline (OcuClear), 371t, 372
Oxyphenbutazone, 248
Oxytetracycline, 244
Oxytocic, 337-338, 337t
Oxytocin challenge test, 337
Oxytocin, 197, 221, 337t

P

PABA. See Para-aminobenzoic acid
Paclitaxel (Taxol), 52t

PAF. See Paroxysmal atrial flutter
Paget's disease, 240, 241
Pain relief, agents used for, 395-406
Pancrease. See Pancrelipase
Pancreatin, 250, 281t
Pancrelipase (Pancrease), 281t
Pancuronium, 73
Pancytopenia, 98, 133
Para-aminobenzoic acid (PABA), 8
Paradoxical effects, 110
Parafon Forte. See Chlorzoxazone
Parasympathetic nervous system agents and antiparkinsonism agents, 69-80
    anticholinergics, 74-78
    cholinesterase inhibitors, 71-74
    direct-acting cholinergic agonists, 69-71
    dopaminergics, 78-80
Parathyroid. See Thyroid and parathyroid agents
Parathyroid hormone (PTH), 239
Paregoric (opium tincture), 295
Parkinson's disease, 69, 75, 76, 78, 128, 129, 374
Parlodel. See Bromocriptine mesylate
Parnate. See Tranylcypromine
Paroxetine (Paxil), 118t
Paroxysmal atrial flutter (PAF), 185
Paroxysmal atrial tachycardia (PAT), 178
Partial thromboplastin time (PTT), 137
PAT. See Paroxysmal atrial tachycardia
Patient-controlled analgesia (PCA), 396
Paveral. See Codeine sulfate
Paxil. See Paroxetine
PBI. See Protein-bound iodine
PBZ-SR. See Tripelennamine
PBZ. See Tripelennamine
PCA. See Patient-controlled analgesia
PCWP. See Pulmonary capillary wedge pressure
PE. See Embolism, pulmonary
Pectin, 174
Pelamine. See Tripelennamine
Pellagra, 360
Penicillamine (Cuprimine), 348t, 361, 365
Penicillin antibiotics, 1-5, 1t
Penicillin G potassium (Megacillin), 1t
Penicillinase, 2
Penicillins, 1-5
Pentamidine, 20
Pentazocine (Talwin), 398t
Pentobarbital, 402
Pentoxifylline, 261
Pepcid. See Famotidine
Peptic ulcers, 157

Pepto-Bismol. See Bismuth subsalicylate
Percodan. See Oxycodone
Pergolide, 78, 79
Periactin. See Cyproheptadine
Peripheral adrenergic neuron antagonists, 156-158, 156t
Peripheral vascular disease, 141
Peripheral vascular resistance (PVR), 140
Peripherally acting muscle relaxants, 89-91, 89t
Persantine. See Dipyridamole
Pertussis, 17
Petechiae, 133, 134, 224
Petit mal seizures, 100
Petrolatum, 369
Pharyngitis, 2
Phenazopyridine (Pyridium), 304t
Phenelzine (Nardil), 120t, 121
Phenergan. See Promethazine
Phenmetrazine (Preludin), 83t
Phenobarbital (Luminal), 73, 98, 93t, 101, 101, 179, 182, 229, 234, 273
Phenolphthalein (Ex-Lax; Correctol), 283t
Phenolsulfonphthalein (PSP), 134
Phenothiazines, 20, 73, 79, 123, 127, 157, 182, 201, 315
Phensuximide (Milontin), 97t
Phentolamine, 65
Phenylamines, 123
Phenylbutazone, 182, 248, 350
Phenylephrine (AK-Dilate), 380t, 381, 402
Phenylephrine hydrochloride (Neo-Synephrine; Sinex), 196t
Phenylpropanolamine, 86
Phenytoin (Dilantin), 9, 37, 73, 79, 91t, 92, 101, 159, 174, 179, 181t, 182, 188, 223, 229, 234, 244, 260, 263, 264, 302, 347, 355
Pheochromocytoma, 270
Phenylbutazone (Butazolidin), 343t
Phlebitis, 4
Phos-Ex. See Calcium acetate
PhosLo. See Calcium acetate
Phosphate-binding agents, 315-317, 315t
Phosphodiesterase, 85
Pholine iodide. See Echothiophate
Phosphorus (Nitro-Phos; K-Phos), 364
Photophobia, 90
Pilocar. See Pilocarpine
Pilocarpine (Pilocar), 373t, 374
Pimozide, 37
Pioglitazone (Actos), 253t
Piperacillin, 191, 223
Piperazines, 128, 201, 206t

Piperidines, 201, 201t, 206t
Pirbuterol, 211
Piroxicam (Feldene), 164, 344t
Pitocin. *See* Oxytocin
Pituitary. *See* Pituitary and adrenal hormones
Plague, 14
Plaquenil. *See* Hydroxychloroquine
Plasminogen, 138
Plastin, 138
Plavix. *See* Clopidogrel
Pneumocystosis carinii, 40
Pneumonia, 2
Pod-Ben-25. *See* Podophyllum resin
Podofilox (Condylox), 392t
Podophyllotoxins, 53
Podophyllum resin (Pod-Ben-25), 392t
Poikilothermia, 129
Polyarteritis, 155
Polycarbophil (FiberCon), 285t, 293t
Polyethylene glycol-electrolyte solution (Golytely), 289t
Polymyxin B, 22
Polyuria, 221
Pork Regular Iletin II, 243t
Posterior pituitary hormone replacement agents, 226-228
Potassium (K-Dur; Micro-K), 364
Potassium iodide solution (SSKI), 235t, 236
Potassium-sparing diuretics, 311-313, 331t
Pramipexole, 78
Pramoxine (Tronothane), 390t
Prandin. *See* Repaglinide
Pravachol. *See* Pravastatin
Pravastatin (Pravachol), 161t
Prazosin, 67, 148
Precose. *See* Acarbose
Prednisone (Deltasone), 60, 228t, 248t
Preludin. *See* Phenmetrazine
Premarin. *See* Estrogens, conjugated
Premature ventricular contractions (PVCs), 178
Prempro. *See* Estrogens/medroxyprogesterone, conjugated, 329t
Prepidil. *See* Dinoprostone
Prevacid. *See* Lansoprazole
Prilosec. *See* Omeprazole
Primacor. *See* Milrinone lactate
Primaxin. *See* Imipenem-cilastatin
Primidone, 101
Priscoline. *See* Tolazoline hydrochloride
Pro-Banthine. *See* Propantheline bromide
Probenecid (Benemid), 6, 19, 22, 56, 125, 133, 165, 216, 248, 356t, 357
Procainamide, 20, 73, 76, 178, 179, 180, 261, 379

Procaine hydrochloride (Novocaine), 4, 103t
Procarbazine (Matulane), 59t, 60
Procardia. *See* Nifedipine
Prochlorperazine (Compazine), 54, 272t, 273
Procyclidine, 76
Progestasert. *See* Progesterone
Progesterone (Progestasert), 326t
Progestin, 326-329, 326t
Prokinetics, 275
Proleukin (Aldesleukin), 44t
Promazine, 128
Promethazine (Phenergan), 201t, 272t
 acute toxicity from, 204
Pronestyl. *See* Procainamide
Propafenone (Rythmol), 184t, 185, 191
Propranolol (Inderal), 147t
Propantheline bromide (Pro-Banthine), 74t
Propine. *See* Dipivefrin
Propionic acid derivatives, 343t
Propofol (Diprivan), 105t
Propoxyphene, 88
Propranolol, 185, 214, 250
Propylthiouracil (PTU), 235, 236, 309
Prostaglandins, 266-267, 266t, 339-340, 339t
Prostaphlin. *See* Oxacillin
Prostigmin. *See* Neostigmine bromide
Protamine sulfate, 137
Protease inhibitor retroviral, 25-26
Protease inhibitors, 37
Protein-bound iodine (PBI), 134
Prothrombin, 360
Prothrombin time (PT), 166, 214, 302
Proton pump inhibitor, 262-264, 262f, 262t
Protropin. *See* Somatrem
Proventil. *See* Albuterol
Provera. *See* Medroxyprogesterone acetate
Prozac. *See* Fluoxetine
Pseudoephedrine (Sudafed; Drixoral), 63t, 64t, 193, 196t
Pseudoparkinsonism, 273
PSP. *See* Phenolsulfonphthalein
Psychosis, 98, 101
Psychotherapeutic agents, 107-130, 108f
 antidepressant agents, 115-127
 antipsychotic agents, 127-130
 anxiolytic agents, 108-113
 sedative-hypnotic agents, 113-115
Psyllium (Metamucil), 285t
PT. *See* Prothrombin time
PTH. *See* Parathyroid hormone
PTT. *See* Partial thromboplastin time

PTU. *See* Propylthiouracil
Pulmonary capillary wedge pressure (PCWP), 176
Pupils, 373
Purified Pork Regular, 243t
Purkinje fibers, 173
PVC. *See* Premature ventricular contractions
PVR. *See* Peripheral vascular resistance
Pyrazolone, 343t
Pyridium. *See* Phenazopyridine
Pyridoxine. *See* Vitamin B$_6$

Q

QRS complex, 180
Quazepam, 109
Questran. *See* Cholestyramine
Quinamm. *See* Quinine
Quinapril (Accupril), 140
Quinidex. *See* Quinidine
Quinidine (Quinidex), 20, 25, 30, 37, 73, 76, 114, 178t, 179, 191, 261, 379
Quinine (Quinamm; Quiphile), 89t, 90
Quinolones, 216, 365

R

RAAS. *See* Renin-angiotensin-aldosterone system
Radiation recall, 58
Ramipril (Altace), 140
Ranitidine (Zantac), 250, 260t
Rapid eye movement (REM) sleep, 81
Rash, morbilliform, 232
Raynaud's disease, 67, 155
Real World Nursing Survival Guide: Drug Calculations and Administration, 23
Receptor sites
 for adrenergic agonists, 64t
 types of, 62
α-Receptors, 62
β$_1$-Receptors, 62
β$_2$-Receptors, 62
Receptors, muscarinic, 70
Recombinant deoxyribonucleic acid, 138
Red man syndrome, 23
Red neck syndrome, 23, 24
Refractoriness, 173
Reglan. *See* Metoclopramide
Relafen. *See* Nabumetone
REM sleep. *See* Rapid eye movement sleep
Renal disorders. *See* Genitourinary tract and renal disorders, drugs affecting
Renal failure
 agents used in, 313-322
 ACE inhibitors, 313

Renal failure—cont'd
 agents used in—cont'd
  cation-exchange resins, 317-318, 317t
  heavy metal antagonists, 319-320, 319t
  iron supplements, 314
  phosphate-binding agents, 315-317, 315t
  vitamin D supplements, 314
 antacids, systemic, 320-322, 320t
 chronic, 362b
Renal function, improvement of
 loop diuretics for, 306-308, 306t
 potassium-sparing diuretics, 311-313, 311t
 thiazides and thiazide-like diuretics for, 308-310, 308t
Renal output, agents used to improve, 300-313
Renin-angiotensin system, 144
Renin-angiotensin-aldosterone system (RAAS), 141, 173, 313
Repaglinide (Prandin), 255t
Reproductive system, drugs affecting, 323-342
 agents affecting uterine motility and infertility, 335-342
 male and female hormones, 323-334
Rescriptor. *See* Delavirdine
Reserpine (Serpasil), 156t, 197
Respiratory system, drugs affecting, 193-220
 antihistamines, 201-208
 upper respiratory disorders, agents affecting, 193-201
Response modifiers, biologic, 38-48.
 See also Specific drugs
 colony-stimulating factor, 46-48, 46t
 immunomodulators, 41-43, 41t
 immunosuppressants, 38-41, 38t
Reteplase, 139
Reticulum, sarcoplasmic, 89
Retinol Cream, 389t
Retrovir. *See* Zidovudine (AZT)
Retrovirus, 24b
Reuptake, 107
Revex. *See* Nalmefene
Revia. *See* Naltrexone
Reye's syndrome, 294
Rhabdomyolysis, 39, 162
Rhinitis, perennial, 134
Rhinyle, 227
Riboflavin. *See* Vitamin B$_2$
Ribonucleic acid (RNA), 8
Rifabutin, 30
Rifampin, 25, 30, 37, 73, 90, 100, 141, 150, 174, 179, 182, 185, 223, 229, 234, 248, 275, 309, 324, 347